Proceedings of the 10th International Symposium on Hearing

ADVANCES IN HEARING RESEARCH

Swabian Conference Centre, Irsee, Bavaria
26 June – 1 July, 1994

Editors

G A Manley, G M Klump, C Köppl, H Fastl & H Oeckinghaus

Technische Universität München

World Scientific
Singapore • New Jersey • London • Hong Kong

Published by

World Scientific Publishing Co. Pte. Ltd.
5 Toh Tuck Link, Singapore 596224
USA office: 27 Warren Street, Suite 401-402, Hackensack, NJ 07601
UK office: 57 Shelton Street, Covent Garden, London WC2H 9HE

British Library Cataloguing-in-Publication Data
A catalogue record for this book is available from the British Library.

ADVANCES IN HEARING RESEARCH

ISBN-13 978-981-02-2260-4
ISBN-10 981-02-2260-2

Preface

The present volume contains the papers presented at the 10th International Symposium on Hearing, which was held at the Swabian Conference Centre in Irsee, Bavaria, between June 26th and July 1st, 1994. The meeting was organized by a team recruited from the Technical University of Munich, from the Departments of Zoology and of Man-Machine Communication. The organizers and a number of participants carry out their research in the cooperative programme funded by the Deutsche Forschungsgemeinschaft as the Sonderforschungsbereich (Special Research Area) "Hearing" (SFB 204) in Munich.

The specific aim of this series of meetings on the hearing system is to provide a forum in which data, ideas and models from both the physiological and psychoacoustical standpoints can be presented and thoroughly discussed. There is great value in striving for an integration of the "top down" and "bottom up" approaches to studying hearing phenomena. We therefore encouraged authors to present papers with review character and gave priority to contributions covering aspects interesting to both Physiologists and Psychoacousticians. Three invited reviews in different fields and adequate discussion time were aimed to encourage interactions between these disciplines and promote discussion. In addition to those areas traditionally covered by these meetings, we added two areas in which there have been very important advances in recent years. These are the new aspects emerging from recent "Comparative studies" and on the recovery of function at both the peripheral and central levels and covered by the title "Development and Regeneration". Insofar as we achieved the goals outlined above, we believe the present volume will be of great interest to all scientists working in the field of audiotry research.

As in previous meetings of this series, a preprint of the manuscripts was circulated to participants two months before the meeting began. We thank the authors for adhering to the strict deadlines; this provided adequate time to study the contributions carefully, which aided greatly in having fruitful discussions.

We gratefully acknowledge the help provided by the two major sponsors of the meeting: the Deutsche Forschungsgemeinschaft and the Bavarian Ministry of Education, Science and Culture. Without this financial support, the cost of the meeting would have been prohibitive for many participants. Our doctoral students Thomas Friedl, Lothar Gallo, Ulrike Hartl, Ulrike Langemann, Andrea Pavusa, Michael Scharmann and Grit Taschenberger helped ease the organizational and administrative load during and after the meeting. As with any meeting, cooperative team work is essential: We thank all those who contributed to the success of this conference. To those whose papers could not be accommodated, we apologise.

Garching, January 1995

G.A. Manley G.M. Klump
C. Köppl H. Fastl
H. Oeckinghaus

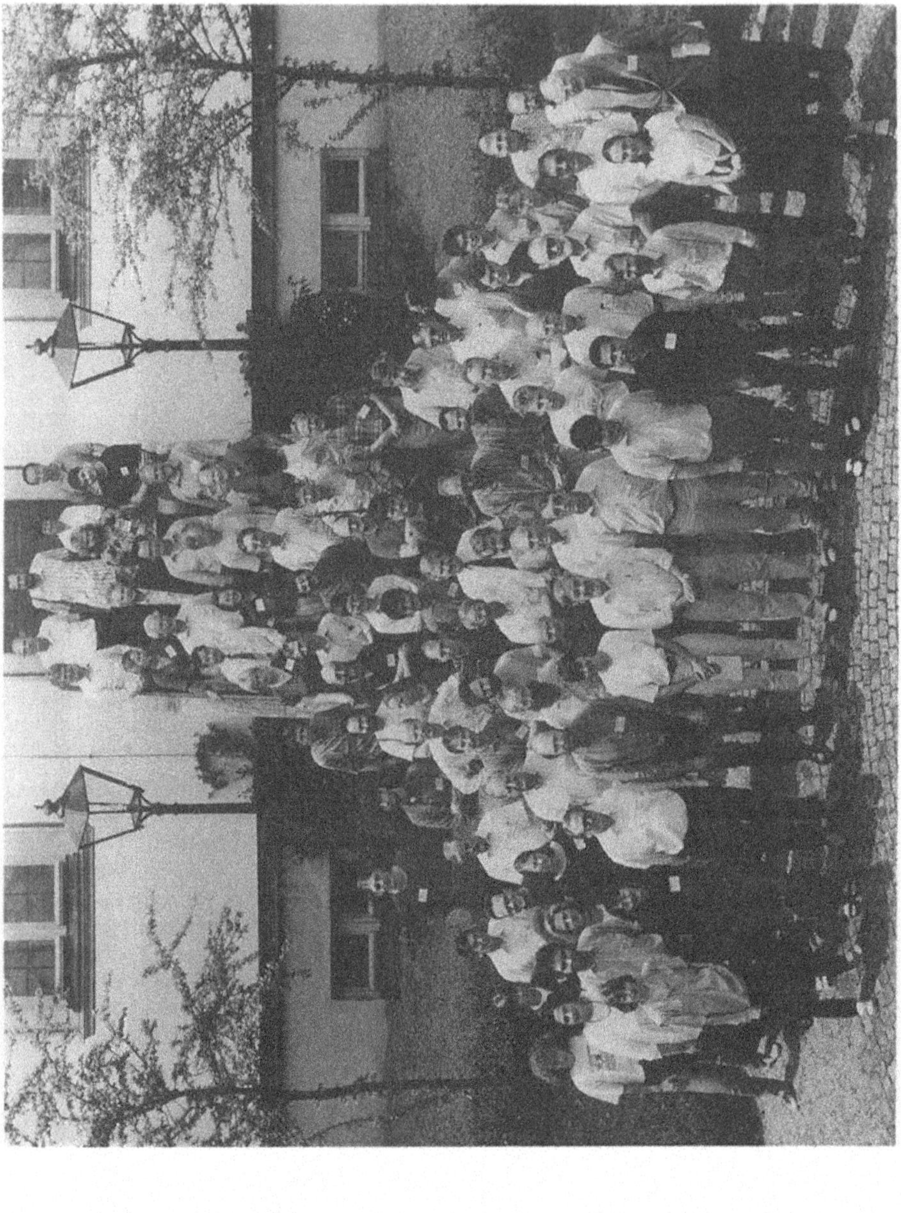

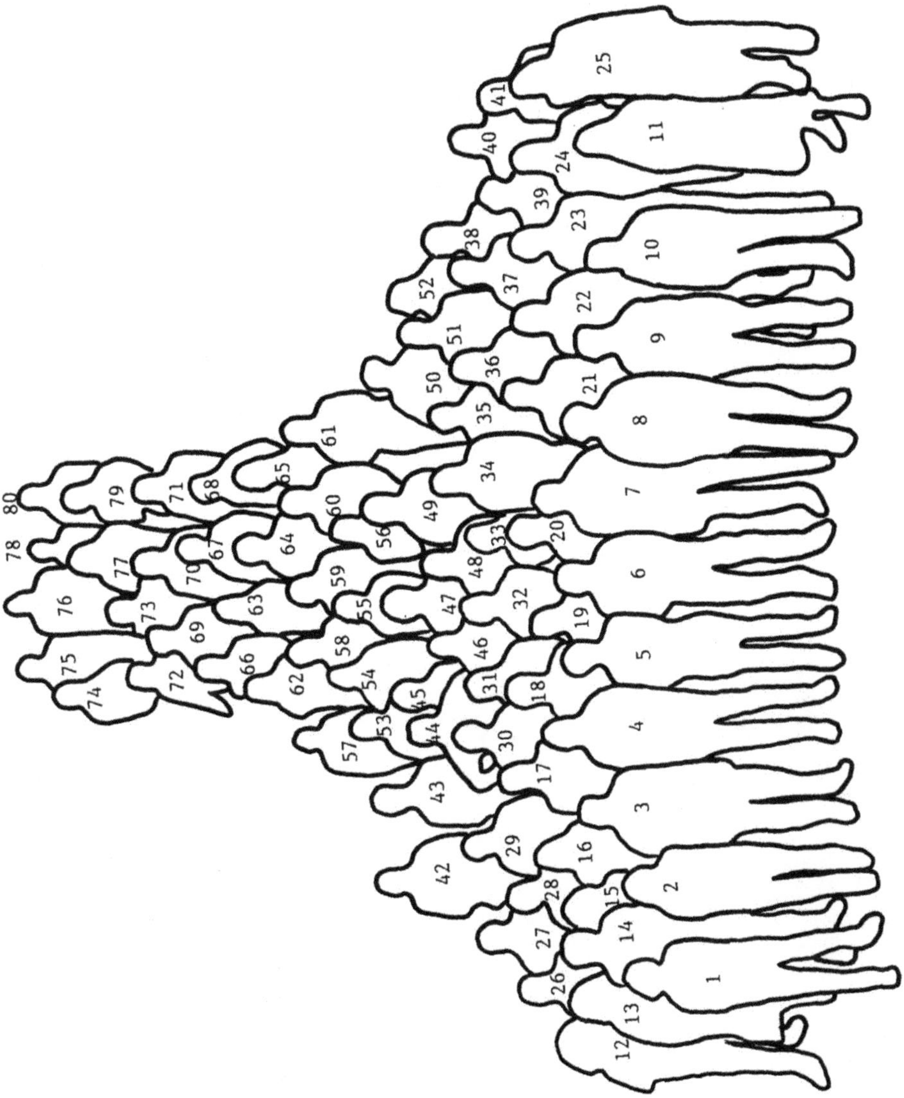

List of participants (numbers refer to photograph)

1. Ulrike Langemann
2. Catherine E. Carr
3. Hugo Fastl
4. Georg M. Klump
5. Christine Köppl
6. Geoffrey A. Manley
7. Horst Oeckinghaus
8. Karl-Heinz Esser
9. Kourosh Saberi
10. John H. Grose
11. Ann Brown
12. Grit Taschenberger
13. Mary Florentine
14. Michael Scharmann
15. Andrea Pavusa
16. Sabine Schmidt
17. Peter Narins
18. Otto Gleich
19. Jozef Zwislocki
20. Bertram Scharf
21. John Culling
22. Bruce Ulrich
23. David Nelson
24. Tino Trahiotis
25. Jens Blauert
26. Ulrike Hartl
27. Tammo Houtgast
28. Lothar Gallo
29. Johan Raatgever
30. Alan Palmer
31. Israel Nelken
32. Tom C.T. Yin
33. Raymond Romand
34. George Spirou
35. William Shofner
36. Joost M. Festen
37. Ben Bonham
38. Tatsuya Hirahara
39. John Hall
40. Leslie Bernstein
41. Neil Viemeister
42. Johannes Lyzenga
43. Peter W.J. van Hengel
44. Birger Kollmeier
45. Esther Wiersinger-Post
46. Bertrand Delgutte
47. Toshio Irino
48. Frans A. Bilsen
49. Jörn Gräbke
50. Richard Salvi
51. Lawrence Feth
52. Virginia M. Richards
53. David Moore
54. Dexter R. Irvine
55. Adrian Rees
56. Jan Wouters
57. Hero Wit
58. J. Wiebe Horst
59. Shihab Shamma
60. Rainer Klinke
61. David Moody
62. Birgitta Gabriel
63. Beverly Wright
64. Günther Ehret
65. Huib Versnel
66. Ted F. Evans
67. Diek Duifhuis
68. David Green
69. Pat Wilson
70. Roy Patterson
71. Richard Fay
72. Mary Ann Cheatham
73. Ray Meddis
74. Søren Buus
75. Adrianus J.M. Houtsma
76. Brian Moore
77. Armin Kohlrausch
78. Katrin Reimer
79. Robert P. Carlyon
80. Huanping Dai

not in photograph: Pim van Dijk and Ian Russell

Contents

Development and regeneration

Peripheral processing

Central neuronal processing

Excitation patterns

Pitch perception

Complex spectral analysis

Development and regeneration

Plasticity in the mature auditory system

D. R. F. Irvine and R. Rajan

Department of Psychology, Monash University, Clayton, Vic. 3168, Australia

1 Introduction

A basic feature of the functional architecture of the major sensory systems is the fact that the receptor surface is topographically represented (or "mapped") in central nervous system structures. Because these maps basically reflect orderly projections from the receptor surface to central structures, they have been termed "projectional" maps. Topographic organizations with respect to other sensory attributes are based on neural processing, and have therefore been termed "centrally synthesized" or "computational" maps (Konishi, 1986). During ontogeny, both types of map change as a result of normal developmental processes and in response to abnormal patterns of input produced by injury or other experimental manipulations. In the auditory system, changes in peripheral and central tonotopy (see Rübsamen (1992) and King and Moore (1991) for reviews) provide examples of normal developmental changes, while changes in the auditory space maps in the mammalian superior colliculus and the homologous optic tectum of the barn owl as a consequence of altered auditory or visual input (see King and Moore (1991) and Knudsen (1988) for reviews) provide examples of developmental changes produced by abnormal sensory experience. Changes of both sorts are commonly referred to as "plasticity", defined in the most general sense as "any persistent change in the functional properties of single neurons or neuronal aggregates" (Tsukuhara, 1981, p. 351).

In contrast to the plasticity exhibited by the developing nervous system, it was for many years generally assumed that representational maps in adult animals were stable and not susceptible to change. Over the last 10-15 years, however, evidence from a number of laboratories has demonstrated in a variety of species that elimination of input from a restricted region of the skin (and a variety of other alterations of sensory input) can result in substantial reorganization of the map of the body surface in the somatosensory cortex of adult animals (see Kaas et al. (1983) and Kaas (1991) for reviews). More recently, analogous reorganization has been demonstrated in adult visual cortex after restricted retinal lesions (e.g., Kaas et al., 1990; Chino et al., 1992; Gilbert and Wiesel, 1992) and in adult auditory cortex after restricted cochlear lesions (Robertson and Irvine, 1989; Rajan et al., 1993). It is now clear that the capacity for such reorganization is a general characteristic of sensory (and motor) cortices in adult mammals, although it is not yet clear whether the same mechanisms are responsible in each case.

This review will focus on plasticity of frequency tuning and organization in the cortical and subcortical auditory system of adult animals as a consequence of various forms of peripheral damage and of procedures that manipulate the significance of specific acoustic stimuli. In examining this evidence, a more restrictive definition of plasticity than that quoted above will be adopted. To take as an example the particular case that will prove to be of particular significance here, it is clear that a restricted cochlear lesion will produce immediate changes in the responses of auditory nerve fibres and central auditory neurons whose input is derived from the damaged region of the cochlea. Although such changes occurring as a direct (or passive) consequence of the removal of input undoubtedly constitute persistent changes in the functional properties of these neurons, and would thus satisfy Tsukahara's definition, they would not generally be considered instances of plasticity. The term "plasticity" will here be reserved for changes in the functional properties of neurons that depend on changes in connections or in synaptic strengths. The term "reorganization" will be used to refer to plastic changes in representational maps.

2 Plasticity in Frequency Organization as a Consequence of Restricted Cochlear Lesions in Adults

2.1 Auditory Cortex

Robertson and Irvine (1989) made restricted mechanical lesions of one cochlea in sexually-mature guinea pigs, and assessed the extent of the resultant hearing loss by recording the compound action potential (CAP) audiogram and by histological examination of the cochleas. The CAP and histological data for a chronically-lesioned animal representative of those with a "notch" hearing loss are presented in Fig. 1A and B. It is apparent from the CAP audiogram (Fig. 1A) that the lesion produced a relatively sharp notch of decreased peripheral sensitivity over a range from approximately 10 to 20 kHz, associated with a discrete region of abnormal (missing or damaged) inner and outer hair cells at the corresponding cochlear place (Fig. 1B).

The frequency organization of auditory cortex in the hemisphere contralateral to the lesioned cochlea was examined using conventional microelectrode mapping techniques 35-81 days after cochlear lesioning. In each of a large number of microelectrode penetrations into auditory cortex, the characteristic frequency (CF; frequency at which threshold is lowest) of a cluster of neurons in the middle cortical layers was determined. Mapping was carried out primarily in the tonotopically-organized rostral field, in which low frequencies are represented ventro-rostrally and high frequencies dorso-caudally. In the frequency map for the chronically-lesioned guinea pig in Fig. 1C, the low-frequency part of the map is like that in normal animals, and this is reflected in the plot of CF against distance for frequencies up to approximately 10 kHz (Fig. 1D). However, the region of cortex that in a normal animal would be occupied by an orderly and continuous representation of frequencies from 10 to 20 kHz is in this case almost entirely occupied by enlarged representations of limited frequency ranges corresponding to the borders of the cochlear lesion (viz., 9.9-10.8 kHz and 20.6-22.0 kHz). As illustrated by this case, the region of cortex deprived of its normal input by the cochlear lesion was partially or wholly occupied

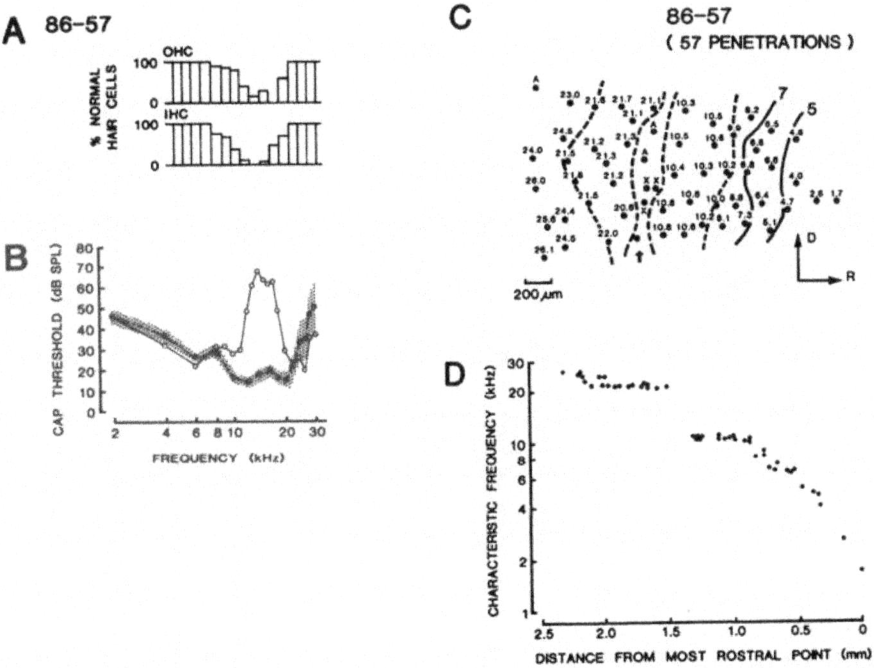

Figure 1. Characteristics of the lesion (A,B) and cortical frequency map (C,D) in a representative chronically-lesioned guinea pig (animal 86-57; survival time 35 days). A, plot showing percentage of normal inner and outer hair cells (IHCs and OHCs) as a function of distance along the organ of Corti; the hair cell counts for 500-μm segments are shown in the vicinity of the lesion. B, Post-recovery CAP audiogram (open circles), compared with the mean CAP audiogram (filled circles) ±1 SD (shading) for normal animals. A and B have been aligned in accordance with the well-established place - frequency map for the guinea pig cochlea. C, D, Frequency organisation of the rostral field. In C, dots represent points at which microelectrode penetrations were made, and the number next to each dot gives the CF at that point. Points marked with letters are those at which no auditory response was obtained ("X") or at which the cluster was acoustically responsive but a CF could not be determined ("A"); the arrow indicates a point at which the cluster had equally low thresholds at 10.6 and 21.4 kHz. The broken lines demarcate the areas of expanded representation (see text); heavy black lines are "iso-frequency contours", (i.e., lines separating points with CF above and below the value indicated at the end of the line) in the normal low-frequency part of the map. In D, the CF at each point in the rostral field is plotted as a function of cortical distance as measured from the most rostral low-frequency point along an axis approximately orthogonal to the predominant orientation of the iso-frequency contours. Modified from Robertson and Irvine (1989).

by expanded representations of lesion-edge frequencies in all chronically-lesioned animals. This form of reorganization is directly analogous to that observed in somatosensory and visual cortices after digit amputation and restricted retinal lesions, respectively.

Two features of the reorganized frequency representations seen in chronically-lesioned guinea pigs are critical to the claim that they should be considered instances of neural plasticity. The first is that the responses of neuron clusters in the reorganized regions of cortex were strong and that their thresholds at their "new" CFs were not significantly different from those of neurons with those CFs in normal animals. The second is that these changes were not seen in experiments in which the cortex was mapped within a few hours immediately following the cochlear lesion. In these acutely-lesioned guinea pigs, the region deprived of its normal input by the cochlear lesion was not silent, but neuron clusters were weakly driven, and had CFs near the low-frequency edge of the lesion with thresholds that were significantly elevated relative to normal. When frequency tuning curves (FTCs) for neuron clusters were obtained at the same cortical loci before and within a few hours after lesioning, the post-lesion FTC fell within the low-frequency, high-intensity region of the pre-lesion FTC. This was interpreted as indicating that the responses seen immediately post-lesion were simply the residue of pre-lesion responses at these frequency-intensity combinations. The existence of such residual responses reflects the fact that the response areas of AI neurons (and of central auditory neurons at subcortical levels) at higher sound pressure levels (SPLs) are derived via convergent input originating from auditory-nerve fibres with CFs other than that of the cortical neuron (e.g., Phillips et al., 1985; Phillips and Hall, 1992).

The contrast between the responses seen immediately post-lesion and after recovery periods of a month or more establishes that the long-term changes reflect a dynamic process of reorganization during the recovery period. These data also make the important point that changes in the frequency map are not in themselves sufficient evidence for the occurrence of reorganization/plasticity. The small "residual" response areas seen in auditory cortex immediately post-lesion are in contrast to the reports from some studies of somatosensory (e.g. Calford and Tweedale, 1988, 1991a,b) and visual (e.g., Gilbert and Wiesel, 1992) cortical plasticity, in which post-lesion recordings have revealed an immediate expansion of the receptive fields of neurons with RFs in, or near the edge of, the peripheral lesion, such that these neurons exhibit large RFs on peri-lesion receptor regions. As discussed below, this difference has implications for the nature of the mechanisms responsible for reorganization.

In these guinea pig experiments, changes in the representation of the lesioned cochlea in the contralateral hemisphere were found using stimulation of the lesioned ear. However, most auditory cortical neurons receive binaural input, i.e., both cochleas are represented in auditory cortex in each hemisphere. One question raised by these data concerns the fate of the representation of the normal ipsilateral cochlea in the cortex in which the representation of the lesioned contralateral cochlea has undergone reorganization. We have examined this issue by determining the effects of unilateral restricted cochlear lesions in adult cats on the representations of the lesioned and normal cochleas in primary auditory cortex (area AI) contralateral to the lesioned cochlea, using the same basic procedures as were used in the guinea pig study (Rajan et al., 1993).

Because the cochlea in the cat is embedded in dense temporal bone, mechanical lesions were made by advancing a micropipette through the round window, and damage was therefore restricted to the basal end of the cochlea. The consequent loss in peripheral sensitivity extended over a broad high-frequency range, as illustrated by data for a representative chronically-lesioned cat in Fig. 2B, where the CAP audiograms for the lesioned (left) and the normal (right) cochleas are shown in comparison with the mean normal audiogram. At frequencies up to 18 kHz, thresholds for both ears are almost identical and within the normal range. Above 18 kHz, however, there is a sharp loss in CAP sensitivity in the lesioned ear, while thresholds in the unlesioned ear remain within the normal range. High-frequency lesions of this sort, with edge frequencies in the range 18-24 kHz, were produced in eight chronically-lesioned cats.

The cortical mapping data for this animal are presented in Figs. 2C and D, based on data obtained in the penetrations whose locations are indicated in Fig. 2A. At frequencies up to about 18 kHz, the map obtained with monaural stimulation of the lesioned contralateral ear (Fig. 2C) shows the caudal-to-rostral, low-to-high-frequency gradient characteristic of normal animals. More rostrally, however, there is an area more than 1000 μm in rostro-caudal extent, demarcated by the broken lines, within which all points have CF in the range 18.5 to 19.0 kHz, corresponding to the edge of the cochlear lesion. That is, there is an enlarged representation of these lesion-edge frequencies. In contrast, the map for stimulation of the ipsilateral ear (Fig. 2D) is of the type seen in normal animals. Most importantly, in the region of cortex occupied by an expanded representation of lesion-edge frequencies in the contralateral map, the ipsilateral map shows a normal progressive increase from 18 to 30 kHz.

Results of the sort presented in Fig. 2 were obtained from all chronically-lesioned cats with broad, high-frequency losses in cochlear sensitivity. Quantitative data on the thresholds and other characteristics of the responses to contralateral stimulation of neuron clusters in the region of the enlarged contralateral representation were compared to data from control normal animals. These data indicated that the expansion of the representation of lesion-edge frequencies reflected a true reorganization during the post-lesion recovery period and that it could not be explained in terms of the residue of pre-lesion responses.

The only other evidence bearing on the effects of experimentally-produced cochlear lesions in adults on the frequency organization of auditory cortex is provided by the study by Schwaber et al. (1993), who mapped AI in three adult macaques before and after inducing a broad high-frequency hearing loss by injection of the ototoxic agents kanamycin and furosemide. When the cortex was remapped 80-90 days after the ototoxic treatment, the high-frequency region of AI was found to be occupied by an enlarged representation of lesion-edge frequencies (i.e., frequencies whose cochlear place was at the edge of the lesion). Unfortunately, Schwaber et al. (1993) presented no data on the thresholds of neuron clusters in the enlarged representation at their "new" CFs. Although it is likely that the changes they described reflect a process of dynamic reorganization, it was noted above that a change in the frequency map alone is not sufficient evidence for the occurrence of such reorganization. As demonstrated by the acute lesion results of Robertson and Irvine (1989) and by the more general arguments developed by Rajan et al. (1993), the fact that auditory cortical neurons respond over a broad frequency range at high SPLs has the consequence that changes in tonotopic maps following peripheral lesions can simply reflect what has been called the residue of pre-lesion responses.

Further evidence for auditory cortical reorganization in adult animals is provided by evidence from studies of animals with naturally-occurring peripheral hearing losses. Willott et al. (1993) have described auditory cortical plasticity in C57BL/6J (C57) mice, which show normal auditory system development up to an age of 1-2 months, then show a progressive sensorineural pathology that begins in the basal turn. These animals therefore suffer a progressive loss of high-frequency hearing, beginning in young adulthood, that is comparable to the (non-progressive) losses produced by mechanical lesions in cats by Rajan et al. (1993). The frequency representation in AI of 3-12-month old C57 mice was characterized by an enlarged representation of a middle-frequency range (10-13 kHz), which occupied the cortical regions that were devoted to higher frequencies in younger C57 mice and in older mice of other strains that do not exhibit this sensorineural pathology. Thresholds in these regions of expanded representation were reported to be "relatively low", indicating that the responses could not be interpreted as the residue of pre-hearing-loss responses at these frequencies.

The reorganization described by Willott et al. (1993) in C57 mice is obviously similar to that seen in adult cats with mechanical lesions of the basal cochlea (Rajan et al., 1993), although there also appear to be some differences. In the cat experiments, the expanded representation was of a relatively limited range of lesion-edge frequencies that differed for each cat, whereas the expanded representation in the C57 mice was always of a range of middle frequencies (viz., 10-13 kHz). Given the progressive nature of the hearing loss in C57 mice, the mechanical lesion data would have led one to expect that the

Figure 2. Effects of unilateral cochlear lesion in adult cat (CML 90-1) on maps of the lesioned (left) and normal (right) cochleas in primary auditory cortex (area AI) in the left hemisphere (i.e., contralateral to the lesioned cochlea). A: Locations of microelectrode penetration relative to sulci defining middle ectosylvian gyrus are indicated by dots on a drawing of the cortical surface made from a photograph taken at the time of the experiment. AES and PES: anterior and posterior ectosylvian sulci; SSS: suprasylvian sulcus. B: Loss in peripheral sensitivity in the left (lesioned) cochlea, as reflected in compound action potential (CAP) audiograms for the lesioned and normal ears obtained at time of cortical mapping (2.5 months post-lesion). Upward-pointing arrows indicate that threshold was higher than highest intensity tested (indicated by base of arrow). The stippled area represents the range ±1SD about the mean normal audiogram, and is based on data obtained from a large sample of normal cats. C and D. Tonotopic organization of AI in the hemisphere contralateral to the lesioned cochlea for stimulation of the contralateral (lesioned) ear (C) and of the ipsilateral (normal) ear (D). In each case, the dots indicate microelectrode penetrations whose locations are shown in A. Conventions as in Fig. 1; points marked with letters are those at which cluster was broadly tuned ("B") or at which stimulation of that ear had a purely inhibitory effect ("I"). "B_{MF}" indicates broad tuning to mid-frequencies (in range 8-20 kHz). In D, the dashed lines indicate the region containing an enlarged representation of lesion-edge frequencies, in the range 18.5 - 19.0 kHz. Modified from Rajan et al. (1993).

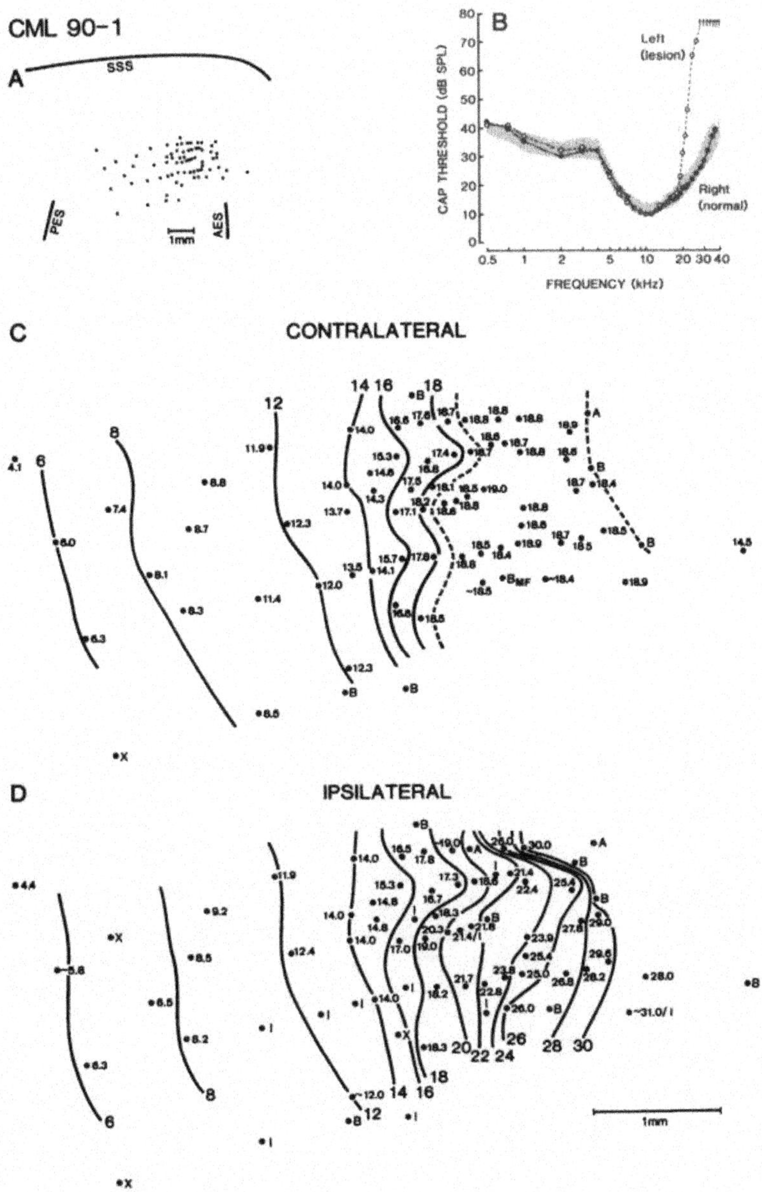
CML 90-1
A
SSS
PES
1mm
AES
B
CAP THRESHOLD (dB SPL)
FREQUENCY (kHz)
Left
(lesion)
Right
(normal)
C
CONTRALATERAL
D
IPSILATERAL
1mm

frequency whose representation was expanded would decrease progressively with age. This apparent contrast might not be real, however, since the extent of hearing loss in Willott et al.'s (1993) study was determined by recording of auditory brainstem responses at 7 or 8 frequencies from 4 to 45 kHz. The edge frequency could therefore not be specified with precision, and the relationship between the edge frequency and those frequencies whose cortical representation was expanded is therefore uncertain.

Auditory cortical reorganization similar to that seen following restricted cochlear lesions in adult animals has also been observed in cat AI as a consequence of neonatal bilateral, high-frequency cochlear lesions produced by ototoxic drugs (Harrison et al., 1991, 1992; R. Rajan, D. R. F. Irvine, L. Z. Wise, and R. Martin, unpublished results). However, it must be emphasised that in both of these studies the lesions were made in neonatal animals and that developmental plasticity of this type could well involve mechanisms (e.g., extensive axonal sprouting) other than those responsible for plasticity in the adult nervous system.

2.2 Subcortical Auditory Centres

The fact that reorganization is observed at the level of the cerebral cortex does not mean that the processes responsible for the reorganization are intrinsic to the cortex. The primary locus of reorganization could be subcortical, and the changes seen at the cortex could simply reflect those at a lower level. In the visual system, there is evidence for reorganization at the level of the lateral geniculate nucleus following restricted retinal lesions (e.g., Eysel et al., 1980, 1981), but the extent of such reorganization is insufficient to account for that at cortex (e.g., Gilbert and Wiesel, 1992). In the somatosensory system, there is also evidence for reorganization at the level of the thalamus (e.g., Garraghty and Kaas, 1991) and at lower levels (see Snow and Wilson (1991) for review), although the extent to which such reorganization contributes to that seen at the cortex is uncertain (e.g., Merzenich et al., 1988; Garraghty and Kaas, 1991).

In adult cats with unilateral cochlear lesions, reorganization of the representation of the lesioned cochlea in contralateral AI occurs without any apparent change in the representation of the normal ipsilateral cochlea. As discussed in detail elsewhere (Rajan et al., 1993), this pattern of results suggests that the primary site of reorganization might be at a subcortical site at or before the locus of binaural interaction. Recordings from the central nucleus of the inferior colliculus (ICC) of adult cats with unilateral basal cochlea lesions (Irvine and Rajan, 1994) have provided evidence of reorganization similar to that seen in AI of cats with the same type of lesion. The reorganization seen at ICC is comparable to that at cortex in that the representation of the contralateral lesioned cochlea is characterized by an expanded representation of lesion-edge frequencies, while the representation of the normal ipsilateral cochlea is apparently unchanged. In contrast to the reorganization seen in the cortex, however, the reorganization in ICC is patchy, in that it is seen in some penetrations through ICC in a given animal but not in others. Furthermore, at some points in those penetrations giving evidence of reorganization, neuron clusters are more broadly tuned than normal, with similar thresholds over a range of frequencies extending below the lesion-edge frequency. These differences between the reorganization seen in ICC and in AI suggest that while the former presumably contributes to the latter, it does not account for it fully.

Whether the reorganization seen in ICC reflects processes intrinsic to the nucleus, or whether it in turn reflects reorganization occurring at lower brain stem levels is unknown. If the latter were the case, the patchy nature of ICC reorganization would suggest that reorganization occurs in only a subset of the multiple brainstem pathways that provide partially segregated input to ICC. Alternatively, reorganization might reflect a process that is intrinsic to ICC but has a patchy distribution.

Reorganization at levels below the colliculus has not yet been examined in adult cats with restricted cochlea lesions. However, Kaltenbach et al. (1992) have reported that there was no evidence of reorganization in the dorsal cochlear nucleus (DCN) of adult hamsters in which restricted cochlear lesions were produced by intense tone exposures. Changes in the DCN frequency map in these animals were explicable in terms of the residue of pre-lesion responses. These data suggest that the pathway from DCN to ICC is not involved in lesion-induced reorganization in the colliculus.

The occurrence of reorganization in the auditory brainstem (at or below the level of the IC) is supported by Willott's (1986) description of reorganization in ICC of C57 mice that is analogous to that seen in the cortex of these mice. In the enlarged representation of the middle-frequency range in the ventral (originally high-frequency) region of ICC the thresholds of multi-neuron clusters were lower than would have been expected had they simply reflected the residue of pre-degeneration responses, and the expansion therefore appears to reflect a dynamic process of reorganization. Willott et al. (1993) have argued that the thresholds in ICC are not as close to normal thresholds as those in AI, and that the ICC reorganization therefore does not appear to account fully for that in AI.

The situation at lower brainstem levels in C57 mice is less clear. Willott et al. (1991) reported an increase in the proportion of neuron clusters and single neurons with CFs in the middle frequency range in both the ventral and dorsal cochlear nuclei (VCN and DCN) of older C57 mice. Thresholds in VCN were significantly elevated relative to those in younger animals, however, suggesting that the change in the frequency organization might simply reflect residual responses. In DCN, in contrast, thresholds were less elevated, by an amount similar to that observed in ICC, which would seem to suggest the occurrence of reorganization in DCN. However, as Willott et al. (1991) note, DCN neurons have much more complex frequency response areas than most VCN neurons. In the absence of quantitative evidence on the thresholds at middle frequencies of high-CF DCN neurons in young C57 mice, it remains a possibility that the enlarged representations of this frequency range in older animals reflect the residue of pre-degeneration input to neurons that were broadly tuned or had complex response areas, and thus had relatively low thresholds at these frequencies.

The data reviewed here indicate that restricted cochlear lesions in adult animals undoubtedly result in some degree of reorganization at the level of the ICC, although the changes at this level do not seem to account fully for the changes seen in auditory cortex. What remains unclear, however, is whether the reorganization seen in ICC reflects processes intrinsic to the colliculus or whether it is wholly or partly the product of changes at lower levels.

2.3 Preliminary Consideration of Functional Significance of Lesion-Induced Plasticity in Central Auditory Pathway of Adults

Given the occurrence of central nervous system reorganization as a consequence of peripheral damage in all of the major sensory systems, it is tempting to think of the reorganization as providing some form of "compensation" for the peripheral loss. In the case of auditory central reorganization, at least, it seems unlikely that this interpretation is appropriate. The critical point in this context is that sensitivity to those frequencies affected by the cochlear lesion is in no way restored by the central reorganization. Nor is there any obvious sense in which an expanded representation of lesion-edge frequencies could be thought of as compensating for the loss of sensitivity to the lesion-affected frequencies. In the case of visual cortical reorganization after a retinal lesion, it has been suggested that such reorganization might be responsible for the perceptual "filling-in" of scotomas associated with retinal degeneration (Chino et al., 1992). While this would be a significant perceptual consequence of reorganization, such filling in does not eliminate the blind spots associated with the scotomas, and is therefore "compensatory" in only a limited sense.

An alternative interpretation of central reorganization after partial deafferentations is that it demonstrates, under the most extreme conditions, the capacity of cortical (and subcortical) sensory structures in adult animals to reorganize when confronted by altered patterns of input. This view is supported by evidence of analogous changes in the cortex as a consequence of altered patterns of input associated with differential use of particular regions of receptor surfaces in the course of normal sensory/perceptual experience. Thus, changes in somatosensory cortical maps have been described in adult monkeys trained in tasks involving either increased stimulation of a restricted skin region or perceptual discrimination of stimuli applied to a restricted region (e.g., Jenkins et al., 1990; Recanzone et al., 1992). In the following section, evidence on learning and use-related changes in the auditory system will be briefly examined, before a more detailed consideration of the functional significance of reorganization.

3 Learning- and Use-related Plasticity in the Adult Auditory System

3.1 Auditory Cortex

Recanzone et al. (1993) trained adult owl monkeys to discriminate small differences in the frequency of sequentially presented tonal stimuli, and found a progressive improvement in discriminative performance with training over a number of weeks. The improvement comprised an initial rapid component, attributed to learning of the task and of task-related strategies, and a second more gradual component. The latter component did not generalise to frequencies at which the monkeys were not trained, and was therefore interpreted as a stimulus-specific change in discriminative capacity, hypothesised to reflect an enhanced central representation of the relevant stimulus parameters. When the frequency organization of AI in the trained monkeys was compared with that in normal (untrained) monkeys and in monkeys given equivalent acoustic stimulation to which they were not required to attend, the representation of frequencies used in discrimination training was found to be larger in the trained monkeys than in either of the control groups. The cortical area of representation of the behaviourally trained frequencies was also found to be correlated with behavioural performance, larger areas of representation being associated with smaller values of the Weber fraction.

Enlarged representations of restricted frequency ranges of the type seen after peripheral lesions and behavioural training obviously reflect the fact that neurons at a larger number of recording sites are tuned to the frequencies in question. The other major line of evidence for plasticity in the adult auditory cortex is provided by studies of changes in the frequency selectivity of cortical neuron clusters as a function of conditioning and other procedures designed to manipulate the significance of specific stimuli. Weinberger and his colleagues have investigated such changes in both primary and secondary auditory cortical fields, in a series of studies that have been reviewed in detail elsewhere (Weinberger, 1993,1995; Weinberger and Diamond, 1987). Only those studies relating to changes in frequency selectivity of neurons in tonotopically organized fields will be considered here.

Single- and multi-unit recordings from the rostral and caudal fields of awake, chronically-implanted guinea pigs have shown that behavioural training with a tonal conditioned stimulus (CS) results in changes in frequency sensitivity at supra-threshold intensities (e.g., Bakin and Weinberger, 1990; Edeline and Weinberger, 1993; Edeline at al., 1993). In these studies, the frequency response area was measured by obtaining iso-intensity response functions at a number of supra-threshold intensities, and the frequency of the CS was selected to be within the response area but at a frequency other than the best frequency (BF; that eliciting maximum discharge). At many (but not all) recording sites, the response to the CS frequency was enhanced while that to the BF and to other non-reinforced frequencies decreased, such that in some cases the CS frequency became the BF (see Fig. 3 for representative data). The specificity of these changes, and the fact that sensitization training (in which equal numbers of stimuli are presented without pairing) results in a general increase in responses to all frequencies within the response area (Bakin and Weinberger, 1990; Bakin et al., 1992; Fig. 3b, panel ii), indicate that the changes reflect the fact that the CS frequency has acquired enhanced significance for the animal as a consequence of conditioning. Habituation training, in which the repeated stimulus loses significance, has been shown to result in a frequency-specific decrement in responsiveness to the repeated frequency in guinea pig auditory cortex (Condon and Weinberger, 1991; Fig. 3b, panel iii).

A difficulty in relating these results to those on injury- and use-related changes in tonotopic maps is that the maps are derived from the spatial distribution of CFs (as determined from threshold FTCs), whereas the conditioning-produced changes in BF are measured at SPLs well above threshold. It is possible that a frequency-specific enhancement of supra-threshold responses to the CS, even to the extent that the CS frequency becomes the BF, could occur without a change in CF. Recently, however, Weinberger et al. (1993) have presented data on changes in the entire frequency response areas of multi-unit clusters in guinea pig auditory cortex, and these data indicate that the

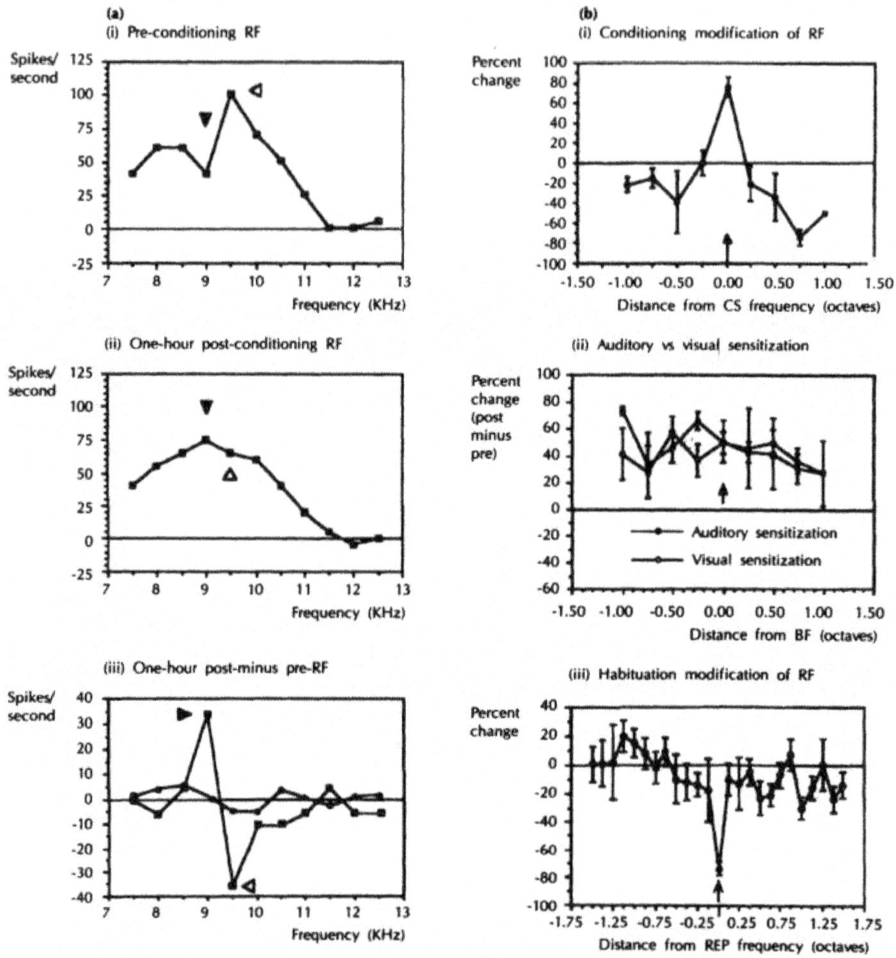

Figure 3. The effects of conditioning and related procedures on the frequency sensitivity of neuron clusters in rostral and caudal fields of awake guinea pigs. (a) Effects of classical conditioning with a tonal stimulus: (i) pre-conditioning iso-intensity function for cluster; BF was 9.5 kHz (open arrowhead) and CS frequency was 9.0 kHz (filled arrowhead). (ii) iso-intensity function 1 hr post-conditioning; response at CS frequency has increased and that at original BF has decreased, so that new BF is at CS frequency. (iii) difference function (post minus pre), showing maximum increase at CS frequency and maximum decrease at original BF. Open circles show lack of systematic effect on spontaneous activity.

BF changes are associated with changes in CF. This study also presented evidence for the long-term retention of learning-induced plasticity, for periods up to 8 weeks after training, and demonstrated that such plasticity was also expressed in the anaesthetized animal. These observations have strengthened the obvious similarities between injury- and learning-related plasticity in the auditory cortex. However, more detailed information on the time course of injury-induced reorganization, and on the mechanisms involved in the two forms of plasticity, is necessary to determine whether they are manifestations of the same processes.

Changes in the cortical area over which neurons respond to a particular frequency, or increases in the strength with which previously-responsive neurons respond, would be expected to be reflected in measures of cortical metabolic activity evoked by that stimulus frequency. Using the 2-deoxyglucose (2DG) method, Gonzalez-Lima and Scheich (1986) reported changes in the pattern of labelling evoked by a narrow-excursion frequency-modulated (FM) tone CS in auditory cortex of the rat as a consequence of conditioning. Although the results of that study are difficult to relate to the neurophysiological data on enlarged frequency representations, recent preliminary reports by Gonzalez-Lima (1992) and by Scheich (1991) have described effects on 2DG labelling that suggest increases in the representational area of particular frequencies as a function of conditioning.

3.2 Subcortical Auditory Centres

Learning-associated changes have been described in the frequency-selectivity of some multi-unit clusters in the ventral division of the medial geniculate body (MG_V) of the awake guinea pig preparation. Although the general form of these changes was similar to that seen in auditory cortex, the changes were transient, being observed only immediately after training, and occurred only if the CS were very close to (within 0.125 octaves of) the BF (Edeline and Weinberger, 1991b). As these authors noted, the changes observed in (MG_V) could account for only a small proportion of the plasticity observed in auditory cortex. In contrast, broadly-tuned neurons in the medial ("magnocellular"; (MG_m) and dorsal (MG_d) divisions of the medial geniculate body showed longer lasting and more robust plasticity (Edeline and Weinberger, 1991a, 1992). The possible contributions of plasticity in medial and dorsal divisions to that seen in auditory cortex have been discussed by Edeline and Weinberger (1992).

The relatively weak and transient conditioning-related plasticity in the subcortical lemniscal-line system suggested by Edeline and Weinberger's (1991) MG_V results is apparently at variance with the report by Gonzalez-Lima and Agudo (1990; Gonzalez-Lima, 1992) of marked changes in frequency representation in ICC as a consequence of conditioning. They used the 2DG technique to measure the regions of activation produced

---

(b) Normalized group difference functions (obtained by averaging difference functions from individual recording sites) ± standard error for three types of training conditions: conditioning (i), sensitization using either a visual or auditory stimulus (ii) and habituation (iii). Frequency axis is distance in octaves from the CS frequency (i), the BF (ii), and the repeated (REP) frequency (iii), respectively. From Weinberger (1993).

by FM tones of small excursion (4-5 kHz and 16-20 kHz) in unanesthetized rats, and reported that the band of increased 2DG uptake produced by either FM signal was enlarged when that signal was paired with an arousing unconditioned stimulus in a differential conditioning paradigm. The many methodological differences between these two studies, and the complexity of the relationships between changes in multi-unit activity and in patterns of 2DG labelling, do not allow any reconciliation of this apparent disagreement. It is clear, however, that further evidence is required to determine the contribution of subcortical changes to conditioning-related plasticity in frequency selectivity in auditory cortex.

A final line of evidence for use-related plasticity in subcortical auditory pathways is provided by Snyder et al.'s (1990) account of the effects of chronic intracochlear electrical stimulation in cats neonatally deafened by injections of neomycin. These animals and those in various control groups were examined electrophysiologically as adults to determine the spatial extent of the activity elicited in ICC by intracochlear stimulation. In control animals that did not receive chronic stimulation, electrical stimulation through intracochlear bipolar electrodes consistently produced activation of a restricted sector of ICC, the location of which was in accordance with the known cochleotopic organization of ICC and with the cochlear location of the electrode pair. In animals chronically stimulated through a given electrode pair, however, the region of ICC activated by stimulation at that cochlear site was approximately twice as large as the region activated in control animals. Although these animals were neonatally deafened, prosthesis implantation and chronic stimulation were not initiated until they were at least 10 weeks old, an age at which the cat's auditory system is in many respects adult. The changes in the representation of the cochlea described in this study would therefore appear to be an instance of adult plasticity.

4 Functional Significance of Lesion- and Use-related Plasticity in the Central Auditory System of Adults

The evidence for conditioning and use-related plasticity in the adult auditory system establishes many points of correspondence between this plasticity and that seen following peripheral lesions. In general, therefore, this evidence supports the view that lesion-induced plasticity can reasonably be considered as the extreme form of a more general plasticity that occurs as a consequence of normal patterns of use and disuse in sensory systems. It should also be noted, however, that identity of the mechanisms involved in injury- and use-related plasticity has not been established, and it remains possible that different mechanisms are involved.

It has been proposed that both forms of plasticity as manifested in the cerebral cortex are manifestations of "self-organizing" mechanisms intrinsic to neocortex that are responsible for the refinement of cortical maps during development and that underlie many higher-order processes such as learning and non-declarative memory (e.g., Edelman and Finkel, 1984; Merzenich et al., 1990a,b; Merzenich and Sameshima, 1993). The possibility that cortical plasticity might underlie at least some aspects of perceptual learning is supported by Recanzone et al.'s data on frequency discrimination, and has also been invoked to explain a form of visual perceptual learning in humans (e.g., Karni and Sagi,

1991). Although the claim that cortical reorganization reflects intrinsically cortical processes must be qualified in the light of evidence for some degree of plasticity at subcortical levels, it remains possible that cortical plasticity differs either qualitatively or quantitatively from that at lower levels.

Although it was argued earlier that cortical reorganization after restricted cochlear lesions does not have a compensatory function, this does not mean that such reorganization would not have functional (i.e., perceptual) consequences. The occurrence of such reorganization in a range of mammals also suggests that it would be likely to occur in humans with noise- or age-related partial hearing losses similar to those seen in experimental animals. If such reorganization does occur in humans, its perceptual consequences are apparently not of a type revealed by standard audiometric testing, as there do not seem to be descriptions in the audiological literature of phenomena that might be thought to reflect such reorganization. One possibility, discussed in more detail elsewhere (Rajan et al., 1993), is that central reorganization after a unilateral hearing loss might contribute to the phenomenon of binaural diplacusis. Recently, there has been speculation in the audiological literature that central reorganization might be a factor in the slow time course of adaptation to a newly-fitted hearing aid (e.g., Gatehouse, 1992; Gatehouse and Killion, 1993). Although such speculations are provocative, identification of any perceptual consequences of presumed central reorganization in humans with partial deafness will depend on studies in which various forms of psychoacoustic performance in the frequency range at the edge of the region of hearing loss are examined in detail.

5 Mechanisms of Plasticity in the Adult Auditory System

Space restrictions preclude a detailed discussion of the possible mechanisms underlying plasticity in the adult auditory system, and only a brief account of current views will be given here. In the absence of compelling evidence for axonal sprouting outside the field of the normal axonal arbor in the adult central nervous system, it is generally assumed that cortical reorganization reflects functional changes within the constraints imposed by existing anatomical connections. The precision of cortical maps is apparently at variance with the extensive arborisation of thalamo-cortical axons in the cortex and the existence of widespread horizontal intracortical connections, which provide a much wider range of potential inputs to neurons at a given cortical locus than is manifested in their receptive fields. Many of these potential inputs are thus thought to be normally unexpressed, either because the synapses involved provide ineffective excitatory input or because the excitatory input they provide is masked by inhibition (e.g., Calford and Tweedale, 1988,1991a,b; Merzenich et al., 1990a; Snow and Wilson, 1991). It is assumed that when the normally dominant input to a cortical region is eliminated by a peripheral lesion, previously unexpressed inputs become effective and their effect is manifested as reorganization. On this view, reorganization after peripheral damage is an extreme manifestation of the processes normally responsible for the refinement of cortical maps within the broad constraints imposed by diffuse neuroanatomical connectivity (e.g., Edelman and Finkel, 1984; Merzenich et al., 1990a).

One of the strongest lines of evidence for the role of release from inhibition in the unmasking of normally unexpressed inputs is the evidence for immediate expansion of cortical receptive fields after peripheral lesions in the somatosensory and visual systems (Calford and Tweedale 1988, 1991a,b; Gilbert and Wiesel, 1992). Reorganization also occurs very rapidly in motor cortex after peripheral lesions (e.g., Donoghue et al., 1990), and there is compelling evidence that this reorganization reflects the unmasking of excitatory intracortical connections that are normally subject to inhibition by local GABAergic interneurons (Jacobs and Donoghue, 1991; see also the general discussion of the role of GABAergic neurons in cortical plasticity by Jones (1993)). The immediate expansion of receptive fields in the visual and somatosensory cortices following peripheral lesions is followed by a gradual contraction of the expanded fields over subsequent weeks (Calford and Tweedale 1988; Gilbert and Wiesel, 1992). This process presumably reflects a re-establishment of excitatory-inhibitory balance in the input to the neurons, possibly based on some form of Hebbian rule of the type thought to be responsible for the strengthening of ineffective synapses (See Merzenich and Sameshima (1993) for discussion).

The available evidence suggests that immediate unmasking of unexpressed inputs is unlikely to be involved in lesion-induced reorganization in the auditory cortex. In acutely-lesioned guinea pigs, there was no evidence of such unmasking. Rather, neuron clusters in the region whose dominant input was eliminated by the cochlear lesion were characterized by high-threshold, "residual" FTCs. These observations suggest that auditory cortical reorganization is more likely to reflect a gradual strengthening of normally ineffective or weakly effective inputs and changes in excitatory and inhibitory synaptic weights. However, more detailed evidence on the time course of changes in the frequency tuning of individual neurons after cochlear lesions will be critical to a better understanding of the mechanisms of lesion induced auditory cortical plasticity.

6 Acknowledgement

Supported by grants from the National Health and Medical Research Council of Australia.

7 References

Bakin, J.S., Lepan, B. and Weinberger, N.M. (1992) Sensitization induced receptive field plasticity in the auditory cortex is independent of CS-modality. Brain Res. 577, 226-235.

Bakin, J.S. and Weinberger, N.M. (1990) Classical conditioning induces CS-specific receptive field plasticity in the auditory cortex of the guinea pig. Brain Res. 536, 271-286.

Calford, M.B. and Tweedale, R. (1988) Immediate and chronic changes in responses of somatosensory cortex in adult flying-fox after digit amputation. Nature. 332, 446-448.

Calford, M.B. and Tweedale, R. (1991a) Acute changes in cutaneous receptive fields in primary somatosensory cortex after digit denervation in adult flying fox. J. Neurophysiol. 65, 178-187.

Calford, M.B. and Tweedale, R. (1991b) Immediate expansion of receptive fields of neurons in area 3b of macaque monkeys after digit denervation. Somatosens. Mot. Res. 8, 249-260.

Chino, Y.M., Kaas, J.H. Smith, III, E.L. Langston, A.L. and Cheng, H. (1992) Rapid reorganization of cortical maps in adult cats following restricted deafferentation in retina. Vision Res. 32, 789-796.

Condon, C.D. and Weinberger, N.M. (1991) Habituation produces frequency-specific plasticity of receptive fields in the auditory cortex. Behav. Neurosci. 105, 416-430.

Donoghue, J.P., Suner, S. and Sanes, J.N. (1990) Dynamic organization of primary motor cortex output to target muscles in adult rats. II. Rapid reorganization following motor nerve lesions. Exp. Brain Res. 79, 492-503.

Edeline, J.-M., Pham, P. and Weinberger, N.M. (1993) Rapid development of learning-induced receptive field plasticity in the auditory cortex. Behav. Neurosci. 107, 539-551.

Edeline, J.-M. and Weinberger, N.M. (1991a) Subcortical adaptive filtering in the auditory system: Associative receptive field plasticity in the dorsal medial geniculate body. Behav. Neurosci. 105, 154-175.

Edeline, J.-M. and Weinberger, N.M. (1991b) Thalamic short-term plasticity in the auditory system: Associative retuning of receptive fields in the ventral medial geniculate body. Behav. Neurosci. 105, 618-639.

Edeline, J.-M. and Weinberger, N.M. (1992) Associative retuning in the thalamic source of input to the amygdala and auditory cortex: Receptive field plasticity in the medial division of the medial geniculate body. Behav. Neurosci. 106, 81-105.

Edeline, J.-M. and Weinberger, N.M. (1993) Receptive field plasticity in the auditory cortex during frequency discrimination training: Selective retuning independent of task difficulty. Behav. Neurosci. 107, 82-103.

Edelman, G.M. and Finkel, L.H. (1984) Neuronal group selection in the cerebral cortex. In: G.M. Edelman, W.E. Gall and W.M. Cowan (Eds.), Dynamic Aspects of Neocortical Function, Wiley, N.Y., pp. 653-695.

Eysel, U.T., Gonzalez-Aguilar, F. and Mayer, U. (1981) Time-dependent decrease in the extent of visual deafferentation in the lateral geniculate nucleus of adult cats with small retinal lesions. Exp. Brain Res. 41, 256-263.

Eysel, U.T., Gonzalez-Aguilar, F. and Mayer, U. (1980) A functional sign of reorganization in the visual system of adult cats: lateral geniculate neurons with displaced receptive fields after lesions of the nasal retina. Brain Res. 181, 285-300.

Garraghty, P.E. and Kaas, J.H. (1991) Functional reorganization in adult monkey thalamus after peripheral nerve injury. NeuroReport. 2, 747-750.

Gatehouse, S. (1992) The time course and magnitude of perceptual acclimatization to frequency responses: Evidence from monaural fitting of hearing aids. J. Acoust. Soc. Am. 92, 1258-1268.

Gatehouse, S. and Killion, M.C. (1993) HABRAT: Hearing aid brain rewiring accommodation time. Hear. Instruments. 44, 29-32.

Gilbert, C.D. and T.N. Wiesel (1992) Receptive field dynamics in adult primary visual cortex, Nature, 356, 150-152.

Gonzalez-Lima, F. (1992) Brain imaging of auditory learning functions in rats: studies with fluorodeoxyglucose autoradiography and cytochrome oxidase histochemistry. In: F. Gonzalez-Lima, Th. Finkenstädt and H. Scheich (Eds.), Advances in Metabolic Mapping Techniques for Brain Imaging of Behavioral and Learning Functions. Dordrecht, Boston. pp. 39-109.

Gonzalez-Lima, F. and Agudo, J. (1990) Functional reorganization of neural auditory maps by differential learning. NeuroReport. 1, 161-164.

Gonzalez-Lima, F. and Scheich, H. (1986) Neural substrates for tone-conditioned bradycardia demonstrated with 2-deoxyglucose. II. Auditory cortex plasticity. Behav. Brain Res. 20, 281-293.

Harrison, R.V., A. Nagasawa, A., Smith, D.W., Stanton, S. and Mount, R.J. (1991) Reorganization of auditory cortex after neonatal high frequency cochlear hearing loss. Hear. Res. 54, 11-19.

Harrison, R.V., Smith, D.W., Nagasawa, A., Stanton, S. and Mount, R.J. (1992) Developmental plasticity of auditory cortex in cochlear hearing loss: physiological and psychophysical findings. In: Y. Cazals, K. Horner and L. Demany (Eds.), Auditory Physiology and Perception, Pergamon, Oxford, pp. 625-633.

Irvine, D.R.F. and Rajan, R. (1994) Plasticity of frequency organization in inferior colliculus of adult cats with unilateral restricted cochlear lesions. In: Abstracts Seventeenth Annual Meeting, Association for Research in Otolaryngology, pp. 21.

Jacobs, K.M. and Donoghue, J.P. (1991) Reshaping the cortical motor map by unmasking latent intracortical connections. Science. 251, 944-947.

Jenkins, W.M., Merzenich, M.M., Ochs, M.T., Allard, T. and Guíc-Robles, E. (1990) Functional reorganization of primary somatosensory cortex in adult owl monkeys after behaviorally controlled tactile stimulation. J. Neurophysiol. 63, 82-104.

Jones, E.G. (1993) GABAergic neurons and their role in cortical plasticity in primates. Cereb. Cortex. 3, 361-372.

Kaas, J.H. (1991) Plasticity of sensory and motor maps in adult mammals. Annu. Rev. Neurosci. 14, 137-167.

Kaas, J.H., Krubitzer, L.A., Chino, Y.M., Langston, A.L., Polley, E.H. and Blair, N. (1990) Reorganization of retinotopic cortical maps in adult mammals after lesions of the retina. Science. 248, 229-231.

Kaas, J.H., Merzenich, M.M., and Killackey, H.P. (1983) The reorganization of somatosensory cortex following peripheral nerve damage in adult and developing mammals. Annu. Rev. Neurosci. 6, 325-356.

Kaltenbach, J.A., Czaja, J.M. and Kaplan, C.R. (1992) Changes in the tonotopic map of the dorsal cochlear nucleus following induction of cochlear lesions by exposure to intense sound. Hear. Res. Res. 59, 213-223.

Karni, A. and Sagi, D. (1991) Where practice makes perfect in texture discrimination: Evidence for primary visual cortex plasticity. Proc. Natl. Acad. Sci. USA. 88, 4966-4970.

King, A.J. and Moore, D.R. (1991) Plasticity of auditory maps in the brain. Trends Neurosci. 14, 31-37.

Knudsen, E.I. (1988) Sensitive and critical periods in the development of sound localization. In: Easter, Barald and Carlson (Eds.), From Message to Mind, Sinauer Assoc., pp. 303-319.

Konishi, M. (1986) Centrally synthesized maps of sensory space. Trends Neurosci. 9, 163-168.

Merzenich, M.M., Recanzone, G., Jenkins, W.M., Allard, T.T. and Nudo, R.J. (1988) Cortical representational plasticity. In: P. Rakic and W. Singer (Eds.), Neurobiology of Neocortex, Wiley, N.Y., pp. 41-67.

Merzenich, M.M., Recanzone, G.H., Jenkins, W.M. and Grajski, K.A. (1990a) Adaptive mechanisms in cortical networks underlying cortical contributions to learning and nondeclarative memory. Cold Spring Harbor Symp. Quant. Biol. 55, 873-887.

Merzenich, M.M., Recanzone, G.H., Jenkins, W.M. and Nudo, R.J. (1990b) How the brain functionally rewires itself, In: M. Arbib and J.A. Robinson (Eds.), Natural and Artificial Parallel Computations. MIT Press, N.Y., pp. 177-210.

Merzenich, M.M. and Sameshima, K. (1993) Cortical plasticity and memory. Curr. Opin. Neurobiol. 3, 187-196.

Phillips, D.P. and Hall, S.E. (1992) Multiplicity of inputs in the afferent path to cat auditory cortex neurons revealed by tone-on-tone masking. Cereb. Cortex. 2, 425-433.

Phillips, D.P., Orman, S.S., Musicant, A.D. and Wilson, G.F. (1985) Neurons in the cat's primary auditory cortex distinguished by their responses to tones and wide-spectrum noise. Hear. Res. 18, 73-86.

Rajan, R., Irvine, D.R.F., Wise, L.Z. and Heil, P. (1993) Effect of unilateral partial cochlear lesions in adult cats on the representation of lesioned and unlesioned cochleas in primary auditory cortex. J. Comp. Neurol. 338, 17-49.

Recanzone, G.H., Merzenich, M.M., Jenkins, W.M., Grajski, K.A. and Dinse, H.R. (1992) Topographic reorganization of the hand representation in cortical area 3b of owl monkeys trained in a frequency- discrimination task. J. Neurophysiol. 67, 1031-1056.

Recanzone, G.H., Schreiner, C.E., and Merzenich, M.M. (1993) Plasticity in the frequency representation of primary auditory cortex following discrimination training in adult owl monkeys. J. Neurosci. 13, 87-103.

Robertson, D. and Irvine, D.R.F (1989) Plasticity of frequency organization in auditory cortex of guinea pigs with partial unilateral deafness. J. Comp. Neurol. 282, 456-471.

Rübsamen, R. (1992) Postnatal development of central auditory frequency maps, J. Comp. Physiol. [A]. 170, 129-143.

Scheich, H. (1991) Auditory cortex: comparative aspects of maps and plasticity, Curr. Opin. Neurobiol. 1, 236-247.

Schwaber, M.K., Garraghty, P.E. and Kaas, J.H. (1993) Neuroplasticity of the adult primate auditory cortex following cochlear hearing loss. Am. J. Otol. 14, 252-258.

Snow, P.J. and Wilson,P. (1991) Plasticity in the somatosensory system of developing and mature mammals - the effects of injury to the central and peripheral nervous system. In: D. Ottoson, (Ed.), Progress in Sensory Physiology 11, Springer-Verlag, Berlin, pp. 482.

Snyder, R.L., Rebscher, S.J., Cao, K., Leake, P.A. and Kelly, K. (1990) Chronic intracochlear electrical stimulation in the neonatally deafened cat. I: Expansion of central representation. Hear. Res. 50, 7-34.

Tsukahara, N. (1981) Synaptic plasticity in the mammalian central nervous system. Annu. Rev. Neurosci. 4, 351-379.

Weinberger, N.M. (1993) Learning-induced changes of auditory receptive fields. Curr. Opin. Neurobiol. 3, 570-577.

Weinberger, N.M. (1995) Dynamic regulation of receptive fields and maps in the adult sensory cortex. Annu. Rev. Neurosci. (In Press)

Weinberger, N.M. and Diamond, D.M. (1987) Physiological plasticity in auditory cortex: rapid induction by learning. Prog. Neurobiol. 29, 1-55.

Weinberger, N.M., Javid, R. and Lepan, B. (1993) Long-term retention of learning-induced receptive-field plasticity in the auditory cortex. Proc. Natl. Acad. Sci. USA. 90, 2394-2398.

Willott, J.F. (1986) Effects of aging, hearing loss, and anatomical location on thresholds of inferior colliculus neurons in C57BL/6 and CBA mice. J. Neurophysiol. 56, 391-408.

Willott, J.F., Aitkin, L.M. and McFadden, S.L. (1993) Plasticity of auditory cortex associated with sensorineural hearing loss in adult C57BL/6J mice. J. Comp. Neurol. 329, 402-411.

Willott, J.F., Parham, K. and Hunter, K.P. (1991) Comparison of the auditory sensitivity of neurons in the cochlear nucleus and inferior colliculus of young and aging C57BL/6J and CBA/J mice. Hear. Res. 53, 78-94.

8 Addendum

Since this manuscript was submitted, Darian-Smith and Gilbert (1994) have presented evidence for the involvement of structural changes in injury-induced reorganization. They reported that cortical reorganization consequent on restricted retinal lesions in adult cats was associated with increased density of axonal fibers in the superficial layers of the reorganized cortex. This was attributed to axon sprouting (presumably associated with synaptic proliferation) of longe-range horizontal fibers. Thus, in the visual system at least, it appears that the increased effectiveness of normally ineffective inputs is due in part to synaptic proliferation.

Darian-Smith, C. and Gilbert, C.D. (1994) Axonal sprouting accompanies functional reorganization in adult cat striate cortex. Nature 368, 737-740.

Comment by G.M. Klump

Some studies of the frequency representation in the brain have demonstrated that changes in the frequency map by the modification of GABAergic inhibition might also be mediated by other neurotransmitters, such as acetylcholine. Acetylcholine is a transmitter that is attributed some function in attentional mechanisms. Studies in the auditory cortex of mammals (e.g., see Metherate and Weinberger 1989) and in the cortex analogue of birds (e.g., see Müller 1987) have shown that acetylcholine changes the neuronal response properties, and to my knowledge, at least in birds these changes may be due to acetylcholine modulating the GABAergic inhibition. Thus, attentional mechanisms may change the frequency map by modifying the strength of lateral inhibition in the frequency domain. This is an additional mechanism that leads to an dynamic modification of the analysing properties of the auditory system.

Metherate, R. and Weinberger, N.M. (1989) Acetylcholine produces stimulus-specific receptive field alterations in cat auditory cortex. Brain Res. 480, 372-377.

Müller, C.M. (1987b) Differential effects of acetylcholine in the chicken auditory neostriatum and hyperstriatum ventrale-studies in vivo and in vitro. J. Comp. Physiol. A 161, 857-866.

Reply

Thank you for this comment, with which I agree entirely. Limitations of time and space prevented me from discussing the evidence for cholinergic modulation of the processes underlying plasticity.

Comment by B. Scharf

First a comment in answer to the last question you posed, and then two questions. Psychoacoustical data do exist on loudness and intensity discrimination near high-frequency hearing losses. Rhona Hellman (JASA 1978, 52, 1113-1119) showed that the dynamic range for loudness at the edge of a high-frequency loss is not reduced even though the spread of excitation to sensitive high-frequency areas is greatly restricted. Could it be that a remapping at higher auditory levels compensates for the loss at the cochlear level thereby restoring--or nearly so--the spread of excitation? However, the fact that a high-pass noise has a similar effect would seem to argue against a remapping explanation. Moreover, discrimination data on the edge of a high-frequency loss seem to argue against any remapping (see Florentine, JASA 1983, 74, 1375-1379).

How long does cortical remapping from behavioral learning remain in effect?
How much do organisms vary in their ability to remap?

Reply

Thank you for the information on the psychoacoustical data. I'm unable to comment on the papers at this stage, but will read them with interest. Since my manuscript was submitted, I've been made aware of some recent data by K. Robinson and S. Gatehouse (in press) on intensity discrimination following long term use of a monaural hearing aid, and on the time course of these effects (ASA, June, 1994). Of course, the connection between these effects and central plasticity within the auditory system itself remains speculative.

With respect to the duration of learning-induced changes, Weinberger et al. (1993) reported that conditioning-produced changes in BF at individual recording sites are still present up to 8 weeks after training. It is not jet known whether such changes are also seen at CF or whether they occur at all recording sites in which the original BF (and adjacent frequencies) were represented. If they are, then learning-induced changes in the frequency map would be expected to be seen for this time period.

Studies of injury-induced reorganization in different species have used different techniques to produce cochlear damage, and it is therefore impossible to determine whether there are species differences in the ability of the auditory CNS to reorganize. In some of our guinea pig experiments (Robertson and Irvine, 1989), we produced broad high frequency losses in sensitivity rather than the notch losses I discussed in my paper here. In these cases, the general characteristics of the reorganization were similar to that seen in cats after basal cochlear lesions. Even in these two cases with mechanical lesions, however both the edge frequencies and the extent of cortex deprived of its normal input by the lesion are different. We are therefore unable to comment on any possible species differences in capacity for reorganization.

With respect to individual differences, these are confounded with differences in lesion characteristics and in recovery times in our studies, so we are unable to draw any conclusions. Recanzone et al. (1993) reported a correlation between perceptual acuity in the frequency discrimination task and the size of the area of cortical representation, and this might reflect individual differences.

The development of Nucleus laminaris in the barn owl

C. E. Carr

*Department of Zoology, University of Maryland,
College Park, MD 20742 USA.*

1 Introduction

Barn owls are nocturnal predators that locate sounds on the basis of auditory cues alone (Payne, 1971; Konishi, 1973). They use interaural time differences (ITDs) to determine the azimuthal location of a sound (Knudsen and Konishi, 1979; Moiseff, 1989). These timing cues are preserved in a specialized pathway in the central auditory system (Takahashi and Konishi, 1984; Carr, 1993). The timing of the auditory stimulus is preserved in the phase locked firing of the auditory nerve. Auditory nerve fibers enter the brain and divide to terminate in the cochlear nucleus angularis and the cochlear nucleus magnocellularis. The projection from the nucleus magnocellularis to the nucleus laminaris supports the encoding and measurement of ITDs. Maps of ITD are formed in the dorso-ventral dimension of the nucleus laminaris by interdigitating axons from the ipsi- and contralateral magnocellular cochlear nuclei. The maps of ITD are tapped by postsynaptic coincidence detectors (Carr and Konishi, 1990).

During the first few weeks of life, the young bird's head more than doubles in size, subjecting it to changing ITD cues. We have analyzed the development of the auditory brainstem to determine how the circuit in the nucleus laminaris adapts to these changing auditory cues. The connections between the nucleus magnocellularis and the nucleus laminaris are formed before the time of hatching (Carr and Boudreau, submitted). The most prominent developmental change in the first month posthatch is in the myelination of the delay line axons within the nucleus laminaris. Delay line myelination occurs late in development, during the period of maximum head growth (Carr and Cheng, 1992). Myelination is significant for development of delay lines, because the amount of delay mapped in the nucleus laminaris depends on the length and conduction velocity of the magnocellular afferents. The timing of the myelination of the delay lines is important because it occurs later than other myelination in this region of the brainstem and at the time when auditory cues stabilize and the head grows to adult size. Since the late myelination of the delay line circuit is functionally significant, we have examined the developmental profile of myelin genes and the factors that regulate their expression in the brainstem auditory nuclei.

In parallel with the studies of myelination, we have also examined the development of time coding during the tuning and assembly of the map of interaural time differences. In the adult bird, nucleus laminaris neurons are maximally excited by the simultaneous activation of their ipsi- and contralateral inputs, via a coincidence detection mechanism.

Since the timing of the presynaptic inputs is critical to coincidence detection, we have measured the neurophonic, or laminaris evoked potential, to determine when the "correct" timing of the inputs is achieved. The mechanism underlying the tuning of these inputs is of general interest, since many models of development depend upon selection of temporally ordered inputs.

2 Methods

This study is based on results from 18 young barn owls (Tyto alba) of both sexes. Most owls were used in parallel studies (Carr and Boudreau, submitted; Cheng and Carr, 1992).

2.1 Anatomical techniques

Immunohistochemical and ultrastructural techniques have been published in detail (see Carr and Boudreau, 1993). For normal ultrastructural studies, animals were anesthetized with Ketamine (33mg/kg IM) followed by an overdose of Nembutal (100mg/kg IV) and perfused transcardially with 2.5% glutaraldehyde, 2% paraformaldehyde. The brainstem is then sectioned and embedded in Araldite resin. Thin sections were taken from areas immediately adjacent to the thick sections. For immunohistochemistry, sections are cut at 30μm and incubated in primary antiserum, then incubated with a biotinylated secondary and processed using the avidin biotin (ABC) technique.

For in situ hybridization studies of proteolipid protein (PLP) mRNA, ^{35}S-cRNA probes were transcribed from chicken PLP cDNA , kindly provided by Dr. K. Nave at the University of Heidelberg. Sections were hybridized with these probes using techniques described in Higgins et al. (1989). After washing and RNAase treatment, slides were air dried and exposed to x-ray film for 24-48 hours, dipped in photographic emulsion, and developed for autoradiography. Selected slides were counterstained for morphometric analysis.

2.2 Electrophysiology

In parallel with the studies of myelination, we have examined the physiological development of the nucleus laminaris. Stimuli were tone or noise bursts of 100msec in duration with rise/fall times of 5msec. The stimuli were generated using the Ariel S-56X DSP coprocessor board with a Sun SPARCstation. Owls are prepared for recording with Ketamine (33mg/kg/hr) and Xylazine (1.7mg/kg/hr) anesthesia, comfortably restrained in a soft leather sling surrounded by a heating pad, and suspended horizontally in a stereotaxic device. All data collection and analyses were done with the SPARCstation using software designed by Mr. J. Mazer. Birds were sacrified after the experiment by injection of a lethal dose of nembutal (100mg/kg IV), and perfused transcardially once deeply anesthetized.

3 Results

We have examined the development of myelination and the development of time coding during the tuning and assembly of the map of ITDs in the nucleus laminaris.

3.1 Normal growth and development

An owl egg takes 5 weeks to hatch. At the time of hatching an owl's skull is about 18 mm wide. It grows to an adult width of about 45 mm at 1 month. The head grows slowly until about 1 week after hatching, then grows rapidly between 8 -20 days of age to reach its adult width by about 25 days (Carr and Boudreau, submitted). Skull width therefore more than doubles in the first month after hatching, subjecting the bird to constantly changing ITDs. The owl experiences stable, adult sound localization cues at the end of two months. These first two months form the sensitive period (Knudsen et al., 1984; Knudsen and Knudsen, 1986).

3.2 Development of myelination in the nucleus laminaris

Myelination was examined using immunohistochemistry, in situ hybridization and ultrastructural techniques. Oligodendrocytes express the major myelin proteins proteolipid protein (PLP), and myelin basic protein (MBP). PLP is the most abundant myelin protein, with MBP second. Both PLP and MBP are required for compaction of myelin lamellae. We have used in situ hybridization to proteolipid protein (PLP) mRNA and antibodies against MBP to describe the progress of myelination during the development of the auditory brainstem (Carr and Higgins, 1990; Cheng and Carr, 1992).

In the week before hatching, large numbers of glial cells and glial precursors have accumulated on the borders of the nucleus laminaris. When the owl hatches at P0, oligodendrocytes have begun to myelinate both the eighth nerve and the magnocellular axons outside the nucleus laminaris (Fig. 1A). In the first week post-hatch, PLP mRNA hybridization characterizes many glial cells on the borders of the nucleus laminaris (Fig. 1B). A wave of glial cell proliferation on the border of the nucleus laminaris is followed by migration of glia into the nucleus laminaris in the first week posthatch. Oligodendrocytes express high levels of PLP mRNA and begin myelination of the magnocellular axons in the nucleus laminaris at the rostral end of the nucleus towards the end of the first week posthatch. Myelination follows the tonotopic gradient within the nucleus laminaris with caudal low best frequency regions myelinated last (Cheng and Carr, 1992).

Oligodendrocytes invade the nucleus laminaris at the time that the eyes open and the head enters a period of maximum growth. Almost all magnocellular axons in the nucleus laminaris are myelinated by P20, although most do not have many myelin wrappings. Myelination proceeds slowly and is almost complete at P30. Thus the delay lines acquire a functional appearance towards the end of the first month of life. Further increases in the degree of myelination, and in fiber diameter continue into the second month posthatch. The maturation of this circuit coincides with the time that the head stops growing, and the bird is no longer subject to changing interaural time cues.

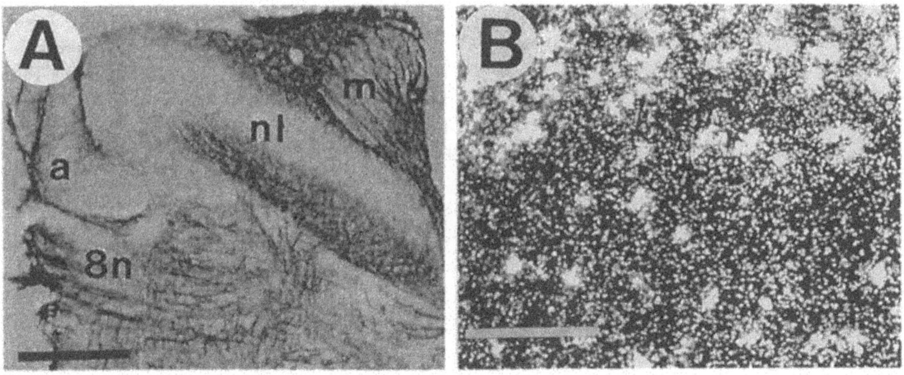

Figure 1. Myelination of the nucleus laminaris. A. Myelin basic protein immunoreactivity on the borders of the nucleus laminaris at P1. a = nucleus angularis, 8n = auditory nerve, nl = nucleus laminaris, m = nucleus magnocellularis. Bar = 1 mm. B. PLP in situ hybridization at P5. The border of the nucleus laminaris is marked by intense hybridization at the top of the photomicrograph. Bar = 200 µm.

3.3 Development of Time Coding

In parallel with the studies of myelination, we have examined the physiological development of the map of ITDs in the nucleus laminaris. The phase locked responses of the delay lines produce a large evoked potential within the nucleus laminaris, called the neurophonic. Neurophonics are found in brain areas where phase locking occurs, and are assumed to represent the phase locked responses of many neurons (Sullivan and Konishi, 1986). When an electrode is lowered through the nucleus laminaris, parallel to the delay lines, the phase of a monaural or binaurally evoked neurophonic shifts in an orderly fashion which reflects the map of delays i.e. with a stimulus of changing interaural phase difference, the optimal binaural delay shifts from far contralateral at the dorsal edge of the nucleus through the zero point to the near ipsilateral location at the ventral edge (Sullivan and Konishi, 1986). Since the afferent delay lines are responsible for the neurophonic (Carr and Konishi, 1988), it can be used to evaluate the development of the maps of delay. In addition, the neurophonic is robust and easy to measure, which is an advantage in young birds. The neurophonic may reveal when the map becomes tuned, and how the tuning changes with changing head size, while a disordered or undeveloped map might be expected to produce a weak or nonexistant neurophonic.

We have investigated the development of the neurophonic to reveal when it acquires adult characteristics. In order to compare responses from birds of different ages, we have recorded the peak amplitude of the neurophonic at the same best frequency (4kHz) and in the same position within the nucleus laminaris. In the adult, the neurophonic response resembles the response of a laminaris neuron: it varies in a cyclic manner with the ITD of a sound stimulus, and the period of the neurophonic response function matches that of the stimulus tone. The response peaks are of similar height and are evoked by the same interaural phase difference (Sullivan and Konishi, 1986). We have measured the peak-to-trough difference between best and worst interaural phase differences, and normalized these changes with respect to neurophonic amplitude in order to calculate the percentage change between peak and trough with age. An increase in peak-trough differences would be expected with maturation of the circuit within the nucleus.

We have measured changes in the binaural neurophonic in the nucleus laminaris for owls between P12 and 2 months of age. The neurophonic amplitude was measured in the 4 kHz best frequency region using a shaped tonal stimulus that varied in interaural time difference between left side leading by 300 µsec and right side leading by 300µsec. In the P12 bird, no ITD-tuned neurophonic could be recorded, although weak frequency tuning was found. The first ITD-tuned neurophonic responses were recorded from a P21 bird (Fig. 2A). In this bird, the overall neurophonic amplitude was small, as was the difference between the peak and the trough of the neurophonic. In a P30 bird, a more recognizably adult neurophonic response was recorded (Fig. 2B). The differences between P21 and P30 may not be due to gross connectional changes within the nucleus laminaris, since frequency response curves were similar for P30 and P21. There are also further changes in the neurophonic after P30. In the P60 bird (data not shown), the peak-trough differences between the maximum and minimum of the neurophonic was larger than in the P30 bird. These results suggest that the emergence of the adult form of the neurophonic may be used to determine when the map of ITDs acquires its functional adult properties.

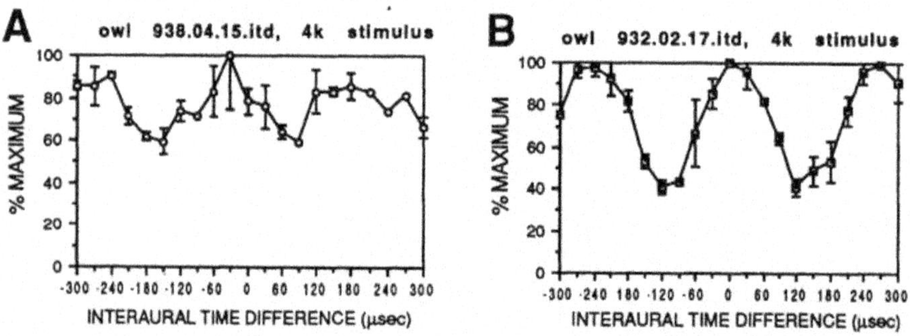

Figure 2. Preliminary data on the development of the neurophonic obtained from experiments on P30 and P21 birds. A. P21 neurophonic amplitude and tuning to an ITD stimulus was weak. B. P30 neurophonic amplitude and tuning to an ITD stimulus is similar in amplitude and ITD sensitivity to the adult neurophonic. Frequency response curves were similar for both birds.

4 Discussion

During the first few weeks of life, the young bird's head more than doubles in size, subjecting it to changing interaural cues. We have shown that the myelination of the magnocellular delay lines within the nucleus laminaris occurs late in development, during this period of maximum head growth. The peak of myelination coincides with the time during which the head experiences maximum growth, and the delay lines acquire a functional appearance towards the end of the first month of life. The anatomical maturation of the delay line axons within the nucleus laminaris coincides with the appearance of an adult neurophonic response. Thus the maturation of this circuit coincides with the time that the head stops growing, and the bird is no longer subject to changing interaural time cues.

In the cat, the central auditory pathways undergo developmental changes which are similar to those of the barn owl. Despite long latency, high threshold responses, some elements of the developing cat auditory system are able to produce characteristic adult responses early in postnatal life (Brugge, 1988). Responses to interaural phase differences were recorded in the auditory cortex of an 18-day old kitten, long before myelination of the auditory brainstem was complete (Brugge, 1988). Robust responses to interaural intensity differences were also recorded in kitten cortex (Brugge et al., 1988). Since the development of the auditory brainstem of the cat and the barn owl is similar, it may be that single unit recordings from the young barn owl may also reveal sensitivity to ITDs before the neurophonic responses acquire their adult characteristics. It may also be that the maturation of the laminaris circuit, and the appearance of synchronous responses in the nucleus laminaris, may be associated with improved sensitivity to ITDs.

5 Acknowledgements

Supported by NIH DCD 00436.

6 References

Brugge, J.F. (1988) Stimulus coding in the developing auditory system. In Brain Function G.M. Edelman, W. Einar Gall and W. Maxwell Cowan, eds. pp. 113-136, John Wiley & Sons, NY.

Brugge, J.F., R. A. Reale and G.F. Wilson (1988) Sensitivity of auditory cortical neurons of kittens to monaural and binaural high frequency sound. Hear.Res. 34:127-140.

Carr, C.E. (1993) Processing of temporal information in the brain. Ann.Rev.Neurosci. 16: 223-243.

Carr, C.E. and M. Konishi (1988) Axonal delay lines for time measurement in the owl's brainstem. Proc.Natl.Acad.Sci. 85:8311-8315.

Carr, C.E. and G.A. Higgins (1990) The role of myelination in the development of the nucleus laminaris in the barn owl. Soc.Neurosci.Abstr. 16:876.

Carr, C.E. and M. Konishi (1990) A circuit for detection of interaural time differences in the brainstem of the barn owl. J.Neurosci. 10:3227-3246.

Carr, C.E. and R. E. Boudreau (1993) Organization of nucleus magnocellularis and nucleus laminaris in the barn owl: encoding and measuring interaural time differences. J. Comp. Neurol. 333:1-19.

Carr, C.E. and R. E. Boudreau (1994) Development of the time coding pathways in the auditory brainstem of the barn owl. Submitted.

Cheng S.-M. and C. E. Carr (1992) The role of myelination in the development of the nucleus laminaris in the barn owl. The molecular biology of hearing and deafness, UCSD, La Jolla.

Haresign, T. and A. Moiseff (1989) Early growth and development of the common barn-owl's facial ruff, The Auk: 105:699-705.

Higgins, G.A., S. Koh, K.S. Chen, and F.H. Gage (1989) Nerve growth factor (NGF) induction of NGF-receptor gene expression and cholinergic neuronal hypertrophy in the basal forebrain of the adult rat. Neuron 3:247-256.

Knudsen, E.I. and M. Konishi (1979) Mechanisms of Sound Localization in the Barn Owl (Tyto alba). J.Comp.Neurol. 133:13-21.

Knudsen, E.I., S.D. Esterly, and P.F. Knudsen (1984) Monaural Occulsion Alters Sound Localization During A Sensitive Period in the barn Owl. J.Comp.Neurol. 4:1001-1011.

Knudsen, E.I. and P.F. Knudsen (1986) The Sensitive Period for Auditory Localization in Barn Owls Is Limited By Age, Not by Experience. J.Neurosci. 6:1918-1924.

Konishi, M. (1973) How the owl tracks its prey. Am.Sci. 61:414-424.

Moiseff, A. (1989) Binaural disparity cues available to the barn owl for sound localization. J.Comp.Physiol. 164:629-636.

Overholt, T., R. Hyson, and E.W. Rubel (1992) A delay-line circuit for coding interaural time differences in the chick brain stem. J.Neurosci. 12:1698-1708

Payne, R.S. (1971) Acoustic localization of prey by barn owls (Tyto alba). J.Exp.Biol. 54:535-573.

Sullivan, W.E and M. Konishi (1986) Neural map of interaural phase difference in the owl's brainstem. Proc.Natl.Acad.Sci. 83:8400-8404.

Takahashi, T., A. Moiseff, and M. Konishi (1984) Time and intensity cues are processed independently in the auditory system of the owl. J.Neurosci. 4:1781-1786.

Comment by E.F. Evans

In connection with the observed improvement in synchrony, is it possible that the system selects or adjusts convergent fibres of differing *length* in the course of development?

Reply

Quite possible but we have not done the experiment to test this hypothesis. It appears, however, that changes in fiber *diameter* are more common.

Comment by R. Romand

What are your myelination criteria for the delay lines to acquire functional characteristics beside timing coincidence between the peak of myelination and appearance of adult neurophonic response?

Reply

We are not yet entirely satisfied by our criteria. This is one reason that it is essential to combine physiological and anatomical studies, since we know adult fibre diameters and conduction velocities. We have already measured the developmental changes in fibre diameter in the delay lines, and we will measure changes in conduction velocity. We hope that these measures will provide the best criterion of delay line function. Obviously measures of safety factor and channel density are important, but they are at present beyond our ability.

Effects of acoustic overstimulation on four species of birds

Robert J. Dooling[1] and Brenda M. Ryals[2]

[1]*Department of Psychology, University of Maryland, College Park, MD 20742, USA*
[2]*Department of Hearing and Speech, James Madison University, Harrisburg, VA 22807, USA*

1 Introduction

The discovery of cochlear hair cell regeneration in birds has spawned a great deal of research into the anatomical and physiological changes associated with this phenomenon. Hair cell regeneration and other anatomical and physiological aspects of cochlear recovery in response to acoustic overstimulation has been described in only two species of birds: chickens (*Gallus domesticus*) and japanese quail (*Coturnix coturnix japonica*) (see, for reviews, Corwin and Warchol, 1991; Cotanche, Lee, Stone, and Picard, 1993; Girod and Rubel, 1991; Saunders, Cohen and Szymko, 1991). Less is known about behavioral recovery of function following acoustic trauma as data are available for only a few species (see, for example, Niemiec, Raphael, and Moody, 1993; Saunders and Dooling, 1974; Hashino, Sokabe, and Miyamoto, 1988). These comparative data were collected in different laboratories by different investigators using different hearing assays and, most importantly, different exposure conditions. Moreover, most of what we know about the time course of functional recovery comes from physiological experiments on very young chicks rather than from behavioral experiments on adult animals. The present experiments were undertaken, in part, to resolve some of these issues. Japanese quail and three other species with similar frequency regions of best hearing, budgerigars (*Melopsittacus undulatus*), canaries (*Serinus canaria*), and zebra finches (*Taeniopygia guttata*), were overstimulated with the same acoustic stimulus and tested in the same behavioral apparatus using the same procedure. The question we asked is whether the same acoustic over-stimulation in different species has similar anatomical and behavioral consequences.

2 Methods

2.1 Subjects and Exposure Conditions

A total of 13 quail, 42 budgerigars, 17 zebra finches, and 15 canaries were continuously exposed from 12-24 hours to either a high-frequency noise band (2-6 kHz) or a high-frequency pure tone (2.86 kHz) at either 112 or 120 dB SPL. The energy spectra of these exposure stimuli were centered within the region of best auditory sensitivity for these four species (Okanoya and Dooling, 1987). The band of noise had skirts of 115 dB/octave and was flat within the passband (+/-3 dB).

2.2 Histology

Some animals were used only for histology while others were tested behaviorally and then sacrificed. Birds for histology were sacrificed either immediately after acoustic overstimulation or at 7, 30, 90, or 365 days later. Basilar papillae were fixed (3.5% glutaraldehyde followed by 1% osmium tetroxide), dehydrated to 70% ethanol, the tectorial membrane removed, dehydrated to 100% and critical point dried using an Autosamdri 814 critical point dryer. Papillae were mounted on aluminum stubs, sputter coated with gold and viewed at 15 kV using a Joel 820 scanning electron microscope (SEM). Estimates were made of the degree of damage in a particular location (ie. whether supporting cells as well as hair cells were damaged) by visual inspection. The extent or area of damage along the papilla was quantified from photomicrographs using digitizing morphometry.

2.3 Behavior

Six budgerigars, two canaries, three japanese quail, and three zebra finches were used for behavioral tests. The apparatus and procedure for training and testing birds has been described previously (Okanoya and Dooling, 1987). The birds were food deprived to approximately 80-90% of their free feeding weight and trained by operant conditioning methods to repeatedly peck one key (observation key) in the absence of sound and to peck another key (report key) whenever a tone was presented. A peck on the report key within two seconds of tone onset resulted in delivery of food. A peck on the report key in the absence of the tone was punished with a 5 second blackout period. The birds were tested in two daily sessions consisting of about 100 trials each. Threshold was determined at 2.86 kHz (center of the exposure stimulus) in one session and 1.0 kHz in the other.

3 Results

3.1 Tone-induced Acoustic Trauma - Behavior

Thresholds at 1.0 kHz and 2.86 kHz were measured in three quail and two budgerigars prior to, and following, exposure to a 112 dB, 2.86 kHz pure tone for 12 hours. A third budgerigar was exposed at a higher intensity (118 dB) and is included in this analysis. Consistent with the species differences in the anatomical response to pure tone overstimulation, there were dramatic differences in behavioral recovery for quail and budgerigars. Thresholds at 1.0 kHz for both quail and budgerigars showed a temporary threshold shift (TTS) which returned to pre-exposure levels within several days and are not shown. Quail showed an initial TTS of 70 dB at 2.86 kHz which remained virtually unchanged for about 8-9 days. From about day 10 post-exposure, thresholds recovered at the rate of about 2 dB/day until about post-exposure day 50 after which no further recovery was observed. This permanent threshold shift (PTS) of about 20 dB was still evident 1 year post-exposure and SEM evaluation of the papillae of these birds at 1 year showed missing hair cells (below). Budgerigars, by contrast, showed an initial TTS of about 40 dB at 2.86 kHz which recovered in three days to within 10 dB of pre-exposure threshold levels. These results are shown in Figure 1 (Top).

3.2 Tone-induced Acoustic Trauma - Histology

The morphology of the basilar papilla as well as hair cell counts are available for budgerigars (Manley, Schwabedissen, and Gleich, 1993), canaries, and zebra finches (Gleich, Manley, Mandl, and Dooling, 1994). Budgerigar papillae contain about 5300 hair cells followed by zebra finches with 3500, and canaries with about 3000. Quail papillae contain about 6400 hair cells. The length of the basilar papilla differs among these species with quail papillae about 10% longer than budgerigar papillae and about 25% longer than canary and zebra finch papillae.

Quail. Immediately following continuous exposure to a 112 dB, 2.86 kHz pure tone for 12 hours, SEM evaluation of the surface of the quail basilar papilla typically revealed a crescent-shaped area of hair cell loss and expanded support cell surface area from approximately 15-30% of the length along the papilla from the basal tip. Hair cell loss extended from the inferior (abneural) edge of the papilla toward, but not reaching, the superior (neural) edge. Birds sacrificed 7 days post-exposure showed extensive hair cell regeneration in this same region of the papilla. Two birds sacrificed 1 year post-exposure showed a normal appearance of hair cells throughout the previously damaged region except for a small area along the abneural edge where no hair cells were present.

Budgerigars. The SEM of budgerigar papillae examined immediately after an identical exposure typically revealed either no damage or a very small finger-like projection of hair cells loss and enlarged support cell surface area from the abneural edge of the papilla at approximately 35% of length from the basal tip. Birds sacrificed 7 days later showed no evidence of missing hair cells.

Canaries and Zebra Finches. SEM evaluation of canary and zebra finch papillae immediately following continuous exposure to the same 112 dB, 2.86 kHz pure tone for 12 hours revealed no obvious missing hair cells or hair cell abnormalities.

In all four species, exposure to a 120 dB, 2.86 kHz pure tone for 24 hours resulted in more extensive damage. For quail and budgerigars, the area of missing hair cells extended further toward the neural edge and slightly more basally. Loss of support cells as well as hair cells was evident in both quail and budgerigar at this intensity. In marked contrast to quail and budgerigars, canaries showed either no damage or a small, crescent-shaped area of hair cell loss approximately 30-35% of the length from the basal tip. SEM evaluation of zebra finch papillae revealed only scattered hair cell loss and expanded support cell surface area over the basal half of the papilla with the damage extending about half-way to the neural edge.

3.3 Noise-induced Acoustic Trauma - Behavior

Two budgerigars, two canaries, and three zebra finches were exposed to bandpass noise (2-6 kHz) at 120 dB SPL for 24 hours. For all three species, thresholds measured at

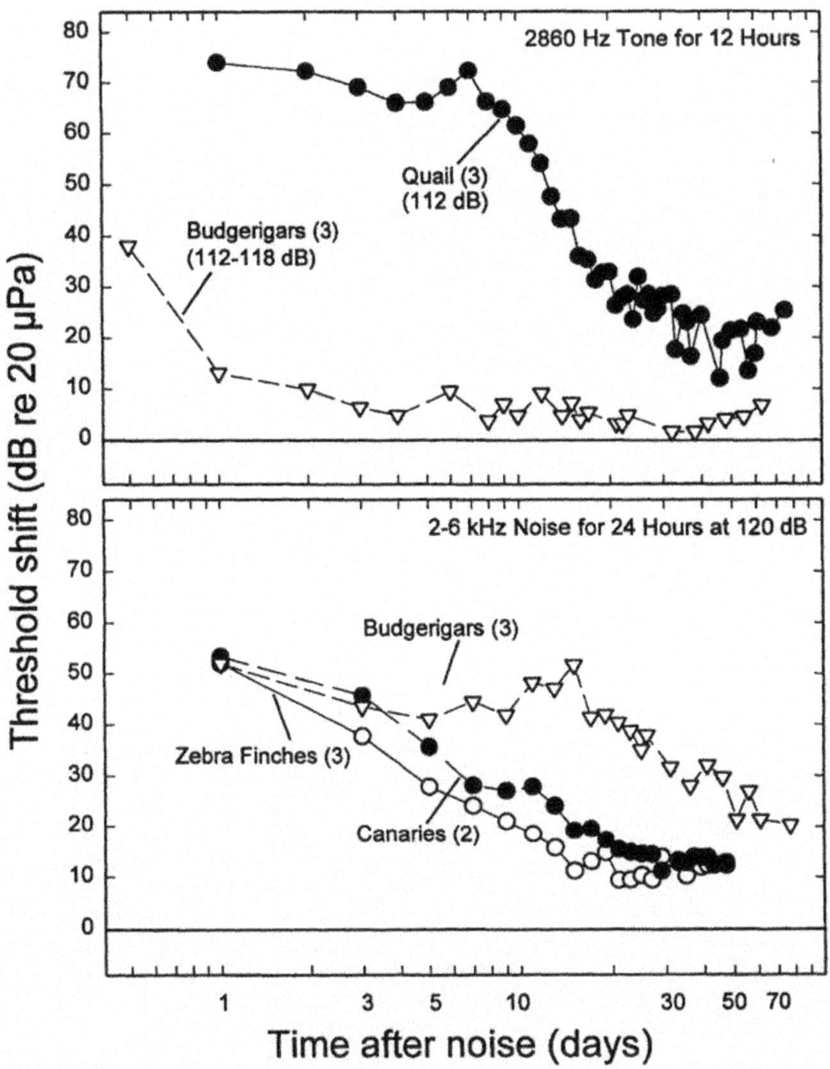

Figure 1. Recovery of absolute thresholds at 2860 Hz in quail and budgerigars following continuous exposure to a 112 dB pure tone at 2860 Hz for 12 hours (Top Panel). Recovery of absolute thresholds at 2860 Hz in budgerigars, canaries, and zebra finches following exposure to 2-6 kHz bandpass noise at 120 dB for 24 hours (Bottom Panel).

1.0 kHz (not shown) indicated an initial TTS of about 10-30 dB which returned to within 10 dB of pre- thresholds at 2.86 kHz exposure levels by 5 days post-exposure. At 2.86 kHz, however, budgerigars showed an initial TTS of about 50 dB which remained unchanged for about 15 days post-exposure. After day 15 post-exposure, thresholds recovered at the rate of about 1 dB/day. No further recovery in threshold was observed beyond 50 days suggesting a PTS of about 20 dB. Canaries and zebra finches also showed an initial TTS of about 50 dB but, in contrast to budgerigars, thresholds in these two species began recovering immediately at the rate of about 1-2 dB/day and came within 10 dB of pre-exposure thresholds by 30 days post-exposure. These results are shown in Figure 1 (Bottom).

3.4 Noise-induced Acoustic Trauma - Histology

Budgerigars. SEM evaluation of the surface of budgerigar papillae typically revealed a crescent-shaped area of hair cell loss and support cell surface expansion at about the same location as that seen following exposure to a 120 dB pure tone (about 35% of the length from the basal tip). The nature of the lesion differed between the tone and noise exposure conditions. Following noise exposure, hair cell loss within the crescent-shaped area was not as severe as in the tone exposure and the area of hair cell loss was bordered on the basal and distal edges by fingers of hair cell loss extending from the abneural edge. Hair cell loss was always greatest on the abneural edge and never fully reached the neural side of the papilla. Budgerigar papillae examined 7 days post-exposure showed a smaller crescent-shaped area of hair cell loss but with no finger-like areas of hair cell loss. The borders of the crescent-shaped lesion in papillae observed at 7 days post-exposure were covered with small, regenerating hair cells. These results are shown schematically in Figure 2 (Top Panel). No hair cell regeneration was seen within the crescent patch at day 7 post-exposure. Examination of budgerigar papillae at 30 and 90 days showed a gradually narrowing (from neural to abneural) and smoothing of the crescent-shaped region of hair cell loss.

Zebra Finch. SEM evaluation of zebra finch papillae after identical exposure revealed a long, narrow region of hair cell loss and support cell surface expansion restricted to the abneural edge of the papillae from about 25-60% of the length from the basal end. Interestingly, compared to the damage caused by a 120 dB pure tone, bandpass noise resulted in hair cell loss that was much less scattered. SEM examination of zebra finch papillae at 7 days post-exposure revealed areas of small, regenerating hair cells but no areas of expanded cell surfaces and no obvious hair cell loss. These results are shown schematically in Figure 2 (Middle Panel).

Canary. SEM evaluation of canary papillae exposed to noise typically revealed two areas of damage at day 0 post-exposure. A narrow region of hair cell loss and support cell surface expansion was evident along the abneural edge of the papillae from 50-75% of the length from the basal end. There was also an area of scattered hair cell loss from 25-35% of the length from the basal end. Surprisingly, overstimulation by bandpass noise resulted in the greatest hair cell damage in the distal half the papilla whereas pure tone overstimulation caused only a small area of scattered hair cell loss toward the basal end of

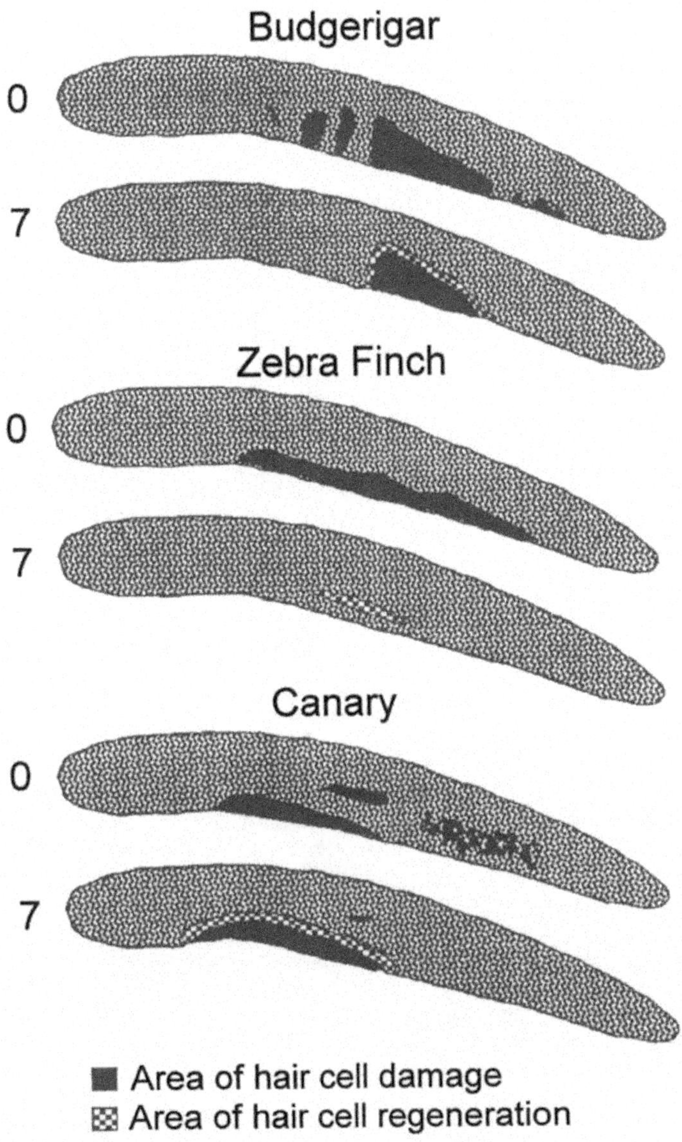

Figure 2. Schematic representations of the typical damage to budgerigar, canary, and zebra finch papillae at 0 days and 7 days post-exposure to a 2-6 kHz bandpass noise at 120 dB for 24 hours.

the papilla. At 7 days post-exposure, the narrow area of contiguous hair cell loss from 50-75% of the length from the basal end of the papilla was still evident. In papillae observed at 7 days post-exposure, however, many small regenerating hair cells were observed along the edges of the lesion. The region of the papilla near the basal tip which showed scattered hair cell loss at 0 days, appeared normal at 7 days. These results are shown schematically in Figure 2 (Bottom Panel).

4 Discussion

The four species examined here show some similarities in response to acoustic overstimulation. When overstimulation was sufficiently intense, all four species showed evidence of an initial and substantial TTS, followed by behavioral recovery, and evidence of hair cell regeneration. Beyond this, however, these species show very different anatomical and behavioral changes to identical overstimulation and very different time courses of recovery. Of the four species, quail were the most sensitive to acoustic overstimulation showing a prolonged period of TTS following a 12-hour exposure to a 112 dB pure tone at 2.86 kHz. On average, budgerigars showed only a small amount of TTS which was resolved in a matter of a few days while canaries and zebra finches showed no evidence of hair cell loss or hair cell abnormalities following identical overstimulation. Quail, on the other hand, not only experienced PTS lasting up to one year but examination of the papillae from these behavioral birds revealed a lesion along the abneural edge which was devoid of hair cells. Interestingly, this lesion observed at 1 year was located in the same area which showed extensive hair cell regeneration in papillae examined at 7 days post-exposure. When overstimulated with identical bandpass noise, budgerigars showed much more prolonged TTS and a larger PTS than canaries or zebra finches with dramatic species differences in the patterns of hair cell loss, regeneration, and anatomical recovery.

Comparing across species and exposure conditions, the data support the notion of two facets of recovery. Quail and budgerigars show a prolonged TTS for up to 8-15 days followed by a 1-2 dB/day recovery in thresholds beyond this point. By comparison, canaries and zebra finches showed a 1-2 dB/day recovery in thresholds which began immediately after cessation of overstimulation. Species similarities in the slope of threshold recovery suggest that similar repair processes may be responsible for recovery. The prolonged TTS observed in quail and budgerigars suggest a more severe initial damage which must be repaired before behavioral recovery can commence. This hypothesis, of course, must be tempered by the fact that these exposure conditions almost certainly alter the micromechanical response of the basilar papilla making it impossible to know which regions of the papilla are contributing to absolute thresholds following acoustic trauma and during recovery.

Finally, it is unlikely that the species differences in response to acoustic overstimulation are due to differences in absolute sensitivity in the region of 2.86 kHz. The pre-exposure thresholds for all species at 2.86 kHz were, on average, between 5-10 dB SPL. Species differences in susceptibility to overstimulation in the face of similar absolute thresholds suggest that there may be species differences in protective mechanisms perhaps involving the middle ear apparatus. On the other hand, the considerable species variation we observed in the pattern of hair cell loss on the basilar papilla following acoustic overstimulation invites speculation about species differences in mechanical events along the basilar papilla during stimulus transduction.

5 Acknowledgements

This work was supported by NIH grant DC-01372 to R.J.D. and B.M.R. and MH-00982 to R.J.D. We thank Winnie Westbrook for assistance with histology and Alison Linzenbold and Micheal Dent for assistance in behavioral testing.

6 References

Corwin, J.T. and Warchol, M.E. (1991). Auditory hair cells: structure, function, development, and regeneration. Ann. Rev. Neurosci. 14, 301-333.

Cotanche, D.A., Lee, K.H., Stone, J.S., and Picard, D.A. (1993). Hair cell regeneration in the bird cochlea following noise damage or ototoxic drug damage. Anat. Embryol. In Press.

Girod, D.A. and Rubel, E.W. (1991). Hair cell regeneration in the avian cochlea: if it works in birds, why not in man? Ear, Nose,Throat J. 70, 343-350.

Gleich, O., Manley, G.A., Mandl, A., and Dooling, R.J. (1994). The basilar papilla of the canary and the zebra finch: A quantitative scanning electron microscopic description. J. Morph. 221, 1-24

Hashino, E., Sokabe, M., and Miyamoto, K. (1988). Frequency-specific susceptibility to acoustic trauma in the budgerigar (*Melopsittacus undulatus*). J. Acoust. Soc. Am. 83, 2450-2453.

Manley, G.A., Schwabedissen, G. and Gleich, O. (1993). Morphology of the basilar papilla of the budgerigar (*Melopsittacus undulatus*). J. Morph., 218, 153-165.

Niemiec, A.J., Raphael, Y., and Moody, D.B. (1993). Return of auditory function following structural regeneration after acoustic trauma: behavioral measures from quail. Abs. Assn. Res. Otolaryngol. 16, 119.

Okanoya, K. and Dooling, R.J. (1987) Hearing in Passerine and Psittacine birds: A comparative study of masked and absolute auditory thresholds. J. Comp. Psych., 101, 7-15.

Saunders, J.C. and Dooling, R.J. (1974). Noise-induced threshold shift in the parakeet (*Melopsittacus undulatus*). Proc. Nat. Acad. Sci., 71, 1962-1965.

Saunders, J.C., Cohen, Y.E., and Szymko, Y.M. (1991). The structural and functional consequences of acoustic injury in the cochlea and peripheral auditory system: a five year update. J. Acoust. Soc. Am., 90, 136-146.

Belgian Waterslager canaries: Morphological and physiological studies of a mutant bird strain showing continuous hair-cell production

Otto Gleich[1] and Robert J. Dooling[2]

[1]*HNO-Klinik Universität Regensburg, Postfach, 93042 Regensburg, Germany*
[2]*Department of Psychology, University of Maryland, College Park, MD 20742, USA*

1 Introduction

Approximately one percent of the population of the United States is affected by deafness (Christiansen, 1991). Loss of cochlear hair cells is responsible for permanent hearing loss in the majority of the patients (Corwin and Warchol, 1991; Richardson, 1993). Animal experiments have also shown that cochlear hair-cell loss is irreversible in several mammalian species (Bohne and Harding, 1992; Gao et al., 1992; Raphael and Altschuler, 1991). In birds, however, the cochlea shows an astounding potential for morphological and functional repair after various insults (e.g. Cotanche et al., 1994; Adler et al., 1993; Marean et al., 1993). This includes even the regeneration of large numbers of lost hair cells (e.g. Cotanche, 1987; Corwin and Cotanche, 1988; Ryals and Rubel, 1988; Cruz et al., 1987; Hashino et al., 1991). Although hair-cell regeneration has been demonstrated for the mammalian vestibular system (Forge et al., 1993; Warchol et al., 1993) it could until now not unequivocally be demonstrated for the organ of Corti.

A lot of effort is currently directed at unraveling the mechanisms of hair-cell regeneration to ultimately develop a therapy for the treatment of cochlear hair-cell loss in humans. In this context we decided to examine the function and morphology of the cochlea in the Waterslager strain of canary, because these birds show a hereditary hearing deficit (Okanoya and Dooling, 1985; Okanoya and Dooling, 1987; Okanoya et al., 1990) despite the powerful cochlear repair mechanisms that have been demonstrated in other avian species. A cochlear origin of the hearing deficit would make Waterslager canaries potentially useful for investigating mechanisms of cochlear hair cell regeneration. While many mutations in humans and other mammals are known to affect hearing, Waterslager canaries are (to our knowledge) the only submammalian example for a hereditary hearing deficit (Steel and Bock, 1983; Steel and Harvey, 1992; Nadeau et al., 1991). Thus a more detailed characterization of the origin of their hearing deficit is necessary for a comparison with genetic hearing disorders described for mammals.

2 Methods

Behavioral thresholds at 1.0, 2.0, 2.86 and 4.0kHz were determined for two Waterslager and one non-Waterslager canary by operant conditioning with food reinforcement as previously described in detail (Okanoya and Dooling, 1990a, b). Measurements of the Compound Action Potential (CAP) and the Cochlear Microphonic (CM) were obtained in 6 Waterslager and 8 (CAP) or 5 (CM) non-Waterslager canaries. The response to tone pips was recorded by a silver wire electrode from the round window or from scala tympani. Test frequencies varied between 0.5 and 6.0 kHz and the levels varied over a 50dB range in 5dB steps starting 10-15dB below the CAP threshold. Stimuli starting with a random phase were used for CAP determination while constant phase stimuli were applied for the CM determination. CAP amplitude was determined as the difference between the largest positive peak and the following largest negative peak within a 5ms time window after the onset of the stimulus. The CM amplitude was determined as the amplitude of the spectral line at the test frequency from a fast fourier transform of the averaged response. CAP and CM thresholds were determined from the respective growth functions using a 6 and 3μV criterion respectively. Choosing these criteria resulted in virtually identical averaged CAP and CM audiograms of the non-Waterslager canary.

We also measured the middle ear reflectance in 4 Waterslager and 4 non-Waterslager canaries. In a closed sound system sealed to the auditory meatus two calibrated microphones were used to determine the phase and the amplitude of the sound signal approximately 5 and 17.15mm from the entrance of the auditory meatus. The pressure reflection coefficient was then calculated from these data (Hudde, 1983).

The morphology of the basilar papilla was analyzed by Scanning Electron Microscopy (SEM) in the 3 birds tested behaviorally and in one non-Waterslager and 2 Waterslager canaries where CAP audiograms had been measured. According to the breeders all these birds were between 1 and 1.5 years old at the time of testing. In addition we examined the basilar papillae of 2 Waterslagers that were only 2 months old without having measured their audiograms. Details of the preparation and the morphological analysis of the avian basilar papilla have been described previously in depth (Gleich and Manley, 1988; Gleich et al., 1994). Briefly, we analyzed the gross papillar dimensions length of the papilla, width of the papilla and number of hair cells from low power photographic reconstructions with a final magnification of 200-300x. The number of stereovilli and the apical hair-cell surface area were analyzed from reconstructions of ≈ 150μm wide strips across the papilla at 2000-4000x magnification.

3 Results

3.1 Threshold measurements

The behavioral thresholds we found confirmed that thresholds in Waterslagers increase with frequency above 1kHz as compared to non-Waterslager canaries (Okanoya and Dooling 1985, 1987). The CAP and CM measurements showed that higher sound pressure levels are necessary to produce a given response in Waterslager canaries especially above 1-2kHz. Thus Waterslager CAP and CM audiograms showed elevated thresholds (Fig.1). The average CAP threshold difference below 1.5kHz was approximately 15dB and increased to more than 40dB at 4kHz. The output of the sound system (≈100dB SPL) was not sufficient to measure a CAP threshold in Waterslagers at

6kHz (Fig. 1a). The difference in CM thresholds between both groups was approximately 5dB below 1kHz. However, for the higher test frequencies above 1kHz the CM threshold difference increased to more than 20dB (Fig. 1b). These data indicate that thresholds in Belgian Waterslagers are elevated at the level of the hair cell and the auditory nerve.

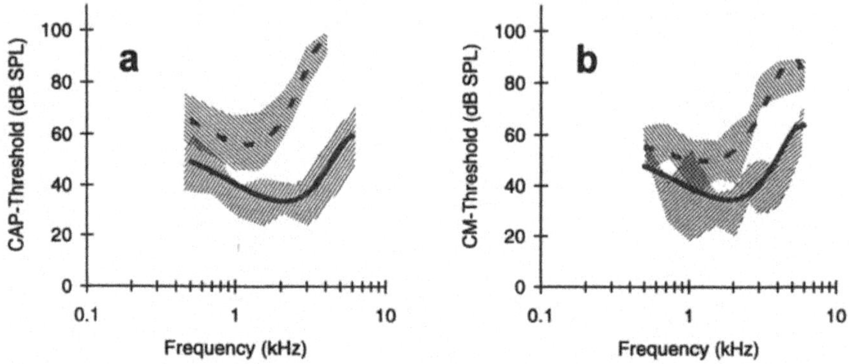

Figure 1. CAP (a) and CM (b) thresholds as a function of test frequency. The heavy continuous and the dotted lines are 3rd order polynomial fits through the raw data from Waterslager and non-Waterslager canaries respectively. The shaded areas indicate the average ± one standard deviation.

3.2 Middle ear measurements

To exclude the possibility that the middle ear was responsible for the elevated thresholds we measured the middle ear reflectance coefficient at 3.0kHz. CAP and CM thresholds at this frequency are on average substantially (>20dB) elevated in Waterslagers. The mean and standard deviation of the reflection coefficient were 0.23± 0.06 in Waterslagers as compared to 0.22±0.15 in the non-Waterslager ears. Filling the middle ear with water significantly increased the reflection coefficient to 0.51±0.15 and 0.44±0.16 in both groups. In addition during the dissection of the specimens we noticed no obvious difference in the external or middle ear structures between both groups

3.3 Morphological measurements

It was very obvious even at low magnification that all investigated basilar papillae from Waterslagers showed at least some degree of pathology as compared to non-Waterslager canaries and other bird species. The total length of the papilla was not affected. However, the regular pattern of the hair cell mosaic and the stereovillar bundles appeared distorted. In addition, most papillae showed a reduction of the basilar papilla width and a reduced number of hair cells. Both of these parameters were quantified (Fig. 2). It is obvious that the width of the papilla is on average reduced in Waterslagers with the difference being most pronounced in the apical half of the papilla (Fig. 2a). Also the number of hair cells across the width of the papilla was reduced in Waterslagers (Fig. 2b). The interindividual variability for both of these parameters was very small among non-Waterslagers, but ranged from almost unaffected to severely affected in Waterslagers. The number of hair cells appeared more affected than the width of the papilla indicating a reduced hair-cell density in Waterslagers.

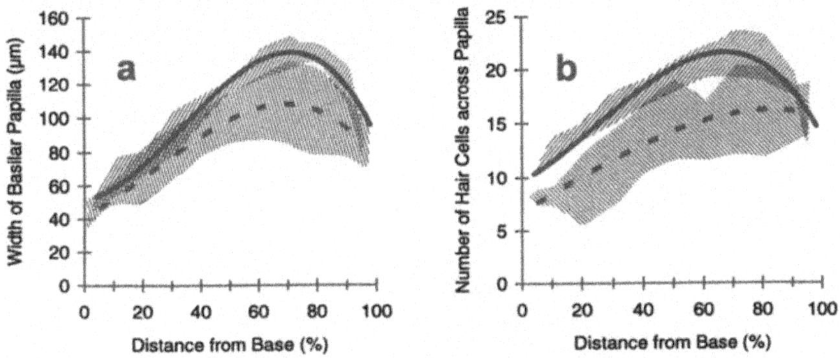

Figure 2. The width of the basilar papilla (a) and the number of hair cells across the papilla (b) as a function of the distance from the base. Non-Waterslager data are shown by the heavy continuous line and data from Waterslagers are shown by the dotted lines. Lines represent 3rd order polynomial fits through the raw data. The shaded areas indicate the average of 10% segments along the papilla ± one standard deviation.

At higher magnifications pathologies at the level of individual hair cells were obvious. The regular appearance of the hair cell mosaic, the elongated shape of the stereovillar bundles and their orderly arrangement on the basilar papilla that were typical for non-Waterslager canaries (Gleich et al., 1994) was severely distorted. The shape of many hair cells as well as that of their stereovillar bundles were abnormal. Less severe pathologies included missing stereovilli in an otherwise normal appearing bundle. Bundles with a very irregularly shaped outline were common. Other abnormalities included the presence of 2-4 sub-bundles on single cells or the almost complete absence of stereovilli combined with a severely enlarged hair-cell surface area. Some hair cells showed gigantic or miniature stereovilli.

In many hair cells from Waterslagers we could not usefully determine several of the parameters used to characterize hair cells in normal canaries and other bird species (Gleich and Manley, 1988; Gleich et al., 1994, Fischer et al., 1988; Manley et al., 1993) because these bundles were severely distorted. Thus we could only quantify the hair-cell surface area and the number of stereovilli (Fig. 3). We included only mature looking hair cells with a smooth apical surface adjacent to their stereovillar bundle in this analysis. We excluded the small, microvilli covered cells (see below) that made up on average 2.5% (range 0.6-3.3% in 4 specimens) of the hair cell population in Waterslagers.

Despite increased variability in the data from the Waterslagers there was a trend for an increased hair-cell surface area as compared to non-Waterslagers (see also Fig. 2). Hair-cell surface area was similar for both groups in neural hair cells and the difference tended to increase towards the abneural edge of the papilla (Fig. 3a). The stereovilli number, however, was reduced in Waterslagers and the reduction was more severe in neural as compared to abneural hair cells (Fig. 3b). In addition the stereovilli number in neighboring hair cells could be very different in Waterslagers. This is in contrast to observations in non-Waterslagers and other birds where stereovilli numbers are very precisely regulated (Tilney and Saunders, 1983; own unpublished observations). The data in Fig. 3 were measured 50% from the base. We performed the same analysis for the 20% and the 80% positions and they indicated that the general basal to apical and neural to abneural gradients described for normal canaries (Gleich et al., 1994) were still present in Waterslagers, despite different absolute numbers and an increased degree of interindividual variability.

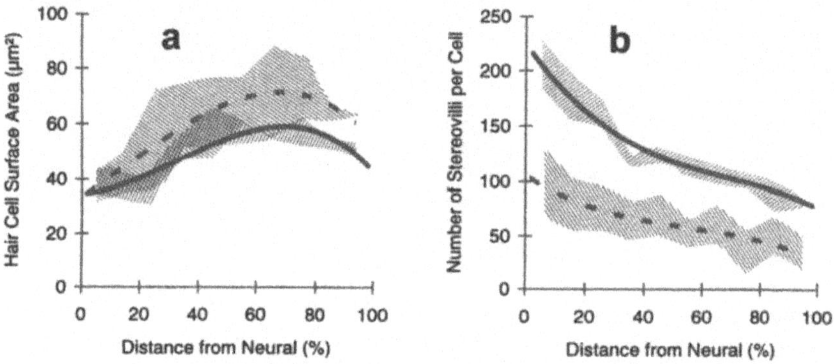

Figure 3. The hair cell surface area (a) and the number of stereovilli per hair cell (b) as a function of the normalized distance from the neural edge of the papilla. Non-Waterslager data are shown by the heavy continuous line and data from Waterslagers are shown by the dotted lines. Lines represent 3rd order polynomial fits through the raw data. The shaded areas indicate the average of 10% segments across the papilla ± one standard deviation.

Another morphological peculiarity that we had never seen in other normal avian basilar papillae consisted of small microvilli covered cells with stereovillar bundles that could be very small or in some cases even be unrecognizable. Even without a recognizable stereovillar bundle these cells differed distinctly from supporting cells that form a narrow border between neighboring hair cells. These small and microvilli covered hair cells were found singly or arranged in pairs intermingled among other more or less damaged hair cells (Fig. 4). In many of these cells with a distinct stereovillar bundle this bundle appeared fairly normal as compared to bundles of other neighboring hair cells (Fig. 4b).

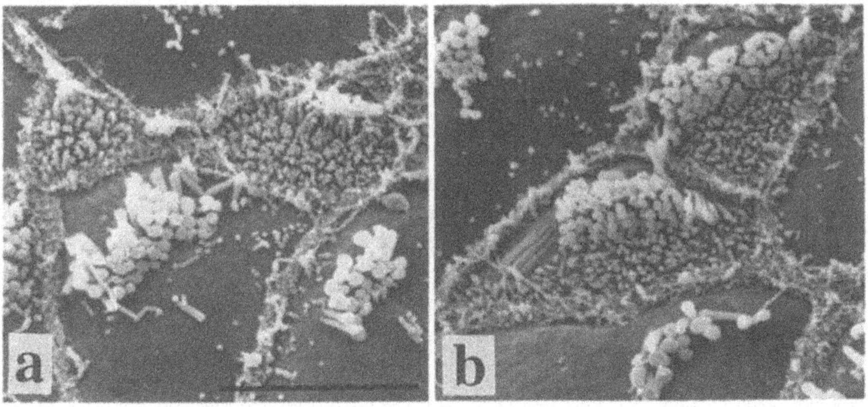

Figure 4. (a) A pair of small microvilli covered cells. The left cell is very small and there is no discernible stereovillar bundle, while the right cell appears slightly more developed. with a very small stereovillar bundle. (b) A pair of small microvilli covered cells with almost mature apearing stereovillar bundles. Note that most neighbors of these small microvilli covered hair cells are other mature hair cells with a varying degree of pathology. Scale Bar = 5μm.

4 Discussion

Our physiological and middle ear measurements clearly demonstrate that the origin of the auditory deficit in Waterslager canaries lies within the cochlea. These observations were confirmed by our morphological findings of severe cochlear and hair-cell pathology in Waterslager canaries.

The hair-cell abnormalities that we found in Waterslagers are very similar to observations made after acoustic over-exposure or aminoglycoside oto-toxicity (Cousillas and Rebillard, 1985, 1988; Cotanche et al., 1987; Hashino et al., 1991, 1992; Marean et al., 1993; Pickles and Rouse, 1991). However, there are several lines of evidence that argue against such external sources for the pathologies that we found in Waterslagers where the whole basilar papilla is affected by the pathologies. In contrast, acoustic over-exposure even at extreme levels and for long periods of time resulted only in a locally restricted damage and was never seen to affect the whole papilla (Cotanche et al., 1987; Dooling and Ryals, in press). Also aminoglycosides even at extremely high doses (at the limit that the animals could tolerate) left apical hair cells undamaged (Cotanche et al., 1994). In addition it has been shown in cross-breeding experiments that the auditory deficit of Waterslagers is hereditary (Okanoya et al., 1990).

The cross breeding experiments showed that intermediate threshold loss can be found in the F1 offspring of Waterslager and Roller canaries. This observation might be related to the large inter-individual variability in cochlear pathology that we observed. We have obtained our Waterslagers from several breeders in the USA and Germany. All of the breeders claimed that their birds were high quality Waterslagers. This strain originates from a very small breeding stock that survived World War I and was bred for its special song characteristics (Pelemann, 1922). The establishment of different breeding lines since then with occasional cross breeds with other canary strains may contribute to the large variability in Waterslager cochlear pathology.

The comparison of the behavioral and the CAP audiograms with the morphological data was somewhat surprising. All the audiograms indicated large threshold increases at high frequencies and no or only small increases below 1kHz in Waterslagers. Based on the known tonotopy in a variety of bird species (Manley et al., 1987; Gleich, 1989; Köppl et al., 1993; Gummer et al., 1987) one might predict that the base of the Waterslager basilar papilla should be much more affected than the apex. However, we found abnormal hair cells along the whole length of the basilar papilla, and indeed some of the morphological parameters even indicated that the apical half was more affected by pathology (Fig. 2). We have no obvious explanation for the "good" thresholds at low frequencies in Waterslagers, despite the observed hair-cell pathologies. However, the reduced number of stereovilli (Fig. 3b) might result in a lowering of the frequencies that are represented on the Waterslager basilar papilla. Lowering the high-frequency cut-off at the base of the papilla might explain the dramatic threshold increases that occurred for frequencies above 1-2kHz.

We have no evidence for a progression of the pathologies with age because the cochleae of the 2 month old birds had very severe pathology and the least affected cochleae were from a bird of the 1-1.5 year old group. This notion is also conform with the earlier observation that high frequency thresholds showed no difference between a group of 6 months old Waterslagers and a group of birds with an average age of 4 years (Okanoya and Dooling, 1987). In two recent abstracts (Park et al., 1993; Weisleder and Park, 1994) it was shown that abnormalities were not only present in the basilar papilla, but also in the sacculus while hair cells in the other vestibular organs appeared normal. These authors have argued that Waterslagers might be affected by Scheibes dysplasia. This type of inner ear abnormality is also classified as cochleo-saccular type and was also found in deaf white cats, dalmatian dogs, white minks and various mouse mutants (Steel, 1983). In contrast to the picture found in several physiologically and morphologically studied mutants with the cochleo-saccular type of abnormality (Steel and Harvey, 1992) Waterslagers do not show signs of pigmentation deficiencies nor a progression of the pathology with age. To more clearly classify the type of abnormality in Waterslagers, an investigation of the tegmentum vasculosum and the endocochlear potential would be desirable.

The small and microvilli covered hair cells illustrated in Fig. 4 are highly reminiscent of developing hair cells as they have been described in the embryonic chicken basilar papilla (Cotanche and Sulik, 1984). We found in our Waterslager specimens all stages from the very immature to almost mature microvilli covered hair cell (Fig. 4). Small microvilli covered hair cells representing different stages of hair-cell development have also been found after various forms of cochlear trauma that caused hair cell loss in a number of avian species (Cotanche, 1987; Cotanche and Corwin, 1991; Dooling and

Ryals, in press; Hashino et al., 1991,1992; Lippe et al., 1991; Saunders et al., 1992). These cells were considered as regenerated hair cells. By application of cell proliferation markers it was shown that in birds with severe cochlear trauma new hair cells are produced as the result of cell division (Corwin and Cotanche, 1988; Ryals and Rubel, 1988; Warchol and Corwin, 1992) and that new hair cells often appear in pairs (Raphael, 1992). By analogy we conclude that the microvilli covered hair cells that we find in Waterslagers (Fig. 4) are newly produced regenerating hair cells. We are currently cooperating with Dr. J. Presson from the Department of Zoology at the University of Maryland to demonstrate with the BrdU technique that these cells are truly regenerating. Preliminary results indicate that a significantly higher rate of cell proliferation occurs in the basilar papilla of Waterslager as compared to non-Waterslager canaries, supporting our conclusions from the SEM observations.

In the SEM we find regenerating hair cells either singly or in pairs surrounded by other mature hair cells, however, we never found larger patches. This observation may be relevant for hypotheses about the stimuli that induce proliferation and differentiation of hair cells (Corwin and Warchol, 1991, Corwin et al., 1993; Richardson, 1993). The observation that stereovillar bundles on fairly mature regenerating hair cells can have a rather normal appearance indicates the possibility that these cells develop normally, and start degenerating only after final maturation. This finding is consistent with reports that regeneration starts even in the presence of an adverse stimulus that caused the loss of hair cells (Pugliano et al., 1993; Hashino et al., 1991, 1992; Marean et al., 1993).

Several questions remain to be clarified: 1) what causes the hair cells to degenerate? 2) why do we find such extensive pathology despite ongoing hair-cell production? 3) can the rate of cell proliferation be increased? The answer to those questions should also contribute to an understanding of the mechanisms of hair-cell regeneration.

5 Acknowledgments

We thank G.M. Klump for help especially with the middle ear measurements. G.A. Manley provided the equipment for physiological and morphological measurements. We are currently cooperating with J. Presson to identify proliferating cells in the basilar papilla with the BrdU technique. We thank J. Strutz for support and discussion and the canary breeder G. Sewing for assistance. A. Linzenboldt measured the behavioral audiograms and K. Bielenberg helped with the morphological analysis. C. Cavanna and G. Niebler helped with photography. Supported by the SFB 204 "Gehör", a Helmholtz grant from the BMFT (OG), the Alexander von Humboldt Foundation and NIH grants DC00198 and MH00982 (RJD).

6 References

Adler, H.J., Poje, C.P. and Saunders, J.C. (1993) Recovery of auditory function and structure in the chick after two intense pure tone exposures. Hear. Res. 71, 214-224.

Bohne, B.A. and Harding, G.W. (1992) Neural regeneration in the noise-damaged chinchilla cochlea. Laryngoscope 102, 693-703.

Christiansen, J.B. (1991) Sociological implications of hearing loss. Ann. N.Y. Acad. Sci. 630, 230-235.

Corwin, J.T. and Cotanche, D.A. (1988) Regeneration of sensory hair cells after acoustic trauma. Science 240, 1772-1774.

Corwin, J.T. and Warchol, M.E. (1991) Auditory hair cells: Structure, function, development and regeneration. Annu. Rev. Neurosci. 14, 301-333.

Corwin, J.T., Warchol, M.E. and Kelley, M.W. (1993) Hair cell development. Curr. Opin. Neurobiol. 3, 32-37.

Cotanche, D.A. (1987) Regeneration of hair cell stereociliary bundles in the chick cochlea following severe acoustic trauma. Hear. Res. 30, 181-196.

Cotanche, D.A. and Corwin, J.T. (1991) Stereociliary bundles reorient during hair cell development and regeneration in the chick cochlea. Hear. Res. 52, 379-402.

Cotanche, D.A. and Sulik, K.K. (1984) The development of stereociliary bundles in the cochlear duct of chick embryos. Hear. Res. 16, 181-193.

Cotanche, D.A., Saunders, J.C. and Tilney, L.G. (1987) Hair cell damage produced by acoustic trauma in the chick cochlea. Hear. Res. 25, 267-286.

Cotanche, D.A., Lee, K.H., Stone, J.S. and Picard, D.A. (1994) Hair cell regeneration in the bird cochlea following noise damage of ototoxic drug damage) Anat. Embryol. 189, 1-18.

Cousillas, H. and Rebillard, G. (1985) Age-dependent effects of a pure tone trauma in the chick basilar papilla: Evidence for a development of the tonotopic organization. Hear. Res. 19, 217-226.

Cousillas, H. and Rebillard, G. (1988) Morphological transformation of hair cells in the chick basilar papilla following an acoustic obverstimulation. Hear. Res. 32, 117-122.

Cruz, R.M., Lambert, P.R. and Rubel, E.W. (1987) Light microscopic evidence of hair cell regeneration after gentamicin toxicity in chick cochlea. Arch. Otolaryngol- Head & Neck Surg. 113, 1058-1062.

Dooling, R.J. and Ryals, B.M. (in press) Effects of acoustic overstimulation of four species of birds. In: Manley, G.A., Klump, G.M., Köppl, C., Fastl, H. and Oeckinghaus, H. (eds.) Advances in Hearing Research Vol. 10. World Scientific Publishers, Singapore.

Fischer, F.P., Köppl, C. and Manley, G.A. (1988) The basilar papilla of the barn owl *Tyto alba*: a quantitative morphological SEM analysis. Hear. Res. 34, 87-102.

Forge, A., Li, L., Corwin, J.T. and Nevill, G. (1993) Ultrastructural evidence for hair cell regeneration in the mammalian inner ear. Science 259, 1616-1619.

Gao, W., Ding, D., Zheng, X., Ruan, F. and Liu, Y. (1993) A comparison in the stereocilia between temporary and permanent hearing losses in acoustic trauma. Hear. Res. 62, 27-41.

Gleich, O. (1989) Auditory primary afferents in the starling: Correlation of function and morphology. Hear. Res. 37, 255-268.

Gleich, O. and Manley, G.A. (1988) Quantitative morphological analysis of the sensory epithelium of the starling and pigeon basilar papilla. Hear. Res. 34, 69-86.

Gleich O., Manley G.A., Mandl, A. and Dooling, R.J. (1994) The basilar papilla of the canary and zebra finch: A quantitative scanning electron microscopical description. J. Morphol. 221, 1-24.

Gummer, A.W., Smolders, J.W.T. and Klinke, R. (1986) Basilar membrane motion in the pigeon measured with the Mössbauer technique. Hear. Res. 29, 63-92.

Hashino, E., Tanaka, Y and Sokabe, M. (1991) Hair cell damage and recovery following chronic application of kanamycin in the chick cochlea. Hear. Res. 52, 356-368.

Hashino, E., Tanaka, Y., Salvi, R.J. and Sokabe, M. (1992) Hair cell regeneration in the adult budgerigar after kanamycin ototoxicity. Hear. Res. 59, 46-58.

Hudde, H. (1983) Measurement of the eardrum impedance of human ears. J. Acoust. Soc. Am. 73, 242-247.

Köppl, C., Gleich, O. and Manley, G.A. (1993) An auditory fovea in the barn owl cochlea. J. Comp. Physiol. A 171,695-704.

Lippe, W.R., Westbrook, E.E. and Ryals, B.M. (1991) Hair cell regeneration in the chicken cochlea following aminoglycoside toxicity. Hear. Res. 52, 203-210.

Manley, G.A., Brix, J. and Kaiser, A. (1987) Developmental stability of the tonotopic organization of the chick's basilar papilla. Science 237, 655-656.

Manley, G.A., Schwabedissen, G. and Gleich, O. (1993) Morphology of the basilar papilla of the budgerigar, *Melopsitacus undulatus*. J. Morphol. 218, 153-165.

Marean G.C., Burt, J.M., Beecher, M.D. and Rubel, E.W. (1993) Hair cell regeneration in the European starling (*Sturnus vulgaris*): Recovery of pure-tone detection thresholds. Hear. Res. 71, 125-136.

Nadeau, J.H., Kosowsky, M. and Steel, K.P. (1991) Comparative gene mapping, genome duplication, and the genetics of hearing. In.: Genetics of hearing impairment. Ann. N.Y. Acad. Sci. 630, 49-67.

Okanoya, K. and Dooling, R.J. (1985) Colony differences in auditory thresholds in the canary (*Serinus canarius*) J. Acoust. Soc. Am. 78, 1170-1176.

Okanoya, K. and Dooling, R.J. (1987) Strain differences in auditory thresholds in the canary (*Serinus canarius*). J. Comp. Psychol. 101, 213-215.

Okanoya, K. and Dooling, R.J. (1990a) Detection of auditory sinusoids of fixed and uncertain frequency by budgerigars (*Melopsitacus undulatus*) and zebra finches (*Poephila guttata*). Hear. Res. 50, 175-184.

Okanoya, K. and Dooling, R.J. (1990b) Detection of gaps in noise by budgerigars (*Melopsitacus undulatus*) and zebra finches (*Poephila guttata*). Hear. Res. 50, 185-192.

Okanoya, K., Dooling, R.J. and Downing, J.D. (1990) Hearing and vocalizations in hybrid Waterslager-Roller canaries (*Serinus canarius*). Hear. Res. 46, 271-276.

Park, T.J., Lu, Y and Weisleder, P. (1993) Vestibular hair cell abnormalities in congenital hearing impaired canaries. Soc. Neurosci. Abstr. 23, 1579.

Pelemann, B. (1922) Broschüre über den Belgischen Wasserschläger. cf. J. Sandfort (1989) Kanarienfreund 42, 470-473.

Pickles, J.O. and Rouse, G.W. (1992) Effects of streptomycin on development of the apical structures of hair cells in the chick basilar papilla. Hear. Res. 55, 244-254.

Pugliano, F.A., Wilcox, T.O., Rossiter, J. and Saunders, J.C. (1993) Recovery of auditory structure and function in neonatal chicks exposed to intense sound for 8 days. Neurosci. Lett. 151, 214-218.

Raphael, Y. (1992) Evidence for supporting cell mitosis in response to acoustic trauma in the avian inner ear. J. Neurocytol. 21, 663-671.

Raphael, Y and Altschuler, R.A. (1991) Scar formation after drug-induced cochlear insult. Hear, Res. 51, 173-184.

Richardson, G. (1993) Keep the noise down. Curr. Biol. 3, 759.762.

Ryals, B.M. and Rubel, E.W. (1988) Hair cell regeneration after acoustic trauma in adult *Coturnix* Quail. Science 240, 1774-1776.

Saunders, J.C., Adler, H.J. and Pugliano, F.A. (1992) The structural and functional aspects of hair cell regeneration in the chick as a result of exposure to intense sound. Exp. Neurol. 115, 13-17.

Steel, K.P. and Bock, G.R. (1983) Hereditary inner-ear abnormalities in animals: Relationship with human abnormalities. Arch. Otolaryngol. 109, 22-29.

Steel, K.P. and Harvey, D. (1992) Development of auditory function in mutant mice. In.: Romand R. (Ed.) Development of auditory and vestibular systems 2. Elsevier Science Publishers, Amsterdam, pp221-242.

Tilney, L.G. and Saunders, J.C. (1983) Actin filaments, stereocilia, and hair cells of the bird cochlea I. length, number, width, and distribution of stereocilia of each hair cell are related to the position of the hair cell on the cochlea. J. Cell Biol. 96, 807-821.

Warchol, M.E. and Corwin, J.T. (1992) Hair cell regeneration in vitro: Determination of the latency and pattern of cell proliferation. Abstr. 15th ARO Midwinter Res. Mtg. p106.

Warchol, M.E., Lambert, P.R., Goldstein, B.J., Forge, A. and Corwin, J.T. (1993) Regenerative proliferation in inner ear sensory epithelia taken from adult guinea pigs and humans. Science 259, 1619-1622.

Weisleder, P. and Park, T.J. (1994) Belgian Waterslager canaries are Scheibe's type dysplasia. Abstr. 17th ARO Midwinter Res. Mtg. p103.

Development, overproduction and regeneration of cochlear hair cells in the rat

R. Romand, M. Abdouh, S. Chardin, and A.-E. Zine

Laboratoire de Neurobiologie, Université Blaise Pascal-Clermont II, 63177 Aubière Cedex, France.

1 Introduction

It is clear at the present time that avian hair cells have the capability to regenerate after being damaged (Corwin and Cotanche 1988, Girod et al. 1989, Rubel 1992, Cotanche et al. 1994). A recent observation in the rat claimed that RA stimulates regeneration of auditory hair cells from cochlea maintained *in vitro* after antibiotic poisoning. (Lefebvre et al. 1993). However, several questions are raised by this experiment, concerning the culture medium used which contained several hormones and the immaturity of the cochlea. Moreover, so far no mitotic activity has been shown related to these 'regenerated' hair cells. Several possibilities can be put forward concerning the regeneration of auditory hair cells beside the action of RA, and other interpretations are possible. For example, it is possible that the aminoglycoside only injured hair cells, and then recovery ensued. This possibility has been put forward by Sobkowicz et al. (1992) after mechanical injury of hair cells. Another possibility is that immature cells of the sensory epithelium, such as supporting cells after hair cell damage, could reenter the cycle of proliferation. Then, cells produced by division could later differentiate into hair cells as this has been shown in amphibians (Balak et al. 1990, Corwin 1992) and in birds (Corwin et al. 1991, Raphael 1993).

In any case, in order to understand the possible cochlear hair cell regeneration in the rat, it is worthwhile to know the temporal and spatial pattern of hair cells development during ontogenesis. Studies by phalloidin staining and scanning electron microscopy (SEM) were undertaken in order to know when hair cells start their differentiation from the progenitor cells of the cochlear sensory epithelium (Romand et al. 1993, Zine et al. 1994). These results served as reference for *in vitro* differentiation of hair cells and later for their modifications by growth factors or other molecules. Surprisingly enough, fetal and neonatal cochlea *in vitro* presented a conspicuous hair cell overproduction independent of growth factors or innervation (Abdouh et al. 1993). With the same technique we investigated the potential of RA for inducing regeneration of hair cells in the postnatal cochlea.

2 Differentiation and development of hair cells

Recent observations on the apical poles of auditory receptors by SEM (Zine et al. 1994) showed that before differentiation of the sensory cells at 16 days of gestation (DG), cells lining the cochlear canal were topped with numerous microvilli and one kinocilium in their center whether they are presumptive hair cells or not. (Fig. 1 A). From phalloidin staining (Romand et al. 1993) it has been shown that the ventral part of the cochlear canal is made of several layers of columnar epithelial cells that give rise to the Kölliker's organ as this has been observed in the mouse (Lim and Rueda 1992).

At the base of the cochlea at 18 DG, the sensory epithelia can be distinguished by cells topped with taller microvilli and a kinocilium. This region is surrounded on the medial side by the Kölliker's organ and on the lateral side by presumptive Hensen and Claudius cells (Fig. 1 B). At this stage, a row of hair cells, presumably inner hair cells (IHCs) as shown by their position and a tuft of cilia, were recognizable (Fig. 1 C). This earliest differentiation of hair cells from the surrounding cells is characterized by short, upright cilia arranged in a round tuft and a short kinocilium in its center (Fig. 1 C). The presumptive region of outer hair cells (OHCs) was visible by a different arrangement of tall microvilli, but no recognizable tufts of cilia were distinguishable from the ubiquitous microvilli on the sensory epithelium surface.

At 20 days of gestation, the prominence of the cilia bundles over the surrounding microvilli permits the identification of IHCs. They start to present cilia arrangement as demonstrated by a gradation in height toward the kinocilium, thus at that time they can be called stereocilia. Moreover, the kinocilium has moved toward the lateral side of the hair cell (Figs. 1 D and E). The cuticular plate can be observed around the kinocilium where cilia have disappeared, leaving a bare region (Fig. 1 E). At this stage, OHCs start to differentiate from the surrounding cells (Fig. 1 D), they look like IHCs observed two days earlier with tall upright cilia organized in round bundles with a kinocilium in the center. Right at the start of their differentiation or later, hair cells present a good spatial organization with one row of IHCs and three rows of OHCs, very seldom one extra row of OHCs is present, and usually when this happens it is for a very short distance.

A few days later, at birth and several days after birth, the main feature of auditory hair cells is present in the basal cochlea, i. e. the U organization of IHCs stereocilia, which will become straight days later and the V shape of OHCs stereocilia which will refine their morphology with maturation. Several days after birth, supporting cells are still topped by numerous tall microvilli and a single kinocilium. Moreover, the internal side of the apical poles of IHCs and OHCs are still filled with numerous small cilia that will disappear first on the OHCs before IHCs. It seems then, that the apical surface of OHCs reaches a mature appearance before IHCs, as this as already been observed by the first disappearance of the kinocilium for OHCs before IHCs (Lenoir et al. 1987).

Both phalloidin staining (Romand et al. 1993) and SEM observations (Zine et al. 1994) showed the same early differentiation of hair cells from the surrounding cells, starting at 18 DG for the IHCs and 2 days later for OHCs. The sensory epithelium differentiates from epithelial cells where the apical surface is covered by microvilli and a kinocilium at 16 DG. Early evidence of cilia is characterized by a round bundle of short upright cilia arranged around a prominent kinocilium that protrude from the apical surface. The same observation was made on the chick embryo (Cotanche and Sulik 1984). In fact, striking similarity can be observed regarding the differentiation of hair cell stereocilia bundles, on the one hand between several species of mammals studied so far, such as the mouse (Lim and Anniko 1985), the guinea pig (Sobin and Anniko 1984), and human (Lavigne-Rebillard and Pujol 1986); and on another hand the chick embryo (Cotanche and Sulik 1984, Cohen and Cotanche 1992).

The sequence following the onset of hair cell differentiation may be the same as described for the chick (Tilney and Tilney 1988, 1992), although no quantitative observations have been made yet in mammals. However, it is interesting to point out that hair cell polarity, as defined by the position of the kinocilium and the orientation of stereocilia bundle, is non-uniform in very young hair cells (see Fig. 1 D) as observed in birds. Early in development, hair cells rapidly acquire a uniform polarity where the kinocilium and the tallest stereocilia are oriented toward the external side of the cochlea.

Figure 1. SEM micrographs from the apical surface of the sensory epithelium of prenatal rats.
A: Ventral part of the cochlear canal in a 16 DG fetus. Cells lining this area are topped with numerous microvilli and one kinocilium (arrows). Scale bar: 2 μm. B: Ventral part of the cochlear canal from a 18 DG fetus. At this stage, three regions can be distinguished by the different development of microvilli and cilia. The medial region correspond to the Kölliker's organ topped with numerous microvilli and kinocilia (1). The central region corresponding to the future sensory epithelium presenting cells topped with a kinocilium and taller microvilli showing different orientations (2). The lateral region is characterized by cells with small microvilli and a kinocilium (3). This region will differentiate later into Hensen and Claudius cells. The central region presents for the first time the differentiation of a row of cells that correspond by their position to future IHCs. These cells are characterized by a round bundle of cilia that differentiate from the surrounding microvilli (arrows). Scale bar: 5 μm. C: Higher magnification of early differentiation of an IHC from a 18 DG fetus. Note the round spatial arrangement of numerous short upright cilia (small arrows) surrounded by taller microvilli (arrow heads) and the central position of the kinocilium (large arrow). Scale bar: 0.5 μm. D: Sensory epithelium from a 20 DG fetus. At the bottom of the micrograph one can observe the IHCs separated from the OHCs by pillar cells (bracket) which are topped by numerous microvilli and a kinocilium (small arrows). On this figure, two rows of OHCs are shown (1, 2). They present different orientations of the kinocilium as well as the IHCs (arrows). OHCs are separated by supporting cells with taller microvilli and a kinocilium. Scale bar: 2 μm. E: One IHC and one OHC from a 20 DG fetus. At this stage the IHC presents a laterally placed kinocilium on the clearly visible cuticular plate devoid of most of its cilia which are still numerous on the medial side (arrow). The bundle of cilia starts to differentiate in a more adult shape with a staircase organization, although not very visible on this micrograph. The OHC on the top left present a typical immature round cilia bundle with a central kinocilium (large arrow). Scale bar: 1 μm.

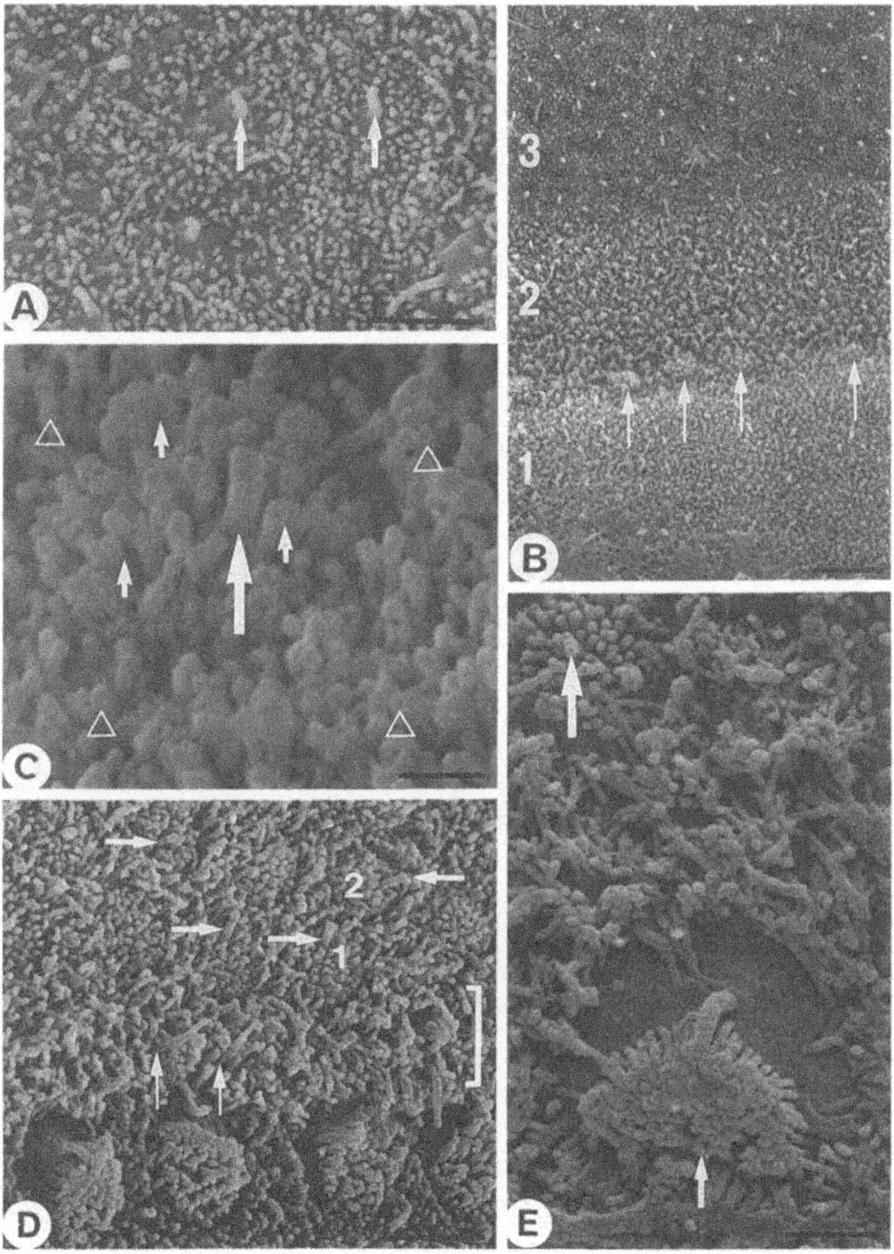
A
3
2
1
B
C
2
1
D
E

3 Ontogenesis of cochlear explants *in vitro*

In normal developing cochlea, hair cells are the most specialized cells in which the cytoskeleton is entirely predictable for a specific region (Tilney and Tilney 1992). It was then, interesting to know, if the cochlea during early *in vitro* ontogenesis would retain the same good spatial structured pattern of organization in several rows and still present a normal development of hair cell apical surface.

In order to determine the degree of differentiation of the apical pole of hair cells from embryonic cochlea maintained *in vitro*, surface preparations with phalloidin staining (Rastel et al. 1993) and SEM preparations were made on these explants. Unexpectedly, fetal and neonatal cochlear explants maintained several days in culture, presented an important overproduction of both types of hair cells (Figs. 2 A and B). It was possible to observe up to 9 rows of OHCs and 3 rows of IHCs. This overproduction of hair cells does not depend on the culture medium or on the innervation of the organ of Corti (Abdouh et al. 1993). Moreover, these supernumerary cells are present without adding mitotic drugs, without previous injury or special manipulation of the explants. In relation to fetal development, younger fetal explants show higher potency for hair cell overproduction than older ones. Close examination of explants after 7 days *in vitro* show that IHCs and OHCs do not present the same regular spatial organization in regular rows. It seems then, that the supernumerary hair cells modified their regular spatial arrangement in rows. Beside this first observation, hair cells are densely packed together and some of them present an aberrant polarity as observed by various positions of the kinocilium. Variation of polarity of hair cells may be different from cell to cell, and some time hair cells may present an opposite orientation between the kinocilium and the tallest stereocilia (Fig. 2 C).

The overproduction of hair cells is observed by extra rows, but also by supernumerary cells between existing hair cells as can be observed by the smaller cuticular plate and less differentiated stereocilia (Figs. 2 A, D and E). In fact, smaller apical surfaces present a central position of the kinocilium which is typical of very immature apical poles of hair cells with a central position of the kinocilium (Figs. 2 A and E). Beside the previous observation, some cells were very close together without any visible separation by supporting cells on their lateral sides. We called these cells 'Siamese twin hair cells' because they presented a common cuticular plate topped with two sets of stereocilia and two kinocilia (Fig. 2 C) and 'twin hair cells' those with two small cells close together, but still separated by supporting cells.

Embryonic organ of Corti in organotypic culture presents for most hair cells a normal development of stereocilia, with a staircase organization, some of them may show a retarded development related to the overproduction of hair cells. It seems that processes governing stereocilia ontogenesis and assembly (reviewed by Tilney and Tilney 1992) are little affected by explantation and *in vitro* conditions. The same observations were made for avian embryonic cochlear explants in short term cultures (Stone and Cotanche 1991). If stereocilia formation is not much modified *in vitro*, this is not the case for cell polarity and spatial organization of the organ of Corti due to supernumerary cells. These differences may come from culture conditions, longer time *in vitro* (7 to 10 days in our case) or a more susceptible mammal cochlea to culture.

The hair cell polarity seems to be very sensitive to explantation and *in vitro* conditions that may lead to modification of epigenetic factors. For instance, intercellular contact may be one of these factors. In fact, it is thought that epithelial cell polarity is a phenotype acquired through a multistage process in early embryonic development and maintained in the adult (Rodriguez-Boulan and Nelson 1989). The polarity of epithelial cells is established once intercellular contacts are formed, conversely, if cell contacts are disrupted or modified, they may loose their normal polarity (Gumbiner 1987).

Another possibility may be put forward regarding the role of the tectorial membrane in shaping the stereocilia and kinocilium orientation during development (Cotanche and Corwin 1991). It is possible that contacts between the apical pole of hair cells and the tectorial membrane after explantation or during culture are modified or lost by retarded growth, then tectorial membrane traction mechanisms may be modified producing aberrant cell polarities.

Supernumerary hair cells inside rows and twin hair cells may be produced by common mechanisms that are responsible for hair cell overproduction. Concerning the key question, Is there cell proliferation through mitotic activity? We do not have a definitive answer yet, although from preliminary observations with bromodeoxyuridine, we did not see enough cells labeled to account for hair cell overproduction observed in our explants. Our hypothesis is that two different mechanisms could be present. One is related to cell overproduction originating from existing cells early in development that will differentiate *in vitro* into hair cells. This hypothesis would suppose that many supernumerary hair cells develop from cells that would have died in normal condition through mechanisms such as programmed cell death (Arends and Wyllie 1991). This would also suggest that cues in cell environment could influence cell fates as well as cell phenotype (Rodriguez-Boulan and Powell 1992, Johnson and Deckwerth 1993).

A recent publication using RA in culture medium with a protocol close to the one we used was able to induce supernumerary hair cells (Kelley et al. 1993). Interestingly enough, tritiated thymidine added to cultures failed to produce labeled hair cells, supporting the role of RA as altering the fate of existing cells, without having mitotic activity. This conclusion would correspond to our first mechanism responsible for hair cell overproduction. This first mechanism, we believe, could be responsible for the production of extra rows of IHCs and OHCs.

However, the disruption of regular alignment inside rows may be due to production of extra cells within each row, thus disrupting their regular arrangement. This phenomena may be due to another mechanism than cell division as suggested by immature hair cells amongst well developed ones, and twin hair cells. Supernumerary cells inside rows could be formed by cells already engaged in differentiation at the time of explantation, that dedifferentiate and reenter the mitotic cycle, as suggested by Corwin (1992) for producing a symmetric set of cells resulting in what we called 'Siamese twin hair cells' and 'twin hair cells'. This observation may be related to a recent finding in the lateral line of some fish where hair cells appear to develop almost exclusively in pairs (Rouse and Pickles 1991). Another possibility may be put forward: division of a progenitor cell which differentiates asymmetrically as a hair cell and a supporting cell, as suggested for the avian vestibular organ (Weisleder and Rubel 1992). Supporting cells, especially when hair cells are already differentiated at 18 DG and later, may be responsible also for overproduction of hair cells. Role of supporting cells in hair cells regeneration from the lateral line of amphibians has been observed (Balak et al. 1990, Jones and Corwin 1993) as well for the avian cochlea (Girod et al. 1989, Corwin et al. 1991, Raphael 1993).

Whatever the exact mechanism for the origin of supernumerary hair cells, it shows that embryonic as well as neonatal cochlea may produce extra hair cells without adding drugs for mitotic activity or for enhancing differentiation of precursor cells. It would be interesting to know what the factors are for triggering this overproduction of hair cells in embryonic explants in order to apply this information to the injured adult cochlea for regeneration purposes.

Figure 2. Overproduction of hair cells from 18 DG cochlear explants maintained several days in vitro. Explants were cultured on a collagen substrate and a feeding solution made of 50% minimum essential medium with 20 mM Hepes, 35% Hanks' balanced salt solution supplemented with glucose and L-glutamine and 15% horse serum.
A: Explant from a 18 DG fetus maintained 7 days in vitro and stained with tetramethyl rhodamine labeled phalloidin. The focus is made on the cuticular plates showing the supernumerary rows of IHCs and OHCs. One can observe the abnormal polarity of hair cells as shown by the position of kinocilia corresponding to the region devoid of actin (arrows). Some OHCs amongst well differentiated cells present smaller cuticular plates with a central position of the kinocilium (large arrows), features typical of immature hair cells. Scale bar: 2 μm. B: SEM micrograph of the apical surface of the sensory epithelium after 10 days in vitro. The overexpression of both types of hair cells show a disrupted regular arrangement compared with in vivo cochlea. Stereocilia show large variations in their orientations. Scale bar: 10 μm. C: SEM micrograph of IHCs showing two sets of twin hair cells from an explant maintained 10 days in vitro. The first set (large arrows) is made of two cells close together, separated by one supporting cell. The second set (arrow head), shows two stereocilia bundles on one cuticular plate, although two kinocilia are present, suggesting they come from two cells that are not well separated, we called them 'Siamese twin hair cells'. On the bottom of the micrograph (arrow), an hair cell present an opposite orientation between the kinocilium and the stereocilia. Scale bar: 2 μm. D: SEM micrograph of OHCs from an explant maintained 10 days in vitro. The regular pattern of OHCs stereocilia is different from cells to cell. Hair cells are well separated by supporting cells topped by microvilli and a kinocilium (arrows). Scale bar: 2 μm. E: SEM micrograph of OHCs from an explant maintained 10 days in vitro. One immature hair cell between well differentiated OHCs is present with its round shaped cilia and its central kinocilium (arrow). Scale bar: 2 μm.

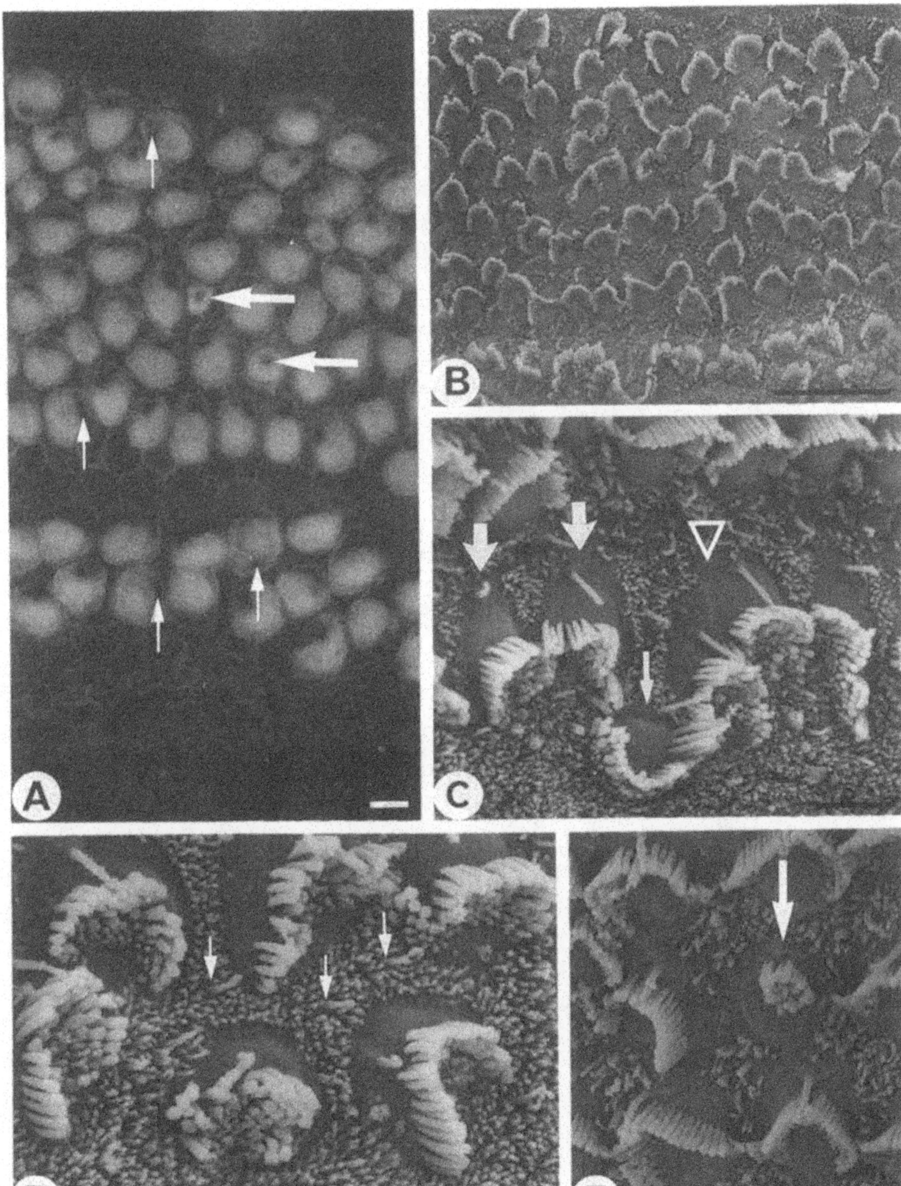
A
B
C
D
E

4 Does RA induce regeneration of hair cells in the neonatal cochlea?

A recent report put forward that RA was able to produce large supernumerary hair cells *in vitro* (Kelley et al. 1993). However, it is worth remembering that we were able to obtain a conspicuous overproduction of hair cells without serum and in a drug free medium (Abdouh et al. 1993). Nevertheless, another report claimed that RA was able to induce hair cell regeneration after antibiotic poisoning (Lefebvre et al. 1993). It is known that RA is a very ubiquitous molecule that plays an important role in the development and homeostasis of vertebrates (Maden 1985, Sive et al. 1990). This molecule has a pleiotropic effect on cultured cells or during development mediated by two classes of receptors (Leroy et al. 1992). Considering these properties, we would not be surprised to find RA and its receptors in the inner ear during development (Represa et al. 1990, Maden et al. 1991, Kelley et al. 1993). However, it is difficult to understand its role in the regeneration of the auditory hair cells since its morphogenetic action is mainly related to inhibitory effects on cell proliferation (Represa et al. 1990, Kennedy and Frank 1993). Moreover, it has been postulated that RA might act as an apoptotic factor (Davies et al. 1992) that could be related to epithelial cell death during early development of the inner ear (Represa et al. 1990).

From the above mentioned observations and from the fact that RA was used in immature cochlea, we decided to replicate the original experiment with our culture technique (Rastel et al. 1993). The main difference between our *in vitro* model and the one used by Lefebvre et al. (1993), is the absence of the N1 medium, although 10% fetal calf serum was present in both protocols.

Explants of 3 day-old cochlea were maintained 10 to 13 days *in vitro*. On surface preparations phalloidin staining showed a good preservation of both types of hair cells (Fig. 3 A). Explants after two days in culture were treated for two days with 10^{-3} M neomycin in order to produce hair cell degeneration and subsequently maintained 7 more days *in vitro*. Surface preparations after phalloidin staining showed the reticular lamina in the form of a reticulum restricted to cell circumference, (Fig. 3 B). However, no stereocilia was visible at the base of the cochlea.

Explants exposed as previously described with neomycin were subsequently treated with 10^{-8} M of RA for 7 days. The phalloidin staining presented the same reticulation as observed with explants treated only with neomycin (Fig. 3 C). The reticular lamina, in both cases of experiment, looks the same as the one described by gentamicin-induced OHC loss (Forge 1985, McDowell et al. 1989) and may correspond to expansion of the adjacent supporting cells. With our culture protocols, we never observed any sign of hair cell regeneration as seen by the absence of stereocilia. The main difference with our protocols compared with the original publication (Lefebvre et al. 1993), is the absence of N1, which is a culture medium for neurons. This medium contains two hormones besides other molecules, progesterone and insulin that may have important effects on hair cell differentiation (Puro and Agardh 1984, Fernihough et al. 1993). One possibility for explaining these contradictory results, may be the fact that hair cells withdraw from the epithelial surface after neomycin treatment, but the cell bodies remain alive and later regenerate. This reparation has been observed *in vitro* after mechanical injury of the sensory epithelium (Sobkowicz et al. 1992). This kind of reparation may be enhanced by hormones present in N1 and fetal calf serum, whereas, RA may have a synergic action with these hormones. Another possibility can be put forward, hormones may induce differentiation of supporting cells into hair cells. In fact, it is known that these cells may be

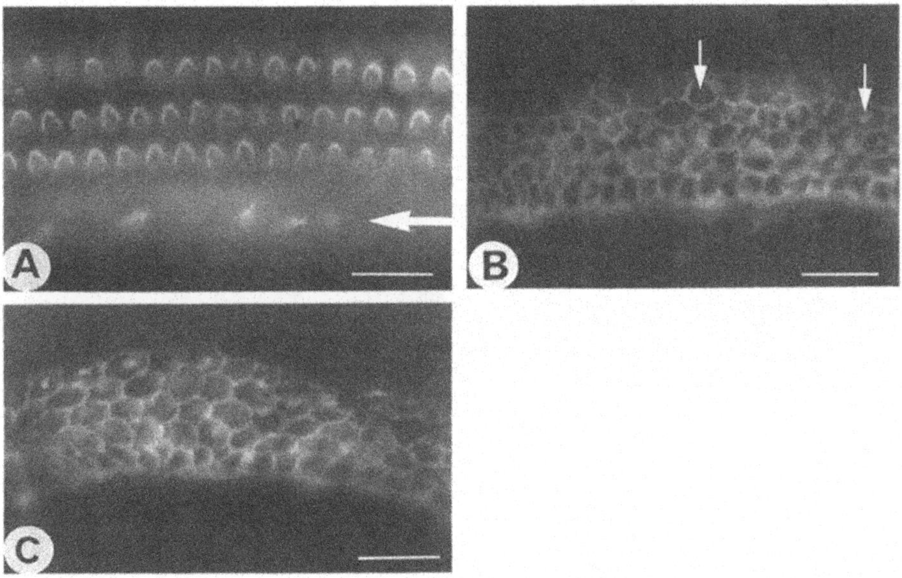

Figure 3. Surface observation of the sensory epithelia of explants from three day-old rats maintained several days in vitro and stained with tetramethyl rhodamine labeled phalloidin. Explants were cultured on a collagen substrate and a feeding solution made of Dulbecco modified Eagle's medium supplemented with 10% fetal bovine serum.
A: Sensory epithelia after 10 days in vitro. The regular organization of the three rows of OHCs' stereocilia is still well preserved. The IHCs are out of focus (arrow). Scale bar: 10 µm. B: Sensory epithelia from an explant after two days in culture, then treated with 10^{-3} M neomycin for two days and maintained for 7 more days in vitro. The reticular lamina presents a reticulation originating from the outline of cells surface by phalloidin staining. No stereocilia is visible, although a small bright spot (arrows) may be present in the center of some cells extending well below the surface. Scale bar: 10 µm. C: Sensory epithelia from an explant treated as for the previous micrograph, with the difference that after the neomycin, the explant was treated for 7 days with 10^{-8} M with RA. The surface of the reticular lamina does not show regeneration after RA treatment. The organization of what is left of the sensory epithelium does not look very different after treatment with neomycin alone. Scale bar: 10 µm.

the progenitor cells for the production of new hair cells during regeneration (Girod et al. 1989, Balak et al. 1990, Corwin et al. 1991, Raphael 1993, Jones and Corwin 1993).

From our observations, we have not seen evidence that RA alone can induce hair cell regeneration in the rat cochlea after ototoxic treatment. Moreover, it is well known that RA is mainly involved in morphogenesis, but not as a mitotic agent as shown for the inner ear (Represa et al. 1990). The addition of RA in chick embryo causes inhibition of cell proliferation in the inner ear and induces differentiation of the sensory epithelium. It is possible that RA enhances immature supporting cells or other cells to transdifferentiate into hair cells as suggested by (Kelley et al. 1993).

Ontogenesis of cochlear receptors *in vivo* produces a structure that is well organized in the temporal and spatial domains. *In vitro*, the spatial organization is more or less disrupted by supernumerary hair cells as well as the cell polarity in some cases. The observation that RA and its receptors are present in the mouse cochlea (Represa et al. 1990, Dollé et al. 1990, Ruberte et al. 1993, Kelley et al. 1993) suggests that RA may act as a polarizing factor or alternatively could induce surrounding cells to acquire a specific morphogenetic activity. In both cases, the question remains open as to how to translate a rather simple and localized signal into a complicated network of positional information required to establish a precise spatial pattern in the cochlea?

It is known that RA influences the expression of Hoxa-1 and Hoxb-1 genes that may be involved in the normal development of the inner ear (Lufkin et al. 1991, Mark et al. 1993). Recent works on genes of the Hox complex have shown that they are used to read a simple morphogenetic signal and to translate it into a more complex pluricellular network of positional information. So, it is possible that RA is involved in the morphogenesis of the sensory epithelium. However, this molecule does not seems to be implicated alone in hair cells regeneration and may only be partially involved in supernumerary hair cells production in fetal explant as shown by the possibility of producing these cells without RA (Abdouh et al. 1993).

In any cases, overproduction of hair cells in fetal cochlea just as the hair cells found after ototoxic drug, whatever the exact causes, shows that mammal cochlea presents potentialities that were unknown in the past recent years, and may be promising for the future in relation to hair cell regeneration in adult mammals.

5 Acknowledgements

This work was supported by La Fondation pour la Recherche Médicale and by l'Association Recherche et Partage.

6 References

Abdouh, M., Després, G. and Romand, R. (1993) Hair cell overproduction in the developing mammalian cochlea in culture. Neuroreport 5, 33-36.

Arends, M.J. and Wyllie, A.H. (1991) Apoptosis: Mechanisms and roles in pathology. Int. Rev. Exp. Pathol. 32, 223-254.

Balak; K.J., Corwin, J.T. and Jones, J.E. (1990) Regenerated hair cells can originate from supporting cell progeny : Evidence from phototoxicity and laser ablation experiments in the lateral line system. J. Neurosci. 10, 2502-2512.

Cohen, G.M. and Cotanche D.A. (1992) Development of the sensory receptors and their innervation in the chick cochlea. In: "Development of auditory and vestibular systems 2", R. Romand (Ed.), Elsevier Science, (Pub), Amsterdam, pp. 101-138.

Corwin, J.T. and Cotanche, D.A. (1988) Regeneration of sensory hair cell after acoustic trauma. Science 240, 1772-1774.

Corwin, J.T. (1992) Regeneration in the auditory system. Exp. Neurol. 115, 7-12.

Corwin, J.T., Jones, J.E., Katayama, A., Kelley, M.W. and Warchol, M.E. (1991) Hair cell regeneration : The identities of progenitor cells potentials triggers and instructive cues. In: Ciba Foundation Symposium, "Regeneration of vertebrate sensory receptors cells", G.R. Bock, J. Whelam, (Eds.), Chichester, Wiley (Pub.), pp. 103-130.

Cotanche, D.A. and Sulik, K.K. (1984) The development of stereocilia bundles in the cochlea duct of chick embryos. Dev. Brain Res. 16, 181-193.

Cotanche, D.A. and Corwin, J.T. (1991) Stereocilia bundles reorient during hair cell development and regeneration in the chick cochlea. Hearing Res. 52, 379-402.

Cotanche, D.A., Lee, K.H., Stone, J.S. and Picard, D.A. (1994). Hair cell regeneration in the bird cochlea following noise damage or ototoxic drug damage. Anat. Embryol., 189 : 1-18.

Dollé, P., Ruberte, E., Leroy, P., Morris-Kay, G. and Chambon, P. (1990) Retinoic acid receptors and cellular retinoic binding protein.I. A systematic study of their differential pattern of transcription during mouse organogenesis. Development 110, 1133-1151.

Fernyhough, P., Willar, G.B., Lindsay, R.M. and Tomlison, D.R. (1993) Insulin and insulin-like growth factor I enhance regeneration in cultured adult rat sensory neurons. Brain Res. 607, 117-124.

Forge, A. (1985). Outer hair cell loss and supporting cell expansion following chronic gentamicin treatment. Hearing Res., 19 :171-182.

Girod, D.A., Duckert, L.G. and Rubel, E.W. (1989) Possible precursor of regenerated hair cells in the avian cochlea following acoustic trauma. Hearing Res. 42, 175-194.

Gumbiner, B. (1987) Structure, biochemistry and assembly of epithelial tight junctions. Am. J. Physiol. 253, C749-C758.

Johnson, E.M. Jr. and Dekwerth, T.L. (1993) Molecular mechanisms of developmental neuronal death. Ann. Rev. Neurosci. 16, 31-46.

Jones, J.E. and Corwin, J.T. (1993) Replacement of lateral line sensory organs during tail regeneration in salamanders: Identification of progenitor cells and analysis of leucocyte activity. J. Neurosci. 13, 1022-1034.

Kelley, M.W., Xu, X.-M., Wagner, M.A., Warchol, M.E. and Corwin, J.T. (1993) The developing organ of Corti contains retinoic acid and forms supernumerary hair cells in response to exogenous retinoic acid in culture. Development 119, 1041-1053.

Kennedy, A. and Frank, R.N. (1993) Cultured ocular cells and extracellular matrices : Role of growth factors, retinoic acid and cell polarity. Current. Eye Res., 12, 693-702.

Lavigne-Rebillard, M. and Pujol, R. (1986) Development of the auditory hair cell surface in human fetuses. A scanning electron microscopic study. Anat. Embryol. 174, 369-377.

Lefebvre, P.P., Malgrange, B., Staeker, H., Moonen, G. and van de Water, T.R. (1993) Retinoic acid stimulates regeneration of mammalian auditory hair cells. Science 260, 692-694.

Lenoir, M., Puel, J.-L. and Pujol, R. (1987) Stereocilia and tectorial membrane development of the rat cochlea. A SEM study. Anat. Embryol. 175, 477-487.

Leroy, P., Krust, A., Kastner, Ph., Mendelsohn, C., Zeleut, A. and Chambon, P. (1992) Retinoic acid receptors. In "Retinoids in normal development and teratogenesis". G. Moriss-Kay (Ed.), Oxford Univ. Press (Pub.), Oxford, U.K. pp. 7-25.

Lim, D.J. and Anniko, M. (1985) Developmental morphology of the mouse inner ear. A scanning electron microscopic observation. Acta Otolaryng.(Stockh.), Suppl. 422, 68p.

Lim, D.J. and Rueda, J. (1992) Structural development of the cochlea. In "Development of auditory and vestibular systems 2", R. Romand (Ed.), Elsevier Science (Pub.), Amsterdam, pp. 33-58.

Lufkin, T., Dierich, A., LeMeur, M., Mark, M. and Chambon, P. (1991) Disruption of the hox -1.6

homeobox gene results to its rostral domain of expression. Cell 66, 1105-1119.

Maden, M. (1985) Retinoids and the control of pattern in limb development and regeneration. Trends Gen. 1, 103-107.

Maden, M., Hunt, P., Eriksson, U., Kuriowa, A., Krumlauf, R. and Summerbell, D. (1991) Retinoic acid-binding protein rhombomeres and the neural crest. Development 111, 35-44.

Mark, M., Lufkin, Th., Vonesch, J.-L., Ruberte, E., Olivo, J.-Ch., Dollé, P., Gorry, Ph., Lumsden, A. and Chambon, P. (1993) Two rhombomeres are altered in Hoxa-1 mutant mice. Development 119, 319-338.

McDowell, B., Davies, S. and Forge, A. (1989). The effect of gentamicin-induced hair cell loss on the tight junctions of the reticular lamina. Hearing Res., 40 : 221-232.

Puro, D.G. and Agardh, E. (1984) Insulin mediated regulation of neuronal maturation. Science 225, 1170-1172.

Raphael, Y. (1993) Reorganization of the chick basilar papilla after acoustic trauma. J. Comp. Neurol. 330, 521-532.

Rastel, D , Abdouh, A., Dahl, D. and Romand, R. (1993) An original organotypic culture method to study the organ of Corti of the newborn rat in vitro. J. Neurosci. Meth. 47, 123-131.

Represa, J., Sanchez, A., Miner, C., Lewis, J. and Giraldez, F. (1990) Retinoic acid modulation of the early development of the inner ear is associated with the control of C-fos expression. Development 110, 1081-1090.

Rodriguez-Boulan, E. and Nelson, W.J. (1989) Morphogenesis of the polarized epithelial cell phenotype. Science 245, 718-725.

Rodriguez-Boulan, E. and Powell, S.K. (1992) Polarity of epithelial and neuronal cells. Ann. Rev. Cell Biol. 8, 395-427.

Romand, R., Zine, A.-E. and Hafidi, A. (1993) Ontogenesis of F-actin in hair cells. Cell Motil. Cytosk. 25, 213-222.

Rouse, G.M. and Pickles, J.O. (1991) Paired development of hair cells in neuroblasts of the teleost lateral line. Proc. C. Soc. Lond. (Biol.) 246, 123-128.

Rubel, E.W. (1992) Regeneration of hair cells in the avian inner ear. In: "Noise-induced hearing loss". A. Dancer, D. Henderson, R.J. Salvi and R.P. Hamernik, (Eds.), Mosby Yearbook, St. Louis, pp. 204-227.

Ruberte, E., Friederich, V., Morris-Kay, G. and Chambon, P. (1993) Differential distribution of CRABP I and CRABP II transcripts during mouse embryogenesis. Development 115, 973-987.

Sive, H.L., Draper, B.W., Harland, R.M. and Weintraub, H. (1990) Identification of retinoic acid-sensitive period during primary axis formation in *Xenopus laevis*. Genes Dev. 4, 932-942.

Sobin, A. and Anniko, M. (1984) Early development of cochlear hair cells stereocilia surface morphology. Arch. Oto-Rhino-Laryng. 241, 53-64.

Sobkowicz, H.M., August, B.K. and Slapnick, S.M. (1992) Epithelial repair following mechanical injury of the developing organ of Corti in culture : An electron microscopic and autoradiographic study. Exp. Neurol. 115, 44-49.

Stone, J.S. and Cotanche, D.A. (1991) Hair cell differentiation in the developing chick cochlea and in embryonic cochlear organ culture. J. Comp. Neurol. 314 : 614-625.

Tilney, L.G. and Tilney, M.S. (1988). Actin and the formation and differentiation of stereocilia. In: "Intrinsic determinants of neuronal form and function". A. R. Liss Inc., New York, pp. 371-383.

Tilney, L.G., Cotanche, D.A. and Tilney, M.S. (1992) Actin filaments, stereocilia and hair cells of the bird cochlea IV. How the number and arrangement of stereocilia are determined. Development 116, 213-226.

Weisleder, P. and Rubel, E.W. (1992) Hair cell regeneration in the avian vestibular epithelium. Exp. Neurol. 115, 2-6.

Zine, E.-A., Després, G. and Romand, R. (1994) Ontogenesis of hair cell stereocilia in the neonatal rat. Assoc. Res. Otolaryng., St. Petersburg, Fl.

Neural regeneration and recovery in the cochlea after excitotoxic injury

J.L. Puel, Christine Gervais d'Aldin, Saaid Saffiedine, Michel Eybalin and Rémy Pujol

INSERM U. 254, Neurobiologie de l'Audition - Plasticité Synaptique, CHU Hôpital St. Charles, 34295 Montpellier cedex 5, France

1 Introduction

It is assumed that mammalian sensory hair cells of the inner ear end organs (cochlea and vestibule) share with neurons an inability to proliferate after their final stage of differentiation. Consequently, loss of hair cells permanently affects the functional properties of these sensory organs. In contrast, the avian cochlea has been reported to regenerate new hair cells after an extensive injury caused by aminoglycoside antibiotics or noise trauma (Corwin and Cotanche, 1988, Ryals and Rubel, 1988). More recently, this capacity to regenerate new hair cells after damage has been suggested for the mammalian inner ear in vitro and in vivo (Forge et al, 1993, Warchol et al., 1993, Lefèbvre et al, 1993). However, in order to restore function, newly differentiated hair cells have to be reconnected to the dendritic terminals of sensory neurons, as it has been observed in the chick cochlea (Duckert and Rubel, 1990). This implies that cochlear neurons, after they have lost their presynaptic targets, have to stop a retrograde degenerative process (Spoendlin, 1975) and undergo regenerative phenomena including sprouting of dendritic neurites, contact with the new targets (newly formed hair cells), and neo-synaptogenesis. Consequently, we have studied the capacity of the auditory nerve dendrites of the guinea-pig cochlea to regenerate *in vivo* and to form new functional synapses with sensory inner hair cells (IHCs). In the experimental model, the IHCs remained both morphologically and functionally unaffected while auditory dendrites were completely destroyed by a strong excitotoxic injury. This excitotoxic model is based upon the implication of glutamate as a neurotransmiter at synapses between IHCs and terminal dendrites of the auditory nerve in the mammalian cochlea (Eybalin, 1993) In previous experiments (Puel et al. 1991), we showed that application into the cochlea of the glutamate agonist AMPA (a-amino-3-hydroxy-5-methyl-4-isoxazole propionic acid) immediately resulted in a dose-dependent loss of electrophysiological responses and concomitant damages to the postsynaptic dendritic terminals of the auditory neurons (i.e. a dendritic swelling followed membrane disruptions). These excitotoxic damages closely mimick those observed after noise trauma (Puel and Pujol, 1993) or ischemia (Pujol et al., 1993, Puel et al, 1994). Furthermore, at low AMPA concentrations (25 µM, corresponding to its EC_{50} in the cochlea) both effects could be immediately reversed by rinses with artificial perilymph (Puel et al., 1994). Thus, the dendritic swelling in the cochlea appears to be, up to a certain extent, a reversible phenomenon. In contrast, at AMPA concentrations of 100 µM and higher, the rupture of postsynaptic membranes with synaptic uncoupling and a complete abolition of the cochlear responses cannot be reversed by artificial perilymph (Puel et al, 1991), indicating that a second stage of injury has been reached. The present paper documents the morphological and functional long term recovery after local exposure to 200 µM of AMPA.

2 Regeneration and Functional Recovery after Excitotoxicity Injury

Guinea pigs of either sex were anesthesized and the right bulla was exposed by a ventral approach, without severing the digastric muscle or the jugular vein. Artificial perilymph with or without AMPA was infused through a hole made in the scala tympani and allowed to exit the cochlea by a second hole in the scala vestibuli. Then, the holes and the bulla was closed and the surgical wound sutured.

- *Functional evaluation of the recovery*

Functional evaluation was performed by recording auditory brainstem responses (ABRs) immediately after the local exposure to artificial perilymph containing 200µM AMPA, and 1, 2, 3 and 5 days after exposure. Recordings were compared to those from a control group in which the right cochlea was perfused with artificial perilymph without AMPA. The absence of ABR changes in this control group (fig.1) rules out the possibility of a non-specific trauma due to the experimental procedure. In contrast, immediately after an intracochlear perfusion of 200µM AMPA, no potentials could be recorded (fig.1 and 2). The physiological follow up of these treated guinea-pigs showed a 30 % recovery of the ABRs one day after the AMPA perfusion, and a return to normal values after 5 days of recovery (fig.1and 2). This is a first demonstration that the cochlea can recover a normal function after a complete disappearance of the cochlear potential due to an excitotoxic event.

- *Histological evaluation of the regeneration*

Electron microscopic analysis was used to assess the morphological correlates of this functional recovery. For clarity, the histological evaluation of the cochleas treated with AMPA is summarized in the shematic drawing in fig.2. While, no structural abnormalities were detected in cochleas perfused with artificial perilymph alone, severe ultrastructural damages were observed after AMPA. The excitotoxicity of 200µM AMPA is already known (Puel et al, 1991, 1994) to cause a massive swelling of auditory neurites which ends in a disruption of membranes and a loss of cytoplasmic content. Indeed, in the cochlea processed immediately after exposure, all the dendrites of the primary auditory neurites below the IHC had disappeared, the IHC itself had a normal appearance apart from mechanical distortions of their basal (synaptic) pole: the membrane being pushed inwards by the swelling of the postsynaptic partners. Normal presynaptic elements facing a remnant of postsynaptic membrane and empty spaces were found. All other sensory and

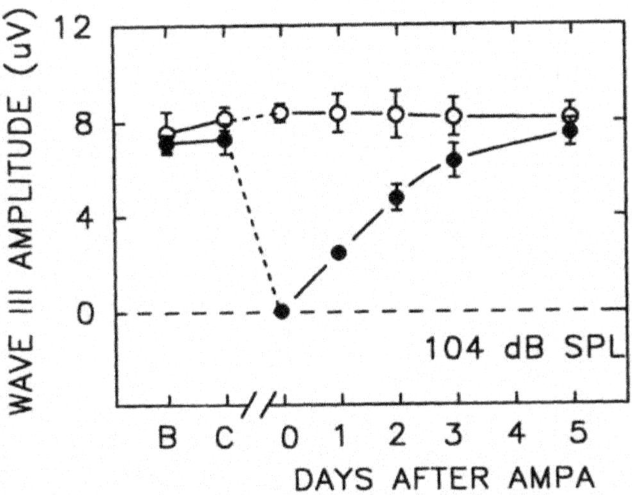

Figure 1. Wave III amplitude of the ABR in μv (means ± SEM) in animals which received an intracochlear perfusion of artificial perilymph alone (control group, open circles, n=6), or artificial perilymph containing 200μM of AMPA (filled circle, n=6). Recordings were done before (B) and after artificial perilymph (C for control), and immediately after (0), and one (1), three (3) and five (5) days after treatment.

neural structures, as well as the supporting cells, in the organ of Corti appeared normal. One day after the AMPA injury, a structural reorganization was clearly evident below the IHCs. The basal pole of the IHC was surrounded by neurites and contacted by some afferent (auditory nerve dendrites) endings. Altough a typical synaptic organization was rarely found in the serial sections examined at this time, some contacts must have been active to account for the partial ABR recovery described above. Some of these contacts were made by thin filopodia of the growing dendrites running up the lateral membrane of the IHC (which sometimes are branching, fig.2), a morphological feature generally found only in early stages of developmental synaptogenesis (Pujol et al., 1978, 1979). A common finding at this stage of the recovery was the presence of an abnormally high number of efferent varicosities bearing an electron dense appearance. Several of them were in close contact with the IHCs in which, sometimes, typical postsynaptic cisternae could be observed. This feature, uncommon in adult cochleas, is also frequently encountered during the normal development. Another feature mimicking early developmental stages was the presence in the IHCs of presynaptic bodies, often multiple, in ectopic positions (not opposite to nerve endings). At 5 days post exposure, the pattern of innervation of the IHC looked normal, thus accounting for the complete recovery of the ABRs. Typical synaptic differentiations were observed at contact between auditory nerve endings and IHCs. The regenerated dendrites were also normally contacted by efferent endings.

These results demonstrate that cochlear neurons are able to regenerate their dendritic neurites and to grow new functional synapses after a strong excitotoxic attack. The time course of regeneration and neo-synaptogenesis in the guinea pig cochlea appears to be relatively fast. Actually, 1 day after the excitotoxic event, cochlear neurons have regenerated their dendritic neurites. Some of these neurites have reached the IHCs and have begun to form functional contacts, as attested by the partial recovery of cochlear potentials. This process seems to be completed 5 days after the excitotoxic event, accounting for the complete functional recovery observed in the ABR recordings.

Figure 2. (see opposite page) Schematic representation of the base of an IHC immediately (day 0) and 1 and 5 days after AMPA. Above each drawing, a representative electrophysiological brain stem response (ABR) is shown. Below each drawing, transmission electron micrographs of the basal pole of an inner hair cell (IHC) taken from animal treatment with AMPA. Note that all dendritic terminals are swollen and blown up immediately after AMPA (empty arrowheads), one day after an auditory dendrite makes a long contact with the IHC (arrows). The IHC is often directly contacted by efferent endings (framed).

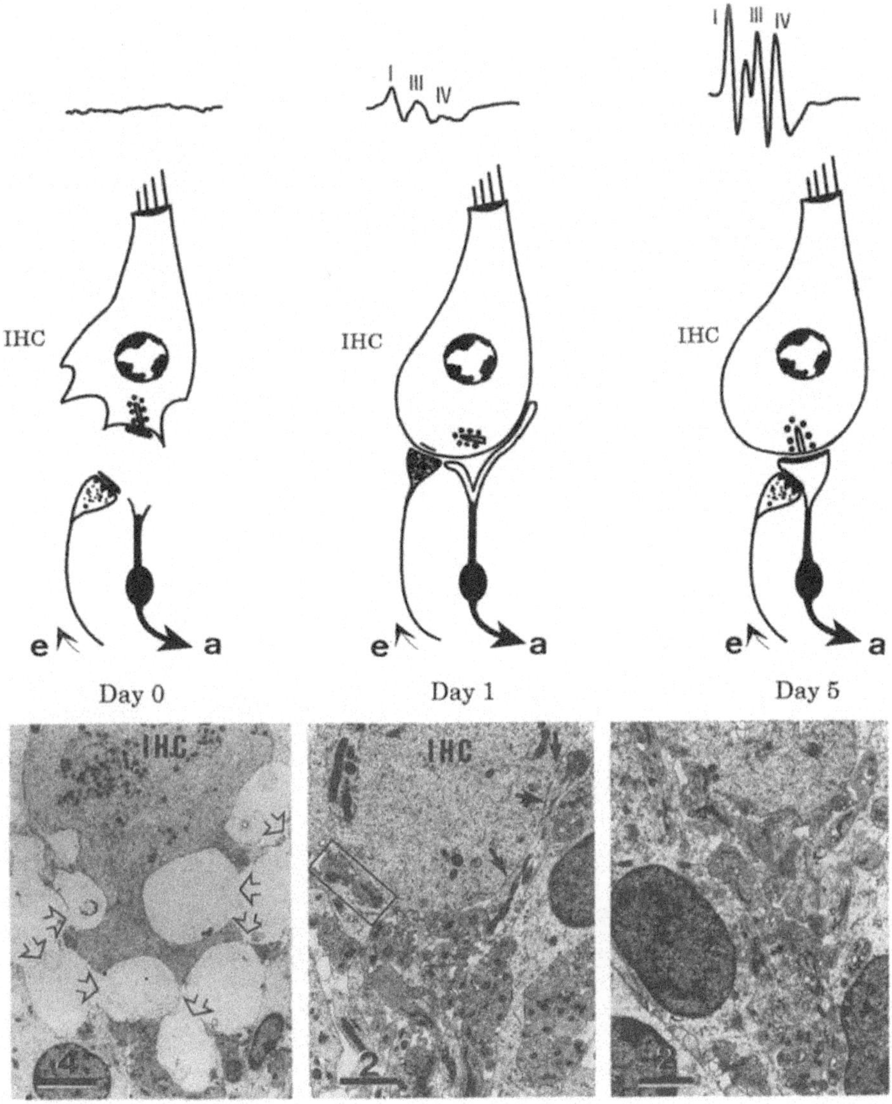
I
III
IV
IHC
e
a
Day 0
Day 1
Day 5
IHC
IHC
4
2
2

3 Molecular Mechanism Leading to the Synaptic Regeneration

This rapid process of regeneration and neo-synaptogenesis should be accompanied by strong metabolic reactions within the auditory neurons. Among the molecular events which could be involved in this process, one should consider the expression of glutamate receptors. Previous *in situ* hybridization data indicated that primary auditory neurons expressed mRNAs encoding GluR2 and GluR3 subunits of AMPA receptors, NMDAR1 subunit of NMDA receptors, and mGluR1 subtype of metabotropic receptors (Ryan et al. 1991, Safieddine and Eybalin, 1992).

Consequently, we used a non-radioactive *in situ* hybridization technique to evaluate variations in the expression of mRNAs encoding these receptors. While the strong expression of the GluR2 (fig.3) and the GluR3 (not shown) mRNAs in primary auditory neurons remained unchanged at any survival time, the expression of mRNAs encoding NMDAR1 and mGluR1 was increased one day after the perfusion of AMPA (fig.3). This enhanced expression decreased slightly two days after the AMPA treatment and returned to a normal value by three days post exposure (fig.3).

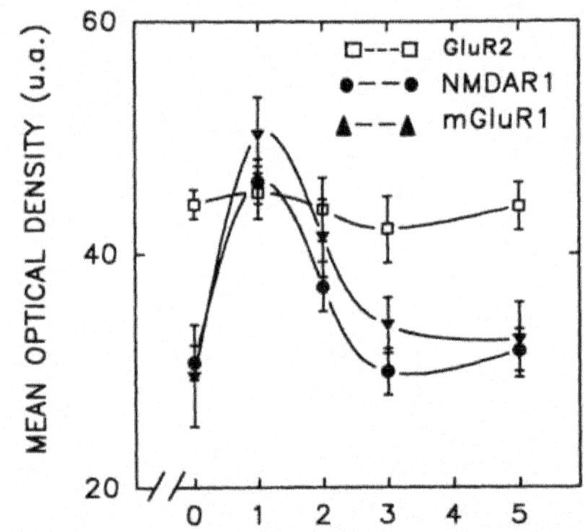

Figure 3. GluR2, NMDAR1 and mGluR1mRNAs variations in primary auditory neurons after AMPA treatment. For each mRNA investigated, the densitometry was done on two non-serial sections per cochlea per each survival stage. The optical density from cochlear regions other than the spiral ganglion was substracted as backround. All the sections were analyzed using the same parameters. The data expressed as means + S.D. a.u.: arbitrary unit.

This pattern of expression excludes a simple process of rebuilding the damaged glutamate receptors on the postsynaptic targets since there was no increased expression of mRNAs coding the AMPA receptors, which are the functionally predominant glutamate receptors in the cochlea (Puel et al., 1991). The increased expression of NMDAR1 and mGluR1 mRNAs agrees with data implicating NMDA and metabotropic glutamate receptors in plastic events. A period of transient overexpression of NMDA receptors in different brain regions generally coincides with the period of synaptogenesis and/or the period of experience-dependent synaptic plasticity (Cline, 1991, Kalb et al, 1992, Burgoyne et al., 1993, Komuro and Rakic, 1993). NMDA receptors are also overexpressed several days after anoxia-induced excitotoxicity CA1 region of rat hippocampus, leading to abnormal bursting discharges in response to synaptic activation (Hori et al., 1991). A similar transient overexpression of metabotropic receptors after excitotoxicity is also suggested by the increased inositol phosphate synthesis stimulated by various glutamate metabotropic agonists which was observed in rat hippocampus days after anoxia (Chen et al, 1988) or, after kainate-induced epilepsy, during the sprouting of mossy fibers (Mayat et al, 1994). This latter finding is consistent with data reporting the implication of metabotropic receptors in postsynaptic protein synthesis in synaptoneurosomes (Weiler and Greenough, 1993). It is thus tempting to hypothesize that the transient increase in the expression of NMDAR1 and mGluR1 mRNAs in spiral ganglion neurons reflects an active role of NMDA receptors and inositol phosphate-coupled metabotropic receptors in regeneration and neo-synaptogenesis in the cochlea.

4 Conclusions

In conclusion, the present study is the first demonstration that the dendrites of the primary auditory neurons postsynaptic to cochlear sensory IHCs can regenerate *in vivo* to form new functional postsynaptic junctions, after they have been disrupted by a strong excitotoxic injury.Understanding the mechanism of the IHC reconnection by the primary auditory dendrites is a very important issue as the dendritic damages linked to glutamate excitotoxicity could be involved in various cochlear pathologies. Auditory dendrites are disrupted after an acoustic trauma (Spoendlin, 1971, 1976, Robertson, 1983) which overstimulates the glutamatergic IHCs (Puel and Pujol, 1993). Consequently, part of the reversibility of the hearing loss observed after noise exposure could be explained by a reconnection of the IHCs by the auditory dendrites (Puel and Pujol, 1993). Similarly, some forms of sudden deafness are possibly due to an ischemia-induced excitotoxicity. Thus, the reversible cases could be accounted for by the regenerative mechanisms described herein. These regenerative phenomenon and restoration of the activity are probably linked to the transient overexpression of NMDA and inositol phosphate-linked glutamate receptors in regenerative phenomena. Our integrative cochlear model could provide a useful tool to further investigate *in vivo* the mechanisms underlying neo-synaptogenesis and functional recovery after excitotoxity.

4 Acknowledgments

The authors wish to thank S. Ladrech, R. Leducq and F. Tribillac for technical assistance and P. Sibleyras for photographic work. Supported by research grant from "Convention CNAMTS-INSERM, 1993".

5 References

Burgoyne, R.D., Graham, M.E. and Cambray-Deakin, M. (1993) Neurotrophic effects of NMDA receptor activation on developing cerebellar granule cells. J. Neurocytol. 22, 689-695.

Chen, C.-K., Silverstein, F., Fisher, S.K., Statman, D. and Johnston M.V. (1988) Perinatal hypoxic-ischemic brain injury enhances quisqualic acid-stimulated phosphoinositide turnover. J. Neurochem. 51, 353-359.

Cline, H T (1991) Activity dependent plasticity in the visual system of frog and fish. Trends Neurosci. 14, 104-111.

Corwin, J.T. and Cotanche, D.A. (1988) Regeneration of sensory hair cells after acoustic trauma. Science 240, 1772-1774.

Dunckert, L.G.and Rubel, E.W. (1990) Ultrastructural observations on regenerating hair cells in the chick basilar papilla, Hear. Res. 48, 161-183

Eybalin, M. (1993) Neurotransmitters and neuromodulators of the mammalian cochlea. Physiol. Rev. 73, 309-373.

Forge, A., Li, L., Corwin, J.T. and Nevill, G. (1993) Ultrastructural evidence of hair cell regeneration in the mammalian inner hair. Science 259, 1616-1619

Hori, N., Doi, N., Miyahara, S., Shinoda, Y. and Carpenter, D.O. (1991) Appearance of NMDA receptors triggered by anoxia independent of voltage in vivo and in vitro. Exp. Neurol. 112, 304-311.

Kalb, R.G., Lidow, M.S., Halsted, M.J. and Hockfield, S. (1992) N-methyl-D-aspartate receptors are transiently expressed in the developing spinal cord ventral horn. Proc Natl Acad Sci USA 89, 8502-8506.

Komuro, H. and Rakic, P. (1993) Modulation of neuronal migration by NMDA receptors. Science 260, 95-97.

Lefebvre, P.P., Malgrange, B., Staecker, H., Moonen, G. and Van De Water, T.R. (1993) Retinoic acid stimulates regeneration of mammalian auditory hair cells. Science 260, 692-695

Mayat, E., Lerner-Natoli, M., Rondouin, G., Lebrun, F., Sassetti, I. and Récasens, M. (1994) Kainate-induced status epilepticus leads to a delayed increase in various specific glutamate metabotropic receptor responses in the hippocampus. Brain Res. 645, 186-200.

Puel, J.-L., Pujol, R., Ladrech, S. and Eybalin, M. (1991) a-amino-3-hydroxy-5-methyl-4-isoxazole propionic acid (AMPA) electrophysiological and neurotoxic effects in the guinea pig cochlea. Neuroscience 45, 63-72.

Puel, J.-L. and Pujol, R. (1993) Recent advances in cochlear neurobiology: Cochlear efferents and acoustic trauma, in Vallet, M. (ed): Noise and Man INRETS, Actes n° 34 , 136-45.

Puel, J.-L., Pujol, R., Tribillac, F., Ladrech, S. and Eybalin, M. (1994) Excitatory amino acid antagonists protect cochlear auditory neurons from excitotoxicity. J Comp Neurol 341, 241-256.

Pujol, R., Carlier, E. and Devigne, C. (1978) Different patterns of cochlear innervation during the development in the kittens. J Comp Neurol 117, 529-536.

Pujol, R., Carlier, E. and Devigne, C. (1979) Significance of presynaptic formations in the very early stages of cochlear synaptogenesis. Neurosci Lett 15, 995-1007.

Robertson, D. (1983). Functional significance of dendrite swelling after loud sounds in the guinea pig cochlea. Hear. Res. 9, 263-278.

Ryals, B.M. and Rubel, E.W. (1988) Hair cell regeneration after acoustic trauma in adult Coturnix quail. Science 240, 1774-1776.

Ryan, A.F., Brumm, D. and Kraft, M. (1991) Occurrence and distribution of non-NMDA glutamate receptor mRNAs in the cochlea. Neuroreport 2, 643-646.

Safieddine, S. and Eybalin, M. (1992) Co-expression of NMDA and AMPA/kainate receptors mRNAs in cochlear neurons. NeuroReport 3, 1145-1148.

Seren, M.S., Aldinio, C., Zanoni, R., Leon, A. and Nicoletti, F. (1989) Stimulation of inositol phospholipid hydrolysis by excitatory amino acids is enhanced in brain slices from vulnerable regions after transient global ischemia. J. Neurochem. 53, 1700-1705.

Spoendlin, H. (1971) Primary structural changes in the organ of Corti after acoustic overstimulation. Acta Otolaryngol 71, 166-176.

Spoendlin, H. (1975) Retrograde degeneration of the cochlear nerve. Acta Otolaryngol 79, 266-275.

Spoendlin, H. (1976) Anatomical changes following various noise exposures. In: Effects of Noise on Hearing, edited by D. Henderson, R.P. Hamernik, D.S. Dosanjh and J.H. Mills. New York: Raven Press, p. 69-89.

Warchol, M.E., Lambert, P.R., Goldstein, B.J., Forge, A. and Corwin, J.T. (1993) Regenerative proliferation in inner ear sensory epithelia from adult guinea pig and humans. Science 259, 1619-1622.

Weiler, I.J. and Greenough, W.T. (1993) Metabotropic glutamate receptors trigger postsynaptic protein synthesis. Proc Natl Acad Sci USA 90; 7168-7171.

Comment by E.F. Evans

We are very interested in your exciting findings in two psychophysical contexts:

a) Recovery of behavioural threshold in guinea pigs treated with kanamycin (Pratt and Evans 1988; Nicol et al. 1992) or gentamycin (Nicol et al., 1993).
In one case, we obtained dissociation between behavioural frequency selectivity and threshold in the sense that substantial recovery of threshold occurred *without* recovery of frequency selectivity (Nicol et al., 1993 and in prep.).

b) Asymptomatic discrete frequency threshold loss in young people exposed to amplified ("pop") music (West and Evans, 1990; and in prep.). Measurements of frequency selectivity or the frequency of the audiometrie notches after compensation for the notch attenuation suggest that the frequency selectivity is normal or above normal.

Both of these phenomena are most easily explained by damage (and recovery in the first case) - restricted to the inner hair cell afferents with damage to the outer hair cells in the first case only.

Pratt, S.R. and Evans, E.F. (1988) Recovery of behavioral threshold in a kanamycin treated guinea pig. Inner Ear Biology Meeting, Nijmegen. (See also Fig. 2 of Nicol et al., 1992).

Nicol, K.M.M., Hackney, C.M., Evans, E.F. and Pratt, S.R. (1992) Behavioral evidence of recovery of auditory function in guinea pigs following kanamycin administration. Hear. Res. 61, 111-131

Nicol, K.M.M., Hackey, C.M., Furness, D.N. and Evans, E.F. (1993) Dissociation between recovery of behaviourally-determined threshold and frequency selectivity following gentamycin administration. British J. Audiol. 27, 359-360.

West, P.D.B. and Evans, E.F. (1990) Early detection of hearing damage in young listeners resulting from exposure to amplified music. British J. Audiol. 24, 89-103.

West, P.D.B. and Evans, E.F. (in prep.) Audiometric notches: their effects on frequency resolution (with and without compensation) and their possible pathological nature.

Reply

This is an interesting point since we know that ototoxic insult induced a dendritic disruption below the IHC (Lenoir, unpublished data). We also saw the same kind of dissociation between CAP threshold and forward masking tuning curves one month after amikacine (300-500 mg/ kg during 5 days) treatment (Puel et al., Hearing Res., 1987). So the neural regeneration reported herein could explain the substantial threshold recovery you observed, while some irreversible outer hair cell damage may be responsible for the absence of frequency selectivity recovery.

Concerning the second point, the absence of frequency selectivity changes attest to the fact that outer hair cells are not damaged.

Regeneration of sensory and supporting cells: Relationship to physiological and anatomical measures

R.J. Salvi, L. Chen, M. Shero, E. Hashino and S.S. Saunders

Hearing Research Lab, Dept. Communicative Disorders & Sciences, 215 Parker Hall, SUNY University at Buffalo, Buffalo, NY 14214, USA

Introduction

Acoustic overstimulation primarily destroys the short hair cells along the abneural edge of the papilla (Saunders and Tilney, 1982; Cotanche et al., 1987). Although most of the hair cells can regenerate after acoustic overstimulation (Cotanche, 1987a; Corwin and Cotanche, 1988; Ryals and Rubel, 1988; Rubel, 1992; Hashino and Salvi, 1993; Henry et al., 1988), it is not clear if this leads to the complete recovery of function because of damage to other cochlear structures. Even when most of the hair cells regenerate, the cochlear ganglion neurons may decrease in number over a period of several months following the exposure (Ryals et al. 1989). Acoustic trauma also destroys the tectorial membrane, but only the lower honeycomb layer regenerates, not the upper fibrous layer (Cotanche, 1987b; Raphael, 1991). In addition, hair cells which survive the traumatizing exposure sometimes have abnormal stereocilia and enlarged apical surfaces which could impair their function (Cotanche, 1987a). Acoustic trauma also damages the tegmentum vasculosum which in turn could affect endolymphatic potential (Ryals et al., 1993). These residual anatomical deficits could conceivably alter the mechanical response of the cochlear partition or the functional characteristics of the hair cells and cochlear ganglion neurons resulting in permanent changes in hearing. The purpose of the present series of investigations was to examine the recovery of function in chickens following acoustic overstimulation using several different physiological and behavioral measures.

2 Methods

Chickens (>12 week of age) were exposed to a 525 Hz pure tone at a sound pressure level of 120 dB for 48 h. This exposure has been shown to produce a crescent shaped patch of hair cell damage along the abneural edge of the papilla, but hair cell counts within the damaged region generally recover to normal levels a few weeks after the exposure (Cotanche et al., 1987). Animals were allowed to recover for various amounts of time after the exposure depending on the experiment.

Behavioral measurements were obtained from one group of animals using a positive reinforcement technique (Saunders et al., 1993). Pure tone (500 ms duration, 10 ms rise/fall cosine ramp) audiograms were obtained from each animal at regular intervals following the exposure. In addition, threshold was measured as a function of stimulus duration at various times following the exposure.

Single unit recordings were obtained from cochlear ganglion neurons of anesthetized (urethane) chickens using techniques similar to those described previously (Salvi et al., 1992; in press). Glass micropipettes were used to record from cochlear ganglion neurons. Measurements were obtained from a group of normal control animals as well as animals that had been exposed to the 525 Hz traumatizing tone and allowed to recover for 0-1, 5, 14 or 28 days.

Prior to the start of the physiological experiments, distortion product otoacoustic emissions (DPOAE) were measured from each animal. DPOAE input/output functions were measured with the F2/F1 ratio set at 1.2. The levels of the primary tones (L1 and L2) were equal. Measurements were made over a range of F1 frequencies ranging from 500 Hz to 4000 Hz.

The cochleas of some of normal and acoustically traumatized animals were removed and evaluated by fluorescence microscopy. Animals were given an overdose of sodium pentobarbital (200 mg/kg) and their cochleas removed and perfused with 3% paraformaldehyde. Cochleas were incubated in Tris-buffered saline (TBS) containing 3% BSA, followed by rhodamine-labeled phalloidin and FITC-labled concanavalin A in TBS-BSA. Specimens were examined with either a rhodamine or FITC filter set.

3 Results

3.1 Behavioral Measures

Figure 1 (left) shows the average threshold shift measured behaviorally from three chickens immediately after the exposure. The average threshold shift ranged from approximately 30 to 45 dB over the range of hearing. Hearing thresholds recovered relatively quickly after the exposure and thresholds were essentially normal 10-15 days after the exposure. The thresholds of all of the animals completely recovered and there was no permanent hearing loss at any frequency (Figure 1, left).

Temporal integration refers to the general improvement in hearing performance that occurs as stimulus duration increases. In normal hearing chickens, pure tone thresholds improved by approximately 10-15 dB as stimulus duration increases from 16 ms to 512 ms (Saunders and Salvi, 1993). An interesting question to ask is, what happens to temporal integration when the hair cells are damaged and after they regenerate? In order to answer this question, threshold-duration functions were measured at several different frequencies before and after the traumatizing exposure. Figure 1 (right) shows the normalized threshold-duration functions measured at 1000 Hz two days after the exposure when the thresholds were significantly elevated and 17 days after the exposure when thresholds were normal. Each threshold was normalized to the threshold measured at 512 ms at a particular post-exposure time. The thresholds were normalized in order to eliminate the overall differences in threshold and to emphasize the differences in temporal integration. Temporal integration was greatly depressed two days after the exposure when

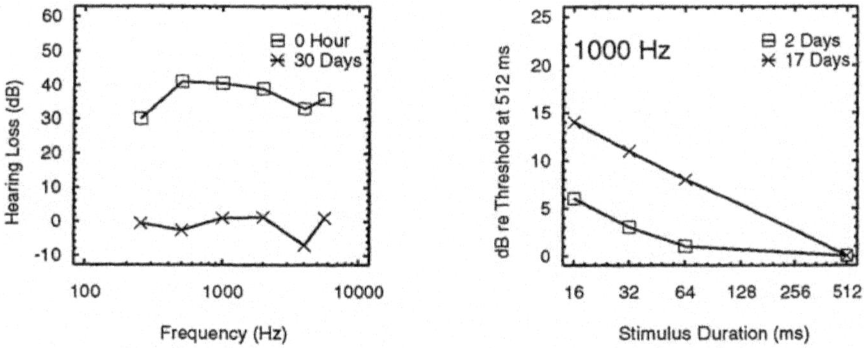

Figure 1. (left) Mean threshold shift immediately after the traumatizing exposure (open square) and approximately 30 days post-exposure (X). (right) Threshold-duration function at 1000 Hz measured two days post-exposure (X) and 17 days post-exposure after threshold had recovered. All thresholds in a given measurement period have been normalized to the threshold measured at 512 ms.

thresholds were elevated significantly. Threshold decreased by less than 6 dB for stimulus durations between 16 and 64 ms, but little improvement was observed at longer durations. However, after 17 days of recovery, hearing was within normal limits and threshold improved approximately 14 dB when stimulus duration was increased from 16 ms to 512 ms. This corresponds to a slope of approximately 3 dB per doubling of stimulus duration which is typical of normal hearing chickens (Saunders and Salvi, 1993).

3.2 Response of Cochlear Ganglion Neurons

Figure 2 (left) shows the typical frequency-threshold tuning curve and the two-tone rate suppression (TTRS) boundaries measured from a cochlear ganglion neuron in a normal chicken. The tuning curves from normal chickens are extremely sharply tuned, relatively symmetrical around the characteristic frequency (CF) and show little evidence of a low-frequency tail.

Most cochlear ganglion neurons show evidence of TTRS. The lower boundaries of the TTRS contours were measured by presenting a continuous tone 20 dB above the threshold at CF. A computer automated threshold tracking procedure was used to determine the frequency-threshold combinations of the suppressor tone (50 ms on/50 ms off) which produced a 1 spike decrease during the two-tone interval (50 ms) compared to the single tone interval when only the continuous tone was on. The lower boundary of the two-tone suppression contours flanked the high and low sides of the tuning curve. The vertical lines at the upper and lower ends of the TTRS boundaries are artifacts of the computer tracking algorithm. Note that the slope of the TTRS boundaries are relatively steep and that the threshold for suppression was generally within 5-15 dB of the threshold at CF.

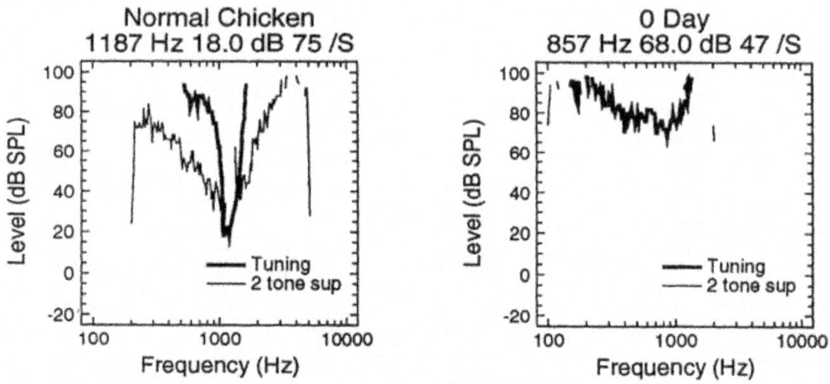

Figure 2. (left) Frequency threshold tuning curve (thick line) and lower boundary of the TTRS contour (thin line) from a normal cochlear ganglion neuron. (right) Tuning curve (thick line) and TTRS contour (thin line) from a cochlear ganglion neuron measured immediately after the exposure.

The effects of the traumatizing exposure are illustrated in Figure 2 (right) which shows the tuning curve from a typical neuron measured a few hours after the traumatizing exposure. The thresholds of the units evaluated at this time were elevated approximately 40-60 dB. Instead of having a narrowly-tuned and relatively symmetrical V-shape, the tuning curves measured at this time were extremely broad, U-shaped and asymmetrical due to a shallow, low-frequency tail. TTRS boundaries were absent from most of the neurons at this time as shown. However, if the TTRS boundaries were present, the slopes of the suppression contours were extremely shallow.

Figure 3 (left) shows a representative tuning curve and the TTRS boundaries obtained 5 days post-exposure. The thresholds for most units were still elevated approximately 20-30 dB at this time. The tuning curves were generally more sharply tuned than those measured immediately after the exposure; however, the tuning curves were generally asymmetrical due to the presence of a broad low-frequency tail below CF. In many cases, the low frequency tail contained a sharply tuned, low-threshold notch below the tip of the tuning curve. This resulted in a tuning curve with a distinct W-shape. In some cases, the threshold near the low-frequency notch was actually lower than the threshold in the tip located near the high frequency cutoff of the tuning curve. Compared to normal units, the thresholds in the tail of the tuning curve were clearly hypersensitive.

TTRS boundaries could be measured in some units at 5 days post-exposure, but the slopes of the TTRS boundaries were generally shallower than those observed in normal animals (Figure 3, left). The threshold of the TTRS boundary was frequently elevated relative to the threshold of the tuning curve tip and the separation between the TTRS boundary and the CF of the unit was abnormally large.

By 28 days post-exposure, the thresholds of most neurons were essentially normal and the tuning curves had regained their sharp tuning and relatively symmetrical shape (Figure 3, right). However, some units showed remnants of a low-frequency tail. In addition, TTRS was present in most neurons and the thresholds and slopes of the TTRS boundaries were similar to those observed in normal animals.

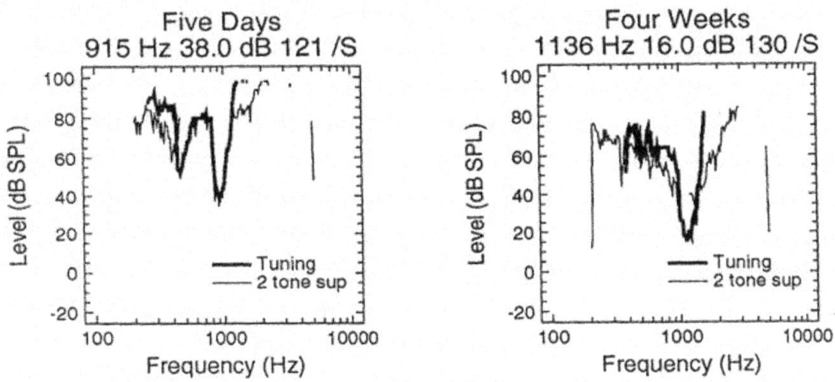

Figure 3. (left) Frequency threshold tuning curve (thick line) and lower boundary of the TTRS contour (thin line) from a cochlear ganglion neuron obtained 5 days post-exposure. (right) Tuning curve (thick line) and TTRS contour (thin line) from a cochlear ganglion neuron obtained 28 days post-exposure.

3.3 DPOAE

DPOAE, which are extremely sensitive to cochlear pathology (Norton and Rubel, 1990; Rubel, 1992), were used to assess the functional integrity of the ears after the traumatizing exposure. DPOAE were measured in a group of normal animals and in animals allowed to recover for 0-1, 5, 14 and 28 days following the exposure. DPOAE input/output functions were shifted to the right approximately 20-25 dB at all frequencies immediately after the exposure (data not shown), but the slopes of the functions were steeper than normal so that there was little reduction in amplitude at high stimulus levels. DPOAE input/output functions showed varying amounts of recovery depending on the test frequency and its relationship to the exposure frequency. Figure 4 (left) shows the DPOAE input/output function measured with F1 at 500 Hz and F2 at 598 Hz, i.e. frequencies near the exposure frequency. The solid line shows the mean DPOAE from normal control animals (N=8) and the dashed line shows the DPOAE from exposed animals allowed to recover for 28 days (N=7). The post-exposure DPOAE input/output function was shifted to the right approximately 10-12 dB, below 75 dB SPL, but the

DPOAE amplitude at 80 dB was normal due to the plateau in the normal input/output function. The input/output functions measured slightly above the exposure frequency (Figure 4, right) were also shifted to the right after the exposure, but to a lesser extent than that seen near the exposure frequency. DPOAE input/output functions measured with F1 at 1600 Hz or higher were essentially normal after 28 days of recovery (data not shown).

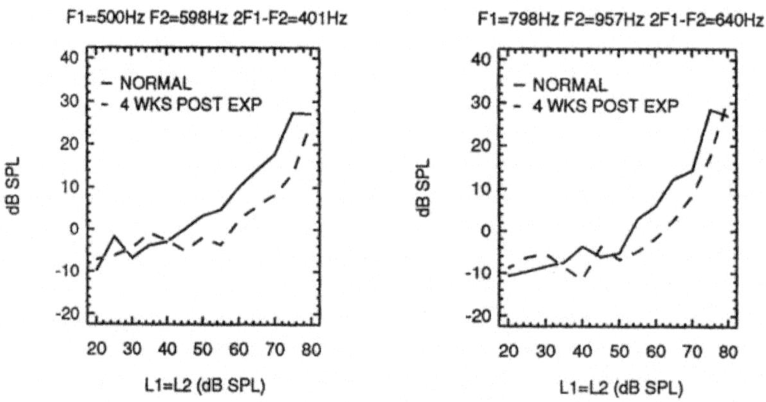

Figure 4. Mean DPOAE input/output functions obtained from normal control animals (N=8, solid line) and from sound exposed chickens that were allowed to recover for 28 days (N=7, dashed line); (left) F1=500 Hz; (right) F1=798 Hz.

3.4 Hair Cells and Tectorial Membrane

The 525 Hz traumatizing stimulus produced a crescent shape patch of hair cell damage along the abneural edge of the basilar papilla where the short hair cells are located. In addition, a crescent shaped patch of the tectorial membrane was destroyed in the same region, but over a section of the cochlea that greatly exceeded the region of hair cell loss. By using a double-labeling technique, it was possible to characterize the extent of damage to both structures in the same ear. The top panel of Figure 5 shows the typical pattern of hair cell damage observed 0-1 day post-exposure. The main region of hair cell loss is located along the abneural edge of the basilar papilla and extends from approximately 30% to 45% of the distance from the apex of the cochlea which corresponds to frequencies between 350 Hz and 700 Hz respectively (Manley et al., 1987). The bottom panel of Figure 5 shows the corresponding pattern of damage to the tectorial membrane. Both the upper fibrous layer and lower honeycomb layer of the tectorial membrane were destroyed along the abneural edge of the papilla. Damage to the tectorial membrane extended from approximately 25% to 65% of the distance from the apex which corresponds to frequencies between 200 Hz and 1500 Hz respectively. In the region of greatest damage, the tectorial membrane was missing across roughly 60-70% of the width of the papilla.

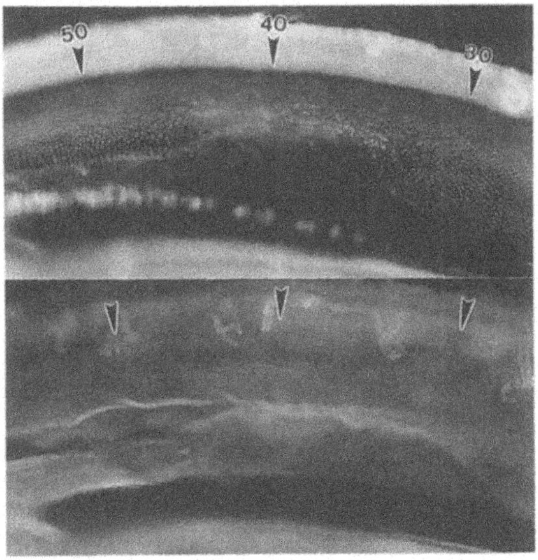

Figure 5. Surface preparation of chicken basilar papilla 1 day post-exposure. Percent distance from apex indicated by arrowheads. Top: Specimen stained with rhodamine-labeled phalloidin which binds to actin in hair cell stereocilia. Bottom: Specimen stained with FITC labeled concanavalin A which labels the tectorial membrane.

After 28 days of recovery, many of the cochleas showed little evidence of hair cell loss as illustrated by the photomicrograph in Figure 6 (top). Although there was a normal compliment of hair cells, the upper fibrous layer of the tectorial membrane (Figure 6, bottom) was absent along the abneural edge of the papilla from approximately 25% to 65% of the distance from the apex (200 Hz-1500 Hz). The lower honeycomb layer of the tectorial membrane completely covered the underlying hair cells and there was no obvious discontinuity between the original honeycomb layer and the newly regenerated segment.

In a few cases, distinct patches of missing hair cells were observed near the 500 Hz region of the cochlea 28 days after the exposure (Figure 7, top). In addition, the upper fibrous layer and lower honeycomb layer of the tectorial membrane failed to regenerate in the region of hair cell loss (Figure 7, bottom); however, the lower honeycomb layer was present in surrounding regions where the hair cells were present. These results suggest that the hair cells and tectorial membrane may not regenerate if the supporting cells, which secrete the tectorial membrane, are destroyed by the exposure.

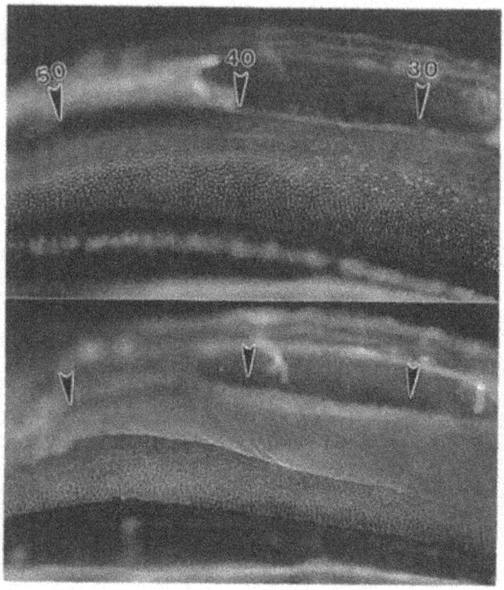

Figure 6. Surface preparation of chicken basilar papilla obtained 28 days post-exposure. Percent distance from apex indicated by arrowheads. Top: Specimen stained with rhodamine-labeled phalloidin which binds to actin in hair cell stereocilia. Bottom: Specimen stained with FITC labeled concanavalin A which labels the tectorial membrane.

4 Discussion

The traumatizing stimulus used in this study produced a crescent shaped patch of missing hair cells along the abneural edge of the papilla, but by 28 days post-exposure most of the cochleas exhibited little or no hair cell loss suggesting that supporting cells in this region had proliferated and differentiated into hair cells to replace those that had been destroyed by the exposure. The exposure also caused extensive damage to the tectorial membrane along the abneural edge of the papilla over a segment of the cochlea that greatly exceeded the region of hair cell loss. The lower honeycomb layer of the tectorial membrane, which is presumably secreted by the supporting cells (Cotanche, 1987b), regenerated in concert with the hair cells and eventually fused with the remainder of the tectorial membrane; however, the upper fibrous layer failed to regenerate and was absent over a considerable length of the cochlea.

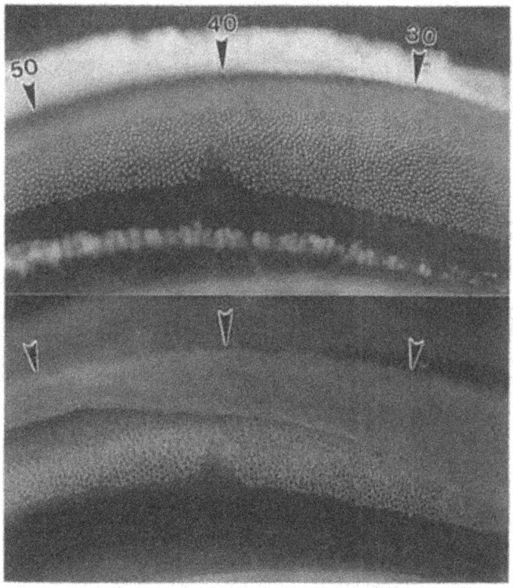

Figure 7. Surface preparation of chicken basilar papilla obtained 28 days post-exposure. Percent distance from apex indicated by arrowheads. Top: Specimen stained with rhodamine-labeled phalloidin which binds to actin in hair cell stereocilia. Bottom: Specimen stained with FITC labeled concanavalin A which labels the tectorial membrane. Note inverted V-shaped patch of missing hair cells and missing honeycomb layer of tectorial membrane approximately 40% of the distance from the apex.

The regeneration of the hair cells and lower honeycomb layer of the tectorial membrane was associated with a rapid and complete recovery of hearing thresholds and temporal integration. Thus, the absence of the upper fibrous layer of the tectorial membrane does not appear to have any effect on threshold or temporal integration. Whether or not other measures of auditory performance fully recover after such exposures is not yet known.

Unlike mammalian tuning curves which have a broad low-frequency tail, avian tuning curves are normally V-shaped, symmetrical and extremely sharply tuned (Salvi et al., 1993). Immediately after the exposure, the tuning curves became extremely broad, asymmetrical and U-shaped with a shallow low-frequency tail, much like those seen in mammals following acoustic overstimulation (Salvi et al., 1983). As the hearing loss began to subside, many W-shaped tuning curves were observed with one tip located near the high frequency edge of the tuning curve and another located in the low-frequency tail of the tuning curve. In many cases, the threshold in the tail of the tuning curve was lower (hypersensitive) than that observed in normal units with the same CF. In mammals, W-shaped tuning curves with hyposensitive tips and hypersensitive tails have been observed when only the outer hair cells (OHC) are damaged (Liberman et al., 1986). By contrast, when OHCs are intact and only the inner hair cells (IHC) are damaged, threshold is elevated throughout the tuning curve. Since hair cell loss was confined to the abneural edge of the papilla, one might speculate that short hair cells in the avian ear serve a function similar to that of mammalian OHCs, i.e., they increase the sensitivity near the tip of the tuning curve and decrease sensitivity in the tail region. This line of reasoning is intriguing given the similarity between the afferent and efferent innervation patterns in avian and mammalian cochleas (von During, 1985).

By 28 days post-exposure, the threshold, tuning and two-tone suppression properties of cochlear ganglion neurons had recovered to normal levels consistent with the behavioral data. However, the DPOAE elicited by stimuli near the exposure frequency were still depressed at frequencies between 500 Hz and 1600 Hz. The deficits observed in the DPOAE could conceivably be related to the incomplete regeneration of the tectorial membrane. However, other factors, such as hair cell loss or damage to surviving hair cells, may contribute to the reduction of DPOAE. Since these residual histopathologies are confined to the short hair cell region, they may have little or no impact on the pattern of neural activity which originates from the tall hair cells, but they nevertheless could influence the DPOAE.

5 Acknowledgment

Research supported in part by NIH grant R01DC001685.

6 References

Cotanche, D.A. (1987a) Regeneration of hair cell stereocilliary bundles in the chick cochlea following severe acoustic trauma. Hear. Res. 30, 181-196.

Cotanche, D.A. (1987b) Regeneration of the tectorial membrane in the chick cochlea following severe acoustic trauma. Hear. Res. 30, 197-206.

Cotanche, D., Saunders, J.C. and Tilney, L.G. (1987) Hair cell damage produced by acoustic trauma in the chick cochlea. Hear. Res. 25, 267-286.

Corwin, J.T. and Cotanche, D.A. (1988). Regeneration of sensory hair cells after acoustic trauma. Sci. 240, 1772-1774.

Hashino, E., Tanaka, Y., Salvi, R.J. and Sokabe, M. (1992b) Hair cell regeneration in the adult budgerigar after kanamycin ototoxicity. Hear. Res. 59, 46-58.

Hashino, E. and Salvi, R.J. (1993) Changing spatial patterns of DNA replication in the noise damaged chick cochlea. J. Cell Sci. 105, 23-31.

Henry, W.J., Makaretz, M., Saunders, J.C., Schneider, M.E. and Vretakos, P. (1988). Hair cell loss and regeneration after exposure to intense sound in neonatal chicks. Otolaryngology Head Neck Surg., 98, 607-611.

Liberman, M.C., Dodds, L.W., and Learson, D.A. (1986). Structure-function correlation in noise-damaged ears: a light and electron microscopic study. In: R.J. Salvi, R.P. Hamernik, D. Henderson, V. Colletti (Eds.) Basic and Applied Aspects of Noise-Induced Hearing Loss, Plenum Press, New York, pp. 163-177.

Manley, G.A., Brix J., Kaiser, A. (1987) Developmental stability of the tonotopic organization of the chick's basilar papilla. Sci. 237, 655-666.

Norton, S.J. and Rubel, E.W. (1990) Active and passive ADP components in mammalian and avian ears. In: D. Geisler, P. Dallos, J. Matthews and M. Ruggero (Eds.) Mechanics and Biophysics of Hearing, Springer-Verlag, New York, pp. 219-226.

Raphael, Y. (1991) Pure-tone overstimulation protects surviving avian hair cells from acoustic trauma. Hear. Res. 53, 173-184.

Ryals, B.M. and Rubel, E. (1988) Hair cell regeneration after acoustic trauma in adult Coturnix Quail. Sci., 240, 1774-1776.

Ryals, B.M., Ten Eyck, B. and Westbrook, E.W. (1989) Ganglion cell loss continues during hair cell regeneration. Hear. Res. 43, 81-90.

Ryals, B.M., Stalford, M.D., Becker, D.G. and Lambert, P.R. (1993) Ultrastructural changes in the tegmentum vasculosum parallel changes in auditory function after acoustic trauma. Abstr. Assoc. Res. Otolaryngol. 171, 43.

Rubel, E.W. (1992) Regeneration of hair cells in the avian inner ear. In: A. Dancer, D. Henderson, R.J. Salvi, and R.P. Hamernik (Eds.), Effects of Noise on the Auditory System. Mosby Year Book, St. Louis, pp. 204-227.

Salvi, R., Henderson, D. and Hamernik, R.P. (1983) Physiological bases of sensorineural hearing loss. In: J.V. Tobias and E.D. Schubert (Eds.), Hearing Research and Theory, Vol. 2., Academic Press, New York, pp. 173-231.

Salvi, R.J., Saunders, S.S., Powers, N.L. and Boettcher, F.A. (1992) Discharge patterns of cochlear ganglion neurons in the chicken. J. Comp. Physiol. A 170, 227-241.

Salvi, R.J., Saunders, S.S., Hashino, E. and Chen, L. (in press). Discharge patterns of chicken cochlear ganglion neurons following kanamycin-induced hair cell loss and regeneration. J. Comp. Physiol. A.

Saunders, J.C. and Tilney, L.G. (1982) Species differences in susceptibility to noise induced hearing loss. In: Hamernik R.P., Henderson D., and Salvi, R.J. (Eds.) New Perspectives on Noise-Induced Hearing Loss, Raven Press, New York, pp. 229-248.

Saunders, S.S., and Salvi, R.J. (1993) Psychoacoustics of normal adult chickens: Thresholds and temporal integration. J. Acoust. Soc. Am. 94, 83-90.

von During, M., Andres, K.H. and Simon, K. (1985) The comparative anatomy of the basilar papillae in birds. Fortschr. Zool. 3, 681-685.

Comment by A. Brown

You found that DPOAE remained depressed while afferent function remained normal at some frequencies. In mammalian ears it has been suggested that the '"odd" behaviour of distortion (reaching a magnitude maximum for a particular frequency rather than for a particular stimulus frequency separation) could be due to filtering of the emission by the tectorial membrane at the site of generation. If the TM has a similar effect in the avian ear, then it is possible that DPOAE would be diminished in the ear canal when the TM fails to cover the sensory epithelium completely. But if the amount of TM coverage is adequate over a critical region of hair cells, then other measures of cochlear and afferent function could appear normal.

Reply

The traumatizing stimulus in our study primarily damaged the hair cells and tectorial membrane along the abneural edge of the basilar papilla; however, most of the afferent neurons contact the tall hair cells along the neural edge of the papilla, thus the "critical region" was not destroyed by the exposure. This may explain why the bahavioral and neurophysiological measures fully recovered. The upper fibrous layer of the tectorial membrane along the abneural edge of the papilla failed to regenerate after the exposure and its absence could affect the reverse transmission of the DPOAE from its site of generation, which some suggest may be in the transduction mechanism. It is conceivable that the absence of the upper fibrous layer of the tectorial membrane could alter its stiffness thereby altering its filtering properties.

Comment by G.A. Manley

I would like to point out that since the early work of Von Düring et al. (1985), much more detailed studies of the innervation of the avian papilla are available - for the chicken, see Fischer (1992).

The tuning curves you show strongly resemble those described by Jones and Jones (1994) from the cochlear ganglion of embryonic chickens. The sequence you demonstrate may thus recapitulate that seen during normal development.

Fischer, F.P. (1992) Quantitative analysis of the innervation of the chicken basilar papilla. Hear. Res. 73, 1-5

Jones, S.M. and Jones, T.A. (1994) Neural tuning characteristics of auditory primary afferents in the chicken embryo. Hear. Res., in press

Von Düring, M., Andres, K.H. and Simon, K. (1985) The comparative anatomy of the basilar papillae in birds. Fortschr. Zool. 30, 681-685

Reply

Fischer's work is obviously quite relevant to our study in chickens. The developmental changes in tuning noted by Jones and Jones fit in quite nicely with the changes in tuning that occur during the time period when the tectorial membrane and hair cells are regenerating following acoustic trauma; however, an important difference is the lack of regeneration in the upper fibrous layer of the tectorial membrane.

Some effects of early hearing loss on auditory perception

David R. Moore

University Laboratory of Physiology
Parks Road, Oxford OX1 3PT

1 Introduction

Experimentally induced sensorineural and conductive hearing loss has been found to produce a variety of anatomical and physiological changes in the central auditory system of several birds and mammals (for reviews see Knudsen, 1988; Moore, 1992; Rubel et al., 1990). However, with the exception of the barn owl (Knudsen, 1988), little is known about the long term consequences of early hearing loss for auditory function. My colleagues and I have been trying to redress this deficiency using two broad approaches. The first is to examine the effects of experimental hearing loss on auditory perception in the ferret. The second is to examine the effects of clinical hearing loss, particularly otitis media with effusion (OME), on the development of human auditory perception. Our long term goal is to understand the biological bases of developmental hearing disorders by comparing these behavioural data with physiological and anatomical data gathered from further studies of experimentally or clinically hearing impaired subjects. In this paper I present the results of our initial attempts to study hearing loss behaviourally and I point to future directions in our work designed to link behavioural and biological research.

2 Hearing in ferrets

2.1 Audiograms

2.1.1 Normals

The ferret is an altricial carnivore with a mature auditory system resembling that of the cat (Moore, 1991). Using standard, positive conditioning procedures, Kelly and his colleagues (Kelly et al., 1986) have shown that the ferret has well developed low frequency hearing, maximum sensitivity in the frequency range 1-10kHz, and an upper frequency limit of about 35kHz. We have used a training and testing procedure identical to that of Kelly. Ferrets were fed dry food and had to work in the test chamber to receive their water. On any trial, the animal was trained to enter a start box and lick a spout. This triggered the presentation of a light and, on 50% of trials, a tone burst (250 or 500ms) from transducers 0.75m in front of the start spout. If the ferret heard a tone it moved to the right to receive further water or, if no tone sounded, the ferret was trained to move to the left. Psychometric functions were obtained using a descending method of limits. The mean thresholds of 4 normal, binaurally-hearing ferrets (Fig. 1) were similar to those reported by Kelly. Note that the interanimal variability was quite large, particularly at the higher frequencies. Further experiments, not shown in Fig. 1, have indicated that this variability is robust and that individual animals really do have different thresholds when tested in this task.

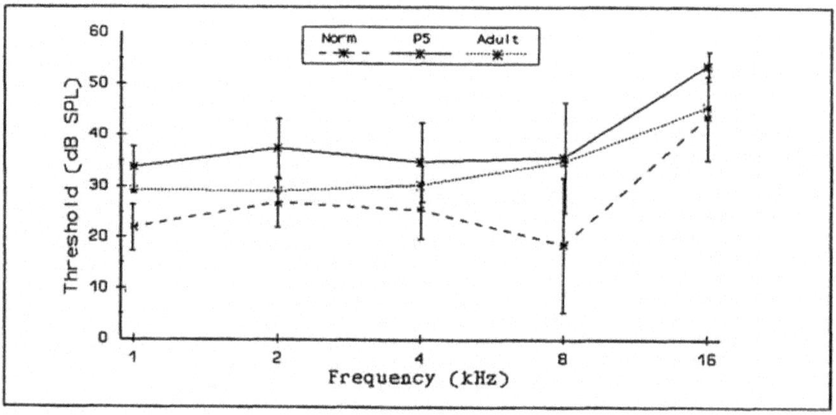

Figure 1. Ferret audiograms. Data points show the mean threshold (±s.d.) for 4 animals in each of the adult, P5 cochlear removal and adult cochlear removal groups.

2.1.2 Effects of cochlear removal

Unilateral cochlear removal produces exuberant neural connections deriving from the cochlear nucleus (CN) on the side of the intact ear (see Moore, 1994) and an increase in the excitatory influence of that ear on single neuron responses in the ipsilateral inferior colliculus (IC; see Moore et al., 1993). These anatomical and physiological effects suggested to us that functional sensitivity in the intact ear might also be enhanced. We have examined the audiograms of 4 ferrets who had one cochlea surgically removed at postnatal day (P)5 and 4 ferrets who had one cochlea removed when they were mature. All animals recovered from surgery for several weeks and, in the case of the neonatally lesioned animals, grew to adulthood before testing. The audiogram test was identical to that used for the normal animals. The results (Fig. 1) showed that, contrary to expectation, neither group of lesioned animals had improved sensitivity . Indeed, there was some indication of poorer sensitivity and in a separate experiment (Hine, 1993), not shown in Fig. 1, we have found that individual adult animals tested before and after unilateral cochlear lesions consistently show a reduction in sensitivity after the lesion.

2.2 Sound localization

2.2.1 Normals

Kavanagh and Kelly (1987, 1992) have shown that, for noise stimuli, ferrets have minimum audible angles (MAAs) in the frontal, mid-sagittal plane (midline) of between 5-20° and MAAs in the lateral field that are typically between 15-30°. Using similar test procedures, we have begun to study minimum audible angles about the midline and in the lateral field (King et al., 1993). Broad band noise stimuli were digitally generated and filtered to compensate for spectral variations between the loudspeakers. The ferrets were trained to lick a water spout that was located on the same side as the speaker from which a sound had been delivered. Minimum audible angles were calculated around the midline using a descending method of limits. The results (Fig. 2) show that, at long stimulus durations (100 or 500ms), performance was high at wide speaker separations. For two of three animals, performance remained above chance levels down to 10°, the minimum separation used. For shorter duration stimuli (40ms), performance was more erratic, but remained above chance level down to 10°. In the lateral field (Fig. 2), MAAs were typically between 15-30°, as previously shown by Kavanagh and Kelly.

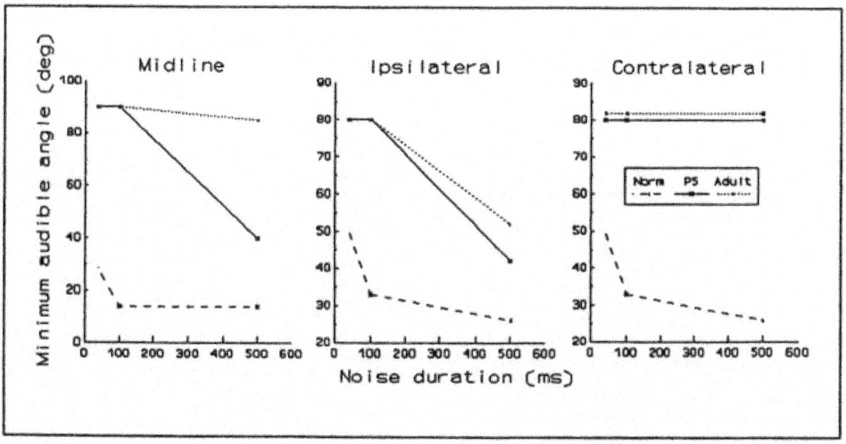

Figure 2. Ferret minimum audible angles. Data points show the mean, 75% levels for 2-4 animals in each group. Note that, for the lateral tasks, the maximum speaker separation was 80°.

2.2.2 Effects of cochlear removal

In the midline task, following either P5 or adult unilateral cochlear removal, ferrets continued to perform above chance level with a 500ms stimulus (Fig. 2). Note that, as for the audiograms (Fig. 1), there was considerable inter-animal variability. One P5 ablated ferret performed above chance level at 10°. However, performance was generally poorer in the one-eared than in the two-eared ferrets and animals lesioned at P5 performed better than ferrets lesioned as adults. For shorter duration stimuli (40 or 100ms), none of the one-eared animals performed above chance level at any speaker separation. Preliminary results from lateral field stimulation (Fig. 2) suggest that one-eared ferrets perform better in the hemifield ipsilateral to their intact ear than in the contralateral field. In both cases their performance was poorer than that of two-eared animals. In the lateral field on the side of the intact ear (ipsilateral), both groups of one-eared ferrets performed normally when a 500ms stimulus was used, but at chance levels for the two shorter duration stimuli. In the contralateral field, only the neonatally lesioned ferrets performed at better than chance levels and only for the 500ms stimulus.

2.3 Binaural unmasking

2.3.1 Normals

We have developed a novel technique for assessing binaural hearing in animals (Hine et al., 1994). Ferrets were trained to detect a 500Hz tone embedded in a narrow-band noise centred at 500Hz. The tone and noise were delivered from a single source positioned 90° to the animal's right. A second noise source was positioned either directly above the tone source ("control" condition), or 90^{0} to the animal's left ("bilateral" condition). Tone thresholds were determined with the method of limits, as for the audiogram test described above. The threshold for detection of the tone (Fig. 3) was about 10dB lower in the bilateral than in the control condition. The noise levels measured at the position of the animal's head were the same (71 dB SPL) in each case. Thus, unmasking (of the tone by the noise) was achieved through a spatial separation of the perceived locus of the tone and the noise.

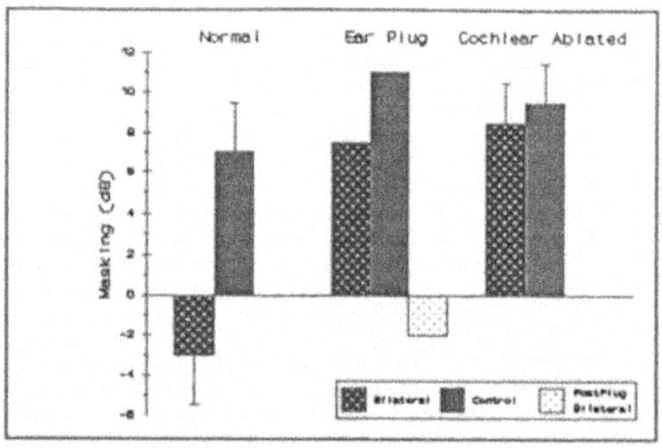

Figure 3: Masking (re. unilateral presentation) provided by control and bilateral noise positions. Each bar is the mean (± s.d.) of 2-4 animals. Signal was presented on side of normal ear.

2.3.2 Effects of hearing loss

To prove that the unmasking shown in Fig. 3 was due to binaural interaction we tested two groups of ferrets that had unilateral hearing impairments. In one case, the impairment was a unilateral cochlear removal. In the other case it was a unilateral conductive loss induced by the insertion of a plug in one ear. In both cases the hearing loss was begun when the animals were adult and was long-lasting. The advantage gained in normal animals by spatial separation of the noise sources was lost in these animals with only a single, normally-hearing ear on the side of the control stimulus presentation (Fig. 3). These results show that the unmasking seen in normal animals in the bilateral condition was due to binaural processing.

2.4 Discussion and future directions

Perhaps unsurprisingly, one-eared animals performed more poorly on all tasks than did animals with two, normally functioning ears. In the audiogram task, both groups of lesioned ferrets were slightly less sensitive than normal. Although this finding is consistent with previous reports of poor sensitivity following unilateral deafening (eg. Masterton et al., 1992), the insensitivity of the neonatally deafened group is in direct contrast to our expectations based on anatomical and physiological data. The failure to find improved sensitivity in this group may be due to a variety of factors. In terms of neural connections, the increased density of afferents to the ipsilateral IC (Moore, 1994) and to the SOC on both sides of the brain (Russell and Moore, 1994) may serve to distort the acoustic signal in some way, or may lead to an increase in both the signal and the noise deriving from the intact ear, with no gain in signal discrimination. Physiologically, the improvement in threshold in the ipsilateral IC and auditory cortex to stimulation of the intact ear may still not improve thresholds beyond those normally recorded in brain structures contralateral to the intact ear. Indeed, recordings from the contralateral IC (McAlpine, 1994) suggest that neural thresholds in that structure are unaffected by neonatal cochlear removal. We have recently measured sensitivity in individual ferrets before and after reversible short-term unilateral hearing loss produced by ear plugging. The results show a decrement in sensitivity in line with that found in the adult lesioned animals.

The detrimental effect of unilateral deafening on tasks based on or requiring binaural processing may seem unexceptional. We believe, however, that there are several points of interest in these studies. The fact that animals with one ear can be trained to localize sounds at all is intriguing, but the suggestion that neonatally deafened animals perform better than animals deafened as adults raises many questions. While it is well-known, for example, that practice produces improved performance, these results suggest that early experience may be particularly beneficial, even in a basic sensory task. At a mechanistic level, the rewiring of the brain following early deafness, shown above to lead to little change in sensitivity, accompanied better sound localization, suggesting that the processes underlying spectrum-based processing may be enhanced by the exuberant afferents of the intact CN. We intend to complete the localization study by running further animals and then go on to see how unilateral conductive loss affects spatial hearing in the ferret. These same animals will also be tested in the binaural unmasking task. We have shown that adult humans wearing unilateral earplugs have poorer than normal unmasking and that several days of experience do nothing to improve this performance (Moore, 1993). We have now begun to ask how unilateral earplugging for longer periods and during the developmental period affects unmasking by using the techniques and control data described here to perform experiments that would be ethically impossible in human subjects.

3 Development and plasticity of human binaural hearing

3.1 Long term effects of otitis media

Based on the known plasticity of the auditory system in experimental animals we hypothesized that the human auditory system might also undergo long term or permanent changes following hearing loss in infancy. Otitis media with effusion (OME), also known as "glue ear", is an accumulation of fluid in the middle ear cavity, producing a flat, 20-40dB fluctuating hearing loss. OME is extremely prevalent in early childhood and its treatment by the insertion of ventilation tubes through the tympanic membrane is the most common reason for childhood surgery in the western world. Although the disease is typically bilateral, it is usually asymmetric to a greater or lesser extent. Thus, both the sensitivity and the binaural processing of the child are compromised during OME episodes.

Our first, retrospective study (Moore et al., 1991) compared binaural unmasking in a group of 6-10 year old children who had multiple recorded episodes of OME before 5 years of age with an age-matched sample of children who had no history of hearing problems. We used standard psychoacoustic methods to measure the amount of unmasking of a 500Hz tone in a narrow band noise centred at 500Hz was produced by inverting the phase, through headphones, of the tone in one ear. The results (Fig. 4)

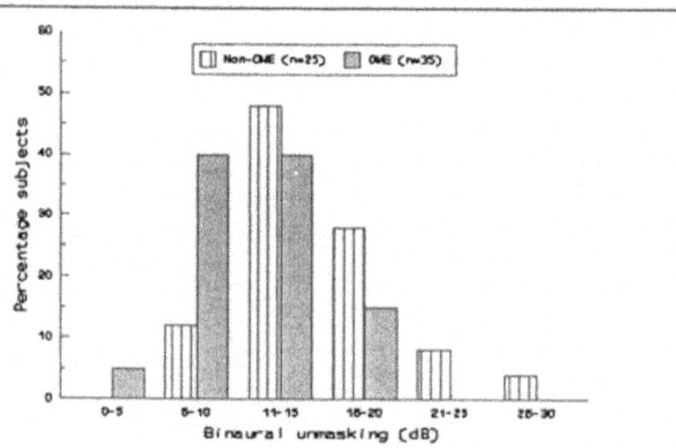

Figure 4. Binaural unmasking in children with and without a history of OME. Histogram bars show the percentage of subjects who had masking level differences in the indicated

range.

showed that, although the performance range of the two groups of children overlapped, the mean unmasking in the OME group (11.5dB) was significantly ($p<0.0005$) lower than the mean unmasking in the non-OME group (15.6dB). Both groups of children had normal audiograms at the time of testing. Given the likelihood that the non-OME group contained children who had, in fact, had the disease on some occasion(s), the results of this study suggest that an early imbalance of binaural input produces long-lasting changes in binaural hearing.

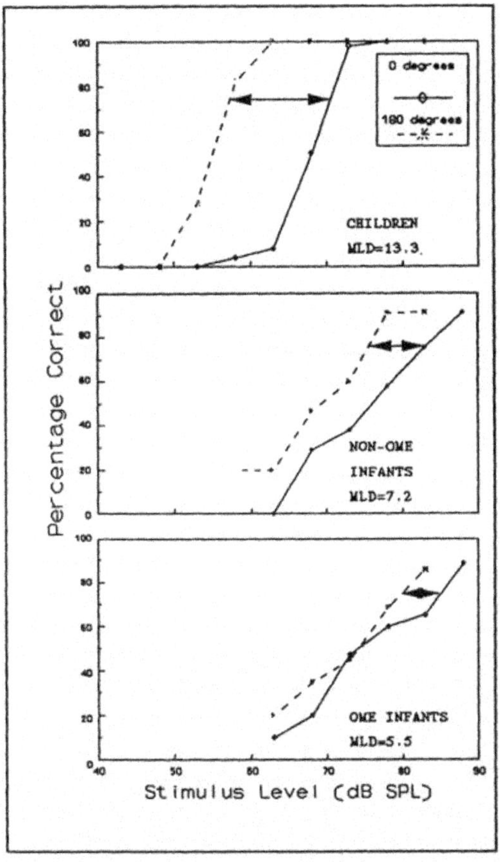

Figure 5. Binaural unmasking in children (7-12 y.o., n=10) and 7 m.o. infants with (n=8) and without (n=9) OME. Dichotic presentation was in-phase (0°) or 180° out of phase.

3.2 Development of binaural hearing

OME is prevalent by 6 months of age (Hogan et al., 1994). Although several studies have shown that binaural hearing is immature at this age, the influence of OME on binaural hearing has not previously been studied. Using headphone delivery of the same tone-in-noise stimuli described above, we have examined (Hutchings et al., 1992) the relationship between the development of binaural unmasking and the occurrence of OME. In these studies, 7-10 month old infants were trained to turn their heads towards a mechanical toy when they heard the tone. The group data (Fig. 5) showed that normally-hearing infants had higher masked thresholds, more irregular psychometric functions, and smaller levels of binaural unmasking than a control group of older children. For the infants who had at least unilateral OME at the time of testing, and a prior history of the disease, the group data were similar to the normally-hearing infants. Thus, during the first year of life when binaural unmasking is small, OME does not appear to compromise this aspect of binaural hearing.

3.3 Prospective analysis of OME

We are now two years into an ambitious project that aims to document fully the OME history of a sample (n=108) of infants over the first five years of life (Hogan et al., 1994). Infants are tested at monthly intervals using otoscopy and tympanometry. At selected ages (7 and 18 months thus far, with a further test planned at 30 months), we have assessed binaural unmasking using a free-field presentation procedure (Schneider et al., 1989) that does not depend on the infants wearing headphones. Some of the preliminary results of this study are shown in Fig. 6. At least 80% of our infants have had at least one episode of OME by the age of 2 years. Binaural unmasking was apparent at both test ages, but we do not yet have a clear picture of either the normal development of unmasking or the effects of OME. Our intention is to test these infants twice more on the free-field unmasking task then, when they are old enough to perform conventional psychoacoustics, give them a wide ranging series of tests including binaural and directional tasks.

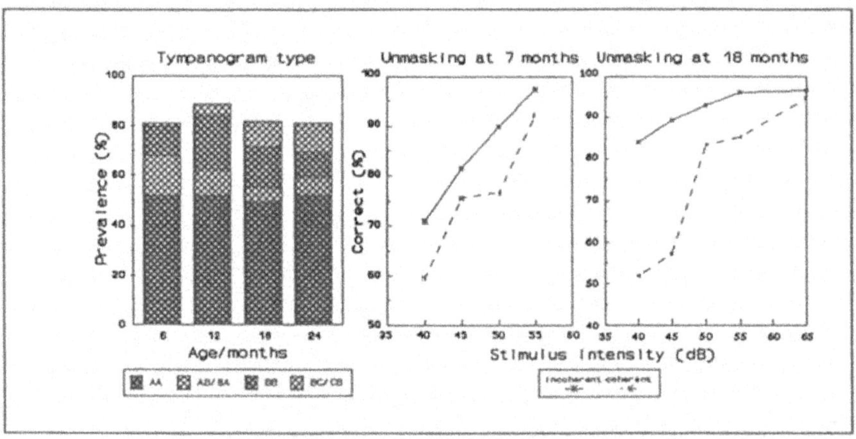

Figure 6: Incidence of normal (AA) and abnormal tympanograms at 6 month intervals and group psychometric functions for binaural unmasking at 7 (n=11) and 18 (n=18) months.

3.4 Discussion and future directions

The quantitative measurement of sensory function in human infants is fraught with methodological and interpretational problems. We have addressed these problems in several ways. In some studies we have avoided the problems of testing young infants behaviourally by examining only objective measures of auditory function (eg. tympanometry) or by performing retrospective analyses. The latter approach is clearly unsatisfactory, but the quality of psychophysical data that we and others have obtained from relatively young children (4-5 years) encourages us to combine these two approaches in our future work. Another feature of our recent work has been to use free-field stimulation techniques. Although light insert earphones have been successfully used by others to test young infants, our experience has been that free-field testing yields an almost complete cooperation rate. Finally, the work we have done with both human infants and ferrets has generated a number of questions that can be addressed by using experimental conductive hearing loss in adult humans. For example, we have already performed studies of the effects of earplugging on binaural unmasking (Moore, 1993) and on the effects of earplugs on phase transformations in the outer ear (S. Hogan and D. Pralong, unpublished observations).

In addition to guiding our future research, the data we have gathered on children has intrinsic interest. The most important result from this work to date is that OME can compromise binaural hearing, possibly resulting in a permanent impairment. In the barn owl, Knudsen and his colleagues (1988) have shown that animals reared with a unilateral earplug until the time of sexual maturation make persistent and systematic mistakes in sound localization. If these phenomena are linked, the results have implications for the treatment of OME and raise the possibility that communicative and educational difficulties associated with persistent OME may have at least a partial basis in central auditory system maladaptation.

4 Acknowledgements

I wish to thank the following past and present members of my laboratory for their contribution to the research reported here: Russell Martin was responsible for setting up animal behavioural research in the laboratory and he contributed to all three ferret hearing projects. Jemma Hine, ZeDong Jiang and Andy King made other, major contributions to the ferret hearing work. The infant psychoacoustics was started by Santie Meyer and has been continued by Sarah Hogan. Mary Hutchings has also been involved with that work since its inception. The work reported in this paper has been primarily supported by the Medical Research Council (U.K.). Additional support has been provided by the Wellcome Trust, the Hearing Research Trust, and the Oxford McDonnell-Pew Centre for Cognitive Neuroscience.

5 References

Hine, J.E. (1993) Free-field binaural unmasking in ferrets and humans. D.Phil. thesis, University of Oxford.

Hine, J.E., Martin, R.L. and Moore, D.R. (1994) Free-field binaural unmasking in ferrets. Behav. Neurosci., in the press.

Hogan, S.C., Moore, D.R. and Hutchings, M.E. (1994) The effect of OME on the development of binaural processing in humans. Ass. Res. Otolaryngol. Abs., 17, 146.

Hutchings, M.E., Meyer, S.E. and Moore, D.R. (1992) Binaural masking level differences in infants with and without otitis media with effusion. Hear Res., 63, 71-78.

Kavanagh, G.L. and Kelly, J.B. (1987) Contribution of auditory cortex to sound localization in the ferret (*Mustela putorius*). J. Neurophysiol., 57, 1746-1766.

Kavanagh, G.L. and Kelly, J.B. (1992) Midline and lateral field sound localization in the ferret (*Mustela putorius*): Contribution of the superior olivary complex. J. Neurophysiol., 67, 1643-1658.

Kelly, J.B., Kavanagh, G.L. and Dalton, J.C.H. (1986) Hearing in the ferret (*Mustela putorius*): thresholds for pure tone detection. Hear Res., 24, 269-275.

King, A.J., Martin, R.L., Jiang, Z.D. and Moore, D.R. (1993) Minimum audible angles in normal and monaurally deafened ferrets. Soc. Neurosci. Abs., 19, 1805.

Knudsen, E.I. (1988) Experience shapes sound localization and auditory unit properties during development in the barn owl. In: G.M. Edelman et al. (Eds.) Auditory Function: Neurobiological bases of hearing. New York: Wiley, 1988, pp. 137-149.

Masterton, R.B., Granger, E.M. and Glendenning, K.K. (1992) Psychoacoustical contribution of each lateral lemniscus. Hear. Res., 63, 57-70.

McAlpine, D. (1994) Binaural influences on the response properties of neurones in the ferret inferior colliculus. D.Phil. thesis, University of Oxford.

Moore, D.R. (1991) Development and plasticity of the ferret auditory system. In: R.A. Altschuler et al. (Eds.) Neurobiology of Hearing: The Central Auditory System, Raven Press, New York, pp. 461-475.

Moore, D.R. (1992) Developmental plasticity of the brainstem and midbrain auditory nuclei. In: R. Romand (Ed.) Development of Auditory and Vestibular Systems 2, Elsevier, Amsterdam, pp. 297-320.

Moore, D.R. (1993) Plasticity of binaural hearing and some possible mechanisms following late-onset deprivation. J. Am. Acad. Audiol., 4, 277-283.

Moore, D.R. (1994) Auditory brainstem of the ferret: Long survival following cochlear removal progressively changes projections from the cochlear nucleus to the inferior colliculus. J. Comp. Neurol. 339, 301-310.

Moore, D.R., Hutchings, M.E. and Meyer, S.E. (1991) Binaural masking level differences in children with a history of otitis media. Audiology, 30, 91-101.

Moore, D.R., King, A.J., McAlpine, D., Martin, R.L. and Hutchings, M.E. (1993) Functional consequences of neonatal unilateral cochlear removal. Prog. Brain Res., 97, 127-133.

Rubel, E.W, Hyson, R.L. and Durham, D. (1990) Afferent regulation of neurons in the brain stem auditory system. J. Neurobiol. 21, 169-196.

Russell, F.A. and Moore, D.R., Afferent reorganisation within the superior olivary complex of the gerbil: Development and induction by neonatal, unilateral cochlear removal. Submitted for publication.

Schneider, B.A., Trehub, S.E., Morrongiello, B.A. and Thorpe, C.A. (1989) Developmental changes in masked thresholds. J. Acoust. Soc. Am., 86, 1733-1742.

Peripheral processing

Developmental effects in complex sound processing

J.H. Grose, J.W. Hall III, & L. Mendoza

Div. Otolaryngology/Head & Neck Surgery, University of North Carolina Medical School, Chapel Hill, NC 27599-7070, USA

1 Introduction

A comparison of the auditory abilities of infants and children with those of adults reveals a complex picture. While many auditory functions develop with age, others appear to be fully developed at infancy. Auditory functions which exhibit changes with age include absolute sensitivity (Trehub et al., 1980; Berg and Smith, 1983; Sinnott et al., 1983; Nozza and Wilson, 1984; Olsho et al., 1988), frequency discrimination (Sinnott and Aslin, 1985; Olsho et al., 1987), temporal resolution (Wightman et al., 1989; Werner et al., 1992; Grose et al., 1993), and the efficiency with which masked signals are detected; i.e., signal-to-noise ratio at threshold (Schneider et al., 1989). Most notable among the functions which appear to be adult-like at infancy is frequency resolution (Olsho, 1985). This finding is consonant with electrophysiologic and otoacoustic measures which suggest that cochlear function is fully developed at term (Werner et al., 1993; Bonfils et al., 1992; Norton and Widen, 1988). While it is reasonable to assume that the developmental effects seen for some auditory functions reflect changes in the geometry and impedance-transforming properties of the external and middle ear, as well as maturation of the neural pathways, other effects suggest the involvement of nonauditory factors such as learning and attention (for review, see Werner and Bargones, 1992).

In addition to charting the course of normal auditory maturation, the study of the development of hearing in children is also bound up with understanding how auditory deprivation in early childhood affects later processing skills. Our own work in childhood hearing originated with the question of how the fluctuating hearing loss associated with otitis media with effusion in early childhood may have enduring effects on complex sound processing even after auditory sensitivity has been restored (Pillsbury et al., 1991; Hall and Grose, 1993). In the course of this work, we became interested in the normal development of complex sound processing in children. Of particular interest was the comparative development of across-frequency processing and binaural (or across-ear) processing.

One method of measuring across-frequency processing is the paradigm of Comodulation Masking Release (CMR) (for review, see Hall and Grose, 1991). The threshold for a signal masked by a narrow band of noise can be reduced if the masking band is accompanied by a set of flanking bands which share the same envelope fluctuation pattern as the masking band. The flanking bands are located well beyond the critical band centered on the signal frequency and can result in a masking release even if presented to the ear contralateral to that containing the signal and masking band. Studies of monaural CMR in children indicate that this across-frequency process is adult-like by at least 4 years of age (Grose et al., 1993).

The development of across-ear processing has been measured primarily with the Masking Level Difference (MLD) (Hirsh, 1948). When masking noise is interaurally in-phase (N_0), a binaural signal can be tracked to a lower level when it is interaurally out-of-phase ($S\pi$) than when it is diotic (S_0). This difference in threshold (N_0S_0 - $N_0S\pi$) is referred to as the MLD. At low frequencies, the MLD appears to be based on interaural differences in the fine-structure of the waveform. At high frequencies, where fine-structure cannot be encoded, MLDs are presumably based on interaural differences in waveform envelope. When the masking noise is relatively broadband (> 300 Hz), the magnitude of the MLD reaches adult levels by about 5-to-6 years of age but, in contrast, when the masking noise has a narrow bandwidth (e.g. 40 Hz), the asymptotic improvement of MLD with age continues beyond 6 years (Hall and Grose, 1990). There is some evidence that at intermediate bandwidths (120 Hz) MLDs are adult-like by, on average, about 9 years of age (Hutchings et al., 1992).

Although the developmental discrepancy between the data for monaural across-frequency processing and broadband across-ear processing is not excessive, the discrepancy for stimuli composed of narrow bands of noise is more striking. That is, the results at first sight suggest that across-frequency processing is adult-like by at least 5-to-6 years of age (e.g. Veloso et al., 1990), but that across-ear, or binaural, processing continues to develop beyond this age (e.g. Hall and Grose, 1990). This difference is notable because the processing of envelope information presumably plays a role in both classes of function for narrow-band stimuli. It is therefore of interest to determine whether actual maturational differences exist between these processes, or whether the differences can be accounted for in terms of dissimilarities in paradigm. To address this, we undertook a developmental study in which MLDs and CMRs were measured in children of various ages. The nature of the stimuli was such that a base set of narrow bands of noise could be combined to yield maskers appropriate for monaural CMRs, dichotic CMRs, MLDs, or combinations of these types of masking release. In addition, two frequency regions were tested: one where both fine-structure and envelope cues were available; and one where only envelope cues were available. The goal of the study was to determine whether real differences existed between the development of binaural processing and across-frequency processing.

2 Method

2.1 Subjects

Twenty-one listeners with normal hearing participated; i.e., audiometric thresholds were better than 20 dB HL bilaterally for the octave frequencies 250 - 8000 Hz. They were divided into 4 groups based on their age: (1) 4 - 5 year olds; (2) 6 - 7 year olds; (3) 8 - 9 year olds; and (4) adults.

2.2 Stimuli

The signal was either a 500-Hz or a 2000-Hz pure tone, 400 ms in duration including a 50-ms cosine-squared rise/fall time. The signal could be presented either to one ear (S_m) or to both; for binaural presentation, the signal could be either homophasic (S_0) or antiphasic (S_π) at the two ears. The signal was always masked by a narrow band of noise, 40-Hz wide, centered at the signal frequency. In some conditions, this masker band was accompanied by a set of comodulated flanking bands. In the 500-Hz region, these 40-Hz wide bands were centered at 200, 300, 400, 600, 700, and 800 Hz; in the 2000-Hz region, they were centered at 800, 1200, 1600, 2400, 2800, and 3200 Hz. The method of generation of the comodulated noise bands is described elsewhere (e.g. Grose and Hall, 1993). Nine conditions were constructed as shown in Table 1. Note that for all conditions expected to yield a masking release, N_0S_0 thresholds were used as the baseline for the sake of expediency even though in some instances N_mS_m threshold references are more traditional (e.g., CMR). In all conditions, the masking noise was presented continuously at a spectrum level of 50 dB/Hz SPL. Stimuli were presented over Sony MDR-V6 headphones.

Table 1. The frequency region and configurations of signal, masker band and flanking bands for the 9 conditions, including the measure derived from that condition.

Cond. #	Signal freq. (Hz)	Signal config.	Masker band	Flanking bands	Resulting measure
1	500	S_0	N_0	-	Baseline
2	500	S_π	N_0	-	MLD
3	500	S_m	N_m	ipsilateral	CMR (monaural)
4	500	S_m	N_m	contralateral	CMR (dichotic)
5	500	S_π	N_0	ipsilateral	MLD + CMR (monaural)
6	500	S_π	N_0	diotic	MLD + CMR (diotic)
7	2000	S_0	N_0	-	Baseline
8	2000	S_π	N_0	-	MLD
9	2000	S_m	N_m	ipsilateral	CMR (monaural)

2.3 Procedure

A 3AFC procedure was used which employed a 3-down, 1-up stepping rule which converged on the 79.4% correct level. The initial step size was 8 dB and this was reduced to 4 dB after two reversals in level direction. Following two more reversals, the step size was reduced to 2 dB. A run continued until a further four reversals had been obtained and the threshold estimate for that run was taken as the mean of the final four reversal levels. At least two threshold estimates were collected for each condition with a further estimate collected if the range of the first two exceeded 3 dB. The threshold for that condition was taken as the mean of the two (or three) estimates. The 3AFC task was embedded in a video game wherein the listener viewed 3 images on the screen (e.g. frogs). Each image in turn opened its mouth to mark the 3 observation intervals. In only one of them, at random, was the signal presented over the headphones. The listener indicated which image was thought to have 'uttered' the signal and visual feedback was provided after each trial in the form of a brief animation sequence which indicated the image associated with the correct choice. The children were provided with a rest/play interval after every two runs; the adult listeners were typically given a break after every six runs.

3 Results

The results for the 500-Hz conditions are shown in Figure 1 and those for the 2000-Hz conditions are shown in Figure 2. In each figure, the upper row of panels depicts the mean masked thresholds for the four groups of listeners under various conditions. Each upper panel pairs the baseline thresholds (N_0S_0) with thresholds for a condition designed to yield some form of masking release, as noted above each panel. The lower row of panels plots the average magnitude of the derived masking release for that condition.

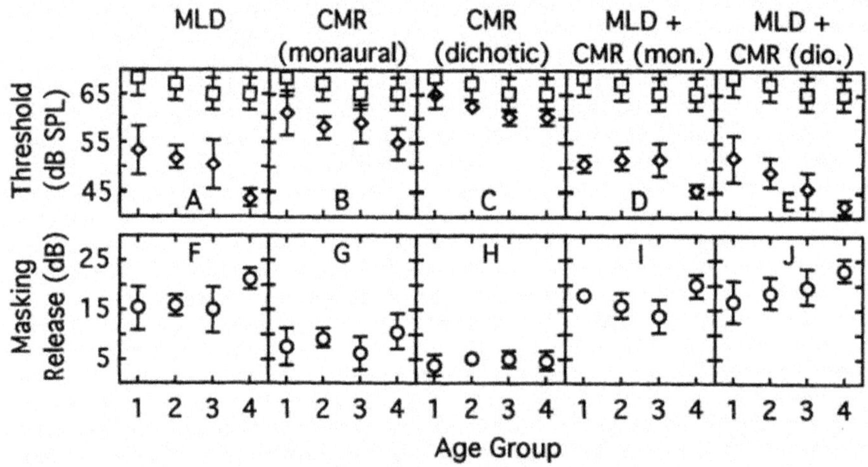

Figure 1. Mean thresholds (upper panels) and derived masking release magnitudes (lower panels) for the 500 Hz region for the four age groups: (1) 4-5 years; (2) 6-7 years; (3) 8-9 years; and (4) adults. Each upper panel contains the baseline N_0S_0 thresholds (squares) plus thresholds for a condition designed to yield the masking release noted above the panel. Error bars are ± 1 standard deviation.

Dealing first with the 500-Hz data (Figure 1), the baseline N_0S_0 thresholds suggest a gradual improvement with age. An analysis of variance (ANOVA) showed this improvement to be significant ($F_{3,17}$=18.6; $p<0.01$), with the children aged 4 - 7 years having higher thresholds than the oldest children and the adults.

The N_0S_π thresholds, shown in Panel A, appear to display a more rapid improvement with age than the N_0S_0 thresholds. An ANOVA assessing the factors of age group and condition (N_0S_0 vs N_0S_π) indicated a significant interaction between group and condition ($F_{3,17}=4.5$; $p=0.02$). The more rapid improvement of N_0S_π thresholds with age relative to the N_0S_0 thresholds translates into a significant increase of MLD with age ($F_{3,17}= 4.5$; $p=0.02$) as can be seen in Panel F. Post-hoc analysis of this effect using the Tukey HSD test indicated that only the 4 - 5 year old group and the 8 - 9 year old group differed reliably from the adults at the p = 0.05 level; the MLDs of the 6 - 7 year old group were smaller than those of the adults, but not significantly so. The three age groups of children did not differ among themselves in terms of MLD magnitude. The average MLD for the adults was about 21 dB; the average MLD across all children was about 15 dB.

Panel B depicts the thresholds for the monaural CMR condition. An ANOVA indicated that there was no significant interaction between age group and condition. Consequently, monaural CMR did not differ as a function of age ($F_{3,17}=1.7$; $p=0.2$). The average monaural CMR across all listeners was about 8 dB, as shown in Panel G.

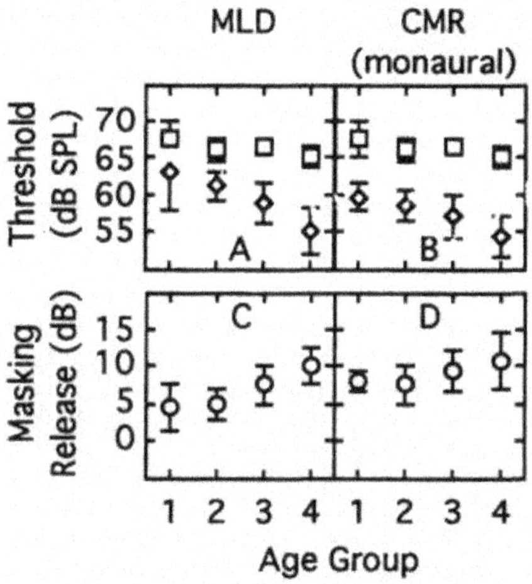

Figure 2. Mean thresholds (upper panels) and derived masking release magnitudes (lower panels) for the 2000 Hz region for the four age groups: (1) 4-5 years; (2) 6-7 years; (3) 8-9 years; and (4) adults. Each upper panel contains the baseline N_0S_0 thresholds (squares) plus thresholds for a condition designed to yield the masking release noted above the panel. Error bars are ± 1 standard deviation.

Panel C depicts the thresholds for the dichotic CMR condition. Again, there was no significant interaction between age group and condition, with the result that dichotic CMR did not differ as a function of age ($F_{3,17}=1.8$; $p=0.6$). The average dichotic CMR across all listeners was just over 4 dB, as shown in Panel H.

Panel D shows the thresholds for the condition where, in addition to the standard N_0S_π configuration, comodulated flanking bands were added to one ear. This condition tested the ability of the auditory system to make use of across-frequency comodulation cues in one ear in addition to binaural difference cues associated with the MLD. A repeated measures ANOVA indicated that there was no overall difference between the N_0S_π thresholds alone and the thresholds with the additional across-frequency cues ($F_{1,17}=0.01$; $p=0.95$). Furthermore, there was no age group by condition interaction indicating that this lack of improvement held across all age groups ($F_{3, 17} = 1.58$; $p = 0.23$).

Panel E shows the thresholds for the condition where, in addition to the standard $N_0S\pi$ configuration, comodulated flanking bands were added to both ears. This condition combines both a modified MLD configuration (more N_0 distributed across frequency) and across-frequency comodulation cues. A repeated measures ANOVA indicated that, overall, the $N_0S\pi$ thresholds alone were higher than the thresholds obtained with the additional across-frequency cues ($F_{1,17}=8.87$; $p<0.01$). In addition, the interaction between age group and condition was not significant, indicating that this improvement held for all age groups ($F_{3,17}=0.76$; $p=0.54$).

Turning now to the 2000-Hz data (Figure 2), the N_0S_0 thresholds did not differ as a function of age group. However, as can be seen in Panel A, the $N_0S\pi$ thresholds did improve rapidly as a function of age. The resulting significant interaction between age group and condition translated into a significant effect of age on the MLD ($F_{3,17}=5.4$; $p=0.01$), as can be seen in Panel C. Post-hoc analysis indicated that the MLDs of the 4 - 7 year olds differed significantly from the older children and the adults.

Panel B depicts the thresholds for the monaural CMR condition. There was no interaction between age group and condition, which translates into a lack of a difference in CMR across age groups, as seen in Panel D. The average CMR across all listeners was about 9 dB.

4 Discussion

The results indicate that monaural across-frequency processing is adult-like by 4- to 5-years of age both at 500 Hz and at 2000 Hz. This is consistent with earlier studies which have reported no differences between adults and young children in this ability (Veloso et al., 1990). The MLD, on the other hand, exhibits developmental effects at both frequency regions. In the 500-Hz region, all of the children (ages 4- to 9-years) performed more poorly than the adults, although the difference for the 6-7 year olds was not significant. In the 2000-Hz region, the 4- to 7-year old children performed more poorly than the adults. Thus, using a standard set of stimuli, the developmental difference between across-frequency processing and across-ear processing has been verified.

The observed pattern of results indicates that the developmental differences between MLDs and CMRs are not simply due to differences in the ability to encode envelope information versus fine structure since the MLD at 2000 Hz presumably is based primarily on envelope information. In addition, the results suggest that the developmental differences between across-frequency processing and across-ear processing are not simply differences in maturation of monaural versus binaural functions since the <u>dichotic</u> CMR did not exhibit any age-effects. That is, the age-dependence which is evident for MLDs but not for CMRs is not a limitation of binaural interaction.

The effects of adding across-frequency cues to a basic MLD configuration are also fairly straightforward. If the comodulated bands are added to one ear only, there is no additional benefit. If the comodulated bands are added diotically, then there <u>is</u> additional benefit. This pattern held across all of the age groups. Such a pattern is consistent with the model put forward by Hall et al. (1988) and modified by Cokely and Hall (1991). The premise of this model is that the residual noise at the output of an equalization/cancellation (E/C) mechanism maintains its original envelope. This allows for an across-frequency comparison of envelope information between the residual noise output from the E/C process fed by the signal channel and the outputs of the non-signal channels. If these envelopes are correlated, then further masking release is possible through a CMR mechanism. Although the model requires modification to include weighting functions to account for 'dip listening' (Buus, 1985; Hall and Grose, 1991), it can nevertheless provide a general account for the present data. When the comodulated flanking bands are added diotically, the envelopes of the residual noise outputs of the E/C mechanism for all channels will be correlated. This permits the functioning of a CMR mechanism, with the result that an additional reduction in signal threshold can be achieved. However, when the comodulated flanking bands are added to only one ear, the predicted outcome is less clear. Two possibilities can be envisioned: In one, the E/C mechanisms for non-signal channels are active but the contralateral inputs to the E/C mechanisms contain only (uncorrelated) internal noise. This is analogous to the presence of dichotic noise in the non-signal channels and this has been shown to result in a worsening of threshold (cf. Cokely and Hall, 1991). The other possible outcome is that the non-signal channel E/C mechanisms are not activated when there is only monaural input. This would generate the prediction that no change in threshold would be observed relative to the base N_0S_π threshold. The present data are supportive of this latter hypothesis.

While this model has the attraction of accounting for the general pattern of the data, it does not lend itself easily to the developmental constraints observed in this study. That is, in the sequence of the model the binaural interaction (E/C mechanism) responsible for the MLD precedes at least some aspect of the CMR process, yet the CMR process appears to mature earlier than the MLD process. It is, of course, simplistic to view complex auditory processing in hierarchical rather than parallel terms, yet is does seem to be the case that real developmental differences exist between aspects of complex auditory processing at presumably central stages. Further research is required to delineate these aspects more precisely and to consider what they may mean in the development of listening skills in real-world environments.

5 Acknowledgments

This work was supported by the National Institute of Deafness and other Communicative Disorders and by the Air Force Office of Scientific Research. We are grateful for assistance in data collection by Madhu Dev and Deb Hatch.

6 References

Berg, K.M. and Smith, M. (1983) Behavioral thresholds for tones during infancy. J. Exp. Child Psych. 35, 409-425.

Bonfils, P., Francois, M., Avan, P., Londero, A., Trotoux, J. and Narcy, P. (1992) Spontaneous and evoked otoacoustic emissions in preterm neonates. Laryngoscope 102, 182-186.

Buus, S. (1985) Release from masking caused by envelope fluctuations. J. Acoust. Soc. Am. 78, 1958-1965.

Cokely, J.A. and Hall, J.W. (1991) Frequency resolution for diotic and dichotic listening conditions compared using the bandlimiting measure and a modified bandlimiting measure. J. Acoust. Soc. Am. 89, 1331-1339.

Grose, J.H. and Hall, J.W. (1993) Comodulation masking release: is comodulation sufficient? J. Acoust. Soc. Am. 93, 2896-2902.

Grose, J.H., Hall, J.W. and Gibbs, C. (1993) Temporal analysis in children. J. Speech Hear. Res. 36, 351-356.

Hall, J.W. and Grose, J.H. (1990) The masking-level difference in children. J. Am. Acad. Audiol. 1, 81-88.

Hall, J.W. and Grose, J.H. (1991) Relative contributions of envelope maxima and minima to comodulation masking release. Quart. J. Exp. Psych. 43A, 349-372.

Hall, J.W. and Grose, J.H. (1993) The effect of otitis media with effusion on the masking level difference and the auditory brainstem response. J. Speech Hear. Res. 36, 210-217.

Hall, J.W., Cokely, J.A. and Grose, J.H. (1988) Combined monaural and binaural masking release. J. Acoust. Soc. Am. 83, 1839-1845.

Hirsh, I.J. (1948) Influence of interaural phase on interaural summation and inhibition. J. Acoust. Soc. Am. 20, 536-544.

Hutchings, M.E., Meyer, S.E. and Moore, D.R. (1992) Binaural masking level differences in infants with and without otitis media with effusion. Hear. Res. 63, 71-78.

Norton, S.J. and Widen, J.E. (1990) Evoked otoacoustic emissions in normal-hearing infants and children: emerging data and issues. Ear Hear. 11, 121-127.

Nozza, R.J. and Wilson, W.R. (1984) Masked and unmasked pure-tone thresholds of infants and adults: development of auditory frequency selectivity and sensitivity. J. Speech Hear. Res. 27, 613-622.

Olsho, L.W. (1985) Infant auditory perception: tonal masking. Infant Behav. Dev. 8, 371-384.

Olsho, L.W., Koch, E.G. and Halpin, C.F. (1987) Level and age effects in infant frequency discrimination. J. Acoust. Soc. Am. 82, 454-464.

Olsho, L.W., Koch, E.G., Carter, E.A., Halpin, C.F. and Spetner, N.B. (1988) Pure-tone sensitivity of human infants. J. Acoust. Soc. Am. 84, 1316-1324.

Pillsbury, H.C., Grose, J.H. and Hall, J.H. (1991) Otitis media with effusion in children. Arch. Otolaryngol. Head Neck Surg. 117, 718-723.

Schneider, B.A., Trehub, S.E., Morrongiello, B.A. and Thorpe, L.A. (1989) Developmental changes in masked thresholds. J. Acoust. Soc. Am. 86, 1733-1742.

Sinnott, J.M., Pisoni, D.B. and Aslin, R.N. (1983) A comparison of pure tone auditory thresholds in human infants and adults. Infant Beh. Dev. 6, 3-17.

Sinnott, J.M. and Aslin, R.N. (1985) Frequency and intensity discrimination in human infants and adults. J. Acoust. Soc. Am. 78, 1986-1992.

Trehub, S.E., Schneider, B.A. and Endman, M. (1980) Developmental changes in infants' sensitivity to octave-band noises. J. Exp. Child Psych. 29, 282-293.

Veloso, K., Hall, J.W. and Grose, J.H. (1990) Frequency selectivity and comodulation masking release in adults and 6-year-old children. J. Speech Hear. Res. 33, 96-102.

Werner, L.W. and Bargones, J.Y. (1992) Psychoacoustic development of human infants. In: C. Rovee-Collier and L.P. Lipsitt (Eds.), Advances in Infancy Research 7, ABLEX, New Jersey, pp. 103-145.

Werner, L.W., Folsom, R.C., and Mancl, L.R. (1993) The relationship between auditory brainstem response and behavioral thresholds in normal hearing infants and adults. Hear. Res. 68, 131-141.

Werner, L.W., Marean, G.C., Halpin, C.F., Spetner, N.B. and Gillenwater, J.M. (1992) Infant auditory temporal acuity: gap detection. Child Dev. 63, 260-272.

Wightman, F., Allen, P., Dolan, T., Kistler, D. and Jamieson, D. (1989) Temporal resolution in children. Child Dev. 60, 611-624.

Speculations on the relation between emission generation and hearing mechanisms in frogs

Pim van Dijk and Hero P. Wit

*Institute of Audiology, University Hospital Groningen, P.O. Box 30.001
9700 RB Groningen, The Netherlands*

1 Introduction

The discovery of otoacoustic emissions (Kemp, 1978) has fundamentally changed the view of hearing research on the function of the inner ear. Before 1978, the ear was believed to be a passive system. The discovery of otoacoustic emissions made research on active signal processing mechanisms in the inner ear a key topic in auditory research.

The possible relation between emission generation and an active filter mechanism in the ear has been pointed out by Gold in 1948. He noted that in order to account for the good frequency resolution of the inner ear, an active filter mechanism in the ear had to be postulated. Although clearly the ear would benefit from an active filtering mechanism, the active filter possibly becomes unstable. As Gold predicted, this would result in emission of acoustical energy from the ear canal.

There is substantial evidence that otoacoustic emission generation is indeed related to hearing mechanisms. For example, spontaneous otoacoustic emissions are primarily found in normal hearing ears, whereas they are an exception in impaired ears (Probst *et al.*, 1991). Moreover, in an individual ear the level of otoacoustic emissions is related to the threshold of hearing: Zwicker (1983) showed that after exposure to loud sound, both emission level is reduced and threshold is increased. Also, the recovery of the hearing threshold and the emission level occur in parallel during several minutes after exposure (Zwicker, 1983). Both these observation comply with the concept that otoacoustic emissions are related to optimal function of the ear.

Although Kemp's discovery of otoacoustic emissions confirms Gold's prediction, it has not yet been shown that otoacoustic emissions indeed result from instabilities in the inner ear filters. Evidence in support of this hypothesis is that suppression tuning curves of spontaneous otoacoustic emissions have a shape similar to that of rate tuning curves of primary auditory fibers. Figure 1 displays both types of tuning curves measured in frogs. Both tuning curve types show a similar asymmetry, which suggests that the interaction between an external tone and an emission involves the auditory filter. On the other hand, the high frequency slope is steeper for the emission tuning curves than for the single fiber tuning curves (Baker *et al.*, 1989). Apparently, additional filtering is involved in the interaction between a suppressor tone and an emission.

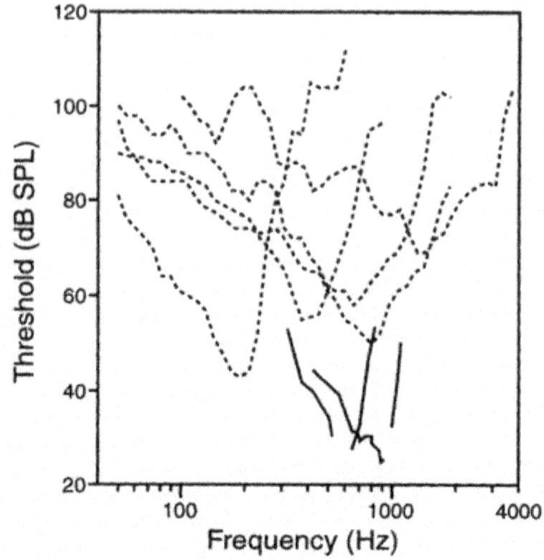

Figure 1: Tuning curves. Solid lines: SOAE suppression tuning curve (Rana temporaria, Baker et al., 1989). Dashed lines: Rate threshold tuning curves of primary auditory fibers in Rana catesbeiana (measured in our lab).

In various species, emission properties depend on body temperature. Figure 2 shows the dependence of spontaneous emission frequency on body temperature for the Bobtail lizard (Manley and Köppl, 1994) and three frog species (Wilson *et al.*, 1986; Genossa, 1989; Van Dijk *et al.*, 1989). The changes observed in the frog and the bobtail are similar. In the guinea pig, for which spontaneous otoacoustic emissions are observed between 0.7 and 2.3 kHz (Ohyama *et al.*, 1991), the average rate of change was 0.04 oct/°C (Ohyama *et al.* 1992). These findings suggest a common origin for emissions, both in warm and cold blooded species.

The neural response properties of the inner ear depend on temperature also. In the frog, best frequency (BF) of primary auditory nerve fibers shifts up with increasing temperature for fibers originating in the amphibian papilla, while no significant changes are observed in the basilar papilla (Moffat and Capranica, 1976; Stiebler and Narins, 1990; Van Dijk *et al.*, 1990; Narins and Benedix, 1994). The temperature dependence of spontaneous emission frequency and BF are not related in a simple way. For example, in *Rana catesbeiana*, Genossa (1989) observed that emission frequency change with 0.04 oct/°C, while best frequency of basilar papilla fibers does not change in the same frequency range (Van Dijk *et al.*, 1990).

In this work we will further elaborate on the relation between spontaneous otoacoustic emissions and filtering in the inner ear. We will present new data on the temperature dependence of neural response properties and compare the results with emission data.

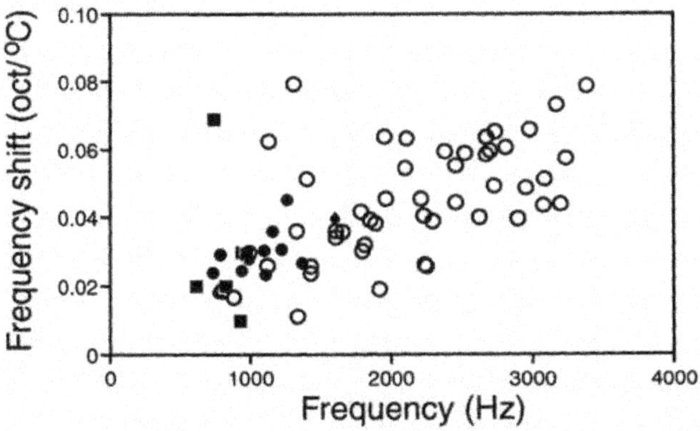

Figure 2: Rate of change of SOAE frequency with temperature. Closed symbols: emissions in frog (squares: R. temporaria, Wilson et al., 1986; circles: R. esculenta, Van Dijk et al., 1989; diamond: R. catesbeiana, Genossa, 1989). Open symbols: emissions in bobtail (Manley and Köppl, 1994).

2 Material and Methods

We measured the response of 12 primary auditory nerve fibers in *Rana esculenta*. The experimental setup used, and the animal preparation technique is described in Van Dijk *et al.* (1994). The body temperature was measured with a small thermocouple placed in the Eustachian tube of the ear being studied. During the experiment, body temperature was consecutively decreased and increased with approximately ±0.5 °C/minute.

When a fiber was contacted by the recording electrode, the ear was stimulated with Gaussian noise. The noise stimulus and the nerve fiber response were recorded on audio DAT tape. Offline, we computed the first- and second-order Wiener kernel by cross correlation of the stimulus and the response. By separately analyzing recording sections of 3 to 4 minutes, we obtained information on the effect of temperature on the kernels. Details on the Wiener kernel analysis are given in Van Dijk *et al.* (1994). In short, the following analyses were performed:

The second-order Wiener kernels of fibers with BF>600 Hz fitted the simple sandwich model shown in Figure 3(a). From the second-order Wiener kernel, we computed the filter functions of both filters $H_a(f)$ and $H_b(f)$ in the model. The best frequency BF(H_a) was defined as the maximum of $H_a(f)$.

The low frequency fibers (BF<600 Hz) could not be fitted with the sandwich model. For these fiber we obtained a frequency response function from the diagonal f_2=-f_1 of the

Fourier transform of the second order kernel. Although not obtained by application of the sandwich model, we will refer to this filter function as $H_a(f)$ also.

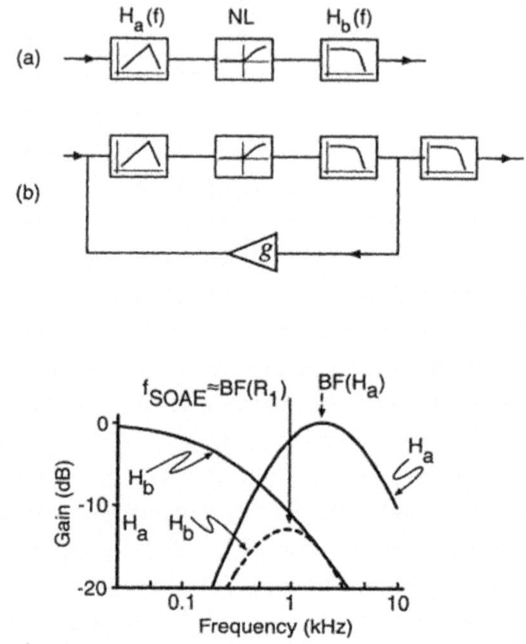

Figure 3: (a) Block diagram of sandwich model. The model consists of two filters with filter functions $H_a(f)$ and $H_b(f)$ and a static nonlinearity NL. The pictograms in the blocks indicate the filter response as function of frequency for the filters, and the input-output curve for the nonlinear element. (b) Sandwich model with a feedback loop. (c) Example of the filter functions $H_a(f)$ and $H_b(f)$ for a basilar papilla nerve fiber. The best frequency $BF(H_a)=2$ kHz of the first filter is well above the cutoff frequency $f_{b(-3dB)}=400$ Hz of the second filter. If the gain in the feedback loop becomes larger then 1, the model system in (b) will oscillate at the frequency where $H_a(f)\cdot H_b(f)$ has a maximum, i.e. at $BF(R_1)$.

3 Results

As an example, Figure 4 shows the temperature dependence of the filter functions H_a and H_b for a high frequency nerve fiber from the basilar papilla. The filter function H_a had bandpass characteristics which did not change with temperature. The second filter H_b was a lowpass filter. Its cutoff frequency increased significantly with increasing temperature. This example was typical for fibers with BF>600 Hz. Figure 4(c) shows the increase of the cutoff frequency for these fibers.

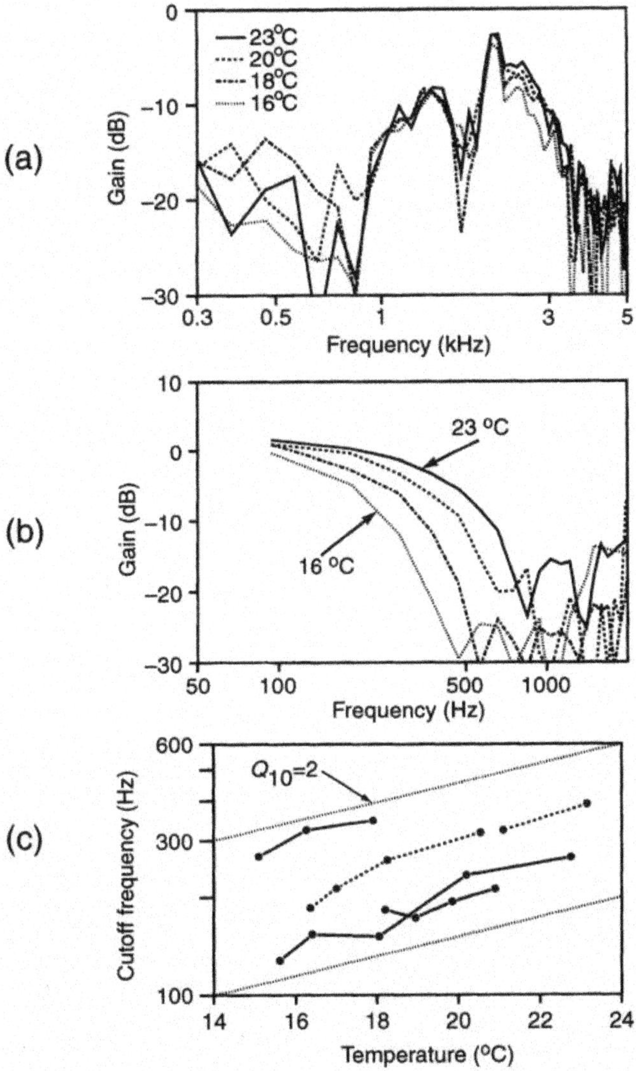

Figure 4: (a) The filter function of the first filter in the sandwich model for a nerve fiber contacting the basilar papilla. Results are shown for 4 different temperatures (b) The same as (a), but for the second filter in the model. (c) The temperature dependence of the cutoff frequency of the filter function $H_b(f)$ for three basilar papilla fibers (solid lines) and two amphibian papilla fibers (dashed lines).

In contrast to the high frequency fibers, BF(H_a) of the low frequency fibers (BF<600 Hz) shifted upwards with increasing temperature at a rate between 0.04 and 0.10 oct/°C. See Figure 5.

For fibers with BF<1000 Hz we measured a significant first-order Wiener kernel (*i.e.* reverse correlation function). In addition to the filter function $H_a(f)$, the Fourier transform $R_1(f)$ of this kernel gives the second estimate of the filter characteristics of the fiber. The maximum BF(R_1) of R_1 changed with temperature in all fibers at a rate between 0.005 and 0.18 oct/°C (see Figure 5).

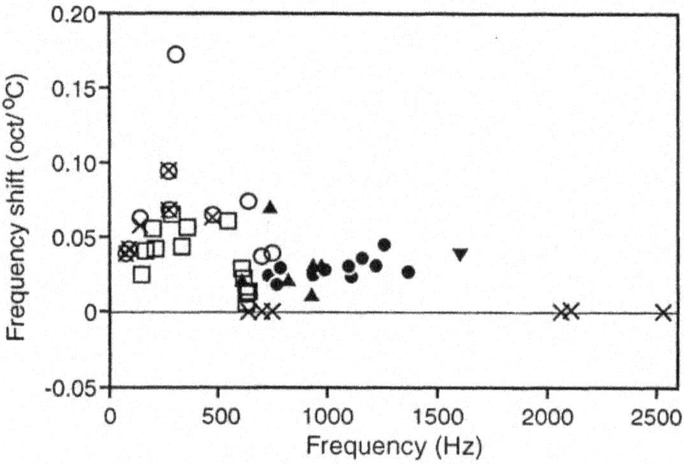

Figure 5:Rate of change with temperature of emission frequencies (closed symbols) and best frequency of nerve fibers (open symbols and X-marks). Emission data are the same as in Fig. 2. The open symbols indicate the rate of change of BF(R_1), the best frequency obtained from the reverse correlation function (open squares: Van Dijk et al., 1990; open circles: this work). The X-marks refer to BF(H_a), the best frequency obtained from the second-order Wiener kernel (this work). For some fibers we determined both BF(R_1) and BF(H_a). This yields two data points in this figure. In some cases the corresponding open circle and X-mark lie on top of each other.

4 Discussion

4.1 Temperature dependence of nerve fiber response

The temperature dependence of best frequency of primary auditory fibers in the frog has been studied by various methods. Before discussing the relation between other reports and our results, we will distinguish the various methods used to estimate best frequency. Moffat and Capranica (1976, *Bufo americanus*) and Stiebler and Narins (1990, *E. coqui* and *H. regilla*) used threshold tuning curves to determine the fiber properties. Van Dijk *et al.* (1990, *R. catesbeiana*) obtained best frequency from revcor functions for amphibian papilla fibers and used constant amplitude tone sweeps for basilar papilla fibers. In this work we also used revcor functions (*i.e.* first-order Wiener kernels) for amphibian papilla fibers. In addition we calculated the second-order Wiener kernel, from which the filter function $H_a(f)$ was obtained.

Regardless of the method being used, all earlier reports describe that best frequency of amphibian papilla fibers changes with temperature. For the basilar papilla no changes with temperature are reported. Stiebler and Narins (1990), who used threshold tuning curves to measure best frequency, find changes of the order of 0.06 oct/°C in the frequency range from 600 to 1000 Hz. Interestingly, using the reverse correlation function, Van Dijk *et al.* (1990) find smaller temperature changes in that frequency range: typically 0.02 oct/°C. Below 600 Hz, Van Dijk *et al.* (1990) and Stiebler and Narins (1990) find a similar effect of temperature on best frequency.

In this work we also present data on the effect of temperature on best frequency BF(R_1) obtained from a revcor function (first-order Wiener kernel). Our results are similar to those of Van Dijk *et al.* (1990), which is not surprising because the same analysis method is used.

Below 600 Hz, the changes observed in BF(H_a), the best frequency obtained from the second-order Wiener kernel, are similar to results from Stiebler and Narins (1990) and Van Dijk *et al.* (1990). However, for best frequencies just above 600 Hz, we found no effect of temperature on BF(H_a), in contrast to the effect on best frequency of revcor functions (Van Dijk *et al.*, 1990; this work) and threshold tuning curves (Stiebler and Narins, 1990). This difference can be interpreted on the basis of the sandwich model (Figure 3): Although $H_a(f)$ did not change with temperature, we did find a significant temperature dependence of the cutoff frequency of the second filter $H_b(f)$ in the model (see Figure 4b). For the sandwich model, the Fourier transform $R_1(f)$ of first-order Wiener kernel (i.e. the revcor function) is proportional to $H_a(f) \times H_b(f)$ (*e.g.* Van Dijk *et al.*, 1994). Thus, if the cutoff frequency of the second filter shifts up with temperature, the maximum BF(R_1) of $R_1(f)$ will shift up, even if the first filter $H_a(f)$ does not change. This accounts for the fact that above 600 Hz, revcor functions do change with temperature (Van Dijk *et al.*, 1990; this work), while the filter function $H_a(f)$ remains unaffected by temperature.

The common interpretation of the sandwich model is that (1) the first filter H_a represents the vibrating inner ear structures which are responsible for the frequency selectivity of the fibers, (2) the nonlinear element represents the hair cell transduction, and (3) the lowpass filter H_b models the dynamics of the baso-lateral hair cell membrane and the synapse. Since the second filter is temperature sensitive (Fig. 4b), its filtering action probably originates from electro-chemical mechanisms (Manley, 1990). For the fibers with BF>600 Hz, the first filter H_a is probably a mechanical filter, because this filter does not change its properties with temperature. Note that our temperature data suggest that the upper frequency range of the basilar papilla (600 Hz<BF<1000 Hz) functions similar to the basilar papilla (BF>1000 Hz). This conclusion is supported by the observation that the nerve fiber responses of fibers contacting these inner ear regions, all comply with the sandwich model (Van Dijk *et al.* 1994).

For fibers with BF below 600 Hz the situation is different. Firstly, their temperature sensitivity differs from the basilar papilla and rest of the amphibian papilla, and secondly, these fibers do not comply with the sandwich model (Van Dijk *et al.*, 1994). Both these observations are not surprising, considering the fact that the hair cells in the low frequency portion of the amphibian papilla are electrically tuned (Pitchford and Ashmore, 1986): firstly, the electrical tuning is expected to depend significantly on temperature, and secondly, an electrically tuned hair cell model would put the bandpass filter after the nonlinear element, in contrast to the situation for the sandwich model in Figure 3(a).

In conclusion, our data suggest that below 600 Hz, the bandpass filter involved in frequency selectivity is governed by electrical hair cell tuning. Above 600 Hz this filter is determined by mechanical tuning in both the amphibian and the basilar papilla.

4.2 Comparison between SOAE and nerve fiber data

Figure 5 displays the rate of change in response to variation of body temperature for (1) the frequency of spontaneous otoacoustic emissions and (2) the best frequency of primary auditory fibers. For the neural data we only show results obtained from Wiener kernels (Van Dijk *et al.*, 1990; this work).

The emission data are limited on the low frequency side at 600 Hz. The 600 Hz border seems to play an important role in the function of the frog's amphibian papilla: below 600 Hz, auditory nerve fibers exhibit nonlinear two-tone interaction, like suppression (Capranica and Moffat, 1980; Narins and Benedix, 1994) and two-tone response (Capranica and Moffat, 1980). In addition, the second-order Wiener kernel of these low frequency fibers has a complex shape compared to the fibers with BF>600 Hz (Van Dijk *et al.*, 1994). Finally, anatomical studies revealed that at the inner ear location sensitive to frequencies around 600 Hz, a tectorial curtain spans across the papillar recess (Lewis *et al.*, 1982).

As can be seen in Figure 5, below 600 Hz the rate of change of the best frequency BF(R_1) is about 0.05 oct/°C. Above 600 Hz the rate of change drops down to 0.02 oct/°C. The latter corresponds well with the rate of change of the emission frequencies. For the fibers in which the low rate of change has been measured, the sandwich model (Figure 3a) gives a good description of the nerve fiber response. We will now discuss how this sandwich model may be adapted in order to model both the temperature dependence of SOAE and best frequency of nerve fibers.

In order to mimic SOAE's with the sandwich model, we have to postulate a mechanism which will cause an unstable (*i.e.* spontaneously oscillating) mode of the model. This can be done by extending the sandwich model with a feedback loop (see Figure 3(b)). The resulting model is similar to the feedback model discussed by Dallos (1992). The Fourier transform of the reverse correlation function (*i.e.* first-order Wiener kernel) of this feedback model is given by $R_1(f)$=constant $x\ H_a(f)\ x\ H_b(f)/[1\text{-}g\ x\ H_a(f)\ x\ H_b(f)]$ (Marmarelis and Marmarelis, 1978), where g is a gain factor. If g is small, the model will essentially be analogue to the simple sandwich model. However, if g increases, an instability will arise at the frequency where $R_1(f)$ has a maximum. This will give rise to a sustained oscillation. If we assume that the oscillating system behaves as a nearly linear system, its oscillation frequency will be equal to the frequency where $R_1(f)$ is maximum. If the maximum changes by a certain amount, for example induced by a change of body temperature, the oscillation frequency will also change by the same amount. Thus, the feedback sandwich model predicts that the frequency of otoacoustic emissions changes at the same rate with temperature as BF(R_1), the best frequency obtained from revcor functions.

Figure 3(c) shows the relation between the various filter functions for a basilar papilla fiber. Although the bandpass filter $H_a(f)$ has its maximum at 2 kHz, $R_1(f)$ has its maximum at 1 kHz. If we would measure the threshold tuning curve for a fiber described by this model, we would find a best frequency equal to 2 kHz. If the gain in the feedback loop becomes larger, the system would start to oscillate at a frequency of 1 kHz. This examples shows how the basilar papilla, tuned to frequencies around 2 kHz might generate an emission at 1 kHz.

The available data (Moffat and Capranica, 1978; Stiebler and Narins, 1990; Van Dijk *et al.*, 1990; this work) show that the filter $H_a(f)$ does not change with temperature for basilar papilla fibers. We showed that the cutoff frequency of the second filter $H_b(f)$ increases significantly with temperature. Consequently, an emission frequency determined by the maximum of $R_1(f)$ will increase with temperature, in qualitative agreement with the experiments.

In qualitative agreement with the feedback model, the experimental data in Figure 5 show that BF(R_1) and emissions frequencies change with temperature at a similar rate. Unfortunately, at present neural data are only available in a limited frequency range around 600 Hz. Further data analysis will have to reveal whether the same applies to higher frequencies.

For the basilar papilla it will not be possible to quantitatively check the theory by measuring a reverse correlation function, because of the poor synchronization observed in these fibers. In other words: because the passbands of the filter functions $H_a(f)$ and $H_b(f)$ do not overlap, the function $R_1(f)$=constant x $H_a(f)$ x $H_b(f)$ will be very small. Thus, we are not able to determine BF(R_1) for these fibers. The reverse correlation function measures the linear response portion of the total system response. The frequency selectivity of the linear response may also be obtained from a synchronization tuning curve (Rose and Weiss, 1988). Measurement of the synchronization tuning curve of basilar papilla fibers may be used to further test the model proposed in this work.

In conclusion, we showed that the relation between the temperature dependence of SOAE frequencies and neural best frequencies may be modelled by a feedback model. This conclusion is preliminary because (1) it is based on a limited amount of data and (2) the implications of the model have to be further elaborated. A test of the model may be performed by measuring the temperature dependence of synchronization tuning curves.

5 Acknowledgements

We thank Hans Segenhout for his assistance during the experiments. The research of Pim van Dijk is supported by the Royal Netherlands Academy of Sciences and Arts. The

Institute of Audiology is part of and supported by the Groningen Centre for Behavioral and Cognitive Neurosciences (BCN).

6 References

Baker, R.J., Wilson, J.P. and Whitehead, M.L.(1989) Otoacoustic evidence for nonlinear behaviour in frogs' hearing: suppression but no distortion products. In: D.T. Kemp and J.P. Wilson (Eds.) Cochlear Mechanisms: Structure, Function and Models, Plenum Press, New York, 349-356.

Capranica, R.R. and Moffat, A.J.M. (1980) Nonlinear properties of the peripheral auditory system of anurans. In: A.N. Popper and R.R. Fay (Eds.) Comparative Studies of Hearing in Vertebrates, Springer Verlag, New York, pp. 139-165.

Dallos, P. (1992) Neurobiology of cochlear hair cells. In: Y. Cazals, L. Demany, and K. Horner (Eds.) Auditory Physiology and Perception, Pergamon, Oxford, pp. 3-16.

Gold, T. (1948) Hearing II. The physical basis of the action of the cochlea. Proc.R.Soc.E. B135, 492-498.

Genossa, T.J., Voigt, H.F. and Burkard, R. (1989) Spontaneous otoacoustic emissions in Rana catesbeiana, the American bullfrog. J. Acoust. Soc. Am. 85, Suppl. 1, S35.

Kemp, D.T. (1978) Stimulated acoustic emissions from within the human auditory system. J.Acoust.Soc.Am. 64, 1386-1391.

Lewis, E.R., Leverenz, E.L. and Koyama, H. (1982) The tonotopic organization of the bullfrog amphibian papilla, an auditory organ lacking a basilar membrane. J. Comp. Physiol. 145, 437-445.

Manley, G.A. (1990) Peripheral Hearing Mechanisms in Reptiles and Birds. Springer, Berlin, pp. 265-267.

Manley, G.A., and Köppl, C. (1994) Spontaneous otoacoustic emissions in the bobtail lizard. III: temperature effects. Hear. Res. 72, 171-180.

Marmarelis, P.Z., and Marmarelis, V.Z. (1978) Analysis of Physiological Systems. The White Noise Approach. Plenum, New York, pp. 394.

Moffat, A.J.M. and Capranica, R.R. (1976) Effects of temperature on the response of the auditory nerve in the American toad Bufo americanus. J. Acoust. Soc. Am. 60, Suppl. 1, S80.

Narins, P.M., and Benedix Jr., J.H. (1994) Temperature dependence of two-tone rate suppression in the northern leopard frog, Rana pipiens pipiens. Abstracts of the 16th midwinter midwinter research meeting of the Association for Research in Otolaryngology. p. 15.

Ohyama, K., Wada, H., Kobayashi, T., and Takasaka, T. (1991) Spontaneous otoacoustic emissions in the guinea pig. Her. Reas. 56, 111-121.

Ohyama, K., Sato, T., Wada, H. and Takasaka, T. (1992) Frequency instability of the spontaneous otoacoustic emissions in the guinea pig. Abstracts of the 15th midwinter research meeting of the Association for Research in Otolaryngology, p. 150.

Pitchford, S., and Ashmore, J.F.(1986) An electrical resonance in hair cells of the amphibian papilla of the frog, Rana temporaria. Hear. Res. 27, 75-83.

Probst, R., Lonsbury-Martin, B.L., and Martin, G.K. (1991) A review of otoacoustic emissions. J.Acoust.Soc.Am. 89, 2027-2067.

Rose, C. and Weiss, T.F. (1988) Frequency dependence of synchronization of cochlear nerve fibers in the alligator lizard: Evidence for a cochlear origin of timing and non-timing neural pathways. Hear. Res. 33, 151-166.

Stiebler I.B.,and Narins P.M. (1990) Temperature-dependence of auditory nerve response properties in the frog. Hear. Res. 46, 63-82.

Van Dijk, P., Lewis E.R.,and Wit H.P. (1990) Temperature effects on auditory nerve fiber response in the American bullfrog. Hear. Res. 44, 231-240.

Van Dijk, P., Wit, H.P. and Segenhout, J.M. (1989) Spontaneous otoacoustic emissions in the European edible frog (Rana esculenta): Spectral details and temperature dependence. Hear. Res. 42, 273-282, 1989.

Van Dijk, P., Wit, H.P. and Segenhout, J.M. (1994) Wiener kernel analysis of frog inner ear function. J.Acoust.Soc.Am. 95, 904-919.

Wilson, J.P., Whitehead, M.L. and Baker, R.J. (1986) The effect of temperature on otoacoustic emission tuning properties. In: B.C.J. Moore and R.D Patterson (Eds.), Auditory Frequency Selectivity, Plenum Press, London, pp. 39-46.

Zwicker, E. (1983) On peripheral processing in human hearing. In: R.Klinke and R. Hartmann (Eds.) Hearing - Physiological Bases and Psychophysics, Springer, Berlin, pp. 104-110.

Comment by J.P. Wilson

Your modelling concerning the different temperature coefficients at different frequencies and in the different papillae is interesting but unfortunately we cannot yet be certain that the BP produces OAEs just because they occur within the appropriate frequency region. To be certain of this it would be desirable to see the effects of ablation of each of the papillae.

Reply

I agree.

Spatial periodicity in the cochlea caused by interaction of spontaneous emissions

P.W.J. van Hengel

Department of Biophysics, and Center for Behavioral and Cognitive Neurosciences, University of Groningen, Nyenborgh 4, Groningen. NL-9747 AG, The Netherlands.

1 Introduction

Since the discovery of evoked otoacoustic emissions, researchers on cochlea models have tried to construct a realistic cochlea model that could simulate these emissions. In 1985 Strube found that his "computationally efficient basilar-membrane model" produced click evoked emissions as an artefact due to the spatial discretisation of the model (Strube, 1985). In a subsequent article (Strube, 1989) he argues that a spatially periodic distribution of reflective properties of the basilar membrane can serve as an explanation for evoked otoacoustic emissions. Such a "spatially periodic" (or "spatially corrugated") cochlea model performs rather well in simulating click evoked and tone burst evoked otoacoustic emissions if the spatial period is approximately 0.4 mm (Strube, 1985, 1989; Fukazawa, 1992; van Hengel and Maat, 1993). Nevertheless, there is considerable opposition to this "spatial periodicity" because a periodic structure with such a long spatial period has not been found in the geometry of the cochlea (e.g., Shera and Zweig, 1993 and 1994). One of the strong arguments in favour of "spatial periodicity" was the fact that the spectra of evoked emissions show regularly spaced peaks. The spacing between these peaks (when computed back to a distance along the basilar membrane using the place-frequency map of the cochlea) corresponds fairly well to a spatial periodicity with the 0.4 mm period. The same regular pattern is seen in the microstructure of the threshold hearing curve and in the spacing between spontaneous otoacoustic emissions (Dallmayr, 1985). Although recently Shera and Zweig (1993 and 1994) have shown that this "spectral periodicity" can also be obtained using a different impedance function for the basilar membrane combined with random inhomogenities of the parameters along the length of the cochlea, a comparison of toneburst evoked emissions as in Fig. 1 clearly shows that a spatially periodic model performs better.

The intention of this paper is to show that there is no need for a specific geometrical basis of spatial periodicity. Spatial periodicity with the required period can be accounted for by the interaction of energy producing sites (spontaneous emissions) and reflection of energy at the oval window in the cochlea.

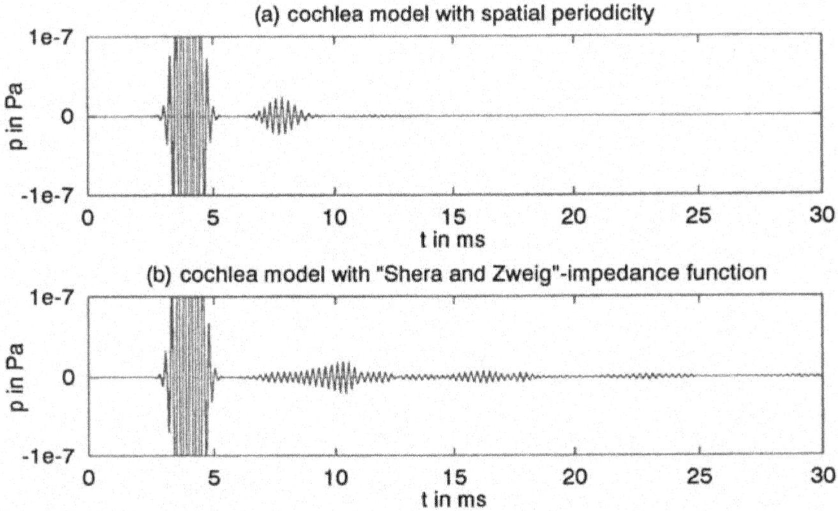

Figure 1. Comparison of toneburst evoked emissions computed with the cochlea model described here using: (a) spatially periodic discontinuities in the stiffness parameter. (b) random fluctuation in the stiffness parameter combined with the impedance function suggested by Shera and Zweig. The (clipped) signal around 4 ms is the 4kHz tone burst stimulus.

2 The model

Since the mathematical description of the model used together with relevant parameter values has already been published before (Duifhuis *et al.*, 1985; van den Raadt and Duifhuis, 1990), the focus of this description will be on the features needed for the simulation of spontaneous and/or evoked otoacoustic emissions.

The model is essentially a transmission line model in which the cochlear partition is divided into 400 sections that are coupled by the fluid in the scalae only. This fluid is assumed to be linear, inviscid, incompressible and it can only move in longitudinal direction (long wave approximation).

The mechanics of a section of the cochlear partition at position x is modelled by mass, damping and stiffness terms, so the equation of its motion becomes:

$$m(x)\ddot{y}(x) + d(x,v)\dot{y}(x) + s(x)y(x) = p(x) \qquad (1)$$

In this equation $y(x)$ is the displacement of the section, $p(x)$ the transpartition pressure and $m(x)$, $d(x,v)$ and $s(x)$ are the mass, damping and stiffness (per unit area) of the section respectively. As shown in previous work (van den Raadt *et al.*, 1993) the damping term $d(x,v)$ can be used to simulate SOAEs by making it dependent on the velocity $v(x)$,

$(v(x) = \dot{y}(x))$. In this model the damping profile consists of two nonlinear parts, multiplied by $\delta\sqrt{s(x)m(x)}$ with $\delta = 0.05$.

$$d(x,v) = [\mathrm{X}\sinh(\alpha v)/\alpha v - \gamma/\cosh(\beta v)]\ \delta\sqrt{s(x)m(x)} \qquad (2)$$

The positive nonlinear part causes saturation at high stimulus levels, and the negative part characterizes an energy supply to the section of the cochlear partition. The parameters χ, α, γ and β can depend on the position x, but following previous work (van den Raadt *et al.*, 1993) χ and α were set at constant values of 1 and 0.01 respectively. The parameters β and γ can both be used to introduce spontaneous emissions and to control their strength. A model section where $d(x,v)$ is negative for some v will be called an emitter.

Solutions have been computed in the time domain on a HP720 workstation. All calculations were performed using the standard fourth order Runge-Kutta method, at a sample frequency of 384 kHz. Dependence of the results on spatial discretisation was checked by recomputing them using 800 sections. No dependence on spatial discretisation was found.

3 Interaction between two emitters

3.1 Method

As described in a previous study (van Hengel and Maat, 1993), the interaction of two emitters in the model was studied in order to examine the suppression of a weak emission by a stronger one in the close proximity. For this purpose at model section 245, corresponding to a resonance frequency of 998 Hz, γ was set to 2 and β to 0.001. This resulted in a 16 dB SPL peak at 988 Hz in the spectrum of the emission computed at the eardrum. A second, weaker emission was introduced by using $\gamma = 2$ and $\beta = 0.05$ for one section within the range of 25 sections around section 245 (resonance frequencies ranging from 1207 Hz down to 879 Hz). Thus, in the spectrum of the emission at the ear drum two peaks can be seen. The level L_2 of the peak corresponding to the weak emission is shown in Fig. 2 as a function of its frequency. In the same way curves were computed for $\beta = 0.04$ and $\beta = 0.03$, which are also shown in Fig.2.

3.2 Results

The curves for $\beta = 0.04$ and $\beta = 0.05$ in Fig.2 clearly show a maximum in L_2 at a frequency of 1.05 kHz. This frequency corresponds to a distance of 0.41 mm between the emitters. Also a clear asymmetry can be observed between the low frequency (weak emitter apical of strong emitter) and the high frequency (weak emitter basal of strong emitter) side. In the region from 960 Hz to 1.02 kHz the emission spectra showed no peak from the weak emitter.

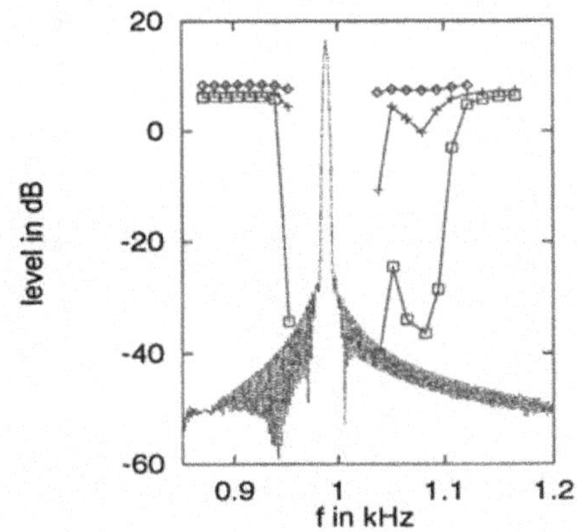

Figure 2. Sound pressure level L_2 of the frequency component in the emission spectrum corresponding to the weak emission, for three values of β: $\beta = 0.03$ (◇), $\beta = 0.04$ (+) and $\beta = 0.05$ (□). For comparison the spectrum of the emission caused by the strong emitter only is also shown (dotted line).

4 Influence of a single strong emitter on a cochlea consisting of weaker emitters

4.1 Method

The effect of increasing the emission level of a single section in a cochlea model in which all sections are emitters, was examined in order to see whether a similar suppression effect as seen in the interaction between two emitters could be observed. Therefore, all sections of the cochlea model were set to emit energy at a low level. For all model sections γ was set to 2 and β to 1, resulting in an emission spectrum in which all frequencies (in the range of the model cochlea) were approximately equal in strength. In this "completely active cochlea model" the emission from one of the sections was increased in strength by decreasing β. For three different values of β (0.4, 0.15 and 0.06) the spectra of the resulting emission at the ear drum was computed. Due to the fact that a cochlea model with all sections emitting energy behaves in a very irregular manner, spectra obtained from a 170 ms time window were not smooth and changed considerably with initial conditions. Therefore 50 spectra were computed, using different initial conditions, and from these an average spectrum was made. In order to investigate the effect of the location of the stronger emission this procedure was carried out for the locations corresponding to resonance frequencies of 0.5, 1, 2, 4 and 8kHz, with $\beta = 0.15$.

4.2 Results

The emission frequencies generated by sections in the direct vicinity of the stronger emitter are suppressed, as shown in the spectra in Fig. 3 (for the stronger emitter at a frequency of 1kHz). This suppression increases both in magnitude and in range as the level of the stronger emitter increases. (In this case there is also a clear asymmetry

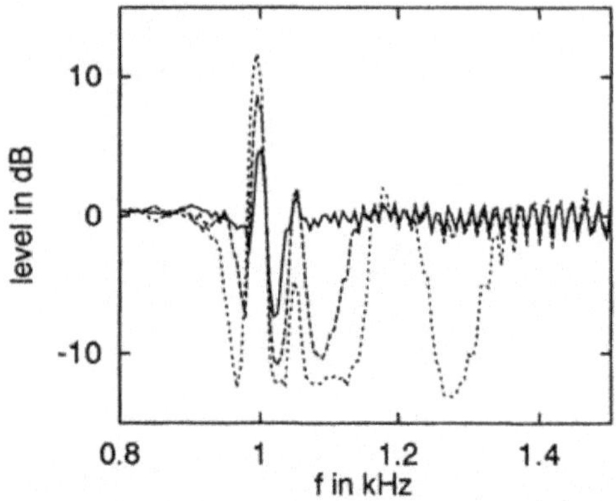

Figure 3. Spectra of sound pressure level computed at the eardrum with the cochlea model using $\gamma = 2$ and $\beta = 1$ for all sections, except section 245 (998 Hz resonance frequency) which has: $\beta = 0.4$ (solid line), $\beta = 0.15$ (dashed line) or $\beta = 0.06$ (dotted line).

between the high frequency (basal) and the low frequency (apical) side of the stronger emitter.) The suppression is strongly non-monotonic. At frequencies 1.05 kHz and 1.18 kHz maxima appear in the spectra, indicating minimum suppression or even enhancement at these frequencies.

Similar spectral features were observed using other frequencies of the stronger emitter. The locations of the maxima in these spectra are given in Table 1 (in frequency as well as in distance between the emitters on the cochlear partition).

f_1 (in kHz)	f_2 (in kHz)	$\Delta x(f_1 - f_2)$ (in mm)	Δx (em.sect - 1st min.) (in mm)
0.51	0.55	0.45	0.47
0.99	1.05	0.38	0.38
1.99	2.07	0.27	0.29
3.97	--	--	0.68
5.97	6.35	0.41	0.42
7.95	8.15	0.17	0.17

Table 1. Frequency of strong emitter (f_1) and frequency of maximum in suppression range (f_2) are shown for 6 different locations of the stronger emitter. From these a distance $\Delta x(f_1 - f_2)$ was computed using the placefrequency map of the cochlea model. The final column shows the distance between the emitter and the closest minimum in the "exitation pattern" along the cochlea (see Discussion for further explanation).

5 Discussion

In 1993 van den Raadt *et al.* showed that the energy dissipated by the cochlear partition in the case of one emitter in the cochlea depends on the distance from the stapes in a non-monotonic manner. This energy dissipation pattern shows a pattern of broad maxima and sharp minima. The explanation of this phenomenon is found in the reflection of the produced energy at the stapes. Due to a mismatch in the impedances of the cochlea and the middle ear / outer ear, part of the generated wave is reflected back into the cochlea, creating this standing wave-like pattern. The suppression (or entrainment) of an emission of course depends in a monotonic way on the level of the suppressor. If the latter shows maxima and minima along the length of the cochlea, so will the suppression. Since the level of the suppressor shows broad maxima and sharp minima (see Fig.4), the level of the suppressed emission will show broad minima and sharp maxima. The distance between the location of the emitter and the first (closest) minimum in the "excitation pattern", is also given in Table I for each of the frequencies used. Clearly, this is equal to the distance between the emitter and the least suppressed emission, given in column 3. (The discretisation of the cochlear partition into 400 sections leads to a spatial resolution of 0.0875 mm. Since this was regarded insufficient, an interpolation technique was used to improve the accuracy in the locations of the minima.)

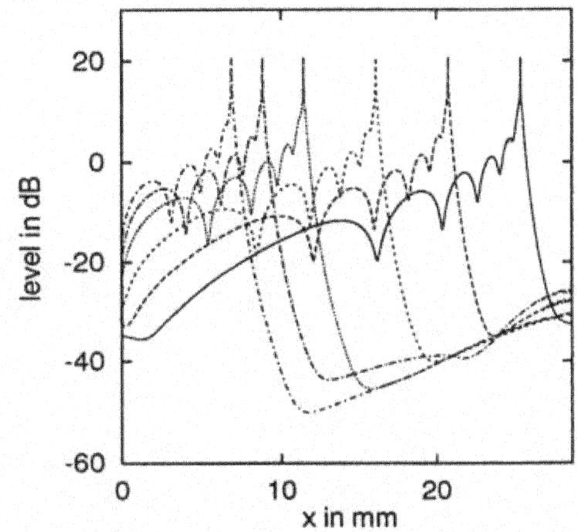

Figure 4. Amplitude of the velocity of the cochlear partition (in dB rel. 1 nm/ms) as a function of distance x along the cochlea ("excitation pattern"), for 6 different locations of a single emitter. The locations correspond to resonance frequencies of: 8kHz, 6kHz, 4kHz, 2kHz, 1kHz and 0.5kHz.

The reflection at the oval window can be removed almost completely for a certain frequency by changing the parameters of the middle ear and the coupling to the outer world (shown by van den Raadt, unpublished data). For a frequency of 1kHz this can be achieved by changing the transformation factor of the middle ear from 30 to 130. The resulting "excitation pattern" of an emitter at 1kHz is shown in Fig.5. Using this new transformation factor the suppression caused by a stronger emission in a "completely active cochlea model", as described in section 4.1, was recomputed. Indeed, the spectra of the resulting emissions, also shown in Fig.5, do not show the profound non-monotonicity seen in Fig.3.

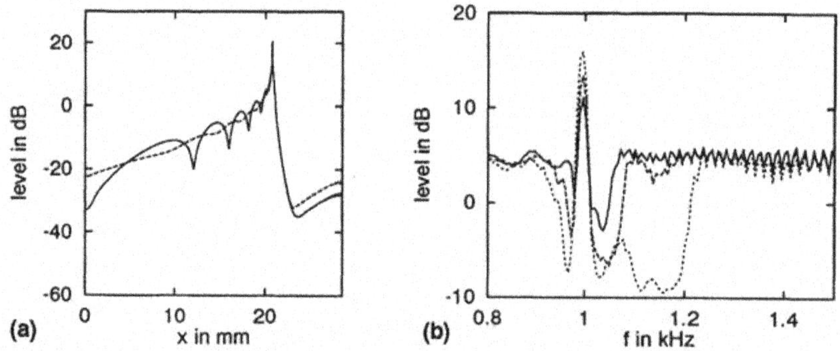

Figure 5. (a) "Excitation pattern" of a single emitter at section 245 (res. freq. ± 1kHz) for a middle ear transformation factor of: 30 (normal situation) (solid line) and 130 (dashed line). (b) Spectra of sound pressure level computed in the same way as described for Fig.3, but with a middle ear transformation factor of 130.

The fact that the distance between the strong emission and the least suppressed emission is not constant can be explained by the fact that the distance between the location of the strong emission and the closest minimum in its "excitation pattern" is not constant. This in turn is due to the fact that the number of periods in the traveling wave caused by an emission is not constant (the same as for an external tone stimulus). Therefore the "excitation pattern" does not only shift in position along the length of the cochlea, but it also changes shape. Figure 4 shows that with normal values for cochlear parameters (mass and stiffness in particular) the number of minima in the "excitation pattern" changes from 4 at 6kHz to 5 at 2kHz. The "excitation pattern" for an emission of 4kHz shows the intermediate stage where the closest minimum is quite far removed from the peak which is probably the reason why no clear maximum could be found in the suppressed region for this frequency at $\beta = 0.15$.

6 Conclusions

It turns out that the interaction of spontaneous emissions in this cochlea model, together with the reflection of energy at the oval window creates "ideal separations" between emitting model sections. These "ideal separations" correspond fairly well to the required spatial period of ±0.4mm which is neccessary in cochlear models to properly simulate evoked otoacoustic emissions. This effect is most probably present in the real cochlea as well, perhaps slightly distorted by minor fluctuations in the cochlear parameters. At present the author is investigating the correspondence between the computed "ideal separations" and measurements of separations of spontaneous otoacoustic emissions in both adults and newborns.

7 Acknowledgements

The author would like to thank prof. H. Duifhuis for the invaluable discussions on this subject, and S. M. van Netten and P. S. Tsang for their comments and corrections on the manuscript.

8 References

Dallmayr, C. (1985) Spontane otoakustische Emissionen, Statistik und Reaktion auf akustische Störtöne. Acustica 59, 67-75.

Duifhuis, H., Hoogstraten, H.W., van Netten, S.M., Diependaal, R.J., and Bialek, W. (1985) Modelling the cochlear partition with coupled van der Pol oscillators. in: Peripheral Auditory Mechanisms, edited by J. B. Allen, J. L. Hall, A. E. Hubbard, S. T. Neely and A. Tubis (Springer, New York) pp. 290-297.

Fukazawa, T. (1992) Evoked otoacoustic emissions in a nonlinear model of the cochlea. Hear. Res. 59, 17-24.

Shera, C.A., and Zweig, G. (1993) Order from chaos: resolving the paradox of periodicity in evoked otoacoustic emissions. in: Biophysics of Hair Cell Sensory Systems, edited by H. Duifhuis, J.W. Horst, P. van Dijk and S.M. van Netten (World Scientific, Singapore) pp. 47-53.

Shera, C.A., and Zweig, G. (1994) Dynamic symmetry creation: The origin of spectral periodicity in evoked otoacoustic emissions. J. Acoust. Soc. Am., submitted.

Strube, H.W. (1985) A computationally efficient basilar-membrane model. Acustica 58, 207-214.

Strube, H.W. (1989) Evoked otoacoustic emissions as cochlear Bragg reflections. Hear. Res. 38, 35-46.

van den Raadt, M.P.M.G., and Duifhuis, H. (1990) A generalized Van der Pol oscillator model. in: The Mechanics and Biophysics of Hearing, edited by P. Dallos, C.D. Geisler, J.W. Matthews, M.A. Ruggero and C.R. Steele (Springer-Verlag, Berlin) pp. 227-234

van den Raadt, M.P.M.G., van Hengel, P.W.J., and Duifhuis, H. (1993) Quantitative evaluation of spontaneous otoacoustic emissions in a one-dimensional macromechanical nonlinear cochlea model. in: Advances in Otoacoustic Emissions - Volume 1, edited by F. Grandori, in press.

van Hengel, P.W.J., and Maat, A. (1993) Periodicity in frequency spectra of click evoked and spontaneous OAE's; theory meets experiment. in: Biophysics of Hair Cell Sensory Systems, edited by H. Duifhuis, J.W. Horst, P. van Dijk and S.M. van Netten (World Scientific, Singapore) pp. 47-53

Comment by J. Blauert

The almost-periodic spacing of otoacoustic emissions along the basilar membrane might be thought of in terms of information reduction in the peripheral auditory system, namely, in that the inner ear may sample the incoming running sound spectra in a discrete way along a log-frequency scale. Has this idea already been considered?

Reply

The spacing of inner hair cells and their afferent innervation in my view give the lower bound on spatial or frequency sampling in the cochlea. Since this lower bound

(10 μm spacing and on average 10 afferent auditory nerve fibres per IHC) is much lower than the +/- 0.4 mm spatial period and because IHCs do not only transmit spectral information, but also locally available temporal information, it seems unlikely to me that frequency sampling in these large sections would occur at this level. Furthermore the almost-periodic spacing of emissions resulting from my model calculation is not due to a periodic structure in the model, but is only caused by the standing-wave like pattern caused by reflection of energy at the stapes. I did not mention this point in my manuscript or presentation, but the "ideal SOAE spacing" effect is independent of spatial discretization in the model. Changing the number of sections in which the cochlea is divided has no effect as long as the size of the sections remains well below 0.4 mm.

Comment by H.P. Wit

In your figure 1b, where you investigate Shera and Zweig's impedance function, the response is repeated approximately every 6 ms. This is, most probably, due to multiple reflections in your model.

Can the parameters in your model be chosen in such way to minimize multiple reflections, or is this phenomenon a fundamental shortcoming of Shera and Zweig's impedance function?

Reply

First of all I would not say that the model with the "Shera and Zweig"-impedance function shows multiple reflections. From the picture in my manuscript it might look like the signal around 16 ms is a copy of the signal around 10 ms, but a larger magnification would reveal differences. The picture was intended to show the difficulties in controlling the model's stability.

But reducing this "after ringing" is possible by reducing the positive feedback. Since this positive feedback is an essential feature of the "Shera and Zweig"-impedance function, at least at low levels of motion of the cochlear partition, introducing a nonlinearity that will make the model essentially passive at higher levels might be a solution.

Acoustic two-tone distortions from the cochlea of echolocating bats

Manfred Kössl and Gerhard Frank

Zoologisches Institut, Universität München, Luisenstr. 14, 80333 München, FRG

1 General properties of high frequency distortion products

To achieve high mechanical sensitivity, low level sound signals are actively amplified in the mammalian cochlea and force generation by the outer hair cells (OHCs) is thought to contribute to this process (e.g. Dallos, 1992). As a byproduct of mechanical amplification, the cochlear response is distinctly nonlinear with increasing sound pressure level and large frequency distortions are generated (e.g. Ruggero, 1993). The hearing range of echolocating bats extends to frequencies beyond 100 kHz and therefore the measurement of acoustic distortions may provide a critical test to which degree active and nonlinear mechanical processes are able to follow high frequencies.

When stimulating with two pure tone primaries of different frequency (f_1, f_2), cubic distortion products at the frequencies of $(n+1)f_1-nf_2$ and $(n+1)f_2-nf_1$ can be measured at the tympanum of mammals. Most prominent is the $2f_1-f_2$ distortion (review: Probst et al., 1991). Substantial $2f_1-f_2$ distortions could be measured up to the frequency limit of the analyzing setup of about 100 kHz in four FM-bat species (*Megaderma lyra, Carollia perspicillata, Tadarida brasiliensis, Eptesicus fuscus*) that use broad band echolocation calls and have a nonspecialized hearing characteristic and in two CF-bats (*Rhinolophus rouxi, Pteronotus parnellii*) that are specialized on an extremely sharply tuned perception of the constant frequency component (CF) of their echolocation calls (Neuweiler, 1990). Similar to the situation in other mammals, to measure maximum distortion level, the level of the f_1 stimulus has to be about 10 dB above that of f_2 and an specific frequency separation between f_1 and f_2 has to be chosen. For frequencies above about 50 kHz, the growth of the $2f_1-f_2$ distortion with increasing stimulus level on average is steeper than for lower

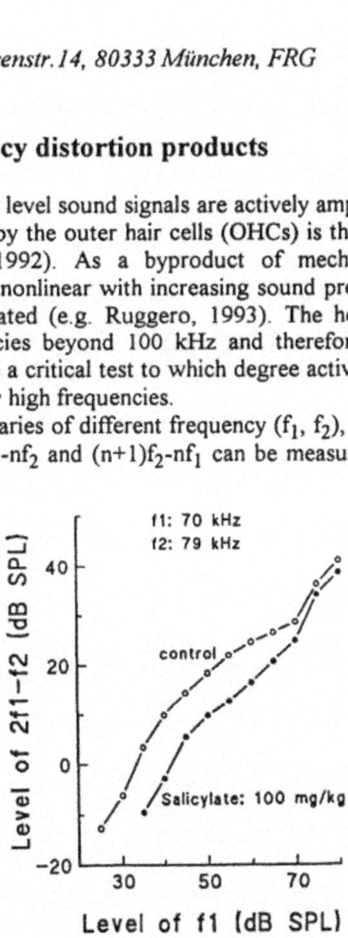

Figure 1. Input/output function for $2f_1-f_2$ in Carollia, the level of f_2 was 10 dB below the f_1 level. After injection of salicylate the distortion level decreases significantly (Kössl, 1992a).

frequencies (slopes of up to 2 dB/dB). This could indicate, that at very high frequencies nonlinear mechanical amplification is even more pronounced. To test if OHC motility is involved in producing high frequency distortions, salicylate that affects fast OHC force generation in vitro (Shehata et al., 1991) was systemically injected in *Carollia* (Fig.1). The level of $2f_1$-f_2 reversibly decreased after injection in dependance of the dose. This may indicate that the speed of fast OHC motility indeed is high enough to follow ultrasonic frequencies. However, it still has to be investigated to which degree slow tonic OHC movenents (e.g. Evans et al., 1991) are involved in nonlinear amplification and how they are influenced by salicylate.

2 Optimum frequency separation and frequency tuning

In normal mammals the frequency separation between the two primaries has to be adjusted such that the ratio f_2/f_1 is about 1.2-1.3 in order to maximize the distortion output (Probst et al., 1991). It is thought that under this condition, the overlap of the two travelling waves produces maximum nonlinearity. This implies that the optimum frequency separation gives an indirect measure of the sharpness of the travelling waves and hence of cochlear tuning. Fig.2 shows the optimum frequency separation Δf for different f_1 frequencies in four bat species. In the FM-bats *Megaderma* and *Carollia*, Δf increases from about 1-10 kHz for f_1 frequencies between 5-95 kHz. The corresponding ratio f_2/f_1 decreases slightly from about 1.2-1.1. This decrease correlates with the general increase of neuronal tuning sharpness (Q10dB values) with increasing frequency as it is known for mammals. In the CF-bats *Rhinolophus* and *Pteronotus*, Δf sharply drops slightly above the frequency of the second harmonic CF (CF2) which is at about 78 and 62 kHz respectively. The frequency of minimum Δf is close to the frequency of the Doppler-shifted CF2-echos. In addition, in *Pteronotus* there is a second minimum of Δf at about 90 kHz which correlates with the range of the third harmonic CF frequency (CF3). The minimum Δf values are between about 30-600 Hz (f_2/f_1: 1.0005- 1.007). In *Pteronotus*, the Δf minimum at about 62 kHz coincides with the frequency of a strong evoked otoacoustic emission (OAE; see Fig2A) that sometimes converts into a spontaneous otoacoustic emission (Fig.3). The emissions are thought to be produced by a mechanical resonance in the cochlea which leads to amplitude amplification and to enhanced tuning. It is imaginable, that if both primary frequencies are close together at the peak frequency of the resonance then they are strongly amplified and any subsequent mechanical processing stage may be saturated easily and hence large distortions are generated. It has to be pointed out that the mechanism of the resonance probably does not rely on micromechanical force generation in the OHCs alone, but may be depend critically on more or less passive reflections and reverberations in the cochlea base that could be produced by structural discontinuities of the basilar membrane (BM). In both CF-bats, the minima of Δf correlate with maximum tuning sharpness and minimum bandwidth of peripheral auditory neurons (Fig.2B: *Pteronotus*). This shows that enhanced tuning to the echolocation frequencies is generated by nonlinear mechanical processes in the cochlea and that the distortion measurement can be used to noninvasively determine components

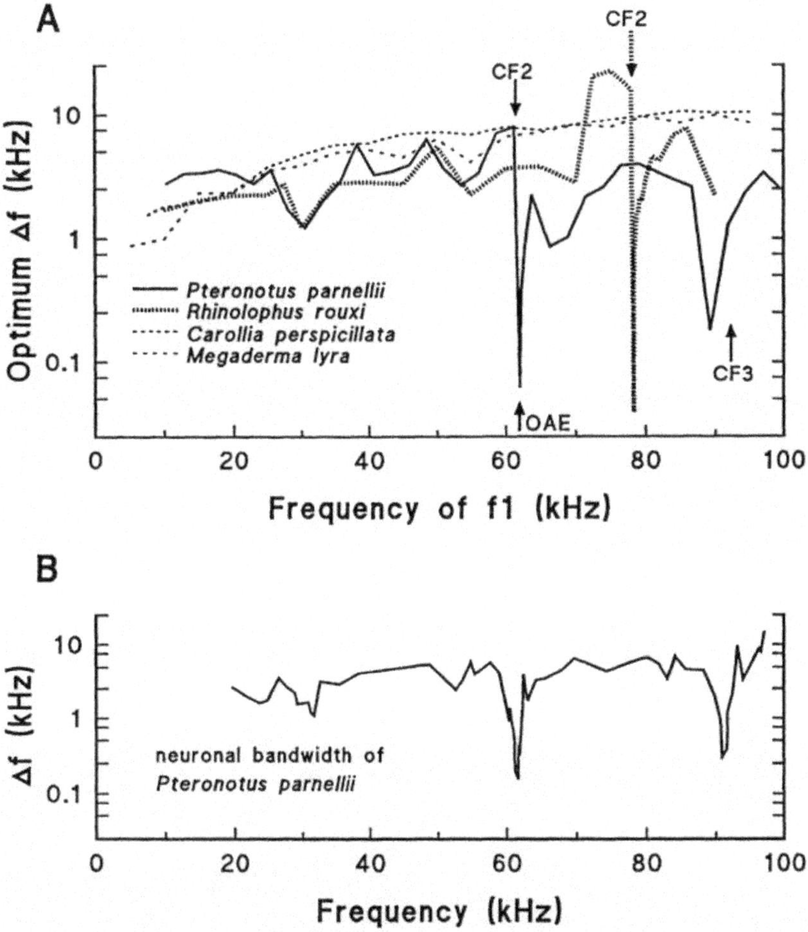

Figure 2. (A) Optimum frequency separation Δf between f_1 and f_2 that produces maximum $2f_1$-f_2 distortion in four bat species. The data were measured for low stimulus levels, at which distortions between -10 to 0 dB SPL were elicited (Kössl, 1992a,b, 1994a). (B) Neuronal bandwidths measured 10 dB above threshold in the cochlear nucleus of Pteronotus (from Kössl and Vater, 1990).

of frequency tuning.

To derive more detailled information about frequency tuning, $2f_1$-f_2 suppression tuning curves were measured in *Pteronotus* by applying a third tone (Fig.4, Frank and

Kössl, 1993a,b). In the low frequency range up to about 60 kHz the shape of the tuning curves resembles that of typical mammals with symmetric slopes or a steep high frequency slope and a shallow low frequency slope (e.g. Brown and Kemp, 1984). For primary frequencies close to the range of the strong evoked OAE and the minimum Δfs at 61-62 kHz, the tuning curves are characterized by a sharp minimum with Q10 dB values up to 177 (Fig.5) and their shape is inverted (Fig.4). The low frequency slope is very steep (up to -89 dB/kHz) and the high frequency slope is shallow. The steep low frequency slope and the sharp minimum are probably due to the mechanical resonance, the shallow high frequency slope may arise from an increased longitudinal coupling of the BM at cochlear places basal to the representation of the OAE. The shapes of normal and inverted suppression tuning curves closely resemble that of neuronal tuning curves (e.g. Kössl and Vater 1990). The degree to which the distortion measurements reflect the detailed characteristics of cochlear tuning, as it is observed in the first neuronal processing stages of the auditory pathway is quite astonishing.

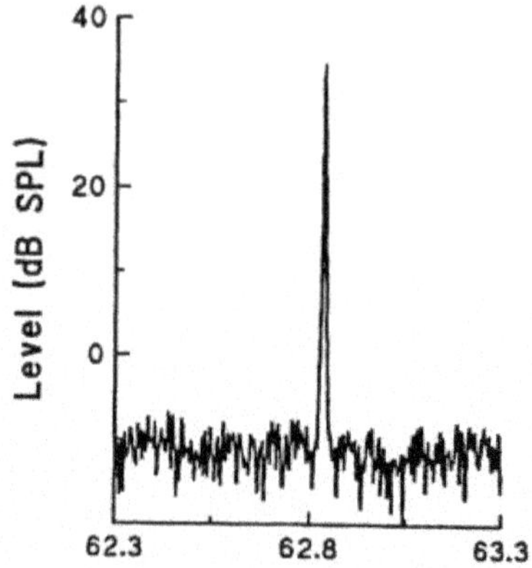

Figure 3. Spontaneous otoacoustic emission in Pteronotus parnellii.

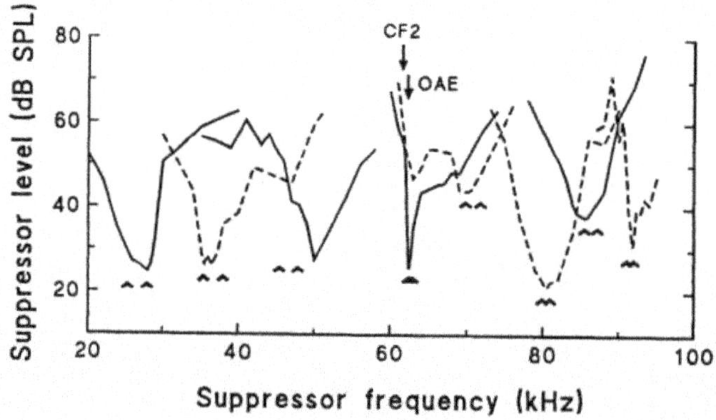

Figure 4. $2f_1$-f_2 supression tuning curves in Pteronotus. In each case the frequencies of the primary stimuli were chosen according the optimum Δf and their level was adjusted to produce a constant distortion of about 10 dB SPL. The frequencies of the primaries are indicated by ^^. Plotted is the level of the third tone f_3 that was sufficient to reduce the distortion by 6 dB for different f_3 frequencies.

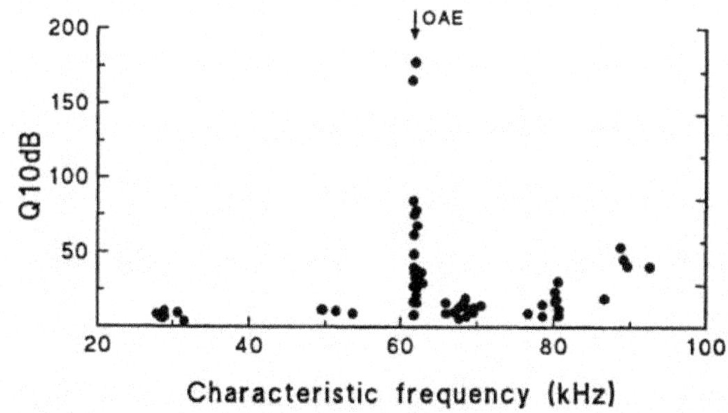

Figure 5. Q10dB values for $2f_1$-f_2 suppression tuning curves from Pteronotus, maximum Q10dB is found close to the frequency of the evoked otoacoustic emission (OAE). In the same frequency range neuronal tuning sharpness is at a maximum; data are normalized to the OAE frequency.

3 Distortion threshold curves

In four bat species it was attempted to derive relative cochlear threshold curves on the basis of distortion measurement. It is known that the level of $2f_1$-f_2 correlates with hearing sensitivity in laboratory mammals and man (Gaskill and Brown, 1990; Brown and Gaskill,1990). Instead of measuring socalled distortion audiograms where the frequency ratio f_2/f_1 and the level of the two primaries is kept constant and the resulting distortion level at different primary frequencies is used as measure of cochlear sensitivity, we determined isoresponse thresholds. For each f_1 frequency, f_2 was adjusted according the optimum Df and by increasing the primary levels, $2f_1$-f_2 input/output functions were measured. From these, the f_1 level that was sufficient to produce a distortion of -10 dB SPL was interpolated. Fig.6 shows the resulting threshold curves. These curves of course are relative thresholds, their vertical position depends on the threshold criterion. Since it is assumed that $2f_1$-f_2 is generated close to the frequency place of the primaries, the threshold curves are plotted against the primary frequencies (f_1).

For *Megaderma* and *Carollia* the thresholds are characterized by a steep decrease at low frequencies between 5-15 kHz. A broad threshold minimum is reached between 15-30 kHz and for higher frequencies the threshold slowly increases. The course of the thresholds is similar to that of neuronal measurements (Rübsamen et al., 1988; Sterbing et al., 1990) and they are elevated by about 20-40 dB compared to the neuronal thresholds. Such shallow threshold curves are typical for nonspecialized mammals, the hearing range of these two bat species enables them to perceive their own broadband echolocation signals and, in the case of the gleaning bat *Megaderma*, also the noise from prey animals.

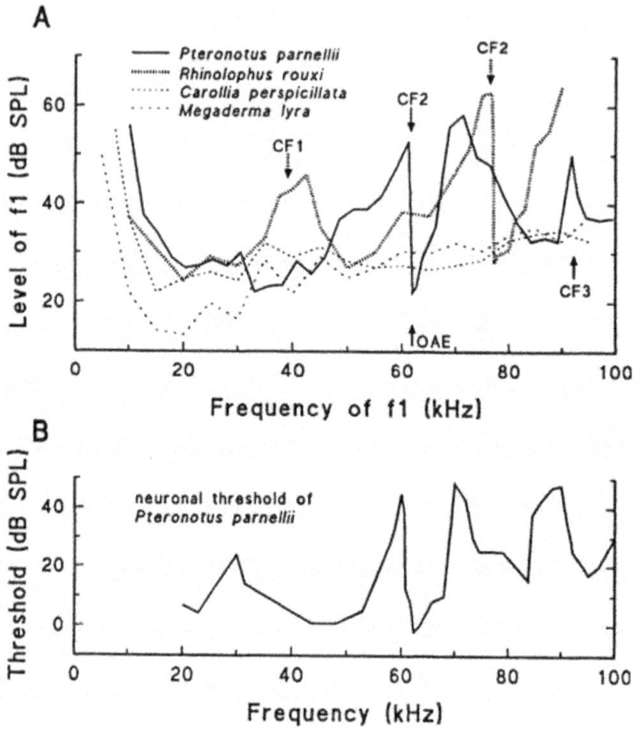

Figure 6. (A) $2f_1$-f_2 threshold curves, plotted is the level of f_1 that elicited a distortion of -10 dB SPL. The level of f_2 was 10 dB below that of f_1 (Kössl, 1992a,b,1994a). (B) Neuronal thresholds from Pteronotus (Kössl and Vater, 1990). The data are normalized to an OAE frequency of 62 kHz (Pteronotus) and to a CF2 of 78 kHz (Rhinolophus).

The thresholds of *Rhinolophus* and *Pteronotus* show distinct maxima and minima in the range of the CF frequencies. In the case of *Pteronotus*, there is a pronounced threshold minimum at the OAE frequency, about 480 Hz above the CF2 frequency of the call. At and slightly below CF2, the threshold is less sensitive by about 30 dB. Additional threshold maxima are at about 70 kHz and just below the CF3 frequency at about 90 kHz. In *Rhinolophus* the situation is similar, within a range of about 0.3-3 kHz above CF2 the threshold is at a minimum. At CF2 and slightly below the threshold is elevated by up to 40 dB. A second threshold maximum is found close to CF1.

When flying towards an object, both CF-bat species compensate the positive Dopplershift of the reflected CF2-echo by lowering the frequency of the CF2-call in order to keep the echo constant a few hundred Hz above the original CF2 frequency. This implicates that during this behavior the CF2 component of the call is shifted even further into the threshold insensitivity. Obviously, the bats are not much interested in their own CF2-call but focus on the sensitive processing of the echoes. This is also evident when recording cochlear microphonics during echolocation, the cochlear response to the bat`s own call is much smaller than that to the Doppler-shifted echoes, even if the level of the call recorded close to the bat is much higher than that of the echo (Henson et al., 1989, 1990).

4 A cochlear notch filter

The BM of *Rhinolophus* and *Pteronotus* shows pronounced thickenings below the OHCs (pars pectinata). Slightly basally to the cochlear frequency representation of CF2, the thickenings abruptly increase in size. In *Pteronotus* this region of maximum BM thickness extends between cochlear places of 62-72 kHz (Kössl and Vater, 1985), In *Rhinolophus*, very large thickenings cover the whole basal halfturn of the cochlea (Bruns, 1976), starting at frequency places about 2-3 kHz above the individual CF2 (Vater et al., 1985).

To explore the function of the thickened BM-regions, the two primary stimuli were adjusted so that either f_2 or both were represented within these regions. Under the assumption that $2f_1$-f_2 is generated close to the frequency place of the primaries, as it is evident from the suppression tuning curves, the behavior of $2f_1$-f_2 should reflect the mechanical processing in the thickened regions. It was found that the distortion level reaches sharp maxima whenever the distortion frequency is equal to or slightly smaller than CF2. In the example shown in Figure 7 for *Rhinolophus*, the frequency of one primary stimulus was fixed at 85 kHz, a frequency that is represented well within the thickened BM-region. Distortion maxima were measured if the second primary was at 81 or 93 kHz, in both cases the $2f_1$-f_2 frequency was at 77 kHz (The bat´s CF2 frequency was at 76.73 kHz). Distortion maxima at a distortion frequency close to CF2 were elicited by any primary combinations as long as f_2 or better both stimuli were more than 2 kHz above CF2. In *Pteronotus*, similar maxima at CF2 were found for primary frequencies between 62 to 72 kHz. It appears as if in the thickened cochlear regions, there are large oscillations at the CF2 frequency that lead to high distortion levels, in spite of the fact that hearing threshold is poor at CF2 (Fig.6). We conclude that the region of maximum BM-thickness strongly reacts to CF2 and therby the respective energy is released into the fluid spaces such that the more apically located frequency place of CF2 is rendered insensitive (see Fig.8).

In the normal echolocation situation, the CF2 component of the call is thought to be absorbed by the cochlear base. During stimulation with two pure tones that are represented in the thickened cochlear base, the CF2 signal is artifically introduced as a distortion that is generated in this region (Fig.8). Fig.9 shows that distortion products of different order ($2f_1$-f_2, $3f_1$-$2f_2$, $4f_1$-$3f_2$) all reach an amplitude maximum when the distortion frequency is at or slightly below CF2. Obviously, the two primary stimuli can be seen as a tool to place a probe signal, which is the distortion, in the thickened region of the cochlea which oscillates when the probe reaches CF2. The data indicate that the bats

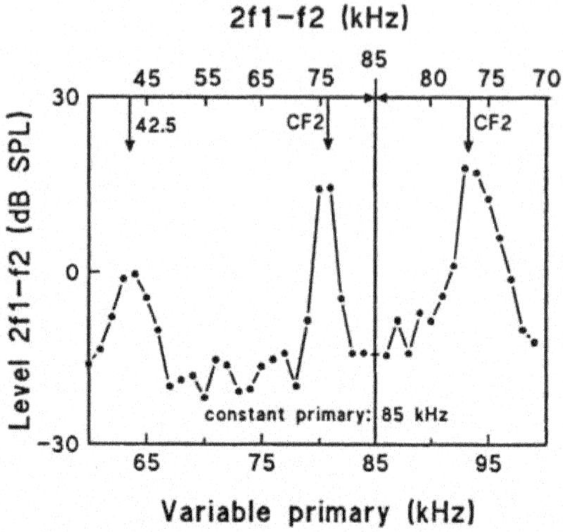

Figure 7. The level of the $2f_1$-f_2 distortion in Rhinolophus elicited by stimulus combinations where the frequency of one primary tone was kept constant at 85 kHz and the frequency of the other primary was varied between 60-100 kHz. The levels of both primaries were at 60 dB SPL. $2f_1$-f_2 refers always to the first lower sideband distortion and at a frequency of the variable primary of 85 kHz, f_1 and f_2 were nominally exchanged. The upper x-axis dislays the $2f_1$-f_2 frequency, at 85 kHz the sign reverses. There are pronounced maxima at primary tone combinations that produce a distortion frequency close to CF2 (76.73 kHz) and at about 42.5 kHz (from Kössl, 1994b). The threshold curve of the same individual is shown in Fig.6A, there are insensitivities at CF2 and at 42.5 kHz (close to CF1).

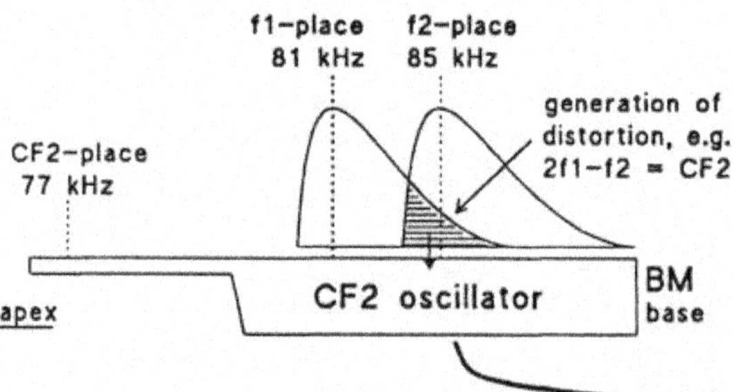

Figure 8. Schematic illustration of the notch filter in Rhinolophus, CF2 energy is absorbed in the basal thickened BM region by resonant oscillations. More apically, at the CF2 place, thresholds are insensitive.

have implemented a specific CF2 notch filter at cochlear regions basally to the CF2 place and to the place of the sensitive processing of the CF2-echos. The notch filter absorbs the CF2 energy such that it does no longer reach the CF2 place where thresholds are high.

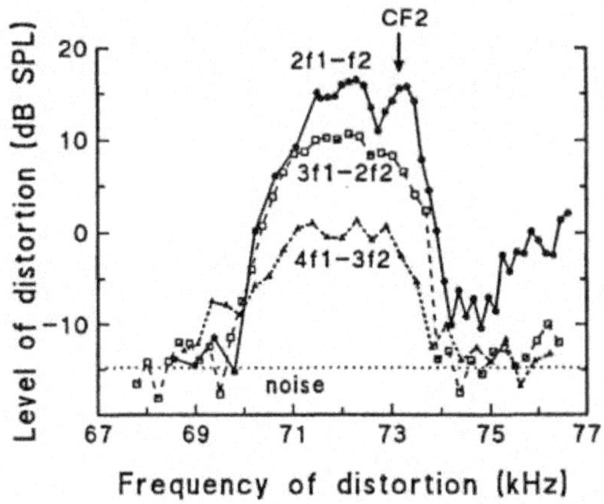

Figure 9. Distortion products of different order elicited by keeping the frequency of f_2 constant at 77 kHz and varying the frequency of f_1. (Levels of $f_1 f_2$: 50,40 dB SPL). CF2 was at 73.22 kHz (Kössl, 1994b).

The concept of using distortion measurement to evaluate cochlear filters is also valid for other mammals. In man, Brown et al. (1992) and Allen and Fahey (1993) measured filter characteristics and attributed them to the tectorial membrane. In the case of CF-bats, the cochlear filter coincides with the place of the thickened BM which does not exclude that other structures in this region participate in the filtering process.

5 Conclusions

The measurement of acoustic distortion products provides a valuable approach for comparative mechanics of the inner ear between different bat species. The measurements can be used to calculate the relative hearing thresholds and, by measuring suppression tuning curves and the optimum Δf, information about the mechanical frequency tuning can be derived.

In contrast to FM-bats, which can be seen as auditory generalists, in CF-bats there are pronounced changes in the distortion properties within a narrow frequency range around the CF-frequencies that are due to specialized mechanical processing in the cochlea. Slightly above CF2 the mechanical frequency resolution is high (Δfs reach minimum values of 30 Hz) and suppression tuning curves have maximum Q10dB values. A mechanical resonator that is evident from large evoked and spontaneous OAEs (*Pteronotus*) may be involved in enhancing the tuning sharpness. As a second specialized feature, in CF-bats there is a remarkable insensitivity of neuronal and distortion thresholds at CF2. The insensitivity reduces the auditory response to the call so that the bat can focus on the Doppler-shifted echos. There is evidence that the insensitivity is produced by a notch filter that is implemented in a region of maximum BM-thickness in the cochlear base of these animals. It is still open if the the sharp tuning slightly above CF2 and the notch filter at CF2 are due to the same resonant mechanism or if different mechanisms are involved.

6 References

Allen, J.B., Fahey, P.F. (1993) A second cochlear frequency map that correlates with distortion product and neural tuning measurements. J. Acoust. Soc. Am. 94:809-816.

Brown, A.M., Kemp, D.T. (1984) Supressibility of the 2f1-f2 stimulated acoustic emission in gerbil and man. Hear. Res. 42:143-156.

Brown, A.M. Gaskill, S.A. (1990) Measurement of acoustic distortion reveals underlying similarities between human and rodent mechanical responses. J. Acoust. Soc. Am. 88:840-849.

Brown, A.M., Gaskill, S.A., Williams, D.M. (1992) Mechanical filtering of sound in the inner ear. Proc. R. Soc. Lond. B 250:29-34.

Bruns, V. (1976) Peripheral auditory tuning for fine frequency analysis by the CF-FM bat *Rhinolophus ferrumequinum*. I. mechanical specializations of the cochlea. J. Comp. Physiol. A 106:77-86.

Dallos, P. (1992) The active cochlea. J Neurosci. 12:4575-4585

Evans, B.N., Hallworth, R., Dallos, P.(1991) Outer hair cell electromotility: the sensitivity and vulnerability of the DC component. Hear. Res. 52:288-304.

Frank, G., Kössl, M. (1993a) Suppression tuning curves of acoustic distortion products in the mustached bat, *Pteronotus parnellii*. Proc. 21th Göttingen Neurobiol. Conf. p 262.

Frank, G., Kössl, M. (1993b) The shape of $2f_1$-f_2 suppression tuning curves reflect basilar membrane specializations in the mustached bat. 30th IEB Abstracts, Budapest p.76.

Gaskill, S.A., Brown, A.M. (1990) The behavior of the acoustic distortion product, $2f_1$-f_2, from the human ear and its relation to auditory sensitivity. J. Acoust. Soc. Am. 88:821-839.

Henson, O.W.jr., Keating, A.W., Henson, M.M. (1989) Evoked potential correlates of echolocation in the mustached bat, *Pteronotus parnellii*. Hear. Res. 38:213-220.

Henson, O.W.jr., Koplas, P.A., Keating, A.W., Huffman, R.F., Henson, M.M. (1990) Cochlear resonance in the mustached bat: Behavioral adaptations. Hear. Res. 50:259-275.

Kössl, M. (1992a) High frequency distortion products from the ears of two bat species, *Megaderma lyra* and *Carollia perpicillata*. Hear. Res. 60:156-164.

Kössl, M. (1992b) High-frequency two-tone distortions from the ear of the mustached bat, *Pteronotus parnellii* reflect enhanced cochlear tuning. Naturwissenschaften 79:425-425.

Kössl, M. (1994a) Otoacoustic emissions from the cochlea of the "constant frequency" bats, *Pteronotus parnellii* and *Rhinolophus rouxi*. Hear. Res. 72:59-72

Kössl, M. (1994b) Evidence for a mechanical filter in the cochlea of the "constant frequency" bats, *Pteronotus parnellii* and *Rhinolophus rouxi*. Hear. Res. 72:73-80.

Kössl, M., Vater, M. (1985) The cochlear frequency map of the mustache bat, *Pteronotus parnellii*. J. Comp. Physiol. A 157:687-697.

Kössl, M., Vater, M. (1990) Resonance phenomena in the cochlea of the mustache bat and their contribution to neuronal response characteristics in the cochlear nucleus. J. Comp. Physiol. A 166:711-720.

Neuweiler, G. (1990) Auditory adaptations for prey capture in echolocating bats. Physiol. Reviews 70:615-641.

Probst, R., Lonsbury-Martin, B.L., Martin, G.K. (1991) A review of otoacoustic emissions. J. Acoust. Soc. Am. 89:2027-2067.

Rübsamen, R., Neuweiler, G., Sripathi., K. (1988) Comparative collicular tonotopy in two bat species adapted to movement detection, *Hipposideros speoris* and *Megaderma lyra*. J Comp Physiol A 163:271-285.

Ruggero, M.A. (1993) Distortion in those good vibrations. Curr. Biol. 3:755-758.

Shehata, W.E., Brownell, W.E., Dieler, R. (1991) Effects of salicylate on shape, electromotility and membrane characteristics of isolated outer hair cells from guinea pig cochlea. Acta Otolaryngol. 111:707-718.

Sterbing, S., Rübsamen, R., Schmidt, U. (1990) Auditory midbrain frequency-place code and audio-vocal interaction during postnatal development in the phyllostomid bat, *Carollia perspicillata.* Proc. 18th Göttingen Neurobiol. Conf. p.140.

Vater, M., Feng, A.S., Betz, M. (1985) An HRP-study of the frequency-place map of the horseshoe bat cochlea: morphological correlates of the sharp tuning to a narrow frequency band. J. Comp. Physiol. A 157:671-686.

A comparison between tone-evoked voltage responses of hair cells and basilar membrane displacements recorded in the basal turn of the guinea pig cochlea

I. J. Russell[1], M. Kössl[2], E. Murugasu[1,3]

[1]*School of Biological Sciences, University of Sussex, Falmer, Brighton, E. Sussex, BN1 9QG, U.K.*
[2] *Zoological Institute, University of Munich, Luisenstrasse, 14, 8000, Germany.*
[3] *ENT Department, Royal Sussex County Hospital, Eastern Road, Brighton, BN2 5BE, U.K.*

1 Introduction

The evidence that outer hair cells (OHCs) play an essential and interactive role in sensory transduction in the cochlea is compelling. Sensitivity to auditory stimulation, the ability to resolve complex sounds into their individual frequency components, and the generation of otoacoustic emissions are all greatly impaired following selective destruction of the OHCs (Liberman and Dodds, 1984, Brown et al, 1989). The reduction of the endocochlear potential, and hence reduction of the driving voltage across the hair cell transducer conductance, reversibly affects the frequency tuning and sensitivity of sound-induced movements of the basilar membrane (BM) (Ruggero and Rich, 1991). Electrical stimulation of the efferent innervation to the OHCs alters acoustic distortion products recorded at the auditory meatus (Mountain, 1980; Siegel and Kim, 1982), and OHCs isolated from the cochlea are capable of both voltage and mechanical-induced motility (Brownell et al., 1985, Canlon et al., 1988). These findings have been taken to indicate that OHCs have a bidirectional mechano-electrical, electro-mechanical role in sensory processing in the cochlea (Davis, 1983) which is also reflected in the sound induced movements of the BM (Sellick et al., 1982). The OHCs are thought to feed-back energy into the cochlear partition to overcome viscous damping, and they are strategically placed to control the relative movements between the two major interacting surfaces of the organ of Corti, the tectorial membrane and reticular lamina. The net mechanical energy resulting from the interaction between the OHCs and the passive mechanical elements of the cochlear partition is detected by the inner hair cells (IHCs), converted into voltage responses, and signalled in the afferent discharges of the auditory nerve.

In this paper we compare the properties and frequency selectivity of sound-induced displacements of the BM with sound-evoked voltage responses recorded from OHCs and IHCs in the basal, high-frequency region of the guinea-pig cochlea.

2 Methods

A detailed description of the methods of preparation, experimental techniques and stimulus presentation is given in Kössl and Russell (1992). Recordings were made from 72 pigmented guinea pigs (230-320 g) anaesthetized with the neurolept anaesthetic technique (0.06 mg atropine sulphate s.c., 30 mg/kg pentobarbitone i.p., 4 mg/kg droperidol i.m.; 1 mg/kg phenoperidine i.m.). The animals were tracheotomized, artificially respired and core temperatures were maintained at 37°C. The cochlear microphonic (CM) and compound action potential (CAP) were recorded through a AG/AgCL electrode placed on the round window. The criterion for a sensitive preparation was one in which the CAP threshold audiogram following exposure of the basilar membrane was less than 10 dB. Intra and extra-cellular recordings were made with micropipettes which were advanced through the basilar membrane in the basal high frequency region of the cochlea. The resistance of the pipettes when filled with 4 M potassium acetate was 180-280 M Ohms. After capacitance compensation the bandwidth of the pipettes extended to 2 - 4 kHz.

In a separate series of experiments, BM displacements were measured by two methods. In early experiments a laboratory constructed fibre-optic Michelson interferometer was used. Light from a laser diode was fed into a single mode quartz fibre, the tip of which was located close to a 10 μm glass sphere (MoSci Corp) which adhered to the BM. Interference between light reflected back from the tip of the fibre and the sphere was measured by a photodiode. The system was calibrated by displacing the tip of the fibre by known amounts with a calibrated piezo-electric crystal. In later experiments, displacements were made using the self-mixing effect of a laser diode. Self-mixing in a laser diode consists of the coupling back of a small part of the laser light into the laser cavity (Koelink et al., 1992). Provided that the frequency of the reflected light remains within the bandwidth of the laser, a mixing of this light with the light actually produced in the cavity is obtained such that there is a cosine dependency between target position and the laser intensity. This technique is similar to a technique first described by O'Neill and Bearden (1993) and is sensitive enough to measure light directly reflected from the BM. The interferometer consisted of a 5mW visible laser diode with an integral photodiode mounted together with a collumating lens and a focussing lens in a small tubular, brass housing about 2 cm in diameter and about 6 cm long. The focussing element formed a spot on the BM about 20 μm in diameter at a distance of about 5 cm from the front surface of the focussing lens. Movements due to respiration and heart beat were minimized by mounting the interferometer on a piezoelement and driving the element via a feedback stabilizing circuit (Fritsch and Adamovsky, 1981) that was fed with a low-pass signal filtered signal (100 Hz) derived from the interferometer. The feedback circuit was fast enough to keep the measurements within the linear operating range of the interferometer. For measuring DC displacements of the BM, the feedback circuit was disconnected.

Low frequency and DC voltages and BM responses were digitized and stored on a microcomputer disc. High frequency AC receptor potentials and BM displacements were analyzed with a two channel lock-in amplifier (EG & G, Princeton, Model 510) set in quadrature. The in-phase and quadrature outputs were digitized and the phase and the magnitude were computed. All sound levels are in dB re 20μPa.

3 Results

3.1 Hair cell DC voltage and BM tonic displacement responses to tones

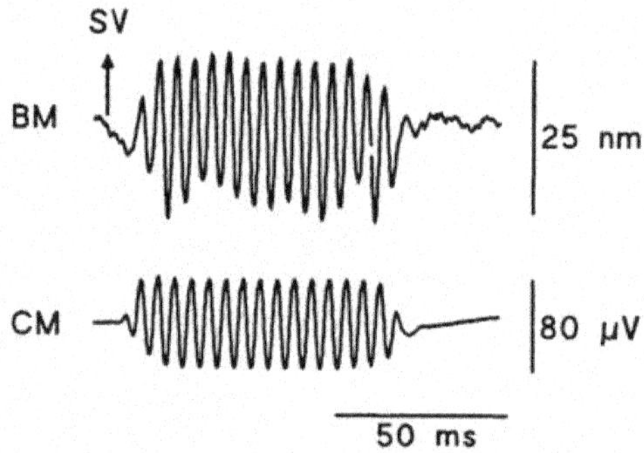

Figure 1. Simultaneous measurements of basilar membrane (BM) displacement and the round window CM to 200 Hz tones at 80 dB SPL recorded in the 15 kHz region of the cochlea. Vertical arrow indicates displacement of the BM towards the scala vestibuli (SV). Each record is the average of 8 presentations.

The mechanically induced displacements of the basilar membrane closely resemble the voltage responses of the OHCs. This is seen in figure 1 where simultaneous measurements of the cochlear microphonic (CM) and BM displacements to a 200 Hz tone are compared. The positive phase of the CM (OHC depolarization, Kössl and Russell, 1992) is associated with displacement of the BM towards scala vestibuli. At the levels and frequencies used for these measurements, the DC voltage component of the round window voltage recordings and tonic elements in the BM displacement responses could not be detected. This characteristic is also seen in responses shown in figure 2 to high frequency tones close to the 18 kHz characteristic frequency (CF) of the recording site. Tonic BM displacements towards scala vestibuli are seen only for high level tones in excess of 90 dB SPL at frequencies below CF (e.g. 13 kHz figure 2) but not at the CF. This is because the threshold for the appearance and the magnitude of both the tonic BM displacements and OHC DC voltage responses are frequency dependent. The threshold increases and the magnitude decreases systematically with frequency for frequencies between one half of an octave below CF and CF. These characteristic are not shared by the DC voltage responses of the IHCs. At all frequencies and levels within their dynamic

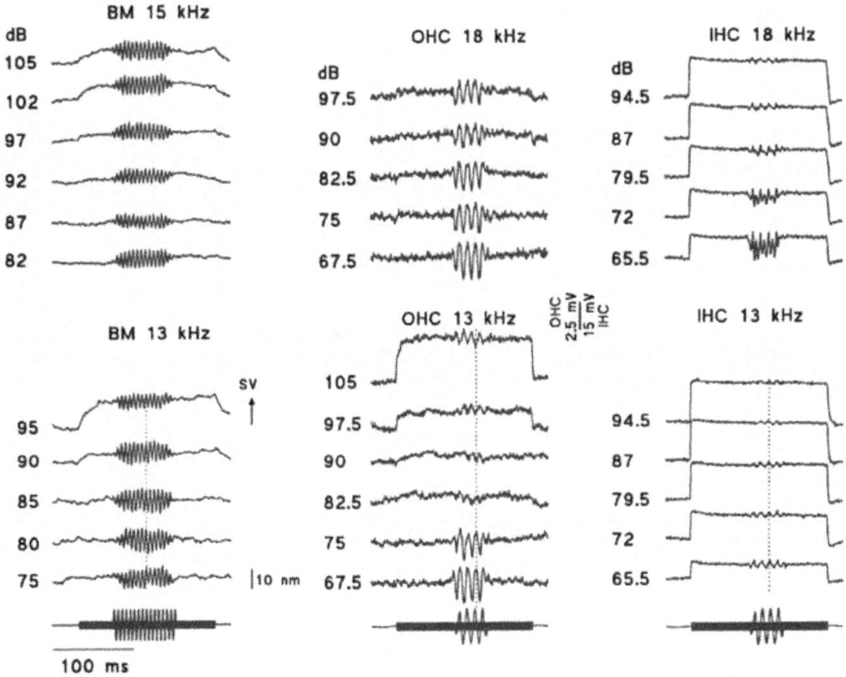

Figure 2. Displacement measurements from the BM and intracellular voltage responses of an OHC and an IHC in the basal turn of the cochlea to combinations of 80 dB SPL, 200 Hz tone (BM), 100 Hz tone (IHC and OHC) and high frequency tones at the frequencies indicated. The waveforms of the low-frequency and high-frequency tones are shown below each pair of records. The IHC (resting potential -45 mV) and OHC (resting potential - 68 mV) are from the 18 kHz region of the same cochlea. The BM recordings are from the 18 kHz region of another cochlea. The voltage responses are low-pass filtered at 3 kHz. Dotted lines drawn through peaks of LF responses during 13 kHz tones show phase reversal of OHC but not BM and IHC responses for levels above 90 dB SPL. The BM measurements are the average of 8 presentations.

range, the DC components of the IHC voltage responses are maximized whilst, for levels below saturation of the AC component of the OHC receptor potential, the DC component of the OHC voltage response and the tonic component of the BM displacement are minimized.

3.2 Frequency and level dependence of hair cell and BM responses

In response to tones over a range of 1 - 30 kHz, it was found that, for frequencies very close to the CF, the level dependency of BM, OHC and IHC responses all resemble each other. This shown in figure 3 for two representative frequencies at 8 kHz and 18 kHz (CF). Responses recorded from sensitive cochleas are very compressive at the CF, although the compression of the IHC response appears to be greater than that of either the OHC and BM. For frequencies of more than about one half of an octave below the CF, the BM response grows linearly and does not saturate while IHC responses are not elicited until the OHC phasic responses reach saturation (figure 3). At a frequency of one half of an octave below the CF (see figure 2, 13 kHz), the excitatory phase of the OHC receptor potential reverses from displacements of the BM towards scala vestibuli to displacements towards scala tympani for levels above about 90 dB. The phase reversal coincides with the appearance of the DC component of the OHC voltage response and with tonic displacements of the BM. However, as can also be seen in figure 2, a level-dependent phase reversal of phasic BM displacements and IHC responses was not observed at 13 kHz.

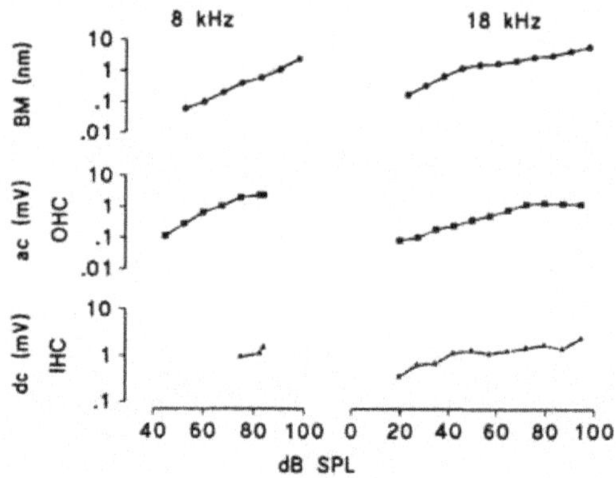

Figure 3. Response-level functions of phasic BM displacement (upper figures), OHC AC responses (middle figures) and IHC DC responses (lower figures) for 8 kHz and 18 kHz (CF) tones measured at the 18 kHz region of the cochlea. The IHC and OHC responses are from the same cochlea. The magnitude of the AC response is corrected by 6 dB/octave from 3.5 kHz to compensate for the low-pass filtering due to the recording system.

3.3 Frequency tuning

The BM, OHC and BM isoresponse frequency tuning curves shown in figure 4 are recorded from the same frequency region of the basilar membrane. The criteria chosen for the isoresponse tuning curves were based on the amplitudes of IHC, OHC and BM responses recorded to tones at the CF at a level which was just sufficient to elicit a compound action potential in the auditory nerve. It can be seen that there is close correspondence between all three curves in the tip region, but that the tails of both the BM and OHC tuning curves are about 20 dB more sensitive than the tail of the IHC tuning curve.

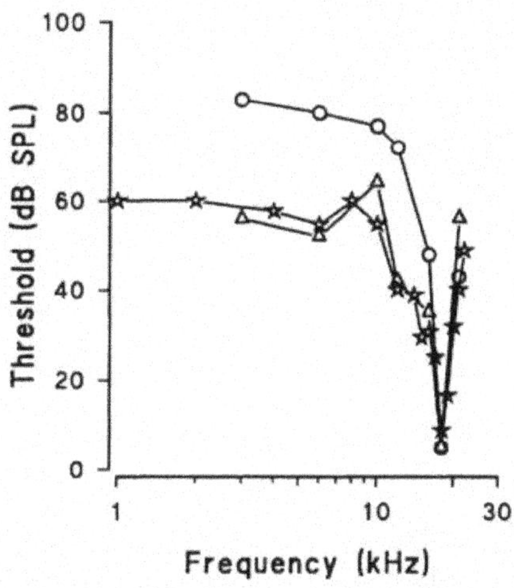

Figure 4. Frequency tuning curves measured intracellularly from an IHC and an OHC in the 18 kHz region of the same cochlea and isoresponse measurements of the displacement of the 18 kHz region of the basilar membrane of a different cochlea. The criteria for the isoresponse tuning curves were 0.5 mV (OHC, AC, triangles), 0.8 mV (IHC, DC, circles), 0.2 nm (BM, displacement, stars). The resting potentials of the IHC and OHC were -45 mV and -65 mV respectively. The OHC AC responses are corrected for the low-pass filtering of the recording system (3.5 kHz) and OHC membrane filter (1 kHz).

4 Discussion

The displacement responses of the BM and the voltage responses of OHCs in the basal turn of the guinea pig cochlea to tones are similar in that for levels below saturation of the OHC transducer conductance, tonic BM displacements and OHC DC voltage responses cannot be detected. The finding that there is not a measurable tonic component in the tone-evoked BM displacements for tones below about 90 dB is in agreement with measurements made by Cooper and Rhode (1992) in the neighbouring hook region of the BM.

It has been proposed that the operating point of the OHC transducer conductance is set so that it operates about its steepest point, and hence at the maximum gain of the input-output function (Russell and Kössl, 1991, 1992). At this point the DC component of the tone-evoked voltage response of the OHC is at a minimum. The appearance of the DC component of the OHC voltage response at high levels may have a protective role in that, during high level tones, it causes the OHC bundle to be moved to a position where more channels are closed at rest and the transducer conductance is operating at lower gain.The gain of the proposed OHC electro-motile feedback system would be reduced and result in a reduction in the amplification of BM displacement.

The phase reversal of OHC voltage responses to high level tones was first observed in the gerbil cochlea by Zwislocki and Smith (1988). Similar observations were made in the guinea pig cochlea for frequencies about one half of an octave below CF of the OHC (Kössl and Russell, 1992; Russell and Kössl, 1992). This is also the optimum frequency for causing temporary threshold shift in hair cells (Cody and Russell, 1985). A theory to account for this observation was first put forward by Zwislocki (1986) and involves a level-dependent change in the coupling between the TM and the OHCs. Zwislocki's proposal that the phase reversal is a result of interaction between the OHCs and the TM rather than as a result of a change in the mode of BM displacement is supported by our finding that BM displacements do not reverse phase at high levels. However, the finding that phase reversal occurs only at frequencies one half of an octave below CF, regardless of the frequency of CF (Kössl and Russell, 1992) lends support to the proposal that the TM may be a resonant structure (Allen,1980; Zwislocki and Kletsky, 1980; Brown et al., 1992) and that the frequency-dependent properties of IHCs and their afferent innervation may be shaped through an interaction between the proposed resonances of the BM and TM which is mediated and amplified by the OHCs.

Support for this idea may also be drawn from the differences in shape of the iso-response tuning curves shown in figure 4 for IHCs, OHCs and BM. The shapes of the OHC and BM tuning curves closely resemble each other and are similar to the 0.35 nm iso-displacement tuning curve derived from the iso-velocity tuning curves of the 18 kHz region of the BM first measured by Sellick et al. (1982). They differ from the IHC tuning curves in that the low frequency tail of the IHC tuning curve is about 20 dB less sensitive. For frequencies below about one half of an octave below CF, the IHCs are not excited until the OHC voltage responses approach saturation. At these frequencies it is suggested that OHCs act to attenuate the net shear displacement between TM and reticular lamina in the region of the IHCs as has been predicted by Allen 1980, Allen and Fahey,1993. For frequencies above the half-octave point, the IHCs are excited in proportion to both the level and the phase of the OHC receptor potential (Kössl and Russell, 1992). With respect to this proposal, it has been shown that in some damaged cochleas (Russell and Sellick, 1978), and in cochleas in which the OHCs have been selectively destroyed (Liberman and Dodds, 1984), the tuning curves of IHCs and afferent nerve fibres become broad and desensitized at the tip but more sensitive at the tail.

5 Acknowledgements

This work is supported by grants from the MRC, Hearing Research Trust and DFG. E. Murugasu is a Lee Kuan Yew fellow. We thank Drs. A.M Brown, C.J Kros and G.P Richardson for stimulating discussion and comments on the manuscript and Mr. J.A. Hartley for designing and building electronic equipment.

6 References

Allen J.B (1980) Cochlear micromechanics- A physical model of transduction. J. Acoust. Soc. Am. 68, 1660- 1670.

Allen J.B. and Fahey, P.F. (1993) Evidence for a second cochlear map. In: H. Duifhuis, J.W. Horst, P. van Dijk, S.M. vanNetten (Eds.), Biophysics of Hair Cell Sensory Systems, World Scientific, Singapore, 219-225.

Brown, A.M., Gaskill, S.A. and Williams, D.M. (1992) Mechanical filtering of sound in the inner ear. Proc. Roy. Soc. Lond. B 250, 29-34.

Brown, A.M., McDowell, B. and Forge, A. (1989) Acoustic distortion products can be used to monitor the effects of chronic gentamyicin treatment. Hear. Res. 42, 143-156.

Brownell, W.E., Bader, C.R., Bertrand, D. and Ribaupirre, Y. (1985) Evoked mechanical responses of isolated cochlear outer hair cells. Science 227, 194-196.

Canlon, B, Brundin, L. and Flock, Å. (1988) Acoustic stimulation causes tonotopic alterations in the length of isolated outer hair cells from the guinea pig hearing organ. Proc. Nat. Acad. Sci. 85, 7033-7035.

Cody A.R. and Russell, I.J. (1985) Outer hair cells in the mammalian cochlea and noise-induced hearing loss. Nature 315, 662-665.

Cooper, N.P. and Rhode, W.S. (1992) Basilar membrane mechanics in the hook region of the cat and the guinea-pig cochleae: sharp tuning and nonlinearity in the absence of baseline position shifts. Hear Res. 63, 163-190.

Davis, H. (1983) An active process in cochlear mechanics. Hear. Res. 9, 79-90.

Fritsch, K and Adamovsky, G., 1981 Simple circuit for feedback stabilization of a single mode optical fibre interferometer. Rev. Sci. Instrum. 52, 996-1000

Koelink, M.H., Slot, M, de Mul, F.F., Greve, J. Graaff, R. Dassel, A.C.M. and Aardnoudse, J.G.(1992) Laser doppler velocimeter based on the self-mixing effect in a fibre-coupled semiconductor laser: theory. Applied Optics, 18, 3401-3408.

Kössl M. and Russell, I.J. (1992) The phase and magnitude of hair cell receptor potentials and frequency tuning in the guinea pig cochlea. J. Neurosci. 12, 1575-1586

Liberman, M.C. and Dodds, L.W. (1984) Single-neuron labelling and chronic cochlear pathology. III. Stereocilia damage and alterations of threshold tuning curves. Hear Res. 16, 55-74.

Mountain, D.C. (1980) Changes in endocochlear potential and crossed olivocochlear bundle stimulation alter cochlear mechanics. Science, 210, 71-72.

O'Neil, M.P. and Beardon, A (1993) The amplitude and phase of basilar membrane motion in the turtle measured with laser-feedback interferometry. In: H. Duifhuis, J.W. Horst, P van Dijk, S.M. van Netten (Eds.), Biophysics of Hair Cell Sensory Systems, World Scientific, Singapore, 398-405.

Ruggero, M.A. and Rich, N.C. (1991) Furosemide alters organ of Corti mechanics: evidence for feedback of outer hair cells upon the basilar membrane. J. Neurosci. 11, 1057-1067

Russell, I.J. and Kössl, M. (1991) The voltage responses of hair cells in the basal turn of the guinea pig cochlea. J. Physiol., Lond. 235, 493-511.

Russell, I.J. and Kössl, M. (1992) Modulation of hair cell responses to tones by low-frequency biassing of the basilar membrane in the guinea pig cochlea. J. Neurosci. 12, 1587-1601.

Russell, I.J. and Sellick, P.M. (1978) Intracellular studies of hair cells in the mammalian cochlea. J. Physiol. (Lond.) 284, 261-290.

Seigel, J.H. and Kim, D.O. (1992) Efferent neural control of cochlear mechanics? Olivo-cochlear bundle affects cochlear biomechanical nonlinearity. Hear Res. 6, 171-182.

Sellick, P.M., Patuzzi, R. and Johnstone, B.M. (1982) Measurements of basilar membrane motion in the guinea pig using the Mössbauer technique. J. Acoust. Soc. Am. 72, 131-141.

Zwislocki, J.J. (1986) Analysis of cochlear mechanics. Hear. Res. 22, 155-169.

Zwislocki, J.J. and Smith, R.L. (1988) Phase reversal of ohc response at high sound intensities. In: J.P. Wilson and D.T. Kemp (Eds.), Cochlear Mechanisms, Plenum Press, New York, London, 163-168.
Zwislocki, J.J. and Kletsky, E.J. (1980) Micromechanics in the theory of cochlear mechanics. Hear. Res. 2, 505-512.

Origins of rate versus synchrony suppression: An evaluation based on two-tone interactions observed in mammalian IHCs

M.A. Cheatham and P. Dallos

Northwestern University, Auditory Physiology Laboratory, Frances Searle Building, 2299 North Campus Drive, Evanston IL 60208 USA

1 Introduction

The phenomenon of two-tone suppression (2TS) has enjoyed a relatively long history and it has now been documented at virtually every recording location in the peripheral auditory system. The literature, however, has been dominated by reports at the single unit level where two aspects of suppression have been investigated. Reductions in discharge rate due to the addition of a second tone to the stimulus (Sachs and Kiang, 1968) are well characterized and referred to as two-tone rate suppression (2TRS). In contrast, changes in the degree to which discharges are synchronized (Javel, 1981) are not as well understood. These studies of two-tone synchrony suppression (2TSS) remain controversial primarily due to the method used for their measurement (Greenwood, 1986). Since the temporal aspects of suppression are poorly defined, it is not known which of several potential sites and/or mechanisms are involved. A short list of candidates may well include nonlinearities associated with cochlear mechanics, the inner hair cell (IHC) transducer, voltage- and time-dependent conductances in the hair cell's basolateral membrane and synaptic and spike-generating processes. The situation is also complicated by the fact that ac components, appearing at any stage, can potentially produce 2TS in succeeding nonlinearites. Hence, as Greenwood (1986) states, there exist an assembly of sources that cannot be ruled out *a priori*. Since recordings from IHCs are not complicated by nonlinearities and time delays inherent in synaptic transmission and neural spike generation, they have advantages over postsynaptic measures of two-tone interactions.

Before evaluating changes in IHC ac and dc receptor potentials (RP) and how they relate to changes in rate and synchrony, methods commonly used at the single unit and hair cell levels are compared. In the neural experiments represented on the left-hand side of Fig. 1, suppression was usually studied using a constant frequency probe placed at the characteristic frequency (CF) of a given auditory nerve fiber. The probe was presented at a low level some 10 dB above rate threshold as shown by the symbol. Shaded areas represent suppressor frequency/level combinations that result in a criterion rate decrease. Regions associated with second tones below CF are referred to as low-side suppression areas; those produced by second tones above CF are called high-side suppression areas.

In contrast, the method we used to collect information from individual inner hair cells is shown on the right. Here the parameter is probe frequency which is varied to map out the response area of the cell. Changes in iso-input functions are measured in the presence of a constant frequency suppressor as represented by the symbol. In this example, a high-side suppressor, i.e., one whose frequency is above CF, is employed. The shaded area highlights magnitude differences between the single- and two-tone conditions. These are largest in the region around CF. Although the iso-output description has dominated the single unit literature, strong arguments can be made that iso-input measures are preferable when studying nonlinear systems such as the auditory periphery (Capranica, 1993).

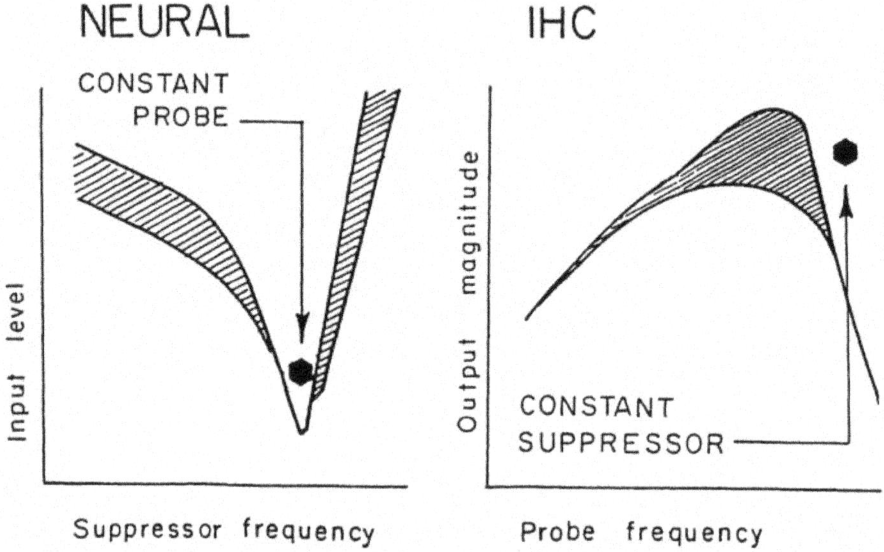

Figure 1. This schematic is used to demonstrate procedural differences between 2TS studied at the single unit and hair cell levels. On the left, a CF probe is usually introduced at a low level. Changes in discharge rate are produced by a suppressor whose frequency and level are varied to generate a predetermined decrease in rate. The shaded regions document these combinations. When presented alone, the suppressor does not produce a rate increase. On the right, an iso-input rather than an iso-response measure is obtained with the parameter being probe rather than suppressor frequency. Although the symbol indicates a high-side suppressor, low-side suppressors with frequencies below CF have also been utilized. In either case, the suppressor is excitatory when presented alone. The frequency response functions used for this schematic are representative of those collected at a relatively low level with the result that magnitude changes are largest at CF as revealed by low-level suppression data (Cheatham and Dallos, 1989, 1990b).

2 Comparisons at the Hair Cell and Single Unit Levels

Initial IHC experiments were difficult to compare with neural studies of rate suppression because the latter employed non-excitatory suppressors to avoid the rate increases produced by second tones inside the response area of the auditory nerve fiber. Since all of our IHC data were obtained using excitatory suppressors, results were supplemented using tones that produced little or no response in the cell. In addition, suppression related magnitude changes were also measured in the dc receptor potential (Cheatham and Dallos, 1990a). The latter is important when considering how changes in IHC receptor potentials relate to alterations in discharge rate. While synchrony suppression probably depends on changes in the ac receptor potential, rate changes are presumably associated with the dc component of the response. Since the ac receptor potential is filtered by the hair cell's basolateral membrane, it is ultimately the dc that sets

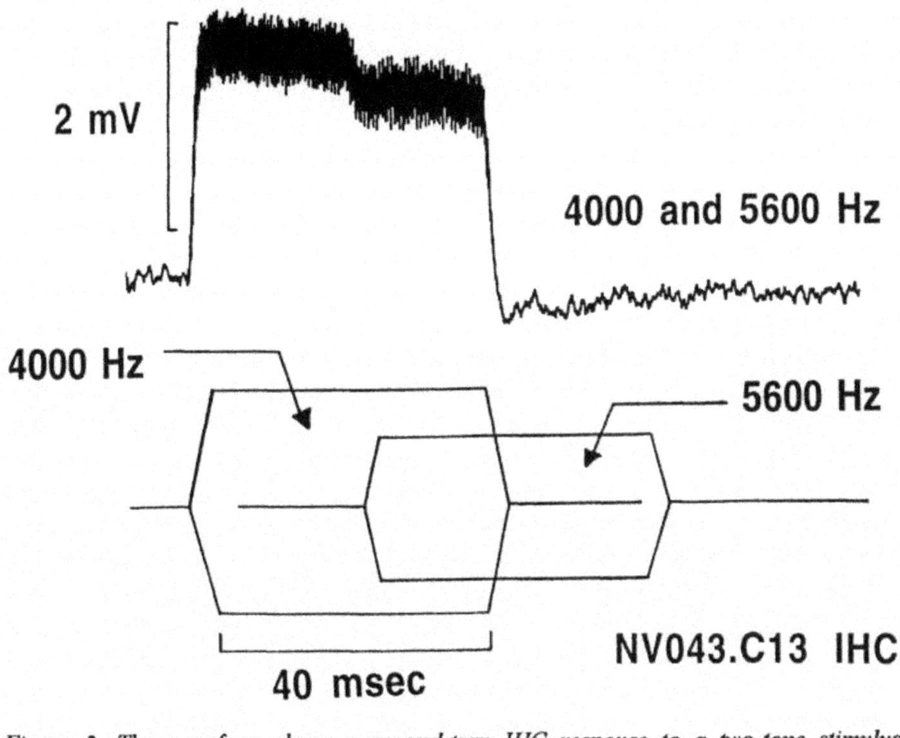

Figure 2. The waveform shows a second-turn IHC response to a two-tone stimulus presented at 50 dB. The timing of the two inputs appears at the bottom of the figure.

the single unit rate response at moderate and high stimulus frequencies (Russell and Sellick, 1978).

In the arrangement illustrated in Fig. 2, two inputs are presented at 50 dB. Stimulus frequencies are shown beside the averaged response waveform and a schematic represents the timing of the two inputs. Notice that the onset of the suppressor at 5600 Hz is delayed relative to the CF probe at 4000 Hz. Inspection of the waveform reveals that the high-side suppressor produces no dc response when presented alone which is indicated on the right during the time when only the higher frequency tone is present. This second input, however, reduces the response produced by the CF probe. Thus, the dc magnitude change, produced in response to the lower frequency tone at 4000 Hz, would probably be reflected in the auditory nerve and rate suppression would be observed.

2.1 Effects of Filtering by the Basolateral Membrane

In an attempt to define the general relations between 2TS in the IHC and in the auditory nerve, it is important to clarify meaning of the term "non-excitatory," i.e., to document responses produced by the suppressor alone. Since the ac response measured in the IHC is filtered by resistances and capacitances associated with the hair cell's basolateral membrane and by the recording electrode (Russell and Sellick, 1978, 1983; Dallos, 1984, 1985; Cheatham and Dallos, 1993, Fig. 3C), it is not a good indicator of the degree to which a tone stimulates the cell or of the signal magnitude present at a preceding mechanical nonlinearity. Consequently, the ac receptor potential measured at 5600 Hz underestimates the ac receptor current and, by inference, the input to the IHC. In other words, the high-side suppressor, which reduces the response at 4000 Hz, may have produced an ac receptor current, but not an ac receptor potential since the latter is subsequently filtered by the hair cell's basolateral membrane.

2.2 Sensitivity Differences Between AC and DC RPs

Although one might argue that the absence of a dc response at 5600 Hz militates against this possibility, differences in sensitivity between ac and dc components of the IHC receptor potential must be considered. For a third-turn IHC whose CF is 1000 Hz, the dc component is approximately 20 dB less sensitive than the ac response (Cheatham and Dallos, 1992, Fig. 8). A similar description also applies to single unit data where phase locking can be detected 10-20 dB below rate threshold (Rose et al. 1971; Evans, 1980; Johnson, 1980). Thus, when iso-rate tuning curves are compared with iso-synchrony curves in low CF units, the latter are displaced to lower levels (Evans, 1975; Rose et al. 1974; Javel, 1981; Javel et al. 1983b). This difference may indicate that rate measures are associated with dc receptor potentials while synchrony depends on ac responses. Consequently, their sensitivity differences may be reflected in the two types of suppression.

2.3 Rates of Growth

It is also remembered that the ac receptor potential rises, as level increases, with a unity slope while the dc grows with a slope of two (Goodman et al. 1982; Smith et al. 1983; Dallos, 1985). Thus, the disparity between the magnitudes of the two IHC response components becomes smaller when comparisons are made at high rather than low input levels. This is not unexpected if one assumes that the hair cell nonlinearity responsible for production of dc responses can be described by a power series where the behavior of individual distortion products is related to their order (Dallos, 1973). Since the dc is associated with the even terms, presumably dominated by the quadratic, it should grow at twice the rate of the fundamental.

3 Implications for Generation of 2TS in the Auditory Nerve

To clarify these considerations, a schematic is presented in Fig. 3 to represent iso-response patterns for idealized IHCs placed at three different locations along the cochlear spiral. The one on the left represents a low frequency region; that on the right, a high frequency region. The representation in the middle is approximately half way between base and apex at about the 5000 Hz location. The latter is used as a point of departure in the following discussion.

Notice that the ac receptor potential is measured only at low stimulus frequencies presumably because of filtering by the cell's basolateral membrane. However, following adjustment for these reductions, the compensated ac function becomes similar in shape to that for the dc and provides an estimate of the ac receptor current and, by inference, the input to the IHC. It is also assumed that this compensated ac function reflects the lower boundary of the region where interactions are possible between two stimulus inputs. Inputs near this boundary, however, do not produce measurable IHC dc receptor potentials since sensitivity differences do exist and a higher input level is required to obtain a just detectable, criterion dc response. Thus, shaded areas represent regions where two excitatory inputs can interact but where no dc receptor potential is produced by the IHC. In other words, the suppressor would be excitatory at the mechanical level but non-excitatory at the neural level. This description is analogous to that of Geisler et al. (1990) who suggested that outer hair cell (OHC) receptor currents become nonlinear at suppressor levels which do not generate significant dc receptor potentials in IHCs.

The shading in Fig. 3 does not extend into the CF region since the "suppressor" itself would probably be reduced by a CF probe due to mutual suppression (Hind et al. 1967; Legouix et al. 1973; Dallos and Cheatham, 1974; Kim et al. 1980; Delgutte, 1989, 1990; Geisler et al. 1990; Nuttall and Dolan, 1991, 1993; Cheatham and Dallos, 1992). Hence, the effect of a suppressor can be decreased or eliminated when it is near CF and when it is presented at a level commensurate with that of a CF probe. Since single unit tuning curves reflect the general character of the dc receptor potential produced by IHCs (Russell and Sellick, 1978), the shaded regions should approximate 2TS areas which emerge above and below CF at the neural level for "non-excitatory" suppressors.

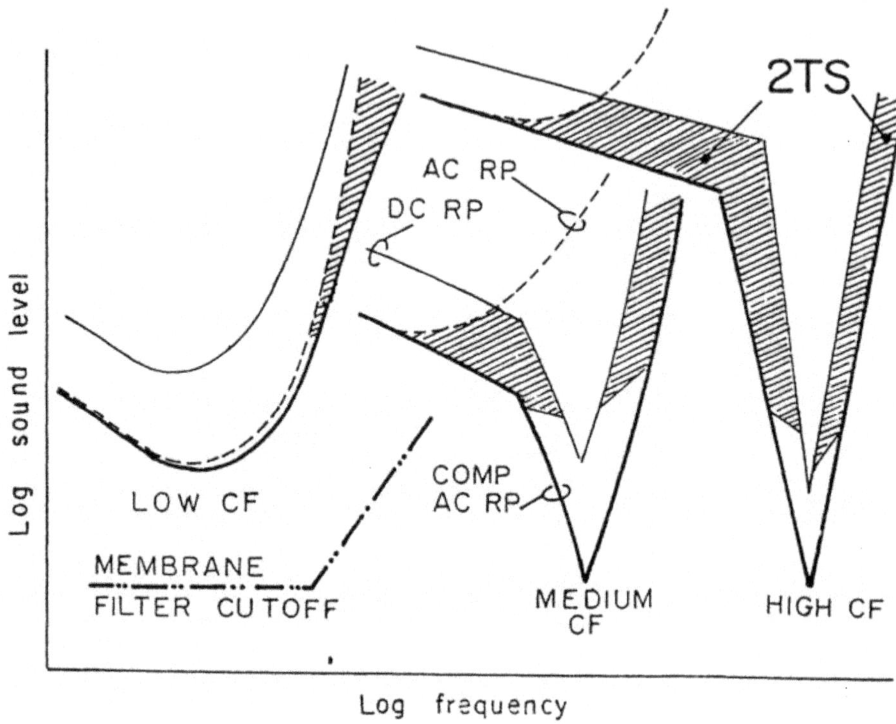

Figure 3. Iso-response functions are plotted for three idealized IHCs with low, medium and high CFs. The ac receptor potential measured from the cell is plotted with dashed lines. Because of filtering by resistances and capacitances associated with the cell's basolateral membrane, there is a measurable ac response at CF only in cells with low and moderate best frequencies. The cutoff of the membrane filter, common to all hair cells, is also provided. Following adjustment for this filtering effect, the compensated ac function (bold solid lines) becomes similar to that for the dc receptor potential (thin solid lines). Shaded regions represent areas where two-tone interactions can occur but where no dc would be produced by the cell. These may relate to similar regions at the single unit level.

It has been shown that auditory nerve fibers exhibit broader low-side suppression areas as CF increases (Arthur et al. 1971; Dallos and Cheatham, 1977; Harris, 1979; Costalupes et al. 1987) which may relate to the following. We propose that low-side suppression areas extend down to a frequency limit determined by the intersection of the high frequency slope of the basolateral membrane filter and the tail of the single unit tuning curve. For example, in the high CF representation in Fig. 3, the membrane filter crosses the tuning curve well below CF allowing a wider low-side suppression region to develop relative to that for the intermediate CF display in the middle of the figure.

Lastly, the reason for the lack of shading at the very lowest probe frequencies requires comment. In these frequency regions below the boundary representing the membrane filter, the unfiltered ac receptor potential may itself produce a dc response as a result of rectification and filtering by the synapse (Allen, 1983). Thus, a very low frequency suppressor would produce an increase in discharge rate and would no longer be considered non-excitatory. However, since rate decreases have been observed at the single unit level for non-excitatory suppressors with frequencies below the cutoff frequency of the basolateral membrane filter (Schmiedt, 1982; Fahey and Allen, 1985), these effects may relate to the velocity dependence of the IHC response for very low frequency inputs (Nuttall et al. 1981; Dallos and Santos-Sacchi, 1983; Russell and Sellick, 1983; Patuzzi and Yates, 1987). For example, the probe would be reduced due to interactions prior to IHC transduction. The very low frequency suppressor, however, would not produce a neural response when presented alone because at low frequencies the IHC responds to the velocity of the basilar membrane and not its displacement.

4 2TRS vs. 2TSS

This overall concept of how two-tone suppression evolves suggests that changes in the IHC's ac receptor potential should be reflected in the auditory nerve as changes in synchrony while changes in the overall dc response should contribute to changes in rate. (However, as noted above, in some circumstances, particularly at low frequencies, the ac receptor potential will produce rate changes via rectification and filtering by the synapse). When this association is valid, suppression-related magnitude changes recorded from individual IHCs should presage neural events. The relationship is useful since a general characterization of two-tone synchrony suppression is lacking in the literature, inasmuch as the method used to assess temporal aspects of the probe-related discharge, vector strength, is inadequate for this purpose (Greenwood, 1986). Due to this complication, measures of IHC ac receptor potentials may provide insights into the ways time-locked responses in the auditory nerve are modified when a second tone is added to the stimulus.

For example, it has been stated that synchrony suppression cannot be produced by non-excitatory suppressors whereas rate suppression can (Javel et al. 1983 a,b). This, however, may not always be the case. Suppose a suppressor and probe interact and reductions in probe response are achieved. In other words, the ac receptor potential produced by the probe is decreased and synchrony at the neural level is compromised. This could be achieved by suppressors higher in frequency than the probe that are subsequently filtered by the hair cell's basolateral membrane or by the synapse. Because of the interleaving of filters and nonlinearities in the peripheral auditory system, the determination of whether or not a suppressor is excitatory at any given stage is not always straightforward. Thus, until 2TSS is characterized further, generalizations may be premature.

A second feature concerns CF specificity. This issue is important because it has been proposed that if 2TSS is independent of probe frequency then basilar membrane mechanics cannot be considered as its potential source (Ruggero et al. 1992b). Relevant data from third turn of the guinea pig cochlea reveal that the largest suppression-related magnitude changes occur around the best frequency of the recording location for the cochlear microphonic (CM) measured in the organ of Corti fluid space (Cheatham and Dallos, 1990b, Fig. 7). Similar observations were made in ac receptor potentials recorded from individual IHCs (Cheatham and Dallos, 1989, Fig. 6). Thus, based on the CF specificity demonstrated in these results, 2TSS may also be frequency dependent, as is rate suppression, provided changes in synchrony are measured in low frequency fibers where CF probes generate phase-locked responses.

While the degree to which CF specificity is reflected in 2TSS at the neural level is controversial, Abbas (1978) did report that synchrony suppression was greatest for tones near CF. Schmiedt (1982) also suggested that results by Javel (1981, Fig. 7b) may not have revealed a frequency dependence simply because the suppressor, whose frequency was near CF, may have shifted the entire tuning curve up by a constant amount as in the data of Kiang and Moxon (1974). Moreover, because measures of 2TSS are complicated by the general use of vector strength as a metric, the CF specificity demonstrated in IHC ac receptor potentials may serve as an indicator in their stead.

A third item relates to vulnerability since it has been reported that 2TSS (Javel et al. 1983a) is less vulnerable to OHC loss than is 2TRS (Schmiedt and Zwislocki, 1980), provided shifts in sensitivity are compensated. In dealing with this issue, it is remembered that the ac receptor potential is more robust than the dc (Schmiedt, 1984; Cody and Russell, 1988), which is produced as a distortion product. This has been demonstrated in countless investigations using various methods and manipulations. Thus, linearizing the system will affect dc-dependent events like rate suppression to a greater degree than synchrony suppression which is associated with the ac component of the response.

The rate of suppression growth also pertains to the issue of vulnerability. If decreases in probe response are plotted versus suppressor level (Cheatham, 1985), the decrease for the fundamental component of the CM response is 1 dB/dB increase in suppressor level. In other words, the function has a slope of -1. This is consistent with measures of basilar membrane mechanics for suppressors below CF (Ruggero et al. 1992a,b) and with measures of 2TSS in single unit responses (Javel et al. 1983b). The decrease for the summating potential, however, is twice that for the CM (Cheatham, 1985). Similar differences between ac and dc responses were also observed in IHC receptor potentials (Cheatham and Dallos, 1990a). The implication is that 2TRS will exhibit greater rates of suppression growth relative to 2TSS because rate suppression depends on the dc rather than the ac component of the IHC response. This has been documented in the single unit literature (Abbas and Sachs, 1976; Fahey and Allen, 1985; Costalupes et al. 1987; Delgutte, 1990) where suppression growth, for rate, exceeds 1 dB/dB increase in suppressor level. The fact that ac and dc responses exhibit different rates of suppression growth suggests that any insult that reduces input to the IHC will affect rate suppression to a greater extent than synchrony suppression.

5 Conclusion

It is suggested that one should exercise caution when evaluating differences between 2TSS and 2TRS which may relate as much to their respective dependence on the IHC's ac and dc receptor potentials as to their place of origin. Thus, it is difficult on the basis of IHC results from the apical part of the cochlea to eliminate any potential sources of 2TSS including cochlear mechanics. In fact, the only situation where basilar membrane mechanics are clearly not involved as a site for 2TS is in the basal, high frequency region of the cochlea when both probe and suppressor are placed on the low frequency tails of single unit tuning curves. In these cases, the basilar membrane response is linear with the result that the IHC and/or the synapse between the IHC and its innervating nerve fiber become likely sources for changes in synchrony. However, in the apex, where CF probes produce time-locked neural responses, generation sites prior to and including IHC transduction should be assessed. Consequently, for the behaviorally relevant low frequencies, cochlear mechanics should not be excluded from "the ensemble of mechanisms" (Greenwood, 1986) that probably underlie 2TSS. Ultimately, of course, the challenge will be to distinguish individual contributors and to define their properties and regions of operation.

6 Acknowledgment

Work supported by the NIDCD grant #DC00089, Studies in Cochlear Hair cell Transduction. The care and use of all animals used in the experiments summarized here were approved by the National Institutes of Health and by the Animal Care and Use Committee of Northwestern University.

7 References

Abbas, P.J. (1978). Effects of stimulus frequency on two-tone suppression: A comparison of physiological and psychophysical results. J. Acoust. Soc. Am. 63, 1878-1886.

Abbas, P.J. and Sachs, M.B. (1976). Two-tone suppression in auditory nerve fibers: Extension of a stimulus-response relationship. J. Acoust. Soc. Am. 59, 112-122.

Allen, J.B. (1983). A hair cell model of neural response. In: E. de Boer and M.A. Viergever (Eds.), Mechanics of Hearing, Delft University Press, The Netherlands, pp. 193-202.

Arthur, R.M., Pfeiffer, R.R. and Suga, N. (1971). Properties of two-tone inhibition in primary auditory neurons. J. Physiol. 212, 21-31.

Capranica, R.R. (1993). The untuning of the tuning curve: is it time? The Neurosciences 4, 401-408.

Cheatham, M.A. (1985). Growth of suppression in the cochlear potentials. Hear. Res. 18, 291-294.

Cheatham, M.A. and Dallos, P. (1989). Two-tone suppression in inner hair cell responses. Hear. Res. 40, 187-196.

Cheatham, M.A. and Dallos, P. (1990a). Two-tone interactions in inner hair cell receptor potentials: AC versus DC effects. Hear. Res. 43, 135-139.

Cheatham, M.A. and Dallos, P. (1990b). Comparison of low- and high-side two-tone suppression in inner hair cell and organ of Corti responses. Hear. Res. 50, 193-210.

Cheatham, M.A. and Dallos, P. (1992). Two-tone suppression in inner hair cell responses: Correlates of rate suppression in the auditory nerve. Hear. Res. 60, 1-12.

Cheatham, M.A. and Dallos, P. (1993). Longitudinal comparisons of IHC ac and dc receptor potentials recorded from the guinea pig cochlea. Hear. Res. 68, 107-114.

Cody, A.R. and Russell, I.J. (1988). Acoustically induced hearing loss: Intracellular studies in the guinea pig cochlea. Hear. Res. 35, 59-70.

Costalupes, J.A., Rich, N.C. and Ruggero, M.A. (1987). Effects of excitatory and non-excitatory suppressor tones on two-tone rate suppression in auditory nerve fibers. Hear. Res. 26, 155-164.

Dallos, P. (1973). The Auditory Periphery. Academic Press, New York NY.

Dallos, P. (1984). Some electrical circuit properties of the organ of Corti. II. Analysis including reactive elements. Hear. Res. 14, 281-291.

Dallos, P. (1985). Response characteristics of mammalian cochlear hair cells. J. Neurosci. 5, 1591-1608.

Dallos, P. and Cheatham, M.A. (1974). Cochlear potential correlates of cubic difference tones. In: E. Zwicker and E. Terhardt (Eds.), Facts and Models in Hearing, Springer-Verlag, Berlin, pp. 312-322.

Dallos, P. and Cheatham, M.A. (1977). Analog of two-tone suppression in whole nerve response. J. Acoust. Soc. Am. 62, 1048-1051.

Dallos, P. and Santos-Sacchi, J. (1983). AC receptor potentials from hair cells in the low-frequency region of the guinea pig cochlea. In: W.R. Webster and L.M. Aitkin (Eds.), Mechanisms of Hearing, Monash University Press, Clayton, Australia, pp. 11-16.

Delgutte, B. (1989). Physiological mechanisms of masking and intensity discrimination. J. Acoust. Soc. Am. 85, S14.

Delgutte, B. (1990). Physiological mechanisms of psychophysical masking: Observations from auditory-nerve fibers. J. Acoust. Soc. Am. 87, 791-809.

Evans, E.F. (1975). The cochlear nerve and cochlear nucleus. In: W.D. Keidel and W.D. Neff (Eds.), Handbook of Sensory Physiology, Springer-Verlag, Heidelberg, Germany, pp. 1-108.

Evans, E.F. (1980). 'Phase-locking' of cochlear fibres and the problem of dynamic range. In: G. van den Brink and F.A. Bilsen (Eds.), Psychophysical, Physiological and Behavioral Studies of Hearing, Delft University Press, Delft, The Netherlands, pp. 300-309.

Fahey, P.F. and Allen, J.B. (1985). Nonlinear phenomena as observed in the ear canal and the auditory nerve. J. Acoust. Soc. Am. 77, 599-612.

Geisler, C.D., Yates, G.K., Patuzzi, R.B. and Johnstone, B.M. (1990). Saturation of hair cell receptor currents causes two-tone suppression. Hear. Res. 44, 241-256.

Goodman, D.A., Smith, R.L. and Chamberlain, S.C. (1982). Intracellular and extracellular responses in the organ of Corti of the gerbil. Hear. Res. 7, 161-179.

Greenwood, D.D. (1986). What is "Synchrony suppression"? J. Acoust. Soc. Am. 79, 1857-1872.

Harris, D.M. (1979). Action potential suppression, tuning curves and thresholds: Comparison with single fiber data. Hear. Res. 1, 133-154.

Hind, J.E., Anderson, D.J., Brugge, J.F. and Rose, J.E. (1967). Coding of information pertaining to paired low-frequency tones in single auditory nerve fibers of the squirrel monkey. J. Neurophysiol.. 30, 794-816.

Javel, E. (1981). Suppression of auditory nerve responses. I. Temporal analysis, intensity effects and suppression contours. J. Acoust. Soc. Am. 69, 1735-1745.

Javel, E., McGee, J.A., Walsh, E.J. and Farley, G.R. (1983a). Studies of "synchrony suppression" in normal and hearing-impaired cats. In: W.R. Webster and L.M. Aitkin (Eds.), Mechanisms of Hearing, Monash University Press, Clayton, Victoria, Australia, pp. 46-51.

Javel, E., McGee, J., Walsh, E.J., Farley, G.R. and Gorga, M.P. (1983b). Suppression and auditory nerve responses. II. Suppression threshold and growth, iso-suppression contours. J. Acoust. Soc. Am. 74, 801-813.

Johnson, D.H. (1980). The relationship between spike rate and synchrony in responses of auditory-nerve fibers to single tones. J. Acoust. Soc. Am. 68, 1115-1122.

Kiang, N.Y.S. and Moxon, E.C. (1974). Tails of tuning curves of auditory nerve fibers. J. Acoust. Soc. Am. 55, 620-630.

Kim, D.O., Molnar, C.E. and Matthews, J.W. (1980). Cochlear mechanics: Nonlinear behavior in two-tone responses as reflected in cochlear-nerve-fiber responses and ear-canal sound pressure. J. Acoust. Soc. Am. 67, 1704-1721.

Legouix, J.P., Remond, N.C. and Greenbaum, H. (1973). Interference and two-tone inhibition. J. Acoust. Soc. Am. 53, 409-419.

Nuttall, A.L., Brown, M.C., Masta, R.I. and Lawrence, M. (1981). Inner hair cell responses to the velocity of basilar membrane motion in the guinea pig. Brain Res. 211, 323-336.

Nuttall, A.L. and Dolan, D.F. (1991). Two-tone suppression in inner hair cell ac and dc receptor potentials. Abst. Assoc. Res. Otolaryngol., p. 132.

Nuttall, A.L. and Dolan, D.F. (1993). Reply to "Comment on 'Two-tone suppression of inner hair cell and basilar membrane responses in the guinea pig' [J. Acoust. Soc. Am. 93, 390-400 (1993)]". J. Acoust. Soc. Am. 94, 3511-3514.

Patuzzi, RB. and Yates, G.K. (1987). Velocity and displacement coupling of mammalian inner hair cells and the mechanical resonance of the stereocilia. Hear. Res. 30, 83-98.

Rose, J.E., Hind, J.E., Anderson, D.J. and Brugge, J.F. (1971). Some effects of stimulus intensity on response of auditory nerve fibers in the squirrel monkey. J. Neurophysiol. 34, 685-699.

Rose, J.E., Kitzies, L.M., Gibson, M.M. and Hind, J.E. (1974). Observations on phase sensitive neurons of anteroventral cochlear nucleus of the cat: Nonlinearity of cochlear output. J. Neurophysiol. 37, 218-253.

Ruggero, M.A., Robles, L., Rich, N.C. and Recio, A. (1992a). Basilar membrane responses to two-tone and broadband stimuli. Phil. Trans. R. Soc. Lond. B 336, 307-315.

Ruggero, M.A., Robles, L. and Rich, N.C. (1992b). Two-tone suppression in the basilar membrane of the chinchilla cochlea: Mechanical basis of auditory-nerve rate suppression. J. Neurophysiol. 68, 1087-1099.

Russell, I.J. and Sellick, P.M. (1978). Intracellular studies of hair cells in the guinea pig cochlea. J. Physiol. 284, 261-290.

Russell, I.J. and Sellick, P.M. (1983). Low-frequency characteristics of intracellularly recorded receptor-potentials in guinea pig cochlear hair cells. J. Physiol. 338, 179-206.

Sachs, M.B. and Kiang, N.Y.S. (1968). Two-tone inhibition in auditory nerve fibers. J. Acoust. Soc. Am. 43, 1120-1128.

Schmiedt, R.A. (1982). Boundaries of two-tone rate suppression of cochlear-nerve activity. Hear. Res. 7, 335-351.

Schmiedt, R.A. (1984). Acoustic injury and the physiology of hearing. J. Acoust. Soc. Am. 76, 1293-1317.

Schmiedt, R.A. and Zwislocki, J.J. (1980). Effects of hair cell lesions on responses of cochlear nerve fibers. II. Single- and two-tone intensity functions in relations to tuning curves. J. Neurophysiol. 43, 1390-1405.

Smith, R.L., Frisina, R.D. and Goodman, D.A. (1983) Intensity functions and dynamic responses from the cochlea to the cochlear nucleus. In: R.Klinke and R.Hartmann (Eds.), Hearing--Physiological Bases and Psychophysics, Springer-Verlag, Berlin, pp. 112-117.

Analysis of pure-tone detection and intensity discrimination in the auditory nerve.

B. W. Edwards and N. F. Viemeister

Department of Psychology, University of Minnesota
75 East River Rd., Minneapolis, MN, USA 55455

1 Introduction

Previous researchers have examined the ability of auditory nerve fibers to encode stimulus intensity with a rate code, for which an increase in intensity is represented by an increase in discharge rate (for a recent review, see Winter and Palmer, 1991). The simplicity of this mechanism is compelling and it has been demonstrated that a small number of fibers is sufficient to produce discrimination performance seen psychoacoustically. In many of these analyses, in order to quantify the ability of an ideal observer to make decisions about stimulus intensity using the discharge rate of a single fiber, the mean and standard deviation of the spike count within a specified time window for both I, the standard, and $I+\Delta I$, the comparison, are estimated. If the standard deviations of the two distributions are equal to , performance can be described using the measure

$$d' = (\mu_c - \mu_s)/\sigma \qquad (1)$$

where μ_c and μ_s are the means of the comparison and standard spike count distributions, respectively. Since the standard deviations are not equal, however, various methods have been used to approximate d' using estimates of σ_c and σ_s (e.g., Young and Barta, 1986; Viemeister, 1988; Kim et al., 1990). Once an estimate of d' is obtained, thresholds for a criterion d' are estimated as a function of discharge rate of the standard.

An implicit assumption underlying Eq. 1, and thus the threshold estimation procedure, is that the distributions of the number of discharges over a given duration are Gaussian. Fig. 1 shows distributions for the number of discharges in a 50-ms window for two different stimulus intensities, and it is clear from the figure that the two distributions are not well-approximated by a discrete Gaussian distribution. Viemeister (1988) compared ROC curves for low, medium, and high spontaneous fibers to those resulting from Gaussian distributions and noted that curves from low spontaneous fibers, particularly at low stimulus levels, were different from those produced with Gaussian distributions. Even though the Gaussian approximation is poor for some conditions, however, it is possible that thresholds estimated from Equation 1 still provide a reasonably accurate measure of discrimination performance.

This paper considers the ability of an auditory fiber to encode intensity without making any assumptions on the form of the distributions. Specifically, using the distributions for the number of discharges during a 50 ms interval resulting from the standard and from the comparison, the area under the ROC curve is calculated, which is equivalent to the percent correct [P(c)] in a 2IFC task (Green and Swets, 1966).

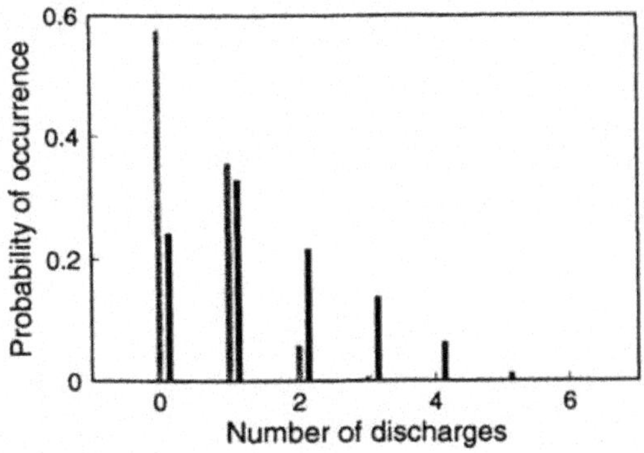

Figure 1. Probability distributions for the number of discharges in a 50 ms window for two stimulus levels. The spontaneous rate was 0 /s.

2 Method

The data were obtained by Dr. Nick L. Powers using techniques described in Powers (1991). Ten seconds of spontaneous activity was recorded for most units. Twenty seconds of activity was recorded during stimulation with pure tones at CF and a fixed intensity. Ten stimulus levels were used per fiber, the lowest level near the beginning of the rate-intensity (R-I) function and the others at successive 5 dB increments.

Spike records were divided into contiguous 50 ms windows: The first 3 windows were discarded so that only steady-state responses were examined. Each record thus consisted of 197, 50- ms spike count samples, and spike count probability distributions were estimated for each unit and stimulus level. Figure 1 shows two such distributions.

For each intensity level as the standard, P(c) for discrimination was estimated for successively higher stimulus levels of that fiber as the comparison. P(c) was also estimated for absolute detection by using spontaneous activity as the standard (subsequently, we will only refer to the discrimination task and the detection task will be implied). Thus, intensity discrimination performance was estimated for intensity differences in multiples of 5 dB. The P(c)'s for a fixed level of the standard produce a neurometric function (Movshon et al., 1982) -- P(c) vs ΔI. Discrimination thresholds were defined as the ΔI necessary for 70% correct performance and were estimated from the neurometric functions.

3 Results

3.1 Intensity Thresholds

Figure 2 shows neurometric functions obtained for two different fibers and are similar to those shown by Viemeister (1988). Discrimination thresholds from four different fibers are shown in Figure 3. Thresholds are plotted as a function of the intensity of the

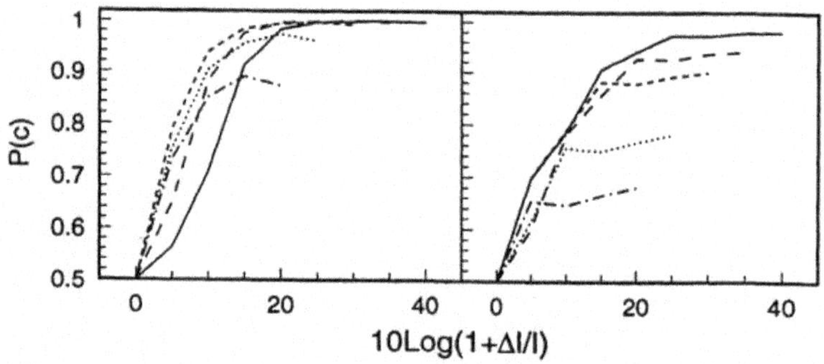

Figure 2. Neurometric functions for five different stimulus levels of the standard, in increments of 5 dB. Each panel represents a different fiber.

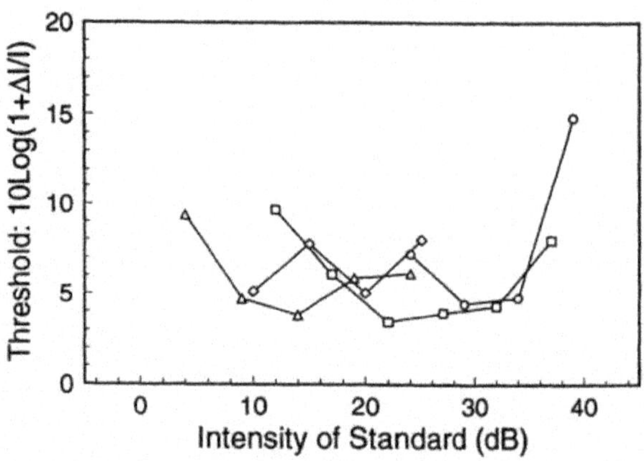

Figure 3. Intensity discrimination thresholds estimated from the neurometric functions of four fibers.

standard and are similar to ones shown by Delgutte (1987), Viemeister (1988) and Geisler et al. (1991). Examination of threshold functions for many units reveal that they all demonstrate a concave-upward form, but have different minima and acceleration rates (see also Delgutte, 1987).

3.2 Rate Thresholds

The same neurometric functions shown in Figure 2 can be replotted as a function of change in rate between the standard and comparison instead of ΔI. These are shown in Figure 4, along with neurometric functions from one other fiber. For example, the five overlapping functions represented by the connected circles are the same data as the five functions shown in the left panel of Figure 2, but with P(c) plotted as a function of rate increase instead of intensity increase. The abscissa of each data point in Figure 2 has effectively been transformed with that unit's R-I function. Unlike the functions in Figure 2, the neurometric functions in Figure 4 are almost identical.

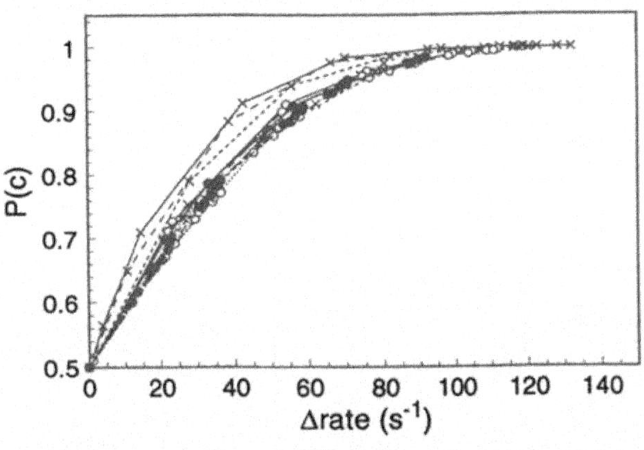

Figure 4. Neurometric functions for three fibers plotted as a function of change in rate instead of ΔI. Five functions are shown for each fiber; different fibers are represented by different connected symbols.

Neurometric functions were obtained for over 200 fibers. Thresholds representing P(c)=70% were estimated from each fiber with different average firing rates as the standard, including spontaneous activity. Instead of plotting thresholds as a function of intensity of the standard as in Figure 3, thresholds in Figure 5 are plotted as a function of the average firing rate of the standard. The different symbols in Figure 5 represent different spontaneous rates categorized by Liberman (1978): circles are low (s.r. < .5/s), crosses are medium (.5/s < s.r. < 18/s), and squares are high (18/s < s.r.). Thresholds are independent of s.r. type and also are independent of the CF of the fiber (not shown). Thus, this representation considerably simplifies analysis of detection and discrimination performance of single fibers.

The data shown in Figure 5 indicate that the threshold change in firing rate does not correspond to either to a fixed Δr, as is frequently assumed, or to a fixed $\Delta r/\sqrt{r}$. For rates above approximately 50 /s. the rate change necessary for P(c)=70% is approximately linear with the standard rate: $\Delta r \approx 0.07r+18$.

The mean and standard deviation of the spike count distributions were estimated for each fiber and discharge rate. An best fit to the data was made and an analytic expression representing mean and standard deviation as a function of average firing rate was obtained. Discrimination thresholds were then estimated using a variation of Equation 1 described by Viemeister et al.(1992). The dash-dot line in Figure 5 shows the prediction. The prediction is seen to be poor for standards with discharge rates less than approximately 50/s, but are relatively accurate for standard rates above that. This is most likely due to the fact that spike count distributions are not Gaussian at low discharge rates but approach a Gaussian shape as the discharge rate increases.

The dashed line represents the thresholds for a Poisson process; the dotted line represents the thresholds for a dead-time modified Poisson process with a 1 ms dead-time

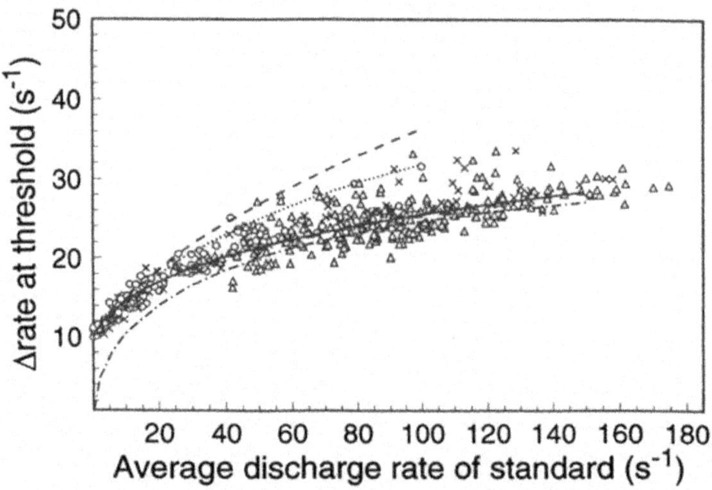

Figure 5. Thresholds as a function average firing rate of the standard for low (circles), medium (crosses) and high (triangles) s.r. fibers. The dash-dot line is the prediction using a technique similar to Equation 1; the dashed line is the prediction for a Poisson process; the dotted line is the prediction for a 1-ms dead-time modified Poisson process; the solid line is the prediction for a modified Poisson process using Gaumond's recovery function.

refractory effect. They were derived analytically, the latter using the probability distributions derived by Möller (1974). Both lines fall well above the thresholds obtained from the data.

A point process simulation was used to create 20 s discharge records at various firing rates, where the point process had a 40-ms recovery function described by Gaumond et al. (1982), i.e., a dead-time of 0.75 ms and a relative recovery function consisting two contiguous exponentials. Thresholds were estimated in the same manner as with the experimental data. The solid line in Figure 5 shows a fit to the simulation data and is consistent with thresholds from the experimental data. This demonstrates that the obtained thresholds are lower than those predicted by a Poisson process because of refractory effects defined by Gaumond's recovery function, which negatively correlate the discharge occurrences and thus reduces the spike count variance. This result is interesting in that the relative portion of the recovery function has more of an effect on lowering the thresholds than does the dead-time.

3.3 Duration Effects

Thresholds for a Poisson process when the rate of the standard is 0/s can be simply calculated using point process theory. The prediction should correspond to that obtained with the data since refractory effects have little impact on discharge statistics at low discharge rates. Defining N as the number of discharges during a counting interval of duration T, and □ as the average firing rate of the Poisson process, the probability of correctly choosing the signal interval in a 2IFC task when the average firing rate in the standard interval is 0/s is:

$$\begin{aligned} 0.7 &= \Pr\{\text{correct decision in 2IFC}\} \\ &= \Pr\{N>0\}+0.5 \cdot \Pr\{N=0\} \\ &= 1-\exp(-\mu T)+0.5 \cdot \exp(-\mu T) \\ &= 1-0.5 \cdot \exp(-\mu T) \qquad (2) \end{aligned}$$

and the firing rate at threshold is

$$\begin{aligned} \mu &= -\ln(0.6)/T \\ &= 10.2\ /\text{s}, \qquad \text{for } T=0.05\ \text{s}. \qquad (3) \end{aligned}$$

This value can be seen to correspond to the thresholds obtained in Figure 5 for standards with average firing rates of 0/s.

Notice that, when the rate of the standard is 0/s, thresholds are inversely proportional to T. For standards at high rates, the Gaussian approximation to the Poisson count distribution and Equation 1 are valid, so that thresholds in this region are inversely proportional to $\sqrt{T}$. Figure 6 shows thresholds derived for 25 ms durations. Also shown by the solid line is $\sqrt{2}$ times the prediction using Gaumond's recovery function from Figure 5. Compared to the thresholds for 50 ms observations, thresholds for 25 ms observations at 0/s have doubled while thresholds approach a $\sqrt{2}$ increase, consistent with $\sqrt{T}$ improvement, at high rates of the standard. Thus, in general, thresholds for observation durations different from 50 ms cannot simply be obtained by scaling the threshold functions for 50 ms since the form of the function will change; one must derive the threshold function for each different duration.

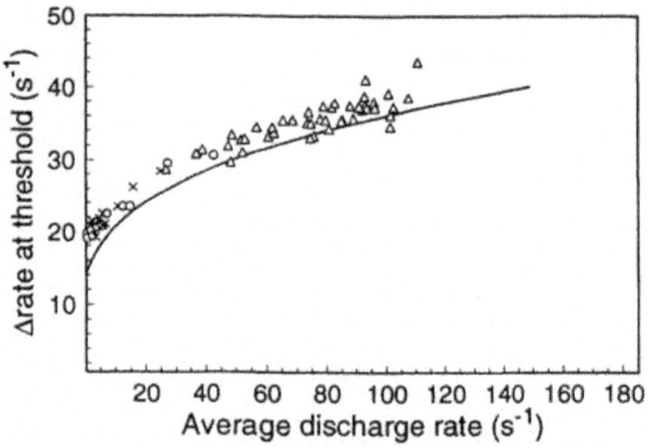

Figure 6. Thresholds estimated from a representative group of fibers using a 25-ms counting window. The solid line is $\sqrt{2}$ times the prediction from the modified Poisson process shown by the solid line in Figure 5. Symbols are the same as in Figure 5.

3.4 Nonrenewal Correlation

Previous research has shown that auditory nerve data has long term correlation indicating fractal behavior (Teich, 1989; Teich et al, 1990). Since refractoriness can be considered short-term correlation and has the effect of reducing thresholds (compare Poisson prediction to prediction for renewal process with Gaumond's recovery function in Fig 5), we investigated whether the long-term correlation affects thresholds. Spike records were shuffled, as described by Perkel et al. (1967). Randomly rearranging the interspike intervals should have no effect on a renewal point process such as the one described by Gaumond's recovery function; any long-term or cross-interval correlation, however, will be disrupted.

The first 150 ms of each 20 s record were removed and the remaining interspike intervals were randomly shuffled. Thresholds from the shuffled data were estimated as before and are shown in the left plot of Figure 7 for a representative group of fibers, while the right plot shows the unshuffled thresholds for the same subset of fibers taken from Figure 5. As can be seen, thresholds have been elevated a significantly simply by shuffling the intervals. Two observations can be made from this result. One is that inter-spike intervals within the 50-ms observations were negatively correlated, thereby reducing the variability of the spike count and reducing thresholds. The other is that a shorter recovery function than estimated by Gaumond is necessary to account for the thresholds once this non-renewal correlation is removed. That is, the predictions in Figure 5 show that thresholds are lowered from those for a Poisson process by the inclusion of a refractory period: the longer the refractory period, the more thresholds are lowered. Since Figure 7 shows a 40-ms refractory period under-predicts thresholds from the shuffled data, a shorter refractory period is necessary to account for the raised thresholds in the left panel of Figure 7, i.e., a more appropriate point process model might be one with a recovery function shorter than Gaumond estimates and with high-order cross-interval correlation.

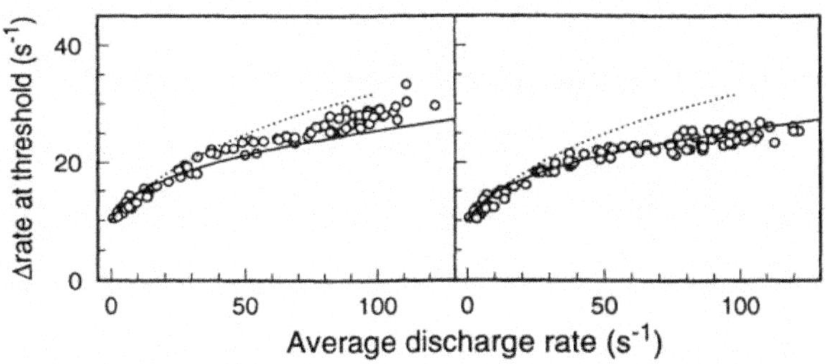

Figure 7. The right panel represents a subset of the thresholds shown in Figure 5, where s.r. has not been distinguished by symbol. The left panel shows the thresholds obtained for the same fibers after the inter-spike intervals within each record were shuffled. The solid line and dotted lines show the predictions for a Poisson process modified by Gaumond's recovery function and a 1-ms dead-time modified Poisson process, respectively, both from Figure 5.

It should be noted that this effect does not seem to be caused by fractal behavior because that phenomenon increases the variance with duration at a greater rate than expected for a renewal process and would cause thresholds to *decrease* when shuffled. Lowen and Teich (1992) have demonstrated that the Fano-factor (the ratio of spike count variance to mean) decreases after the inter-spike intervals are shuffled for counting times greater than approximately 100 ms, a characteristic of the fractal behavior. They also demonstrated,however, that the Fano-factor *increases* after shuffling for counting intervals less than 100 ms, a characteristic not accounted for by fractal behavior. An increase in variance after shuffling would increase the thresholds, as seen in Figure 7. When Lowen and Teich attempted to measure first order cross-interval correlation, however, no clear trend was evident in the data, indicating that the results may be caused by higher order correlation, consistent with the findings of Teich and Khanna (1985).

3.5 Weber's Law

Pure tone intensity discrimination thresholds obtained psychoacoustically produce a nearly constant Weber fraction when spread of excitation is limited (Viemeister, 1974). Consider, for example, discrimination performance with a Weber fraction of 1, i.e., $\Delta I/I = 1$ for P(c) = 70%. This means that the level of the comparison at threshold is 3 dB greater than the level of the standard.

For 50-ms observation intervals,the amount the discharge rate must be incremented to reach threshold as a function of rate of the standard is defined by the solid line in Figure 5 -- call this r(R). For a fiber to produce a discrimination threshold with a Weber fraction of 1 when firing at a rate R, the rate must increase exactly $\Delta r(R)$ in 3 dB. If $R(I)$ is the R-I function with I in dB, then the following must hold everywhere in the R-I function for the fiber to produce discrimination performance with $\Delta I/I = 1$:

$$R(I{+}3\mathrm{dB}) = R(I){+}\Delta r(R(I)). \qquad (4)$$

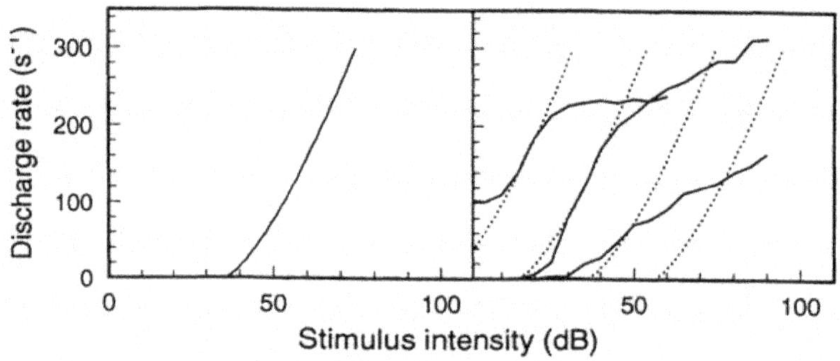

Figure 8. The left panel shows the hypothetical R-I function necessary for a single fiber to give intensity discrimination performance with ΔI/I = 1 using 50-ms counting windows. The right panel shows duplicates of the hypothetical function shifted along the intensity axis, along with R-I functions for a high, medium, and low s.r fiber.

The left panel of Figure 8 shows a R-I function derived using Equation 4 and the ; the starting point along the abscissa is arbitrary. We can now compare R-I functions for typical auditory nerve fibers with that of the ideal to examine each fiber's performance.

The right panel of Figure 8 shows R-I functions for high, medium, and low s.r. fibers taken from Möller et al (1991). Also plotted are shifted versions of the ideal R-I function from the left panel. A fiber achieves $\Delta I/I = 1$ performance wherever the slope of its R-I function equals that of the ideal function. As can be seen, both the high and medium s.r. fibers achieve this at the point where their R-I slope is maximal, but the low s.r. fiber does not, except perhaps just above 0/s. In fact, approximately four low s.r. fibers must be grouped in order to achieve the appropriate R-I slope. These results are in concurrence with those shown by others (e.g., Viemeister, 1983; Young and Barta,1986).

4 Summary

—Thresholds as a function of average firing rate, when estimated using a distribution-free measure, are independent of CF and s.r. of the fiber;
—Thresholds derived using variations of Equation 1 do not hold for small discharge rates of the standard due to the inappropriateness of the Gaussian assumption of the spike count distribution;
—Thresholds are predicted by a Poisson process modified by Gaumond's recovery function;
—The threshold function does not simply scale as a function of observation duration T: for very low standard discharge rates thresholds are inversely proportional to T, and for very high standard discharge rates thresholds are inversely proportional to $\sqrt{T}$;
—Thresholds increase when interspike intervals are shuffled, indicating that interspike intervals are negatively correlated in a non-renewal manner not accounted for by fractal behavior;
—To compare intensity coding performance of different fibers, the slopes of their R-I functions must be compared at the same discharge rate; using this technique, low s.r. fibers encode intensity poorer than medium or high s.r. fibers.

5 Acknowledgements

The authors would like to thank Dr. Nick L. Powers for allowing us to use his data. This research was supported by NIDCD grant DC00683.

6 References

Delgutte, B. (1987) Peripheral auditory processing of speech information: Implications from a physiological study of intensity discrimination. In: M.E.H. Schouten (ed.), The Psychophysics of Speech Perception, Nijhot, Dordrecht, The Netherlands, 333-353.

Gaumond, R.P., Molnar, C.E. and Kim, D.O. (1982) Stimulus and recovery dependence of cat cochlear nerve fiber spike discharge probability. J. Neurophysiol. 48, 856-873.

Geisler, W.S., Albrect, D.G., Salvi, R.J. and Saunders, S.S. (1991) Discrimination performance of single neurons: rate and temporal-pattern information. J. Neurophysiol., 66, 334-362.

Green, D.M. and Swets, J.A. (1966) Signal detection theory and psychophysics. Wiley, New York.

Kim, D.O., Chang, S.O. and Dirianni, J.G. (1990) A population study of auditory nerve fibers in unanesthetized decerebrate cats: Response to pure tones. J. Acoust. Soc. Am. 87, 1648-1655.

Liberman, M.C. (1978) Auditory-nerve response from cats raised in a low-noise chamber. J. Acoust. Soc. Am. 63, 442-455.

Lowen, S.B. and Teich, M.C. (1992) Auditory-nerve action potentials form a nonrenewal point process over short as well as long time scales. J. Acoust. Soc. Am. 92, 803-806.

Movshon, J.A., Tolhurst, D.J. and Dean, A.F. (1982) How many neurons are involved in perceptual decisions? Invest. Ophthalmol. Vis. Sci. 22, 207.

Müller, J.W. (1974) Some formulae for a dead-time-distorted Poisson process. Nucl. Instrum. and Meth. 117, 401- 404.

Müller, M., Robertson, D. and Yates, G.K. (1991) Rate-versus-level functions of primary auditory nerve fibres: Evidence for square law behaviour of all fibre categories in the guinea pig. Hear. Res., 55, 50-56.

Perkel, D.H., Gerstein, G.L. and Moore, G.P. (1967) Neuronal spike trains and stochastic point processes: I. the single spike train. Biophys. J. 7, 391-418.

Powers, N.L. (1991) Discharge rate fluctuations in the auditory nerve of the chinchilla. Ph.D. thesis, State University of New York, Buffalo.

Teich, M.C. and Khanna, S.M. (1985) Pulse-number distribution for the neural spike train in the cat's auditory nerve. J. Acoust. Soc. Am. 77, 1110-1128.

Teich, M.C. (1989) Fractal character of the auditory nerve spike train. IEEE Trans. Biomed. Eng. 36, 150-160.

Teich, M.C., Johnson, D.H., Kumar, A.R. and Turcott, R.G. (1990) Rate fluctuations and fractional power-law noise recorded from cells in the lower auditory pathway of the cat. Hear. Res. 46, 41-52.

Viemeister, N.F. (1974) Intensity discrimination of noise in the presence of band-reject noise. J. Acoust. Soc. Am. 56, 1594-1600.

Viemeister, N.F. (1983) Auditory intensity discrimination at high frequencies in the presence of noise. Science 221, 1206-1208.

Viemeister, N.F. (1988) Psychophysical aspects of auditory intensity coding. In: G. M. Edelman, W. E. Gall and W. M. Cowan (eds.), Auditory Function: Neurobiological Bases of Hearing, Wiley, New York, 213-241.

Viemeister, N.F., Shivapuja, B.G. and Recio, A. (1992) Physiological correlates of temporal integration. In: Y.Cazals, L. Demany and K. Horner (eds.), Auditory Physiology and Perception, Pergamon, Oxford, 323-329.

Winter, I.M. and Palmer, A.R. (1991) Intensity coding in low-frequency auditory-nerve fibers of the guinea pig. J. Acoust. Soc. Am. 90, 1958-1967.

Young, E.D. and Barta, P.E. (1986) Rate responses of auditory nerve fibers to tones in noise near masked threshold. J. Acoust. Soc. Am. 79, 426-442.

Comment by E.F. Evans

Have you separated duration from position within a long-term stimulus? The dynamic range for rate measures is much longer for short duration stimuli or for short duration analyses at the onset of the stimulus, compared with durations in the later (adapted) portion (e.g. Evans 1981).

Evans E.F. (1981) The dynamic range problem: place and time coding at the level of cochlear nerve and nucleus In: J. Syka and L. Aitkin (eds.), Neuronal Mechanisms of Hearing, Plenum Press, NY, 69-85

Reply

We are currently analysing data obtained with gated, 50 ms tone bursts at CF. Preliminary results are in agreement with the "steady-state" data shown in Figure 5 except at moderately low values of r (e.g. 50/s) where the threshold values are elevated. At present we have no compelling explanation for the similarities and differences between the results obtained with gated and continuous tones but we conjecture that they reflect the effects of long-term refractoriness.

The effects of aspirin and of intense low-frequency tones on human hearing: The psychophysics of the outer hair cell?

Robert P. Carlyon[1] and Hazel A. Beveridge[2]

[1] *MRC Applied Psychology Unit, 15 Chancer Rd., Cambridge CB2 2EF, England*
[2] *Laboratory of Experimental Psychology, Sussex University, Brighton BN1 9QG, England.*

1 Introduction

An important goal of hearing research is to explain human hearing in terms of underlying physiological mechanisms. Unfortunately, many of the physiological manipulations available to researchers cannot, for ethical reasons, be applied to human subjects, and so we are often faced with the problem of relating physiological data obtained in animals to psychophysical findings obtained in humans. In addition to possible species differences, there are additional complications in that procedures such as the administration of anaesthetic or the invasion of the cochlea might affect peripheral auditory processes in an unknown way. The experiments described here use two techniques, the administration of aspirin and the presentation of low-frequency biasing tones, which produce a reversible effect on human hearing. Both techniques have been used in animal experiments, the results of which indicate that they both affect the operation of cochlear outer hair cells (OHCs).

2 Effects of aspirin on psychophysical tuning curves (PTCs)

2.1 Background

It has been known for at least 50 years that aspirin (acetylsalicylic acid, or "salicylate") produces a reversible reduction in auditory sensitivity (Falbe-Hansen, 1941). A number of physiological experiments indicate that it affects hearing via changes in OHC motility. First, Tunstall, Ashmore, and Gale (1994) have recently shown *in vitro* that salicylate reduces the non-linear component of OHC membrane capacitance, indicating a reduction in OHC motility. Second, salicylate administered *in vivo* reduces the amplitude of cochlear distortion products (Stypulkowski, 1990), which are widely believed to be mediated by OHCs. Third, salicylate removes the sharp tips of frequency threshold curves (FTCs: Evans and Borerwe, 1982; Stypulkowski, 1990) , a change also observed in other manipulations believed to affect OHCs, such as the production of temporary threshold shifts by exposure to intense sound (Cody and Johnstone, 1980) and the stimulation of the efferent fibers innervating OHCs (Guinan and Gifford, 1988).

In an earlier study, Carlyon and Butt (1993) showed that moderate doses of aspirin can affect human auditory filter shapes. Although that study showed a clear reduction in frequency selectivity, it did not reveal whether the reduction occurred in the tip of the underlying FTC, as seen in physiological experiments, or in the skirts. In our first experiment, we clarified this issue by measuring the effects of aspirin on the psychophysical analogue of the FTC, the "psychophysical tuning curve (PTC)". A second aim was to see whether the effects of aspirin interacted with those of two-tone suppression, a phenomenon which some authors (Geissler *et al.*, 1990) have also attributed to the operation of OHCs. Two approaches were used to achieve this second aim. First, we investigated the effect of aspirin on PTCs, measured both in forward and in simultaneous masking. PTCs are typically sharper in forward than in simultaneous masking, a difference which is at least partly due to suppression enhancing frequency selectivity in forward, but not in simultaneous masking (Moore, 1978). Thus, if aspirin reduces the effects of suppression, it should impair tuning more in forward than in simultaneous masking. Another way of measuring suppression comes from the reduction in the forward-masked threshold of a brief signal, caused by presenting a high-frequency suppressor tone concurrently with the masker (Houtgast, 1972). We therefore also compared the size of this reduction in the aspirin and placebo conditions.

2.2 Method

Eight male listeners took part in a double-blind, placebo-controlled study. Details of the drug schedule (three 320 mg aspirin tablets, or placebo, every six hours for 72 hours) were as described by Carlyon and Butt (1993). All testing took place one hour after the last dose, and started with absolute threshold measurements for 300-ms signals at all audiometric frequencies plus 6000 Hz, and for a 10-ms 4-kHz signal.

PTCs were measured for a 10-ms, 4-kHz signal presented 15 dB above its absolute threshold in the drug condition being tested (aspirin or placebo). The masker was a 100-Hz- wide multiplied noise with a center frequency (f_m) of, in forward masking, 2400, 3200, 3800, 4000, 4200, 4300, or 4400 Hz. In simultaneous masking an additional f_m of 4800 Hz was included. The masker duration was 200 ms; all stimuli were turned on and off with 5-ms raised-cosine ramps. A white noise, lowpass filtered at $0.375f_s$ and with a spectrum level 20 dB below that of the masker, was gated on and off with the masker in all conditions: this was done in order to help "cue" the end of the masker in forward masking (Moore *et al.*, 1984). In forward masking the signal was presented 1 ms (zero-voltage points) after the end of the masker; in simultaneous masking it was presented during the last 10 ms of the masker. In order to measure two-tone suppression, in one condition a 4.8-kHz sinusoidal "suppressor" was presented simultaneously with a masker centered on 4 kHz: in this condition the level of the suppressor was always 30 dB above the masker's spectrum level. In all conditions, the masker level at threshold was determined using a two-down, one-up adaptive procedure. Stimuli were presented through one earpiece of a Sennheiser HD414 headset.

2.3 Results

No blood samples were taken from our listeners, and we had to rely on absolute threshold shifts at 4 kHz for evidence that they had taken sufficient aspirin to affect the region of the cochlea tuned to the signal frequency. We applied an arbitrary criterion of a minimum 4 dB threshold shift for the 4-kHz 10-ms signal, and analysed the data from the five listeners who met this criterion. PTCs obtained from three of them are shown in the left- and right-hand columns of Fig. 1 for simultaneous and forward masking respectively. It can be seen that the effect of aspirin is broadly similar to that obtained in neural data, in that the sharp tip of the PTC is partially removed. A two-way ANOVA (drug * "forward vs simultaneous masking") revealed a strong effect of aspirin on the level of a 4-kHz masker at signal threshold ($F_{1,4} = 22.4$; $p < 0.01$), but the size of this effect did not depend on whether the signal was presented in forward, or simultaneous, masking.

To evaluate the effect of aspirin on the slopes of the PTCs, straight lines were fitted to each side, and a three-way ANOVA (drug * forward vs. simultaneous masking * low vs high side) applied to the absolute values of the obtained slopes. The most important result of the ANOVA was that slopes were signicantly reduced in the aspirin condition ($F_{1,4} = 31.07$; $p < 0.01$). The absence of any significant interactions indicated that, overall, the reduction in slope caused by aspirin did not differ significantly between the two sides of the PTC, or between forward and simultaneous masking. However, a two-way ANOVA (drug * "low vs. high side") applied separately to the simultaneous-masking data *did* reveal an interaction between drug and "high vs. low side" ($F_{1,4} = 38.29$; $p<0.01$), providing tentative evidence that, for simultaneous masking, the effects of aspirin were greatest on the high-frequency side of the PTC.

If aspirin reduced frequency selectivity as a result of a reduction in suppression, then it should have a greater effect on PTC slopes in forward than in simultaneous masking. As mentioned above, this was not the case. A more direct test of the effect of aspirin on suppression comes from the reduction in forward masking produced by a 4.8-kHz suppressor tone. Inspection of Fig. 2 reveals that this, too, did not differ significantly between the aspirin and placebo conditions.

3 Masking period patterns, low-frequency biasing tones, aspirin, and PTCs

3.1 Background

In the 1970s, Zwicker (1976b; 1977) measured the threshold for a brief high-frequency tone ("HFT": e.g., 2 ms, 1500 Hz) presented with an intense low-frequency tone ("LFT": e.g., 40 Hz, 100 dB SPL), as a function of the phase of the LFT at which the HFT was presented. These "masking period patterns (MPPs)" typically showed a large threshold maximum at a phase corresponding to a rarefaction at the eardrum, and a smaller maximum at a phase corresponding to a pressure condensation; thresholds were generally lowest near zero-crossings of the LFT waveform. Explanations of the

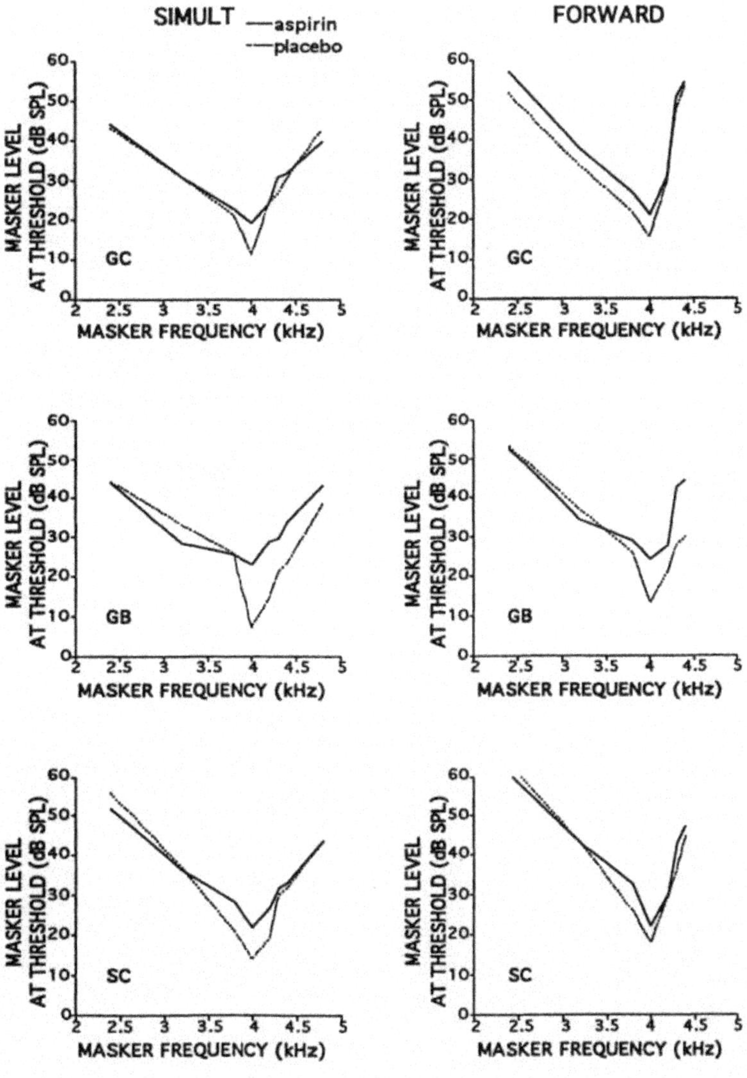

Figure 1. PTCs obtained in simultaneous masking (left-hand column) and in forward masking (right-hand column). Solid lines: aspirin. Dotted lines: placebo.

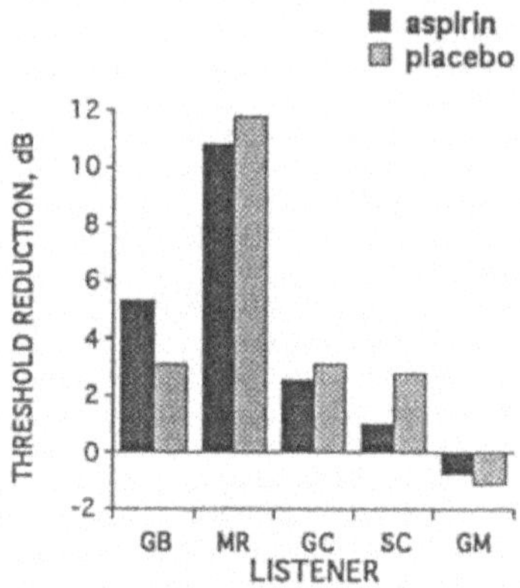

Figure 2. Reduction in threshold caused by the addition of a "suppressor" tone, for the aspirin (darker bars) and placebo (lighter bars) conditions.

phenomenon at the time usually assumed that one maximum was due to the LFT moving the basilar membrane in a manner opposite to that which normally gives rise to auditory-nerve (AN) activity, resulting in the signal level having to be increased in order to overcome this motion. The other maximum was attributed to the LFT producing excitatory BM motion, thereby "swamping" the activity in IHCs and AN fibers tuned to the signal. There was some debate as to which of these two processes corresponded to the larger of the two maxima, but the models proposed by Zwicker (1976a) and by Schwartz and Escudier (1985) both assumed, at least for very brief signals and sinusoidal LFTs, that the larger maximum was due to "inhibitory" motion of the BM,.

In the 1980s and 1990s, physiological experiments revealed a seemingly analagous phenomenon, in which an intense LFT could modulate the response to an HFT of the basilar membrane (BM), inner hair cells (IHCs), OHCs, and auditory nerve fibers (Schmiedt, 1982; Patuzzi and Sellick, 1984; Patuzzi *et al.*, 1984; Schwartz and Escudier, 1985; Russell and Kössl, 1992). As with MPPs, a sinusoidal LFT reduced the response to the HFT at two phases roughly 180° apart, and again there was an asymmetry in the size of the effect between these two maxima. However, the explanation for this phenomenon differs from that previously proposed to account for MPPs: the consensus seems to be that the biasing introduced by the LFT reduces the "positive feedback" into BM vibration that results from OHC motility - one appealing explanation is that it shifts the OHC "input-output" function away from its steepest point (Patuzzi *et al.*, 1984). Unfortunately, as is the case for MPPs, there is some controversy over which phase of BM vibration produces the maximum effect (Schmiedt, 1982; Patuzzi and Sellick, 1984; Ruggero *et al.*, 1992 ; Russell and Kössl, 1992).

We tested two predictions of the hypothesis that the peaks in the MPP occur at LFT phases at which the OHCs are maximally "biased". First, ingestion of aspirin, which reduces OHC motility, should raise thresholds in the MPP "valleys": the hypothesis assumes that sensitivity at these LFT phases is normally enhanced by OHC motility, and so aspirin should increase these thresholds so that they are more similar to those at MPP maxima The second prediction stems from the finding that the largest reduction in sensitivity caused by biasing the OHCs occurs for HFTs at the characteristic frequency (CF) of the unit, with smaller reductions for HFTs remote from the CF (Schmiedt, 1982; Patuzzi and Sellick, 1984; Klis *et al.*, 1988). This results in tuning being broader than when the OHCs are not biased . If the peaks in the MPP occur for HFTs presented at a "biasing" phase of the LFT, then the frequency selectivity of the auditory system to those HFTs should be poorer than that to HFTs presented at other phases. We tested this prediction by measuring PTCs for a 1500-Hz signal, forward masked by a train of tone pips that were presented against an intense LFT, for various phase relationships between the masker pips and the LFT. In order to do this, we needed to choose a duration for the tone pips which was short enough to produce marked peaks in the MPP, but long enough to have a narrow frequency spectrum. By using the computer program described by Glasberg and Moore (1990), we determined that the width of a 12-ms tone's excitation pattern was determined mainly by auditory frequency selectivity, rather than by physical splatter. However, this signal duration is rather longer than those usually used in MPP experiments, and so we performed a preliminary experiment to verify that the resulting MPPs would not be significantly "flattened", relative to those obtained with the shorter signals more commonly used to measure MPPs.

3.2 Method

3.2.1 MPPs and Aspirin

MPPs for 1500-Hz tones, turned on and off with raised-cosine ramps (no steady-state), were measured in the presence of a 300-ms 40-Hz LFT with a level of 101 dB SPL. The total duration (zero-voltage points) of the signal was either 4 ms or 12 ms. Thresholds were obtained using a one-up two-down adaptive procedure in a two-interval forced-choice task. The effects of aspirin were measured using a similar drug schedule to that described in section 2, with the exception that administration was neither double-blind nor placebo-controlled. Instead, MPPs were simply measured before, immediately after, and one week after aspirin ingestion. As the aspirin raised the detection threshold for the LFT, we also measured MPPs in the "no drug" condition with the sensation level of the LFT reduced to equal that in the aspirin condition.

3.2.2 MPPs and PTCs

PTCs were measured for a 12-ms 1500-Hz signal presented at a fixed level of 10 dB SL *after* the offset of the LFT (which, by itself, produced less than 4 dB of forward masking). This was done by measuring the level of a train of eleven 12-ms tone pips necessary to mask the signal. The pips were presented during an LFT, and were separated by one LFT period (25 ms): this meant that, in each condition, all masker pips occurred at the same LFT phase. The value of this phase differed across conditions, and the phase values were chosen to match salient features of each listener's MPP. The temporal structure of the LFT, masker pips, and signal are shown schematically for three conditions in Fig. 3. In each condition, a PTC was obtained by varying the frequency of the masker pips: as the Fig. shows, the delay between the center of the final masking pip and the center of the signal was always 27.875 ms. In order to help cue the end of the masker,

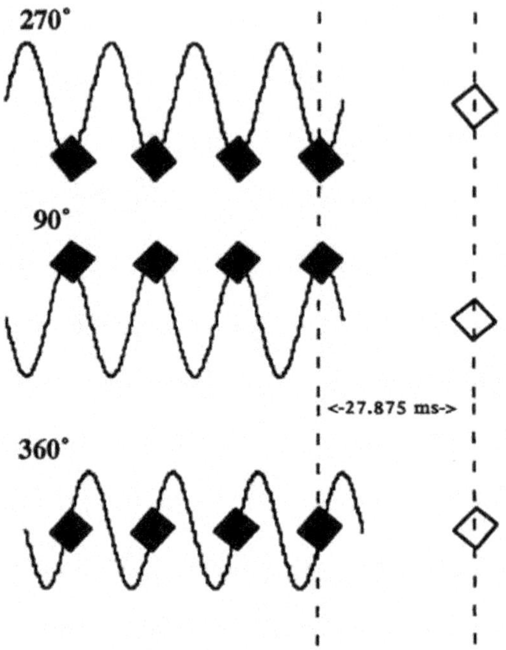

Figure 3 Schematic diagram of the LFT, masker pips (solid diamonds) and signals (open diamonds) used to measure PTCs. Three conditions are shown, differing in the LFT phase at which the maskers were presented, but all with a 27.875-ms delay between the final masker pip and the signal. (see dashed lines)

each masker pip was accompanied by a second, synchronous tone burst, with a level equal to that of the masker but with a frequency remote from f_S: for masker frequencies of 1500 Hz and below the frequency of the added tone was 2500 Hz, whereas for masker frequencies above 1500 Hz it was 500 Hz.

3.2.3 Headset

All stimuli described in this section were presented using a headset developed by the MRC Institute of Hearing Research Clinical Outstation, and kindly loaned to us. It consisted of a TDH-49 earpiece clamped into a metal cavity via foam washers, with an otoscope tip sealed to the face of the earpiece using epoxy putty at one end, and connected to a length of plastic tubing at the other. We connected the tubing to the input port of an E-A-R microphone; this was essentially an E-A-R plug with a plastic tube through the center. In order to calibrate our stimuli at the eardrum, we inserted a second piece of tubing through the plug, to which we attached a third tube containing a Knowles BT-1754 microphone. Calibration was carried out using an HP3561A spectrum analyser; special care was taken to check that the LFT did not produce any non-linearities in the headset response to the signal or masker.

3.3 Results

3.3.1 MPPs and Aspirin

Fig. 4 shows MPPs for four listeners at signal durations of 4 ms (upper trace) and 12 ms (lower trace): it can be seen that the shape of the MPP does not differ markedly between the two durations. All listeners show a large maximum at an LFT phase of either 270° or 225°, whereas the size and location of the secondary peak shows a greater variation across listeners: for example, listener GC shows almost no secondary peak, whereas the MPP for listener AC shows two peaks of almost equal size.

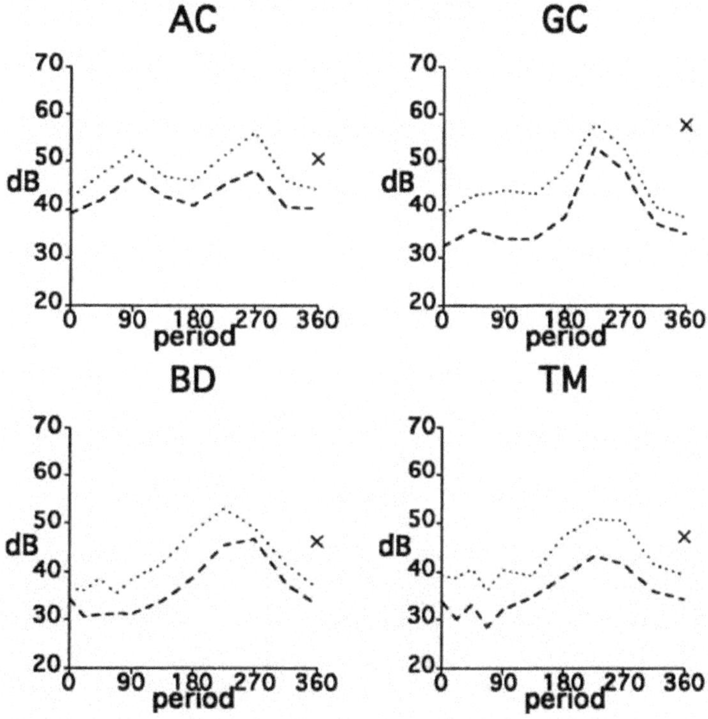

Figure 4. MPPs for signal durations of 4 ms (dotted lines) and 12 ms (dashed lines). The crosses show absolute thresholds for the 40-Hz LFT.

The MPPs for two listeners obtained with a 101-dB masker and a 4-ms signal are shown in Fig. 5 for the aspirin (solid line) and "pre drug" (dotted line) conditions. Listener

TM's MPP was not greatly affected by the aspirin, whereas that of listener BD was considerably flattened. However, the flattening was not mainly due to thresholds being "levelled up" to that obtained at the maximum, as would be expected if aspirin were reducing the positive feedback provided by the OHCs; rather, much of the effect is due to thresholds at the MPP maximum (225°) being *lowered* by aspirin. An alternative explanation is that aspirin somehow attenuated the BM response to the LFT, thereby reducing the amount by which it masked the signal. This explanation is supported by two findings. First, the unconnected symbols to the right of each plot show that listener BD's absolute threshold for the 40-Hz LFT was higher in the aspirin condition (circle) than in the pre-drug condition (cross), but that this difference was much smaller for TM, whose MPPs were also less affected. Second, when BD was tested several weeks after his last aspirin dose, with the LFT's sensation level reduced (dashed line) to equal that in the aspirin condition, his MPP flattened and acquired a shape similar to that seen with aspirin. This conclusion should be qualified by the observation that recent data obtained with three further listeners indicate that the pattern of results varies markedly across subjects.

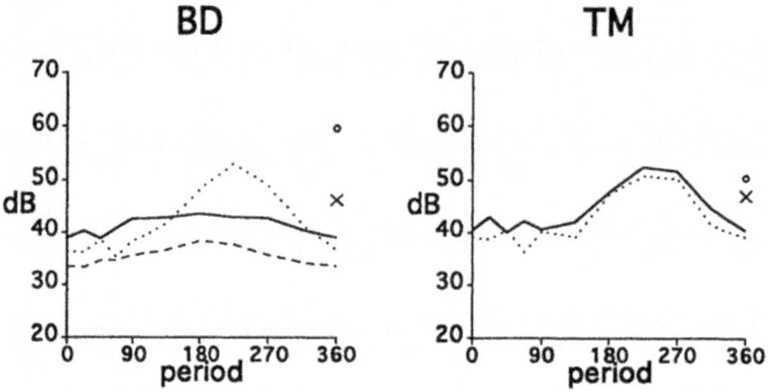

Figure 5. MPPs for the pre-drug (dotted lines) and aspirin (solid lines) conditions. The dashed line shows listener BD's MPP several weeks after his last aspirin dose, but with the LFT sensation level reduced to equal that in the aspirin condition. The crosses and circles show absolute thresholds for the LFT in the pre-drug and aspirin conditions respectively.

A finding of secondary interest, not shown in the Figs., is that thresholds for the 4-ms 1500-Hz signals in the absence of the LFT were not affected by aspirin, but that those for 300-ms signals were raised by approximately 8 dB for both listeners. This means that temporal integration, defined as the threshold difference between the two signal durations, was decreased by aspirin consumption, a finding previously reported by McFadden (1984).

3.3.2 MPPs and PTCs

Fig. 6 shows PTCs obtained in three conditions. Although there was considerable variability across listeners, it is clear that PTCs were not broadest for maskers presented at the major peak in the MPP (solid lines). Thus, the data do not support the hypothesis that the peaks in the MPP occur at those phases of the LFT which produce maximum biasing of the OHCs.

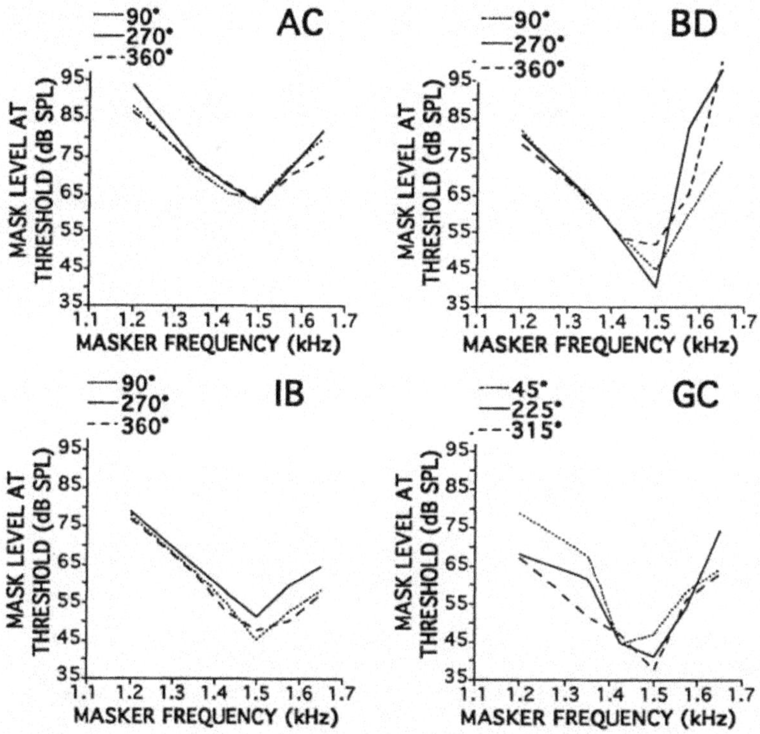

Fig. 6. PTCs measured for four listeners, where the masker pips were presented at LFT phases corresponding to the larger MPP maximum (solid lines), the smaller maximum (dotted lines), and a region of low thresholds (dashed lines).

4 Discussion

We have measured the effects of two manipulations believed to influence the operation of OHCs in the human cochlea. Administration of aspirin raised the tips of human PTCs, a finding similar to the effect of salicylate on neural and BM tuning curves obtained in anaesthetised animals. There was some tentative evidence that, in simultaneous masking, aspirin had a greater effect on the high-frequency side of the PTC than on the low-frequency side. We could not find any evidence that aspirin affects suppression, although this does not preclude the possibility that, had our listeners taken larger doses of aspirin, such an effect could have been observed.

The results of our experiments using intense low-frequency tones do not support the idea that the maxima in psychophysically measured MPPs correspond to those phases of BM motion at which the OHCs are maximally biased away from the steep part of their input-output functions. The strongest evidence against the hypothesis comes from the PTCs obtained with masker pips presented at various phases of the LFT: when the LFT phase corresponded to the largest peak in the MPP, the PTCs were, if anything, *sharper* than those obtained at other phases. Our data are consistent with the shape of the MPP being dominated by the "excitatory" and "inhibitory" effect of the LFT on IHC and AN responses, in much the same way as originally envisaged by Zwicker (1976a; 1977) and by Schwartz and Escudier (1985). However, it is interesting to note that, although the LFT itself did not mask the signal, it could affect PTCs in a way which depended on the phase at which the masker pips were presented. This would be consistent with the idea that the effects of the LFT on OHCs can be measured psychophysically, but that the maximum biasing occurs at LFT phases other than those corresponding to MPP maxima. One way in which this could happen would be if MPP maxima corresponded to maximal BM velocity (which is what drives the IHC response to 40-Hz tones), but that the broadest tuning corresponded to maximal BM displacement (which is what drives the OHCs). However, we should stress that our data are not yet sufficiently complete to determine whether or not this is the case, and restrict our conclusions to the statement that MPP maxima are unlikely to be due to OHC biasing.

5 References

Carlyon, R. P. and Butt, M. (1993). Effect of aspirin on human auditory filters. Hearing Research 66, 233-244.

Cody, A. R. and Johnstone, B. M. (1980). Single auditory neuron response during acute acoustic trauma. Hearing Research 3, 3-16.

Evans, E. F. and Borerwe, T. A. (1982). Ototoxic effects of salicylates on the responses of single cochlear nerve fibres and on cochlear potentials. Brit. J. Audiol. 16, 101-108.

Falbe-Hansen, J. (1941). Clinical and experimental histological studies on effects of salicylate and quinine on the ear. Acta Otolaryngol. Supp. 44,

Geissler, C. D., Yates, G. K., Patuzzi, R. B. and Johnstone, B. M. (1990). Saturation of outer hair cell receptor currents causes two-tone suppression. Hearing Research 44, 241-256.

Glasberg, B. R. and Moore, B. C. J. (1990). Derivation of auditory filter shapes from notched-noise data. Hearing Research 47, 103-138.

Guinan, J. J. and Gifford, M. L. (1988). Effects of electrical stimulation of efferent olivocochlear neurons on cat auditory-nerve fibers. Hearing Research 37, 29-46.

Houtgast, T. (1972). Psychophysical evidence for lateral inhibition in hearing. J. Acoust. Soc. Am. 51, 1885-1894.

Klis, J.F.L., Prijs, V.F., Latour, J.B., and Smoorenburg, G.F. (1988) Modulation of cochlear tuning by low-frequency sound. Hearing Research 36, 163-174.

McFadden, D., Plattsmier, H. S. and Pasanen, E. G. (1984). Aspirin-induced hearing loss as a model of sensorineural hearing loss. Hearing Research 16, 251-260.

Moore, B. C. J. (1978). Psychophysical tuning curves measured in simultaneous and forward masking. J. Acoust. Soc. Am. 63, 524-532.

Moore, B. C. J., Glasberg, B. R. and Roberts, B. (1984). Refining the measurement of psychophysical tuning curves. J. Acoust. Soc. Am. 76, 1057-1066.

Patuzzi, R. P. and Sellick, P. M. (1984). The modulation of the sensitivity of the mammalian cochlea by low frequency tones. II.Inner hair cell receptor potentials. Hearing Research 13, 9-18.

Patuzzi, R. P., Sellick, P. M. and Johnstone, B. M. (1984). The modulation of the sensitivity of the mammalian cochlea by low frequency tones. III. Basilar membrane motion. Hearing Research 13, 19-27.

Ruggero, M. A., Robles, L. and Rich, N. C. (1992). Two-tone suppression in the basilar membrane of the cochlea: mechanical basis of auditory-nerve rate suppression. Journal of Neurophysiology 4, 1087-1099.

Russell, I. J. and Kössl, M. (1992). Modulation of hair cell voltage responses to tones by low-frequency biasing of the basilar membrane in the guinea pig cochlea. Journal of Neuroscience 12, 1587-1601.

Schmiedt, R. A. (1982). Effects of low-frequency biasing tones on auditory-nerve activity. J. Acoust. Soc. Am. 72, 142-150.

Schwartz, J.-L. and Escudier, P. (1985). Masking-period patterns: presentation of a model compatible with an enlarged set of psychophysical and physiological results. J. Acoust. Soc. Am. 78, 474-487.

Stypulkowski, P. H. (1990). Mechanisms of salicylate ototoxicity. Hear.Res. 46, 113-146.

Tunstall, M. J., Ashmore, J. F. and Gale, J. E. (1994). The effect of salicylate on properties of isolated outer hair cells from the guinea-pig cochlea. British Journal of Audiology 27, 332-333.

Zwicker, E. (1976a). A model for predicting masking period patterns. Biol. Cybernetics 23, 49-60.

Zwicker, E. (1976b). Psychoacoustic equivalent of period histograms [in memoriam Dr. Russell Pfeiffer]. J. Acoust. Soc. Am. 59, 166-175.

Zwicker, E. (1977). Masking-period patterns produced by very-low-frequency maskers and their possible relation to basilar-membrane displacement. J. Acoust. Soc. Am. 61, 1031-1040.

Comparative studies

Comparative studies of sound source perception

Richard R. Fay

Department of Psychology and Parmly Hearing Institute, Loyola University of Chicago, 6525 North Sheridan Road, Chicago, IL 60626

1 Introduction

The usual working definitions of the sense of hearing arises from introspection and experiments on human listeners. It is probably inevitable, and even proper, that the sense of hearing in which we are most interested, and the one we understand best (our own), provides the conceptual framework that guides experimental design and interpretation in comparative auditory research. It is interesting, however, that our introspections and common sense can lead to a general view of the biological significance of hearing that does not often drive research. For the most part, hearing research investigates the relations between the acoustic variables characterizing sounds and the responses of mechanical structures, biological membranes, cells, cell groups, and whole organisms. Introspection on the roles of hearing in everyday life, on the other hand, suggests that hearing is a process by which we become aware of the identities and locations of the objects around us that produce and scatter sound. While it is clear that the auditory system operates on the sounds reaching the ears, the sense of hearing informs us not so much about sounds, but about their sources, out in the world.

The notion that our auditory system is organized to determine the sources of sounds, although perhaps intuitively obvious, has only recently begun to guide thinking and experiment in auditory research on humans (e.g., McAdams, 1989, Bregman, 1990; Hartmann, 1988; Yost, 1991). It has begun to become popular to study analytic and synthetic listening, and to investigate the acoustic features that lead to the perceptual grouping and segregation of acoustic components. It seems clear, in general, that components tend to be grouped in perception if it is likely that they could arise from a single sound source, and that groups of components tend to be segregated if it is unlikely that the groups arose from a single source. It seems that hypotheses about the nature of sound sources in general determine, in part at least, how information is grouped and segregated to synthesize auditory perceptions. These and other considerations have led to a general acceptance of the idea that an important aspect of hearing is in the analysis and synthesis of auditory scenes (Bregman, 1990). The phrase "auditory scene" implies an image, possibly analogous to a visual image, of the objects in the environment that produce and scatter sound. Perhaps the most fundamental function of the human sense of hearing, then, is the synthesis of auditory scenes in perception so that we may act appropriately with respect to their causes.

Research on this aspect of the sense of hearing has required methods, paradigms, and stimuli that are somewhat different from those used in traditional psychoacoustics. In general, these paradigms don't so much ask about the acuity of sound discrimination as they ask about the distinctions we normally make when listening to sounds complex enough to seem almost natural, or usual, in everyday experience. It is not surprising that much of the experimental work on these aspects of auditory perception has focused on human speech and music (e.g., Handel, 1989). There is no question of the "biological significance" of speech, or of the intrinsic interest that musical sounds hold for us. Both are complex, more or less natural kinds of sounds having sources that have been well studied acoustically. Even in research on more arbitrary complex sounds, such as in the work on complex pitch perception (e.g., de Boer, 1976), co-modulation masking release (Hall and Grose, 1990), profile analysis (Green, 1988), and modulation detection interference (Yost et al., 1989), results tend to be interpreted and applied with respect to speech and music perception.

If we can accept the foregoing as a broad sketch of the biological significance of human hearing and of some recent psychoacoustic research, we can now turn to questions in comparative hearing research. Two scientific traditions have shaped much of the auditory research on nonhuman animals (from now on referred to simply as animals). The first, American behaviorism, has focused on the relations between simple acoustic variables and conditioned responses in a wide variety of species, including fishes, amphibians, reptiles, birds, and mammals. The second, European ethology and more recently, neuroethology, has concentrated on the relations between "biologically significant" complex sounds (often communication sounds) and the ways in which animals in a natural or simulated natural setting usually respond to these sounds without being conditioned to do so. The behaviorist tradition has produced a wealth of psychoacoustic data that allow quantitative comparisons among distantly related species of their capacities to detect and discriminate sounds (Fay, 1988).

The ethological tradition has produced a number of specific, detailed stories focusing on the ways in which a given species may be adapted or specialized to acquire and process specific information from sound sources of known biological significance. One example of the success of the ethological approach is our present understanding of sound source localization in the barn owl (e.g., Knudsen and Konishi, 1979). In this case, a naturally occurring behavior (flying from a perch to the ground, or turning the head toward a sound source) was used to study the processing of brief broadband sounds similar to those caused by a mouse moving over leaves. Following initial observations of this type with neurophysiological studies of neural response properties to loudspeakers arrayed in real space led to the discovery of a neural map of auditory space within the inferior and superior colliculi. In addition, a combination of anatomical, physiological, and behavioral studies led to the discovery that a sound source's azimuth is computed using interaural time differences while its elevation is computed using interaural differences in spectrum shape. This impressive example of comparative auditory research included the following ingredients: thoughtful selection of the species and problem for study, careful initial observation of the acoustic behavior of interest (successful hunting based on auditory cues), use of complex naturally occurring sounds presented as real sources in space, and use of naturally-occurring responses of the animal in a context that has obvious biological significance (hunting and feeding). The neuroethological approach seems like a natural and valuable one for investigating the most fundamental functions of hearing in animals.

The ethological approach has its problems, however. Foremost is the problem that species are chosen for study that display the behavior (or solve the particular problem) of interest, and not all or even many species can be studied similarly. Each species tends to be viewed as a special case, each with its own characteristic behavior, problem to be solved, processing strategy, and biologically significant sound sources. The notion that "[human] speech is special" is another example of an essentially ethological approach. If a successful ethological research program must begin with the observation of a clearly specialized acoustic behavior or an observation of a species-specific use of the sense of hearing, then ethology may begin to convince us that the fundamental biological functions of hearing, the reasons we all have ears and an auditory system, are somehow different for each species. For example, my undergraduate students begin (and sometimes end) the semester believing that speech perception somehow explains human hearing.

Another problem with the ethological paradigm, one that touches my own research on hearing in fishes more closely, is that the absence of any obvious natural response to sound in a species, or the absence of deliberate vocalizations, tends to suggest that the species has an impoverished, or at least unexplained, sense of hearing, and prompts questions such as "What do goldfish or lizards listen to, anyhow?" An answer that would be accepted most of the time could include something like, "To escape predators," or "To detect prey," as if our understanding of hearing in animals reduces to the notion that sound simply acts as a trigger for one or two stereotyped behaviors. It is clear that many species do, in fact, show orientation and other stereotyped responses to sound, but it is probably an error to believe that these behaviors define or explain their ears, central auditory system, or their sense of hearing.

The question "What does the goldfish (or any animal) look at?" is usually not asked. Although visual cues (behavior, body patterns, and colors) may function in communication, we generally do not attempt to explain structures of the retina, response properties of ganglion cells, or the ability to see simply as adaptations for receiving visual communication signals. The functional significance of seeing must be more general and important than this. It makes intuitive sense that vision informs the organism about objects that produce and scatter visible light. One could suggest that animals "look at" everything visible and probably form an image representing these objects and their spatial relationships. Perhaps we should view the sense of hearing similarly. Perhaps the most general, primitive function of hearing is to obtain information on the identities and locations of the objects that produce or scatter sound so that the listener can draw the right conclusions about them and act appropriately. The organisms best able to draw the right conclusions about objects in the environment would probably be more fit than those that fail to apprehend reality, and would probably live longer and reproduce more successfully.

Viewing the sense of hearing among animals in this way, one could argue that all sources that may produce or scatter sound are to some degree "biologically significant" in the sense that no single source can be determined without processing the sounds from all sources that are simultaneously audible. In a further analogy with vision, a "figure" or visual object is defined and perceived with respect to its background, or "ground." In the auditory world, both "signals" and "noise" require analysis because the sources of both have to be determined to some degree before the source of interest (the "signal") can be identified and located in the presence of competing sources (the "noise"). Thus, one could hypothesize that the sense of hearing among all animals functions, perhaps to varying degrees, to characterize the acoustic ambience and its perturbations created by all audible sources and scatterers (e.g., Rogers et. al. 1989). It makes sense that once such a perceptual system had evolved, it also would be recruited for communication purposes. However, an understanding of hearing as a biological phenomenon could be increased by recognizing what is probably its most primitive, or shared, role; the identification and localization of sound sources within the "auditory scene" (Bregman 1990), and the representation of objects within the scene during the passage of time and during relative movements between the perceiver and the perceived.

Traditional human and animal psychoacoustical studies have not focused on describing and analyzing the sense of hearing as described above, and there are few experimental psychoacoustical paradigms designed to study sound source perception within auditory scenes. Furthermore, most of the paradigms reviewed in Bregman (1990) and Handel (1989) for studying scene analysis in humans seem difficult to adapt for use with subjects who do not speak or understand language, and who do not listen to human speech and music. This may be one of the reasons why the notion that animals perhaps also perceive the auditory scene is not more generally held; it is not clear how to study auditory scene analysis in animals using traditional conditioning methods. After all, if behaviorist methods can't measure it, the "it" in question just might not exist (or at least behaviorists might behave as if "it" didn't exist).

Should we look to the ethological paradigm for ways to study auditory scene analysis in animals? This would be worth exploring, but there are some initial problem to overcome. One is the hypothesis that scene analysis, as outlined above, is probably a primitive, shared character of all vertebrate auditory systems, and as such may not be easily revealed in species with specialized sensory processing and acoustic behaviors. In these species, recognizing scene analysis in their behavior might be "masked" by their specializations. For example, while we are now certain that auditory space maps exist in the midbrain nuclei of barn owls, and that these are responsible, in part, for rapid head orientation and prey-catching behavior. However, it is not clear whether the neural maps are available for other more general functions such as helping to form something like a cognitive map of auditory space, or whether these functions (if they exist) depend on other processing mechanisms, in parallel with the sensory-motor space maps. Similarly, in studies of the Mauthner cell "C-start" response in fishes (e.g., Zottoli, 1977; Canfield and Eaton, 1990), we do not know whether or not the presumed underlying binaural processing is made available for the formation of auditory scenes in perception. In both cases, the specialized orientation behaviors may be taken to somehow explain the existence of the responsible mechanisms, and the question of the role these may play in the more general sense of hearing is usually not asked.

In one case, at least, some traditional behaviorist paradigms have been successful in analyzing specialized, naturally occurring acoustic behaviors. Simmons and his colleagues (e.g., Simmons, Moss, and Ferragamo, 1990) have used simple conditioning methods to study the perception of target characteristics by some bat species using echolocation. Although echolocation and its underlying mechanisms are highly specialized adaptations among mammals, this work has led to provocative hypotheses on the "acoustic images," analogous to visual images, some bats may form of echolocation targets in perception. This is one of the few hearing research programs that has studied anything like auditory scene perception in animals. Even though the animals studied are highly specialized acoustically, the hypotheses advanced and evaluated are rather general, at least not species-specific. It could be suggested, for example, that previously existing scene-forming functions of the auditory system were recruited for echolocation in bats, and in whales as well.

2 Sound Perception in the Goldfish

There are a wealth of methods used with a variety of species that could possibly be adapted to the study of sound source determination and auditory scene analysis (e.g., Dooling, 1989; Dooling and Hulse, 1989; Moody and Stebbins, 1989). These sorts of studies will not be reviewed here. Rather, a general approach to studying sound source determination is outlined that has been used in studies on goldfish. These methods were initially developed (Fay, 1969, Fay and MacKinnon, 1969) as a way to carry out psychophysical studies on sound detection and discrimination in restrained animals. Recently, they have been used in a new way that might permit assessment of the capacities of the goldfish to determine sound sources and to perceive the auditory scene. These methods and data, by themselves, only begin to approach some of the simplest questions, and are presented primarily to be suggestive and possibly encouraging about future studies on sound source perception.

The primary method is classical conditioning of respiratory suppression (Fay and MacKinnon, 1969) in a stimulus generalization paradigm (see Malott and Malott, 1970). Briefly, a common goldfish is gently restrained in a cloth bag in an acoustic test tank. A mild electric shock (unconditioned stimulus, or UCS) through the body causes a brief suppression of respiration lasting several seconds. A six-second auditory signal coterminating with the shock becomes a conditioned stimulus after several conditioning trials, evoking a conditioned respiratory suppression. Respiration is measured with a thermistor near the fish's mouth that responds to the cooling effects of respiratory water flow. The voltage signal from the thermistor bridge circuit is digitally recorded. Respiratory activity (L) is quantified as the length of the voltage waveform in arbitrary units minus the length expected for no respiratory activity. A respiratory suppression ratio (SR) is defined as B/(A+B), where B is the L value for the last 4 sec of the 6-sec conditioned stimulus (CS) period, and A is the L value for the 4 sec period immediately preceding the CS. The SR is thus a continuous quantity that varies between 0, indicating complete respiratory suppression, and about 0.5, indicating no respiratory suppression.

2.1 Perception of Pure Tones

It was discovered by accident that goldfish conditioned to a pure tone failed to respond robustly when the frequency of the tone was changed slightly (Fay, 1969b). In other words, the animals failed to generalize to tones with frequencies differing from that of the initial conditioning stimulus. A systematic study of pure tone frequency generalization (Fay, 1970a) began with 40 conditioning trials (2-3 min intertrial intervals) using a pure tone fixed in frequency. In the same session, 40 additional test trials were presented consisting of eight novel stimuli (having different frequencies but the same levels above threshold) presented four times each in random order, without the UCS. On

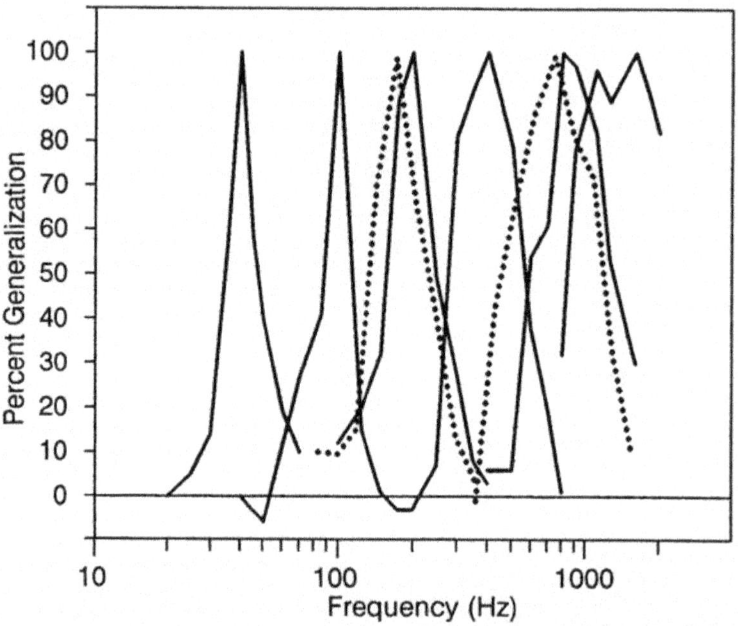

Figure 1. Pure tone generalization gradients. Eight groups of four animals were conditioned to one frequency and tested at novel frequencies. Gradient peaked at 40 Hz from Fay (1969b); other solid lines from Fay (1972); dotted lines from Fay (1992).

every fifth trial, the conditioning stimulus was presented with the UCS in order to help maintain the conditioned response magnitude. For each trial, the magnitude of the respiratory suppression response (the SR value) was measured. Figure 1 shows pure tone generalization gradients from two studies (Fay, 1970a; 1992). In general, animals responded only to test tones close in frequency to the conditioning stimulus, and responses to novel tones above and below the conditioning frequencies reached chance levels along monotonic and symmetrical gradients.

These studies were interpreted as indications that tone frequency corresponds to a salient perceptual dimension for the goldfish, possibly analogous to pitch for human listeners. Significant responses to the novel frequencies (i.e., generalization) were interpreted to indicate the equivalence of the novel and conditioning stimuli under the conditions of the experiment. A failure to generalize was interpreted to indicate that the test stimuli lack at least one important feature of the conditioning stimulus that had become salient during initial conditioning. Since goldfish can be conditioned to discriminate between the conditioning and all test frequencies of Figure 1 (Fay, 1970b), the generalization that occurs can't be explained as a lack of acuity. The ability to discriminate is necessary but not sufficient to explain the generalization failure. This type of experiment appears to reveal similarities and differences between the sensory effects of stimuli that are salient without explicit differential conditioning, and may be analogous to similarity judgements in humans. Thus, generalization studies may point to stimulus dimensions or features that are normally meaningful to the animal (see Nelson and Marler, 1989), and could possibly be used in a more subjective animal psychophysics analogous to, for example, pitch matching (Burns, 1982), and scaling complex sound quality (Freed, 1990).

2.2 Perception of Amplitude-Modulated Tones

Stimulus generalization was used next in nine experiments on the perception of amplitude modulated tones by the goldfish (Fay, 1972). Eight groups of goldfish were conditioned to respond to pure tones sinusoidally amplitude modulated (SAM) at 40 Hz. Animals conditioned to SAM signals failed to generalize to any pure tone, including those at the carrier frequenciès (400 and 1000 Hz), but responded to varying degrees to other SAM stimuli (Figure 2). In general, the responses to novel SAM signals were strongly controlled by the SAM carrier and modulation depth, and more weakly controlled by modulation rate. This multidimensional control of the conditioned response suggested that goldfish independently acquired information about envelope and waveform fine structure from these complex sounds.

The ninth group of animals was conditioned to a 40 Hz pure tone and then tested for response to a 1 kHz tone amplitude modulated at a range of rates above and below 40 Hz. Responses were greatest to a 40 Hz modulation, and declined for modulation rates above and below 40 Hz. This generalization gradient demonstrated the near equivalence of pure tone and envelope periodicity, and was interpreted as a demonstration of something like periodicity pitch in fish. The results of these experiments indicate that information is acquired about both temporal envelopes and waveform fine structures independently, and that this information can be integrated so that features common across spectral regions can be recognized and can control behavior.

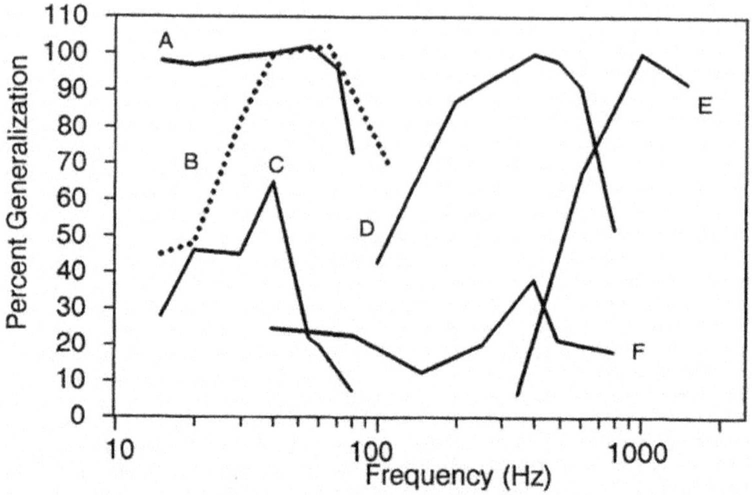

Figure 2. Generalization gradients in a study of the perception of amplitude modulated (AM) tones. Group A conditioned to 400 Hz modulated at 40 Hz and tested at different modulation frequencies. Group B conditioned to 1 kHz carrier modulated at 40 Hz, and tested as in A. Group D conditioned to a carrier of 400 Hz modulated at 40 Hz, and tested at different carrier frequencies. Group E conditioned to a 1 kHz carrier and tested as in D. Group F conditioned to 400 Hz modulated at 40 Hz, and tested to pure tones. Group C conditioned to a 40 Hz tone and tested with a 1 kHz tone AM at various rates (from Fay, 1972).

2.3 Analytic Listening

The stimulus generalization paradigm was used next in a simple study of analytic listening (Fay, 1992). Although goldfish (and all other vertebrates investigated) are able to discriminate between successive sounds of different frequency or spectral pattern (reviewed by Fay, 1988), there had been little direct evidence that any animal is able to identify the individual frequency components of complex sounds; that is, to listen analytically. Analytic listening is a prerequisite for auditory scene analysis, since simultaneous sources must be segregated to some degree before they are resolved and identified. In these experiments, animals were conditioned to respond to a two-tone complex, and then tested for response to novel pure tones, including those making up the conditioning complex. If animals generalize to the pure tone frequencies making up the conditioning complex more than to others, the goldfish can be said to have acquired independent information about the simultaneous frequency components of the complex, and thus to have listened analytically.

Figure 3 shows mean results in which eight animals were conditioned to respond to the two-tone complex (166 plus 724 Hz) and tested for their response to individual pure tones. The generalization gradient shows relatively robust responses to the 166 and 724 Hz tones, as would be expected if they had listened analytically. Clearly, goldfish acquired and used independent information about the frequencies of both components of the complex sound.

The unexpectedly large response at 1500 Hz cannot be readily explained. An essentially similar gradient, including the large response to 1500 Hz, was obtained by conditioning animals to pure tones of 166 Hz and 724 Hz alternately on successive trials rather than simultaneously on each trial (Fig. 3, dotted line). Since this unexpected response occurred in both experiments, it cannot be explained in terms of an additional dimension evoked by the complex conditioning stimulus. Moreover, since the effect also did not appear when animals were conditioned either to 166 or 724 Hz alone, it cannot be explained as a "near octave" confusion in processing one or both of the components. In any case, the response to 1514 Hz in both experiments are interpreted as a real perceptual effect deserving further study.

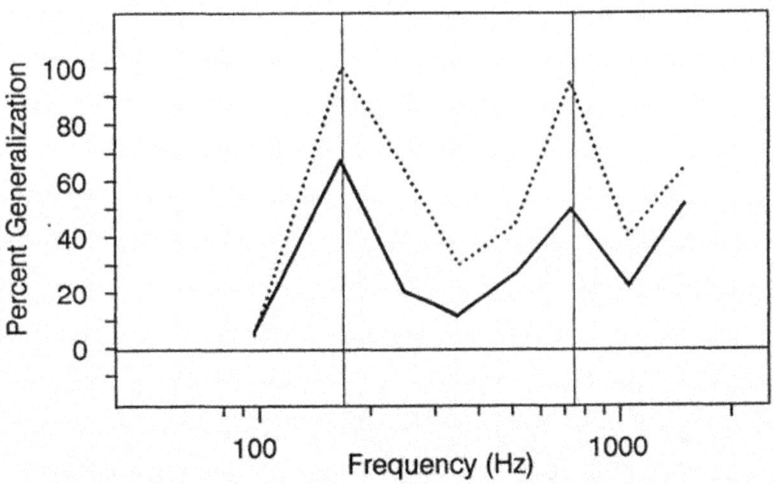

Figure 3. Generalization gradients for two groups of animals in a study of analytic listening from Fay (1992). Solid line: Animals conditioned to a two-tone mixture (indicated by thin vertical lines), and tested to pure tones. Dotted line: Animals conditioned to two pure tones presented singly, alternating on successive trials, and tested to pure tones.

2.4 Pitch and Synthetic Listening

More recent experiments have focused on the perceptual dimensions revealed in response to complex, periodic stimuli. If sound sources are to be correctly identified or recognized, it is necessary that the individual frequency components belonging to a single source be grouped or fused in perception. Pitch perception is one example of synthetic listening because a unitary perception is derived from the presence of multiple frequency components in an harmonic series. The relationships among the harmonics determines that the pitch is equal to the frequency of the common fundamental. In one recent experiment on pitch perception (Fay, 1994a), goldfish were conditioned to an harmonic series consisting of 250, 500, 750, 1000, and 1250 Hz, and having a pitch that human listeners would match to the fundamental frequency of 250 Hz. Animals were then tested for their response to pure tones between 150 and 1000 Hz. The generalization gradient, shown in Figure 4, has a peak at 250 Hz, indicating that there is an essential similarity between the perception evoked by the broadband, multicomponent stimulus and a pure tone of 250 Hz. This result cannot be interpreted with any confidence yet because the possibility has not been ruled out that the animals listened analytically, and selectively, to the 250 Hz component of the complex.

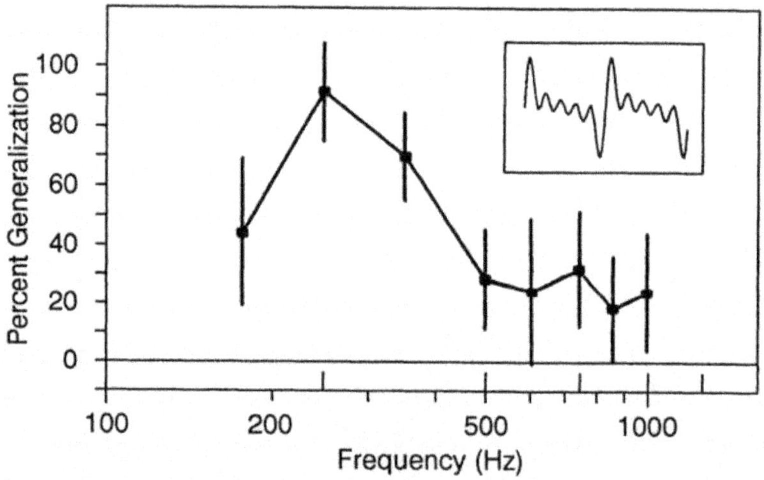

Figure 4. Generalization gradient for eight animals conditioned to first five harmonics of 250 Hz (producing waveform with 4 ms period in inset), and tested to pure tones (from Fay, 1994a). Vertical lines through data points are plus and minus one standard deviation.

2.5 Perception of Temporal Pattern

The results shown in Figure 1 above indicate that goldfish have a monotonic perceptual dimension corresponding with tone frequency that seems analogous to pitch perception in humans. Given the suggestion in Figs. 2 and 4 above that goldfish also have a perceptual dimension something like periodicity pitch in humans (de Boer, 1976), new experiments were designed to investigate its properties. In these experiments (Fay, 1994b), animals were conditioned to a periodic pulse train with a particular interpulse interval (IPI) and then tested to novel pulse trains with different IPIs. Figure 5 shows that generalization gradients tend to be symmetric and monotonic with the difference in repetition rate between conditioning and test stimuli. It appears that pulse trains are judged similar to one another to the extent that they have similar repetition rates. These data support the idea that there is a perceptual dimension, perhaps similar to periodicity pitch, that is monotonic with stimulus pulse repetition rate.

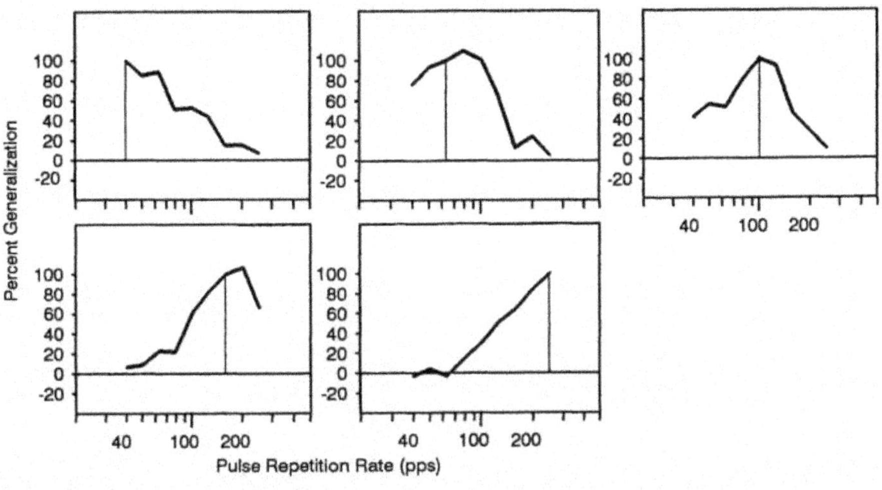

Figure 5. Generalization gradients for five groups of animals conditioned to a high-pass (above 500 Hz) click repeated at the rates indicated by thin vertical lines in each panel, and then tested with the same click repeated at different rates (from Fay, 1994b).

3 Conclusions

The series of stimulus generalization experiments reviewed here have only indirectly addressed the question of auditory scene analysis in a nonhuman animal. Analytic and synthetic listening, the fundamental functions required for sound source determination, have been demonstrated to exist to some degree in goldfish. However, it is not yet clear whether fish are capable of a scene analysis of the type demonstrated for human listeners. The methods and representative results outlined in this paper illustrate the potential usefulness of these and related methods for investigating these kinds of questions. In future studies, these methods will be applied to help determine what aspects of human hearing are specialized or derived, and what aspects are generalized, primitive, and shared with other vertebrates.

4 Acknowledgments

The writing of this paper and the author's research discussed was supported by a Program Project Grant to the Parmly Hearing Institute from the NIH, NIDCD.

5 References

Bregman, A.S. (1990) *Auditory Scene Analysis*. MIT Press: Cambridge.

Burns, E.M. (1982) Pure tone pitch anomalies I: Pitch-intensity effects and diplacusis in normal ears. J. Acoust. Soc. Amer. 72, 1394-1402.

Canfield, J.G., and R.C. Eaton (1990) Swimbladder acoustic pressure transduction initiates Mauthner-mediated escape. Nature 347, 760-762.

de Boer, E. (1976) On the "residue" and auditory pitch perception. In W.D. Keidel and W.D. Neff (Eds.) *Handbook of Sensory Physiology* vol V/3. Springer-Verlag: Berlin, pp. 479-583.

Dooling, R.J. (1989) Perception of complex, species-specific vocalizations by bird and humans. In R.J. Dooling and S.H. Hulse (Eds.) *The Comparative Psychology of Audition: Perceiving Complex Sounds*. Hilldale, NJ: Lawrence Earlbaum Associates, pp. 423-444.

Dooling, R.J. and Hulse, S.H. (Eds.) (1989) *The Comparative Psychology of Audition: Perceiving Complex Sounds*. Hilldale, NJ: Lawrence Earlbaum Associates, pp. 423-444.

Fay, R.R. (1969) Auditory sensitivity of the goldfish within the acoustic nearfield. U.S. Naval Submarine Medical Center, Submarine Base, Groton, Connecticut, Report No. 605, 1-11.

Fay, R.R. (1970a) Auditory frequency generalization in the goldfish. J. Exp. Anal. Behav. 14, 353-360.

Fay, R.R. (1970b) Auditory frequency discrimination in the goldfish. J.Comp. Physiol. Psychol. 73, 175-180.

Fay, R.R. (1972) Perception of amplitude modulated auditory signals by the goldfish. J. Acoust. Soc. Amer. 52, 660-666.

Fay, R.R. (1988) *Hearing in Vertebrates: A Psychophysics Databook*. Hill-Fay Associates: Winnetka, IL.

Fay, R.R. (1992) Analytic listening by the goldfish. Hearing Research 59, 101-107.

Fay, R.R. (1994a) The sense of hearing in fishes: Psychophysics and neurophysiology. Sensory Systems, in press.

Fay, R.R. (1994b) Perception of Temporal acoustic patterns by the goldfish (*Carassius auratus*). Hearing Research, in press.

Fay, R.R. and MacKinnon, J.R. (1969) A simplified technique for conditioning respiratory mouth movements in fish. Behav. Res. Meth. & Instru. 1, 123-124.

Freed, D.J. (1990) Auditory correlates of perceived mallet hardness for a set of recorded percussive sound events. J. Acoust. Soc. Amer. 87, 311-322.

Green, D.M. (1988) *Profile Analysis*. Oxford University Press: Oxford.

Hall, J.W. III, and Grose, J.H. (1990) Comodulation masking release and auditory grouping. J. Acoust. Soc. Amer. 88, 119-125.

Handel, S.J. (1989) *Listening: An Introduction to the Perception of Auditory Events.* MIT Press: Cambridge.

Hartman, W.M. (1988) Pitch perception and the segregation and integration of auditory entities. In Edelman, G.M., Gall, W.E., and Cowan, W.M. (Eds.) *Auditory Function: Neurological Bases of Hearing*. New York: Wiley, pp. 623-645.

Knudsen, E.I., and Knonisi, M. (1979) Mechanisms of sound localization in the barn owl (*Tyto alba*). J. Comp. Physiol. A 133, 13-21

Malott, R.W., and Malott, M.K. (1970) Perception and stimulus generalization. In W.C. Stebbins (Ed.) *Animal Psychophysics: the Design and Conduct of Sensory Experiments.* Appleton-Century-Crofts: New York, pp. 363-400.

McAdams, S. (1989) Segregation of concurrent sounds. I: Effects of frequency modulation coherence. J. Acoust. Soc. Amer. 86, 2148-2159.

Moody, D.B., and Stebbins, W.C. (1989) Salience of frequency modulation in primate communication. In R.J. Dooling and S.H. Hulse (Eds.) *The Comparative Psychology of Audition: Perceiving Complex Sounds.* Hilldale, NJ: Lawrence Earlbaum Associates, pp. 353-376.

Nelson, D.A., and Marler, P. (1989) Categorical perception of a natural stimulus continuum: Birdsong. Science 244, 976-978.

Rogers, P., Lewis, P.N., Willis, M.J., and Abrahamson, S. (1989) Scattered ambient noise as an auditory stimulus for fish. J. Acoust. Soc. Amer. 85, S35 (abstract).

Simmons, J.A., Moss, C.F., and Ferragamo, M. (1990) Convergence of temporal and spectral information into acoustic images of complex sonar targets perceived by the echolocating bat, *Eptesicus fuscus.* J. Comp. Physiol. A 166, 449-470.

Yost, W.A., Sheft, S., and Opie, J. (1989) Modulation detection interference: effect of modulation frequency, J. Acoust. Soc. Amer. 86, 2138-2148.

Yost, W. A. (1991) Auditory image perception and analysis, Hearing Research 56, 8-19.

Zottoli, S.J. (1977) Correlation of the startle reflex and Mauthner cell auditory responses in the unrestrained goldfish. J. Exp. Biol. 66, 243-254.

Comment by E.F. Evans

In the slide you showed of respiration traces across stimuli, it was clear that the fish did gereralize across stimuli in terms of its initial response (i.e: immediately after signal onset compared with the later epoch you chose to use). The early response looks more like the generalization obtained in mammals (e.g. in a positive reinforcement procedure). If you used the early response instead and employed classical discrimination paradigms would you obtain different results from those you presented?

Reply

It's quite true that the respiration wave forms illustrated many trials for one animal (also published in Fay, 1992) show an initial suppression of respiration lasting about 1 sec. at stimulus onset to most all stimuli. If this initial response were used to define the generalization gradients (as in Fig. 2) they would be much wider and show little selecitvity. I believe that this early response is in fact generalization to an acoustic feature shared by all stimuli; thus onset against a silent background. However, the responses occurring later in each trial reflect, I think, the processing of stimulus frequency, sometimes that may take more time to occur than the awareness of stimulus onset. In any case, this generalization paradigm apppears to be sensitive to multiple features of even rather simple stimuli.

As I pointed out in the papers all stimuli used in the generalization test are easily discriminable (Fay, 1970) when goldfish are conditioned to discriminate.

Comment by B. Scharf

In the "detection" task, what were the levels at which sounds were presented? How does the width of the generalization curve compare to the critical band in the goldfish?

Reply

All generalization test stimuli were presented at a sensation level of about 30-40 dB, and thus were clearly detectable.

In general, the width of the generalization gradients (Fig. 2) are many times wider than frequency discrimination thresholds (Fay, 1970), and conform to a parallel function of conditioning frequency. Although we do not have good estimates of critical bandwidths in fish, we do know fish exhibit critical band behaviour and at least have a set of psychophysically defined auditory filters of relatively narrow width (see Fay, 1988 for review).

In general, I believe that the width of generalization gradients will approximate the width of critical bands when they are properly measured, and their functions of frequency will be similar.

Comment by J.P. Wilson

You mentioned that fish were able to discriminate between different delay times in comb-filtered noise. This cue, impressed on environmental noises by reflection, is used by blind people in avoiding obstacles. The human auditory system appears to be well adapted to use this cue (Wilson, 1966) with optimal sensitivity in the 1-10 ms range (reflecting surface distances 0.15-1.5 m). In fish, however, owing to the greater speed of sound in water these distances may be 0.75-7.5 m. These strike me as being greater than that in which fish would be interested. In particular they presumably have adaquate depth information from hydrostatic pressure.

Wilson, J.P. (1966) Obstacle detection using ambient or self generated noise. Nature 211, 218.

Reply

Fay, Yost and Loombs (1983) showed that goldfish are able to discriminate between repetition noise delays of about 1 to 20 ms with about 5 % accuracy. So it is true that goldfish seems to be nearly as well adapted to this cue as humans. It is true that the corresponding distances in water will be over four times greater than in air. Although there are often many good sound reflections underwater (e.g. the surface, bottom, bottom features and other fish with swimbladders) and presumably there will be value to the animal in knowing about their presence and distances, we don't know enough about normal acoustic behavior in usual environments to decide whether or not these distances will be out of a behaviorally significant range.

Fay, R.R., Yost, W.A. and Coombs, S. (1983) Repetition noise processing by a vertebrate auditory system. Hear. Res. 12, 31-35.

Inspiration for a Neuroethologist
by Peter Narins

Though I may hail from another camp
I fully appreciate your damp and ramp.
They lit my lamp and with little cramp,
I intend to tramp through the heat and damp
to playback through my speaker-amp
both the ramp and the damp to a vamp-
ire bat and a frog,
to discover if stimulus generalization
obtains in general.

Reply

Thanks for the lovely poem! [Note that the "ramp" and "damps" experiments Peter refers to here were presented at the meeting but were not incluced in the chapter. An abstract of this work appears in Fay, R.R. and Patterson, R. (1994).

Fay, R.R. and Patterson, R.D.. (1994) Perception of sinusoid "ramps" and "damps" by the goldfish. Abstr. 127th Meet. Acoust. Soc. Am., J. Acoust. Soc. Amer. 95, 2941

Temperature dependence of auditory function in the frog

P.M. Narins

University of California at Los Angeles, Dept. of Biology 405 Hilgard Avenue, Los Angeles, CA 90024, USA

1 Introduction

The inner ear of anurans (frogs and toads) is unusual in that it contains at least two organs which are specialized for the reception of airborne sounds. The amphibian papilla (AP) and the basilar papilla (BP) are anatomically distinct, spatially separate organs each with its own complement of sensory hair cells and overlying tectorium. The AP is the anatomically more complex of the two structures, containing roughly 1000 tonotopically-arranged hair cells, stimulated by the tectorial membrane which presumably supports a travelling wave. The AP is innervated by fibers tuned to low (<500 Hz) and mid (500-1000 Hz) frequencies, although the actual frequency boundaries are species-specific (Zakon and Wilczynski, 1988). In contrast, the BP is thought to be a simply-tuned structure containing roughly 100 hair cells, which are innervated by auditory nerve fibers all tuned to roughly the same high frequency in an individual (the particular frequency is again species-specific). Although these organs have been well-described anatomically (see Lewis *et al.*, 1985 for review) and physiologically (see Fritzsch *et al.*, 1988) quantitative data on the temperature-sensitivity of the response properties of the auditory nerve fibers originating from the two organs has only recently become available. This review is an attempt to describe the effects of temperature changes on the ability of the peripheral auditory system of anuran amphibians to perform spectral and temporal analyses of incoming sounds.

2 Methods

Species chosen for this study were the Pacific tree frog (*Hyla regilla*) and the Puerto Rican coqui (*Eleutherodactylus coqui*), primarily because of the different range of temperatures to which each species is normally exposed. Although *E. coqui* is subjected to a wide range of temperatures in its natural habitat along an altitudinal gradient of over 1000m (Narins and Smith, 1986), local populations at a given altitude experience little temperature variation during the course of the year. Males of this arboreal species produce a two-note advertisement call (Co-Qui). At the higher elevations the 'Co' note is a 100 ms, constant-frequency tone of about 1.1 kHz, and functions in male-male territorial interactions (Narins and Capranica, 1978). The 'Co' note is followed by a pause of 150-200 ms and a second ('Qui') note which sweeps upward in frequency from about 1.8 kHz to 2.1 kHz in about 170 ms. The 'Co' note functions in male-male territorial encounters whereas the 'Qui' note serves to attract females (Narins and Capranica, 1976, 1978).

The Pacific tree frog is found in western North America, from southern British Columbia to Baja California (Stebbins, 1966). Populations of this species occur from sea level up to 7000 feet in areas which experience large temperature variations throughout the year. Males of *H. regilla* produce three distinct calls, as described by Snyder and Jameson (1965): (1) a two-part (diphasic) call consisting of 5-11 frequency-modulated chirps followed by a pause and 2-5 additional chirps. This is the species' advertisement call; (2) a one-part, slightly higher-pitched call consisting of 11-23 chirps repeated at a higher rate than the advertisement call. This vocalization is given in response to movements of other frogs in the vicinity of a calling male; and (3) a prolonged series of staccato notes given in response to the approach of another male. Playback experiments with females have shown that the species-specificity of the call obtains from its temporal parameters (Snyder and Jameson, 1965).

2.1 Animal Preparation

Adult animals were anesthetized 24-48 hrs prior to recording with an intramuscular injection of 1.5-2.0 µl/g of sodium pentobarbital (Nembutal, 50 mg/ml). The eighth nerve was exposed using either a ventral or dorsal surgical approach. Details of the surgical procedure have been described elsewhere (Narins and Wagner, 1989). Animals were only used for experiments if they exhibited normal post-operative behavior, that is, if they could sit upright, and hop in a straight line without circling or listing. About one hour prior to the experiment, the animal was lightly anesthetized (Nembutal) and immobilized with an i.m. injection of curare (1.75-2.5 µl/g). For the recordings the frog was wrapped in wet gauze and placed in a sound insulated chamber (IAC 1202-A) on a Peltier plate located on a vibration-attenuating table.

2.2 Temperature Control

The body temperature of the animal was regulated by a Peltier plate (Cambion, fluidcooled microscope stage) the surface of which could be heated or cooled with an accuracy of ± 0.1°C. Both the core temperature and that of the upper jaw close to the nerve were monitored using a 2-channel thermocouple thermometer (Sensortek BAT-10). Several calibrations were made with one thermistor placed at the location of the nerve and the second one either in the cloaca, beneath the tongue or on the roof of the mouth covered by wet gauze. During the experiments the thermistor was placed on the roof of the mouth, since previous calibrations (Stiebler and Narins 1990) had shown that this location showed the minimum deviation from auditory nerve temperature (Fig. 1) .

During experiments, body temperatures were kept within a range of 12-25°C, and most of the data were collected at temperatures in this range. Starting temperatures varied, as did the direction in which temperature was changed. As a general rule, when the starting temperature was >20°C, the frog was cooled on successive trials, and when starting temperature was <20°C, the frog was warmed. Temperature was changed at a rate of approximately 0.5°C/min, which did not appear to introduce error as similar results were obtained on repeated measures taken on single cells at a single temperature during a heating cycle, a cooling cycle and thermal stasis. Temperature increments between successive trials were 1-3°C.

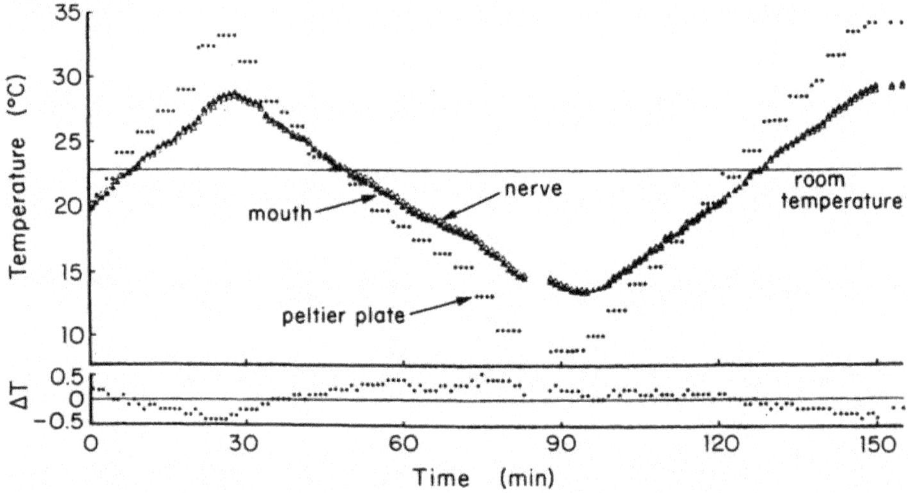

Figure 1. Temperature calibration experiment. The anesthetized frog was placed on a Peltier plate which was subject to a control temperature shift of 24°C/hr. The temperature of a sensor placed on the roof of the mouth with its tip covered with four layers of wet gauze differed from a sensor at the location of the auditory nerve by less than any other sensor position tested (± 0.2°C mean discrepancy).

3 Results

In all frog species tested to date, increasing the temperature results in an upward shift in the CF and a concomitant reduction in CF-threshold of the tuning curves for fibers innervating the amphibian papilla (low- and mid-frequency fibers). In contrast, basilar papilla (high-frequency) fibers appear to have temperature-independent CFs and CF-thresholds (Fig. 2).

Temperature induced shifts of CFs varied from 0.08 octaves/°C for low-frequency fibers to no CF shift for high-frequency BP fibers. The frequency shift/°C may be expressed as a thermal Q_{10} value to simplify comparisons with other temperature-dependent processes (Eatock and Manley, 1981). The thermal Q_{10} for a frequency shift of s octaves may be calculated by:

$$Q_{10} = e^{s\,(10/\Delta T)\ln 2} \qquad (1)$$

where ΔT is the induced temperature shift. From this relationship, the mean Q_{10} for AP fibers of *H. regilla* and *E. coqui* at 300 Hz is 1.74, while the mean Q_{10} for AP fibers for these species at 1000 Hz is 1.45. Clearly, BP fibers have thermal Q_{10} values approximating 1.

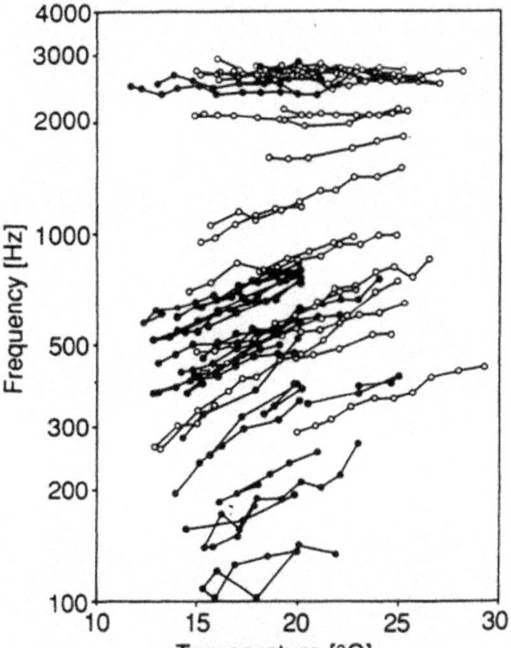

Figure 2. Temperature-induced shift of the CF from all neurons that could be recorded over a range of 5°C or more [24 neurons in H. regilla (●) and 27 neurons in E. coqui (○)]. Data points from the same neurons are connected by lines. The amount of frequency shift decreases with increasing temperature and with increasing CF (from Stiebler and Narins, 1990).

Other response properties of auditory neurons also illustrate pronounced temperature dependence. For example, cooling the fibers results in an increase in CF-thresholds, a progressive phase lead in the preferred phase of firing, an overall diminishing in the strength of phase locking, especially rapidly below 13.0°C, and an increased latency in the response to short duration clicks. All of these changes are illustrated for a representative afferent fiber from *E. coqui* in Fig. 3.

Recently, the temperature dependence of two-tone rate suppression (TTRS) was determined for a population of AP fibers in the northern leopard frog, *Rana pipiens pipiens* (Benedix *et al.*, 1994). The existence region of two-tone rate suppression in frog low-frequency auditory nerve fibers was found to include a suppressive region below a fiber's characteristic frequency, contrary to previous reports. In response to a 3°C temperature rise, the area and the best suppressive frequency (BSF) of the low-side suppressive region significantly increased. Increasing core temperature of the frog by 6°C

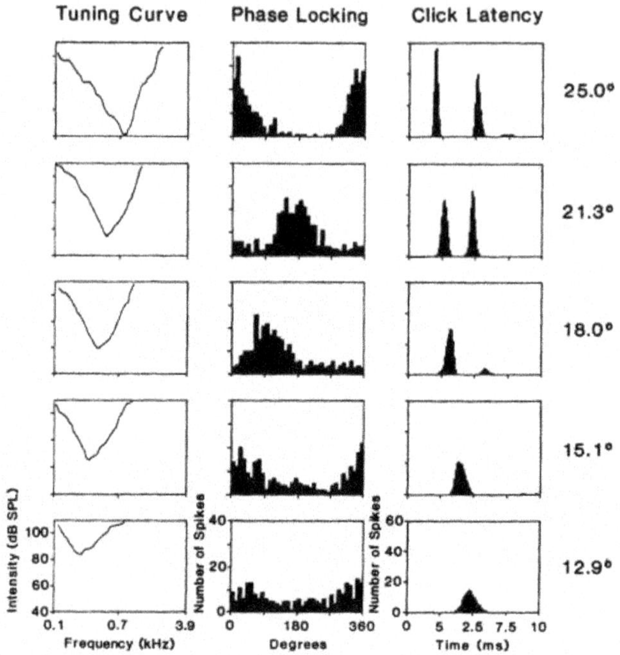

Figure 3. An example of tuning curve displacement, preferred firing phase shift, and click latency change in response to decreasing temperature from an AP neuron in E. coqui. This fiber had a CF at 25°C of 751 Hz; at 12.9°C the CF was reduced to 239 Hz.

resulted in significant changes in the high-side suppressive region: its area decreased, and its BSF and best suppressive threshold (BST) increased. Fig. 4 shows the responses of two AP fibers in *Rana pipiens pipiens* to core temperature changes of 3°C and 6°C. In each case the excitatory tuning curve shifts to higher frequency and the best threshold decreases in response to heating the fiber. The high-side suppressive region decreases in area and its best suppressive threshold increases, while the low-side suppressive area shifts to higher CFs without a concomitant shift in best suppressive threshold.

4 Discussion

Tuning in the peripheral auditory system is a process that depends on the integrity of the inner ear metabolism. Controlled temperature shifts offer the possibility to assess the metabolic dependency of the tuning process in a reversible way, especially in ectothermic animals for which daily core temperature changes of 20°C are not uncommon (Huey,

1982). Data on temperature effects on response properties of single auditory fibers are relatively scarce. In the cat, eighth nerve fibers with characteristic frequencies (CFs) near 20 kHz exhibited increased thresholds at lower temperatures with little change in CF (Klinke and Smolders, 1977). Primary auditory fibers in the tokay gecko (Eatock and Manley, 1981), the caiman (Smolders and Klinke, 1984) and the pigeon (Schermuly and

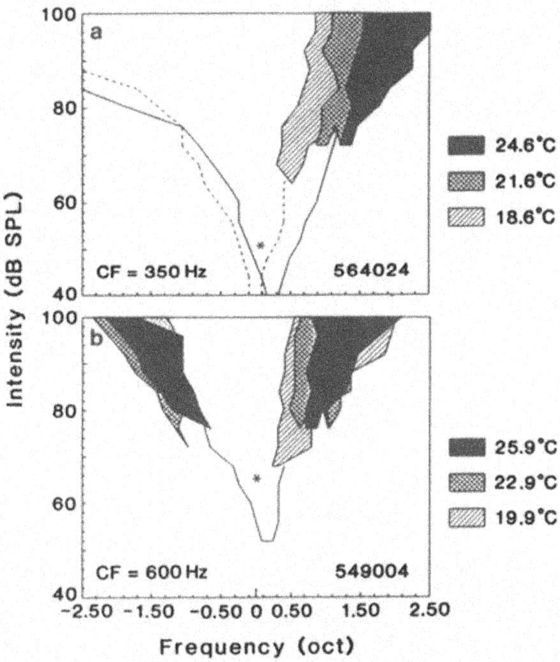

*Figure 4. Shifts in suppression areas resulting from changes in frog body temperature for two AP fibers. In (a), two excitatory tuning curves (FTCs) are given; the dashed line is the FTC taken at the lowest of the three temperatures tested, while the solid line is the FTC obtained at the highest temperature tested. The only FTC obtained in (b) was for the highest temperature tested. The ID number of the fiber is indicated in the lower right of each panel, while the CFs given refer to the '0' (reference) points on the frequency axis. All other frequencies on this axis are relative to the reference point. The frequency and intensity of the excitatory tones are marked by the *'s. As temperature increases, the high-side suppressive regions are generally reduced in area, elevated in threshold and shifted to higher frequencies. Low-side suppressive areas (b) increase, shift to higher frequencies, but thresholds remain unchanged in response to temperature increases. All suppression areas indicate 100% suppression.*

Klinke, 1985) showed decreases in CF and concomitant elevations in CF-thresholds upon cooling. In a brief report, Moffat and Capranica (1976) stated that similar temperature-dependent CF-shifts occur in fibers innervating the amphibian papilla of the American toad (*Bufo americanus*) but not the basilar papilla.

The frequency of otoacoustic emissions in frogs has been shown to be temperature-dependent (van Dijk and Wit, 1987), suggesting a metabolic dependence for their production. Interestingly, the higher frequency emissions appear to show a greater frequency shift for a given temperature change than do the lower frequency emissions. Thus, the relationship between otacoustic emissions and auditory nerve responses in the frog is still unclear, and needs to be explored further.

We and others have demonstrated the temperature-dependence of auditory fiber frequency selectivity, CF and CF-threshold. Moreover, we have showed that the preferred firing phase and precision of phase-locked neural responses are susceptible to temperature variation in the range of that experienced by the animal in its natural habitat (Stiebler and Narins, 1990). Such clear temperature dependence of auditory nerve function strongly implies a metabolic, possibly membrane-related process in the mechanisms underlying temporal coding as opposed to a purely mechanical process (Ashmore and Atwell, 1985).

The facts that (1) the low-side and high-side suppression areas shift differentially in response to small temperature shifts (as small as 3°C, and certainly 6°C), and (2) the excitatory and suppressive areas exhibit quite distinct behaviors in the face of a temperature shift suggest the possibility that the two suppression areas are independently generated. Moreover, the uncoupling of excitation and suppression under conditions of temperature shift implies that separate mechanisms might be responsible for their generation.

There is some precedent for these observations in mammals. Evans (1980) showed that in pathological guinea pig cochleas the BST for the high-side suppressive area can increase by more than 40 dB above the low-side suppressive area. In addition, following intra-arterial application of 2.5 ml of furosemide in the cat, the time constant for recovery of excitation of auditory nerve fibers appears to be longer than that for suppression (Narins and Evans, unpublished data). Robertson and Johnstone (1981) demonstrated that in guinea pigs exposed to a high-intensity tone in the vicinity of the high-side suppression region, the excitatory tuning curve remained unchanged while the area of the high-side suppressive region decreased (no effect was observed on the low-side suppressive areas).

Decreasing body temperature has been shown to decrease the CFs and increase the thresholds of anuran AP fibers (Moffat and Capranica 1976; Stiebler and Narins 1990; van Dijk *et al.* 1990). Two factors that may contribute to these shifts are mechanical changes in the overlying tectorial membrane and changes in the kinetics of ion-specific channels in the hair cell membranes. The observed shifts in the tuning curve in response to a reduction in temperature are consistent with an increase in the stiffness of the tectorial membrane. This simple change in a single mechanical property of the tectorial membrane would result in a smaller displacement in response to a given force, and a shift in the position of the maximum displacement caudalward (toward higher frequencies). We assume that at a fiber's CF the hair cells innervated by that fiber are being maximally stimulated. Thus, from the perspective of a given auditory nerve fiber, after a temperature decrease and a concomitant caudal shift of the position of maximum displacement, the stimulus frequency would need to be lowered in order to once again produce maximum displacement at the locus of that fiber's distal synapse. Similarly and consistently, an increase in temperature results in an upward CF-shift and a threshold decrease for AP fibers. Moreover, changes (with temperature) in the stiffness of the stereociliary bundle may affect the mechanical motion of the tectorial membrane (Benser *et al.*, 1993) and thus contribute to the observed changes in eighth nerve fiber responses. However, we believe that it is unlikely that temperature shifts as small as 3°C could change these mechanical properties enough to account for the observed changes in TTRS. Direct measurements of the tectorial membrane motion as a function of temperature would be needed to resolve this question.

Lability of excitatory (and suppressive) tuning curves is more likely due to electrical changes in hair cell membranes. One possible explanation for the CF shift may be found in the mechanism underlying electrical tuning in sensory hair cells such as that reported in the turtle cochlea (Crawford and Fettiplace, 1981) and for low-frequency hair cells of the frog's AP (Pitchford and Ashmore, 1987). Since the kinetics of whole cell currents are known to be temperature dependent (Hodgkin and Huxley, 1952), it is at least plausible that the hair cell resonance frequency would increase with increasing temperature. Hair cell resonances are thought to arise from the interplay between a voltage-activated Ca^{++} conductance and a Ca^{++} -activated K^{+} conductance in the hair cell membrane (Lewis and Hudspeth, 1983). Little direct evidence is available to date implicating the temperature-lability of specific channel currents as the biophysical underpinning of the observed auditory nerve fiber CF-shifts evoked by warming or cooling the auditory system (see Serrano and Narins, 1989 for an exception). We are presently conducting experiments in our lab to elucidate the extent to which specific ionic hair cell membrane currents are temperature-dependent, and how this dependence contributes to CF, threshold and tuning shifts observed at the level of the auditory nerve.

5 Acknowledgments

The author gratefully acknowledges the contributions of Jim Benedix, Imme Stiebler, Marisa Pedemonte and Ricardo Velluti to this work. Supported by NIH grant no. DC-00222.

6 References

Ashmore, J.F. and Attwell, D. (1985) Models for electrical tuning in hair cells. Proc. R. Soc. Lond. B 226, 325-344.

Benedix, J.H., Jr., Pedemonte, M., Velluti, R., and Narins, P.M. (1994) Temperature dependence of two-tone suppression in the northern leopard frog, *Rana pipiens pipiens*. J. Acoust. Soc. Am. (In press).

Benser, M. E., Issa, N. P., and Hudspeth, A. J. (1993) Hair-bundle stiffness dominates the elastic reactance to otolithic-membrane shear. Hearing Res. 68, 243-252.

Crawford, A.C. and Fettiplace, R. (1981) An electrical tuning mechanism in turtle cochlear hair cells. J. Physiol. 312, 377-412.

Eatock, R.A. and Manley, G.A. (1981) Auditory nerve fibre activity in the Tokay Gecko II. Temperature effect on tuning. J. Comp. Physiol. 142, 219-226.

Evans, E. F. (1980) Comment on "Two-tone suppression and intermodulation distortion in the cochlea: effect of outer hair cell lesions," (P. Dallos et al.) In: Psychophysical, Physiological and Behavioural Studies in Hearing, (G. van den Brink and F. A. Bilsen, eds.) Delft University Press, Delft, 250.

Fritzsch, B., Ryan, M., Wilczynski, W., Hetherington T., and Walkowiak, W. (1988) The Evolution of the Amphibian Auditory System. John Wiley & Sons, New York.

Hodgkin, A.L. and Huxley, A.F. (1952) A quantitative description of membrane current and its application to conduction and excitation in nerve. J. Physiol. 117, 500-544.

Huey, R.B. (1982) Temperature, physiology, and the ecology of reptiles. In: Biology of the Reptilia. C. Gans and F.H. Pough, Eds. Acad. Press, London. pp. 25-91.

Klinke, R. and Smolders J. (1977) Effect of temperature shift on tuning properties. Addendum to: Klinke, R., Pause, M.: The performance of a primitive hearing organ of the cochlea type: Primary fibre studies in the caiman. In: Psychophysics and Physiology of Hearing, (E.F. Evans and J.P. Wilson, eds.) Academic Press, London, 100-112.

Lewis, E.R., Leverenz, E. L., and Bialek, W. S. (1985) The Vertebrate Inner Ear (CRC Press, Boca Raton, Florida).

Lewis, R. S., and Hudspeth, A. J. (1983) Voltage- and ion-dependent conductances in solitary vertebrate hair cells. Nature 304, 358-541.

Moffat, A. J. M., and Capranica, R. R. (1976). Effects of temperature on the response of the auditory nerve in the American toad (*Bufo americanus*). J. Acoust. Soc. Am. 60, Suppl. 1, S80.

Narins, P.M., and Capranica, R. R. (1976) Sexual differences in the auditory system of the tree frog *Eleutherodactylus coqui*. Science 192, 378-380.

Narins, P.M. and Capranica, R.R. (1978) Communicative significance of the two-note call of the treefrog *Eleutherodactylus coqui*. J. Comp. Physiol. 127, 1-9.

Narins, P.M. and Smith, S.L. (1986) Clinal variation in anuran advertisement calls: basis for acoustic isolation? Behav. Ecol. Sociobiol. 19: 135-141.

Narins, P.M. and Wagner, I. (1989) Noise susceptibility and immunity of phaselocking in amphibian auditory nerve fibers. J. Acoust. Soc. Am. 85, 1255-1265.

Pitchford, S. and Ashmore, J.F. (1987) An electrical resonance in hair cells of the amphibian papilla of the frog *Rana temporaria*. Hearing Res. 27, 75-83.

Robertson, D., and Johnstone, B. M. (1981). Primary auditory neurons: Nonlinear responses altered without changes in sharp tuning. J. Acoust. Soc. Am. 69, 1096-1098.

Schermuly, L. and Klinke, R. (1985) Change of characteristic frequency of pigeon primary auditory afferents with temperature. J. Comp. Physiol. 156, 209-211.

Serrano, E.E. and Narins, P.M. (1989) Membrane currents in dissociated hair cells from the inner ear of *Rana pipiens*. Abstr. of presentation at 19th meeting of the Society for Neuroscience 207.

Smolders, J.W.T and Klinke, R. (1984) Effects of temperature on the properties of primary auditory fibres of the spectacled caiman, *Caiman crocodilus* (L.). J. Comp. Physiol. 155, 19-30.

Snyder, W.F. and Jameson, D.L. (1965) Multivariate geographic variation of mating call in populations of the Pacific Tree Frog (*Hyla regilla*). Copeia 1965, 129-142.

Stebbins, R.C. (1966) A Field Guide to Western Reptiles and Amphibians. Houghton Mifflin Co., Boston.

Stiebler, I.B. and Narins, P.M. (1990) Temperature-dependence of auditory nerve response properties in the frog. Hearing Res. 46, 63-82.

van Dijk, P., Lewis, E.R., and Wit, H.P. (1990) Temperature effects on auditory nerve fiber response in the American bullfrog. Hearing Res. 44, 231-240.

van Dijk, P. and Wit, H.P. (1987) Temperature dependence of frog spontaneous otoacoustic emissions. J. Acoust. Soc. Am. 82, 2147-2150.

Zakon, H.H. and Wilczynski, W. (1988) The physiology of the anuran eighth nerve. In: The Evolution of the Amphibian Auditory System, (B. Fritzsch, M..J. Ryan, W. Wilczynski, T.E. Hetherington, W. Walkowiak, eds.) John Wiley & Sons, New York, 125-155.

Otoacoustic emissions as an indicator for active cochlear mechanics: A primitive property of vertebrate auditory organs

Christine Köppl

Institut für Zoologie, Technische Universität München, Lichtenbergstraße 4, 85747 Garching, Germany

1 Introduction

It is generally believed that otoacoustic emissions represent mechanical energy actively produced by the hair cells of the auditory organ and transmitted via the middle ear to the external world. This is especially true for spontaneous otoacoustic emissions, that are faint tonal sounds emitted without any external stimulation, to provide a primary source of energy. Models based on a self-sustaining sinusoidal oscillator (e.g. Talmadge et al., 1991) are able to reproduce some important properties of spontaneous emissions, although the physical realization of this oscillator in the auditory organ still remains to be established.

Spontaneous as well as evoked otoacoustic emissions have been measured in all major groups of land vertebrates, including frogs, reptiles, birds and mammals. It may thus be assumed that the ability to generate otoacoustic emissions is a primitive property of vertebrate hearing organs. The present paper provides a brief overview of otoacoustic emissions, with special emphasis on spontaneous emissions and non-mammalian species, and discusses the possible mechanisms generating these emissions in the different vertebrates.

2 Which species show otoacoustic emissions?

There are two basic classes of otoacoustic emissions, spontaneous and evoked. The latter are commonly categorized with respect to the stimulus evoking them, i.e. click-evoked or delayed-evoked emissions, simultaneously-evoked or stimulus-frequency emissions (in response to a continuously-swept tone) and distortion-product emissions (in response to two simultaneously-presented tones).

All of these different kinds of emissions were originally described in humans and have subsequently been found with varying success in other mammalian and non-mammalian species. Distortion-product emissions can be reliably evoked in most healthy ears (Rosowski et al., 1984; Norton and Rubel, 1990; Probst, 1990; Kettembeil and Manley, 1992; Manley et al., 1993), but they are appear to be absent in frogs (Baker et al., 1989). Click-evoked emissions are only known from mammals (Probst, 1990). However, the failure to detect them in non-mammalian species may be due to technical limitations:

the short emission latency that may be expected from those auditory organs (which are mostly significantly shorter than a mammalian cochlea) possibly precludes a clear separation of stimulus and emission (Manley et al., 1987). Stimulus-frequency emissions have been found in all non-mammalian species where they were looked for (frog: Whitehead et al., 1986; caiman: Klinke and Smolders, 1984; starling: Manley et al., 1987).

Spontaneous otoacoustic emissions (SOAE) also seem to be universal, being described in several species of frogs and lizards, a bird (the barn owl) and several species of mammals. Since they are also the most obvious and least disputed indicator for an active production of mechanical energy by the auditory organ, their characteristics will be briefly reviewed and compared between the different species.

Frogs: SOAE in amphibians have been looked for and found in three closely-related frog species (review in Wilson et al., 1990): *Rana temporaria* (grass frog; Baker et al., 1989), *Rana catesbeiana* (the American bullfrog; Genossa et al., 1989) and *Rana esculenta* (the European edible frog; Palmer and Wilson, 1981; van Dijk et al., 1989), where the most detailed data exist. The frequency of occurrence seems to be seasonally dependent and was as high as 71% of ears at the best time of year (van Dijk et al., 1989). SOAE frequencies show a bimodal distribution in *R. esculenta*, with peaks around 0.8 and 1-1.2 kHz respectively, reflecting the common pattern of 1 or 2 SOAE per ear (van Dijk et al., 1989; Long et al., 1993). In *R. temporaria* and *R. catesbeiana* (Whitehead et al., 1986; Baker et al., 1989; Genossa et al., 1989), SOAE frequencies are below 1 kHz. Suppression of SOAE with external tones is most sensitive around the SOAEs' own frequency (Baker et al., 1989), suggesting that the SOAE originate at the place in the auditory organ with the highest sensitivity to their centre frequency. According to frequency maps and other information about tonotopic organization in mostly other frog species (review in Zakon and Wilczynski, 1988), the SOAE thus probably originate in the amphibian papilla and not in the basilar papilla.

Frog SOAE are often relatively broad-band, with spectral widths ranging between 1 and 200 Hz (van Dijk et al., 1989). The amplitude distributions of large SOAE (providing a sufficient signal-to-noise ratio) are two-peaked, indicating that they are a truly sinusoidal signal and not narrow-band noise (van Dijk et al., 1989; van Dijk and Wit, 1990). External tones placed close to an SOAE in frequency and not loud enough to suppress it, induce a shift of the SOAE's frequency away from the tone, up to 80 Hz in two cases tested (Baker et al., 1989). Frog SOAE are temperature-sensitive, shifting up in frequency with an increase in temperature (Whitehead et al., 1986; van Dijk et al., 1989; Genossa et al., 1989). The rate of shift is larger for higher-frequency SOAE and at lower temperatures, ranging between 0.02 and 0.055 octaves/°C and corresponding to a thermal Q_{10} of 1.1 to 1.4 (van Dijk et al., 1989).

Lizards: SOAE in lizards have been found to date in several species of different families with very different structures of the auditory organ: *Tiliqua rugosa* (the Australian bobtail lizard; Köppl and Manley, 1993), *Gekko gecko* (the Tokay gecko), *Eublepharis macularius* (the leopard gecko) and *Callopistes maculatus* (the Chile teju; Manley et al., 1994a). Preliminary, unpublished data also exist for *Cnemidophorus* *lemniscatus* (spotted racerunner) and *Varanus exanthimaticus* (Bosc's monitor). All lizards show SOAE with a very high probability; between 72 and 100% of ears were found to emit in different species (Köppl and Manley, 1993; Manley et al., 1994a). The SOAE are always rather broad-band, with spectral widths between 7 and 225 Hz (Köppl and Manley, 1993; Manley et al., 1994a). As in frogs, the amplitude distribution of large SOAE suggests a sinusoidal generator (van Dijk and Manley, pers. comm.).

The emission pattern, i.e. number and frequencies of SOAE per ear, is clearly species-specific and shows some correlation with the anatomy of the auditory organ, the basilar papilla (Manley et al., 1994b). Thus the SOAE patterns of the bobtail lizard and the geckos are similar to each other, typically showing many SOAE between 1 and 4.5 kHz. The pattern seen in the chile teju, the racerunner and the monitor lizard on the other hand is quite distinct from this, typically showing 2 SOAE at species-specific frequencies with little inter-individual variation. Unfortunately, the bobtail lizard is currently the only species where sufficient physiological data are available to infer the place of origin of SOAE within the papilla. In this species, the frequency range of SOAE (0.93-4.6 kHz) overlaps perfectly with the range coded by the high-frequency segment of the papilla, whereas frequencies appropriate for the low-frequency segment are missing in the SOAE (Köppl and Manley, 1993). Also, the shape of SOAE suppression tuning curves strongly suggests an origin of SOAE in the high-frequency segment only (Köppl and Manley, 1994). A division of the basilar papilla into two distinct segments is typical for lizards and indirect evidence indicates that micromechanical tuning mechanisms are much more important in the high-frequency segment (Köppl and Manley, 1992).

Lizard SOAE are easily shifted in frequency by external tones placed near them. Shifts of 100-200 Hz directed away from the external tone are regularly observed, maximal shifts exceeded 300 Hz (Köppl and Manley, 1994 and unpublished observations). Lizard SOAE are also temperature-sensitive in a way qualitatively similar to that described in frogs (Manley and Köppl, 1994). However, the rates of change of frequency per degree temperature change seem to be significantly faster in the Chile teju (0.08 to 0.19 octaves/°C; Pavusa, pers. comm.) compared to the bobtail lizard and the geckos (0.01 to 0.1 octaves/°C; Manley and Köppl, 1994; Gallo, pers. comm.).

Birds: In birds, SOAE have only recently been reported for the first time, in the barn owl, *Tyto alba* (Manley and Taschenberger, 1993). Several chickens (*Gallus gallus*) and starlings (*Sturnus vulgaris*) have also been screened, but so far showed no indication of SOAE (Taschenberger and Kettembeil, pers. comm.). In the owl, SOAE are fairly common (65 to 75% of ears), but low in amplitude (mostly below 0 dB SPL) and often unstable. Most SOAE frequencies cluster at the upper end of this bird's hearing range (7.5 to 10.3 kHz). They are suppressed most easily with external tones of a frequency very close to their own. Assuming therefore that they are generated at the place on the basilar papilla most sensitive to their frequency, most SOAE probably originate from a very specialized region of the owl's papilla, termed the auditory fovea (Köppl et al., 1993). Here, the frequency band behaviorally most relevant for the owl in acoustic prey localization (5 to 10 kHz), is represented over an enormously expanded space and many morphological specializations are seen compared to other birds. The spectral bandwidths of the larger owl SOAE ranged between 4.5 and 22 Hz. As in frogs and lizards, SOAE are temperature sensitive, with rates of change of 0.023 to 0.044 octaves/°C (Taschenberger, pers. comm.).

Mammals: SOAE in mammals have been most intensively studied in humans, which seem to show by far the highest incidence of SOAE (at best about 55% of ears; Talmadge et al., 1993) compared to other mammalian species (Martin et al., 1985; Ohyama et al., 1991; review in Probst, 1990). SOAE are mostly within the same frequency range as seen in non-mammals, i.e. up to 10 kHz. However, reports on rare SOAE in the mustached bat, *Pteronotus parnellii* (Kössl and Vater, 1985; Kössl, 1994) show that they can occur at frequencies as high as 63 kHz. Mammalian SOAE often reach larger amplitudes than those seen in non-mammalian species, sometimes as high as 40 or 50 dB SPL (review in Probst, 1990). In addition, they seem to be much narrower in bandwidth, typical values for large SOAE being below 1 Hz (van Dijk and Wit, 1990). However, as in non-mammals (van Dijk et al., 1989; Köppl and Manley, 1993), a dependence of bandwidth on the level of the SOAE is observed, such that low-level SOAE (more comparable to non-mammalian SOAE) have bandwidths up to 30 Hz (Talmadge et al., 1993).

SOAE shift in frequency in response to external tones placed near them, but only up to 15 Hz (Rabinowitz and Widin, 1984; Long et al., 1991). They are most sensitive to suppression by external tones at a frequency systematically higher than their own, by between 10 and 150 Hz (von Dallmayr, 1985; Martin et al., 1988). Interestingly, experiments on guinea pigs in which the body temperature was varied over a 6° range showed the SOAE to be temperature-sensitive (Ohyama et al., 1992). The rate of change of frequency with temperature was within the range of values observed in non-mammals.

3 How do spontaneous otoacoustic emissions compare across species?

Several fundamental properties of SOAE are universal across all species:

a) Each spontaneously-emitting ear shows an individual pattern of SOAE frequencies, which is stable over both short and long time periods.

b) SOAE are physiologically vulnerable, e.g. they vanish reversibly under brief hypoxia.

c) As indicated by their amplitude distribution, SOAE are sinusoidal signals, generated by some active oscillator.

d) SOAE can be suppressed by external tones. This effect is strongly frequency-selective, requiring higher sound pressures for tones further away in frequency from the SOAE.

e) SOAE frequency is temperature-dependent. This is even true in the case of mammals, where a temperature dependency of tuning frequency is not seen any more at the level of the cochlear nucleus (Gummer and Klinke, 1983).

Differences between SOAE in different species are:

a) The prevalence of SOAE varies widely, with the lizards showing the highest probability (up to 100% of ears), closely followed by frogs (at least at their active time of year). In birds and mammals, the probability of SOAE being found seems to be extremely species-dependent. However, the consistently reported and so far unexplained difference in human SOAE prevalence between men and women suggests that a problem may also lie in the detectability of SOAE, tiny differences in e.g. the sizes of inner- middle- and outer ear structures possibly having a large influence.

b) The typical number of SOAE per ear and their frequency range are largely species-specific, sometimes correlating with extreme specializations in the inner ear, as in the barn owl and the mustached bat.

c) The spectral bandwidths of SOAE seem at first glance to be far smaller in mammals. Considering that non-mammalian SOAE are mostly smaller in amplitude, however, and that the bandwidth depends on the level of the SOAE, this difference diminishes. Remaining smaller differences, also between the non-mammalian species, could be due to different intrinsic cochlear noise levels perturbing the presumed oscillatory emission generator. Also, or in addition, they could reflect different inherent stabilities of the generator itself.

d) SOAE generally shift their frequency in response to an external tone, however, to a very varying extent. Lizard SOAE often shift several hundred Hz, frog SOAE about 80 Hz, but mammalian SOAE only up to 15 Hz.

e) The shapes of iso-suppression tuning curves of SOAE differ in a species-specific manner, corresponding to the shapes of neural tuning curves typical for the respective species. In non-mammals, the tips of such tuning curves correspond, on average, to the SOAE's own frequency, whereas in mammals, a small but consistent deviation to higher frequencies is present.

In conclusion, SOAE are a wide-spread phenomenon among vertebrate auditory organs. The differences seen between SOAE are to a large extent species-specific in nature. Apparent differences between mammalian and non-mammalian SOAE (e.g. in amplitude, spectral bandwidth and frequency shifting) are mostly of a gradual type and are also seen, to a lesser extent, between the various non-mammalian species. The only genuine difference so far seems to be that the most effective suppressor frequency and the SOAE frequency do not coincide in mammals, whereas they do in the non-mammals. This contrast, however, does not necessarily imply a genuine difference in the SOAE generator mechanism. It may instead be associated with the introduction of a sharply-tuned mechanical travelling wave in the mammalian cochlea, a mechanism of less (Gummer et al., 1987) or no importance (Peake and Ling, 1980; Manley et al., 1988) in non-mammalian auditory organs.

4 Is OHC-like electromotility a likely universal mechanism?

SOAE almost undoubtly reflect the active production of mechanical activity within the auditory organ. In mammals, the concept of a cochlear amplifier or active feedback mechanism actively enhancing vibration amplitudes in response to near-threshold stimuli, is now well established (e.g. Dallos, 1992; Yates et al., 1992; Pickles, 1993). SOAE are generally thought to be an epiphenomenon of this cochlear amplifier. The fast electromotility of guinea pig outer hair cells (OHC) *in vitro*, discovered about a decade ago (Brownell et al., 1985) and intensively studied since then, is regarded as a possible physical basis of such an active mechanism. However, active cochlear mechanisms, if SOAE are any indication, are obviously a primitive property, present in many vertebrate auditory organs. Given the fundamental similarities between SOAE of different species, we may ask whether fast electromotility of the hair-cell body, similar to that observed for OHC, is a likely general mechanism.

To date, there have been virtually no attempts to directly reproduce the *in vitro* electromotile responses of guinea pig OHC with hair cells from non-mammalian species. Preliminary experiments with isolated hair cells of the pigeon basilar papilla showed no cycle-by-cycle contraction to current injection (Zimmermann et al., 1989). Lacking physiological data, there are also morphological correlates of fast electromotility that may serve as indicators for its presence or absence. The motor mechanism itself, located within the plasma membrane of OHC, is correlated with an unusually high density of intramembrane particles (Kalinec et al., 1992). A highly-organized cortical cytoskeleton, like that of OHC, consisting of the cortical lattice and associated lateral cisternae (Holley, 1991), is probably necessary to maintain cell shape and direct the forces produced in the membrane. Also, mammalian OHC in the intact organ of Corti are only loosely surrounded by supporting cells, with prominent spaces theoretically providing enough freedom for the OHC cell body to move. With the exception of the density of intramembrane particles, whose visualization requires freeze-fracturing (Kalinec et al., 1992), these anatomical characteristics can be recognized by standard histological techniques. Despite a large body of morphological data, including many studies at the TEM level, however, *none* of these features has been identified to date in non-mammalian auditory organs (e.g. Takasaka and Smith, 1971; Lewis and Lombard, 1988; Miller and Beck, 1988; Sneary, 1988; Fischer, 1992, 1994).

Mostly indirect, but abundant, evidence therefore suggests that OHC-like fast electromotility of the cell body is not likely to be a universal mechanism, but something mammals developed either in addition to or instead of a previously existing active mechanism. It is important in this context that doubts about the presumed role of OHC motility as the cochlear amplifier in the mammalian cochlea have been raised, the chief question invariably being its feasability as a cycle-by-cycle amplifier at high frequencies. The cut-off frequency of the actual motor mechanism may still be uncertain due to technical limitations (Santos-Sacchi, 1992). However, it has often been pointed out (e.g. Dallos, 1992; Santos-Sacchi, 1992; Pickles, 1993) that its dependance on transmembrane voltage will in effect mean a low-pass characteristic following the hair cell's receptor potential. Above several kHz, the potential cycle-by-cycle effect of electromotility would therefore be negligible. Experiments with isolated OHC or cochlear explants from the bat *Carollia perspicillata* corroborate this sceptical view: even in this high-frequency specialist, no electromotiliy was detectable above a stimulation frequency of 1 kHz (Kössl et al., 1993). It is also worth noting that spontaneous oscillatory motility of isolated OHC has never been reported to occur under the wide range of electrical and chemical conditions employed *in vitro*.

5 Are there alternative mechanisms?

If we assume that electromotility is unique to mammalian hair cells, this means that another active mechanism must be operative in non-mammals and possibly in mammals as well. A well-known alternative is oscillatory movements of the hair cell's stereovillar bundle, as observed spontaneously or in response to step displacements or current injections in papillar hair cells of the red-eared turtle (Crawford and Fettiplace, 1985), in saccular hair cells of frogs (Denk and Webb, 1992) and in ampullary hair cells of eels (Rüsch and Thurm, 1990). The underlying mechanism and its upper frequency limit are not known. These bundle motions, however, have been observed at frequencies of several hundred Hz (Crawford and Fettiplace, 1985; Denk and Webb, 1992). For the frog saccular hair cells, Denk and Webb (1992) concluded that the membrane potential drives bundle motion. In the turtle, a tight correlation of membrane potential and bundle motion was also observed (Crawford and Fettiplace, 1985).

The dependence on membrane potential, however, raises the same argument as given above for electromotility with regard to the efficiency of such a mechanism at high frequencies: it would not work on a cycle-by-cycle basis above several kHz. While a mechanism with an upper limit of several kHz would be sufficient for non-mammals, it clearly would not do for mammals, remembering the strong suggestion of mechanical activity at 63 kHz by SOAE in the mustached bat (Kössl and Vater, 1985; Kössl, 1994).

It seems that a universal mechanism for the cochlear amplifier in vertebrates, covering the high frequencies in mammals as well, would ideally be independent of the AC membrane potential. Possible force-generating mechanisms that are directly associated with the transduction channels are of interest in this context. Hudspeth and Gillespie (1994) have recently suggested that hair-bundle myosin, thought to mediate adaptation, may also be involved in active amplification. Markin and Tsong (1991) suggested, on theoretical grounds, a mechanism possibly involving only the transduction channels. Their model showed that an ion-transporting protein undergoing conformational changes that produce stretch in the membrane possesses bidirectional transduction properties. It makes several predictions, one of which, a stiffness decrease during protein conformational transition, is reminiscent of the change in stiffness shown by stereovillar bundles of frog saccular hair cells as they are displaced. This has been interpreted as reflecting forces generated by the mechanoreceptive gates switching states (Howard and Hudspeth, 1988). A suggestion along similar lines, directly linking the active mechanism to the transduction channels, is made by Manley (this volume).

In conclusion, SOAE are a strong indication that active cochlear feedback is operating in most or all vertebrate auditory organs. From an evolutionary point of view and considering the fundamental similarities between SOAE in different species, the same basic generator mechanism may be assumed. Convincing evidence for such a mechanism, however, is still lacking. The main problem for any possible mechanism remains the effective generation of the very high frequency oscillations shown and required in the mammalian cochlea.

6 References

Baker, R.J., Wilson, J.P. and Whitehead, M.L. (1989) Otoacoustic evidence for nonlinear behaviour in frogs' hearing: Suppression but no distortion products. In: J.P. Wilson and D.T. Kemp (Eds.) Cochlear mechanisms: Structure, functions and models. Plenum Press, London, pp. 349-356

Brownell, W.E., Bader, C.R., Bertrand, D. and de Ribaupierre, Y. (1985) Evoked mechanical responses of isolated cochlear outer hair cells. Science 227, 194-196.

Crawford, A.C. and Fettiplace, R. (1985) The mechanical properties of ciliary bundles of turtle cochlear hair cells. J. Physiol. 364, 359-379.

von Dallmayr, C. (1985) Spontane oto-akustische Emissionen: Statistik und Reaktion auf akustische Störtöne. Acustica 59, 67-75.

Dallos, P. (1992) The active cochlea. J. Neurosci. 12, 4575-4585.

Denk, W. and Webb, W.W. (1992) Forward and reverse transduction at the limit of sensitivity studied by correlating electrical and mechanical fluctuations in frog saccular hair cells. Hear. Res. 60, 89-102.

van Dijk, P. and Wit, H.P. (1990) Amplitude and frequency fluctuations of spontaneous otoacoustic emissions. J. Acoust. Soc. Am. 88, 1779-1793.

van Dijk, P., Wit, H.P. and Segenhout, J.M. (1989) Spontaneous otoacoustic emissions in the European edible frog (*Rana esculenta*): Spectral details and temperature dependence. Hear. Res. 42, 273-282.

Fischer, F.P. (1992) Quantitative analysis of the innervation of the chicken basilar papilla. Hear. Res. 61, 167-178.

Fischer, F.P. (1994) Quantitative TEM analysis of the barn owl basilar papilla. Hear. Res. 73, 1-15.

Genossa, T.J., Voigt, H.F. and Burkard, R. (1989) Spontaneous otoacoustic emissions in *Rana catesbiana*, the American bullfrog. J. Acoust. Soc. Am. 85(Suppl. 1), S35.

Gummer, A.W. and Klinke, R. (1983) Influence of temperature on tuning of primary-like units in the guinea pig cochlear nucleus. Hear. Res. 12, 367-380.

Gummer, A.W., Smolders, J.W.T. and Klinke, R. (1987) Basilar membrane motion in the pigeon measured with the Mössbauer technique. Hear. Res. 29, 63-92.

Holley, M. (1991) High frequency force generation in outer hair cells from the mammalian ear. BioEssays. 13, 115-120.

Howard, J. and Hudspeth, A.J. (1988) Compliance of the hair bundle associated with gating of mechanoelectrical transduction channels in the bullfrog's saccular hair cell. Neuron 1, 189-199.

Hudspeth, A.J. and Gillespie, P.G. (1994) Pulling springs to tune transduction: Adaptation by hair cells. Neuron 12, 1-9.

Kalinec, F., Holley, M.C., Iwasa, K.H., Lim, D.J. and Kachar, B. (1992) A membrane-based force generation mechanism in auditory sensory cells. Proc. Natl. Acad. Sci. USA. 89, 8671-8675.

Kettembeil, S. and Manley, G.A. (1992) Anesthesia effects on the distortion-product emission 2f1-f2 in birds. Abstr. 15th Midw. Meetg. ARO, St. Petersburg Bch., Fla., 153.

Klinke, R. and Smolders, J.W.T. (1984) Hearing mechanisms in caiman and pigeon. In: L. Bolis, R.D. Keynes and S.H.P. Maddrell (Eds.) Comparative physiology of sensory systems. Cambridge Univ. Press, Cambridge, pp. 195-211

Köppl, C. and Manley, G.A. (1992) Functional consequences of morphological trends in the evolution of lizard hearing organs. In: D.B. Webster, R.R. Fay and A.N. Popper (Eds.) The Evolutionary Biology of Hearing, 1st edn. Springer Verlag, New York, pp. 489-510

Köppl, C. and Manley, G.A. (1993) Spontaneous otoacoustic emissions in the bobtail lizard. I: General characteristics. Hear. Res. 71, 157-169.

Köppl, C. and Manley, G.A. (1994) Spontaeous otoacoustic emissions in the bobtail lizard. II: Interactions with external tones. Hear. Res. 72, 159-170.

Köppl, C., Gleich, O. and Manley, G.A. (1993) An auditory fovea in the barn owl cochlea. J. Comp. Physiol. A 171, 695-704.

Kössl, M. (1994) Otoacoustic emissions from the cochlea of the 'constant frequency' bats, *Pteronotus parnellii* and *Rhinolophus rouxi*. Hear. Res. 72, 59-72.

Kössl, M. and Vater, M. (1985) Evoked acoustic emissions and cochlear microphonics in the mustache bat, *Pteronotus parnellii*. Hear. Res. 19, 157-170.

Kössl, M., Reuter, G., Hemmert, W., Preyer, S., Zimmermann, U. and Zenner, H.-P. (1993) Motility of outer hair cells in the organ of Corti of the bat, *Carollia perspicillata*. In: N. Elsner and M. Heisenberg (Eds.) Gene - Brain - Behaviour (Proc. 21st Göttingen Neurobiol. Conf.). Georg Thieme Verlag, Stuttgart, New York, p. 264

Lewis, E.R. and Lombard, R.E. (1988) The amphibian inner ear. In: B. Fritzsch, M.J. Ryan, W. Wilczynski, T.E. Hetherington and W. Walkowiak (Eds.) The Evolution of the Amphibian Auditory System. John Wiley & Sons, New York, Toronto, p. 93-123.

Long, G.R., Tubis, A. and Jones, K.L. (1991) Modeling synchronization and suppression of spontaneous otoacoustic emissions using Van der Pol oscillators: Effects of aspirin administration. J. Acoust. Soc. Am. 89, 1201-1212.

Long, G.R., van Dijk, P. and Wit, H.P. (1993) Modification of the frequency and bandwidth of spontaneous otoacoustic emissions in the European edible frog. Abstr. 16th Midw. Meetg. ARO, St. Petersburg Bch., Fla., 98.

Manley, G.A. and Köppl, C. (1994) Spontaneous otoacoustic emissions in the bobtail lizard. III: Temperature effects. Hear. Res. 72, 171-180.

Manley, G.A. and Taschenberger, G. (1993) Spontaneous otoacoustic emissions from a bird: a preliminary report. In: H. Duifhuis, J.W. Horst, P. van Dijk and S.M. van Netten (Eds.) Biophysics of Hair Cell Sensory Systems. World Scientific Publishing Co., Singapore, pp. 33-39

Manley, G.A., Schulze, M. and Oeckinghaus, H. (1987) Otoacoustic emissions in a song bird. Hear. Res. 26, 257-266.

Manley, G.A., Yates, G.K. and Köppl, C. (1988) Auditory peripheral tuning: evidence for a simple resonance phenomenon in the lizard *Tiliqua*. Hear. Res. 33, 181-190.

Manley, G.A., Köppl, C. and Johnstone, B.M. (1993) Distortion-product otoacoustic emissions in the bobtail lizard. I: General characteristics. J. Acoust. Soc. Am. 93, 2820-2833.

Manley, G.A., Gallo, L., Pavusa, A. and Köppl, C. (1994a) Spontaneous otoacoustic emissions in three lizard species. Abstr. 17th Midw. Meetg. ARO, St. Petersburg Bch., Fla., 53.

Manley, G.A., Pavusa, A., Gallo, L. and Köppl, C. (1994b) Otoacoustic emissions patterns in lizards correlate with hearing-organ structure. In: N. Elsner and H. Breer (Eds.) Sensory Transduction (Proc. 22nd Göttingen Neurobiol. Conf.). Georg Thieme Verlag, Stuttgart, New York, p. in press

Markin, V.S. and Tsong, T.Y. (1991) Reversible mechanosensitive ion pumping as a part of mechanoelectrical transduction. Biophys. J. 59, 1317-1324.

Martin, G.K., Lonsbury-Martin, B.L., Probst, R. and Coats, A.C. (1985) Spontaneous otoacoustic emisions in the nonhuman primate: A survey. Hear. Res. 20, 91-95.

Martin, G.K., Lonsbury-Martin, B.L., Probst, R. and Coats, A.C. (1988) Spontaneous otoacoustic emissions in a nonhuman primate. I. Basic features and relations to other emissions. Hear. Res. 33, 49-68.

Miller, M.R. and Beck, J. (1988) Auditory hair cell innervational patterns in lizards. J. Comp. Neurol. 271, 604-628.

Norton, S.J. and Rubel, E.W. (1990) Active and passive ADP components in mammalian and avian ears. In: P. Dallos, C.D. Geisler, J.W. Matthews, M.A. Ruggero and C.R. Steele (Eds.) The Mechanics and Biophysics of Hearing. Springer Verlag, Berlin Heidelberg, pp. 219-226

Ohyama, K., Wada, H., Kobayashi, T. and Takasaka, T. (1991) Spontaneous otoacoustic emissions in the guinea pig. Hear. Res. 56, 111-121.

Ohyama, K., Sato, T., Wada, H. and Takasaka, T. (1992) Frequency instability of spontaneous otoacoustic emissions in the guinea pig. Abstr. 15th Midw. Meetg. ARO, St. Petersburg Bch., Fla., 150.

Palmer, A.R. and Wilson, J.P. (1981) Spontaneous and evoked acoustic emissions in the frog *Rana esculenta*. J. Physiol. 324, 66.

Peake, W.T. and Ling, A. (1980) Basilar-membrane motion in the alligator lizard: its relation to tonotopic organization and frequency selectivity. J. Acoust. Soc. Am. 67, 1736-1745.
Pickles, J.O. (1993) Early events in auditory processing. Curr. Opin. Neurobiol. 3, 558-562.
Probst, R. (1990) Otoacoustic emissions: An overview. In: C.R. Pfaltz (Ed.) New aspects of cochlear mechanics and inner ear pathophysiology, vol 44. Adv. Otorhinolaryngol., Karger, Basel, pp. 1-91
Rabinowitz, W.M. and Widin, G.P. (1984) Interaction of spontaneous oto-acoustic emissions and external sounds. J. Acoust. Soc. Am. 76, 1713-1720.
Rosowski, J.J., Peake, W.T. and White, J.R. (1984) Cochlear nonlinearities inferred from two-tone distortion products in the ear canal of the alligator lizard. Hear. Res. 13, 141-158.
Rüsch, A. and Thurm, U. (1990) Spontaneous and electrically induced movements of ampullary kinocilia and stereovilli. Hear. Res. 48, 247-264.
Santos-Sacchi, J. (1992) On the frequency limit and phase of outer hair cell motility: Effects of the membrane filter. J. Neurosci. 12, 1906-1916.
Sneary, M.G. (1988) Auditory receptor of the red-eared turtle: I. General ultrastructure. J. Comp. Neurol. 276, 573-587.
Takasaka, T. and Smith, C.A. (1971) The structure and innervation of the pigeon's basilar papilla. J Ultrastructure 35, 20-65.
Talmadge, C.L., Tubis, A., Wit, H.P. and Long, G.R. (1991) Are spontaneous otoacoustic emissions generated by self-sustained cochlear oscillators? J. Acoust. Soc. Am. 89, 2391-2399.
Talmadge, C.L., Long, G.R., Murphy, W.J. and Tubis, A. (1993) New off-line method for detecting spontaneous otoacoustic emissions in human subjects. Hear. Res. 71, 170-182.
Whitehead, M.L., Wilson, J.P. and Baker, R.J. (1986) The effects of temperature on otoacoustic emission tuning properties. In: B.C.J. Moore and R.D. Patterson (Eds.) Auditory Frequency Selectivity. Plenum Press, London, pp. 39-48
Wilson, J.P., Baker, R.J. and Whitehead, M.L. (1990) Otoacoustic emissions in frogs. In: F. Grandori, G. Cianfrone and D.T. Kemp (Eds.) Cochlear mechanisms and otoacoustic emissions, vol 7. Adv. Audiol., Karger, Basel, pp. 47-56
Yates, G.K., Johnstone, B.M., Patuzzi, R.B. and Robertson, D. (1992) Mechanical preprocessing in the mammalian cochlea. Trends Neurosci. 15, 57-61.
Zakon, H.H. and Wilczynski, W. (1988) The physiology of the anuran eighth nerve. In: B. Fritzsch, M.J. Ryan, W. Wilczynski, T.E. Hetherington and W. Walkowiak (Eds.) The Evolution of the Amphibian Auditory System. John Wiley & Sons, New York, Toronto, p. 125-155.
Zimmermann, U., Reuter, G., Gitter, A.H., Zenner, H.P. and Klinke, R. (1989) Isolation and short-term culture of pigeon hair cells. In: N. Elsner and W. Singer (Eds.) Dynamics and Plasticity in Neuronal Systems (Proc. 17th Göttingen Neurobiol. Conf.). Georg Thieme, Stuttgart, New York, p. 286

Comment by J. P. Wilson

You quote the data of Ohyama et al. (1992) in the guinea pig as evidence that mammals have a comparable sensitivity to temperature change of SOAE frequency as the other classes of animals that you discuss. This is, however, quite different from humans where the temperature dependence is certainly very much smaller. Wit (1985) found diurnal changes of -4.2 ± 0.83 Hz at an SOAE frequency of 1.09 kHz and -2.9 ± 1.1 Hz at 1.41 kHz in the afternoon compared with the morning. Assuming that this would relate to a less than maximum change of say 0.5°C, this would imply temperature coefficients of

-0.01 and -0.003 oct/°C respectively. He found negligible changes of 0 and -2 Hz for head temperature increases of 1°C and 1.8°C induced by room heating. Wilson (1986) found changes of +0.0007 ± 0.0008 oct/°C over the diurnal cycle and -0.006 ± 0.001 oct/°C over the menstrual cycle for several frequency components in one subject. Irrigation of the ear canal in this and another subject at 30°C and 44°C failed to give any consistent trend of temperature dependence. Thus, not only are the above changes much smaller than found in other animals but they are predominantly in the opposite direction. Thus, it appears that one cannot generalise across mammals.

Another interesting point is that even with the animals showing a very large temperature coefficient there appears to be a variability greatly exceeding the likely measurement errors of temperature and frequency. In the study of Whitehead et al. (1986) in frogs the coefficient ranged between 0.01 oct/°C and 0.07 oct/°C. Perhaps biological factors such as muscle tone are induced by large temperature shifts altering the phase of the internal reflection from the middle ear and therefore the frequency of the SOAE.

Whitehead, M.L., Wilson, J.P. and Baker, R.J. (1986) The effects of temperature on otoacoustic emission tuning properties. In: B.C.J. Moore and R.D. Patterson (Eds.) Auditory Frequency Selectivity. Plenum Press, London, pp. 39-48

Wilson, J.P. (1986) The influence of temperature on frequency tuning mechanisms. In: Peripheral Auditory Mechanisms, eds J.B. Allen, J.L. Hall, A. Hubbard, S.T. Neely and A. Tatis, Springer Berlin, pp. 229-236.

Wit, H.P. (1985) Diurnal cycle for spontaneous otoacoustic emission frequency. Hear. Res. 18:197-199.

Reply

In my view, the data on temperature effects on human spontaneous emissions that you cite are not conclusive for two reasons. Firstly, the ranges of natural temperature fluctuations were very small (below 1°C); in the case of ear canal irrigation there was no control of cochlear temperature and presumably it took a variable amount of time to insert the measurement probe after the irrigation. Secondly, the variations occurred over a relatively large time scale of days or weeks. Both factors would increase the influence of measurement errors and temperature-unrelated variation in emission frequency, possibly even masking any consistent temperature-related shifts.

With regard to the large variation of the temperature coefficients in a given species, it is worth pointing out two major factors of variability in pooled data. In addition to relative temperature, the temperature coefficient is also systematically dependent on absolute temperature, i.e. it will be different when measured around 20°C as compared to e.g. around 30°C. It is also dependent on the emissions frequency, i.e. lower-frequency emissions shift less with temperature than higher-frequency ones (vanDijk et al., 1989; Manley and Köppl, 1994).

van Dijk, P., Wit, H.P. and Segenhout, J.M. (1989) Spontaneous otoacoustic emissions in the European edible frog (*Rana esculenta*): Spectral details and temperature dependence. Hear. Res. 42, 273-282.

Manley, G.A. and Köppl, C. (1994) Spontaneous otoacoustic emissions in the bobtail lizard. III: Temperature effects. Hear. Res. 72, 171-180.

Reply by J.P. Wilson

I certainly accept your later points that temperature coefficient is temperature and frequency dependent but not the earlier ones concerned with small temperature emissions or time scale. In the cases quoted long and short term stability were quite adequate to have shown consistent temperature dependence had it been comparable in magnitude to that of frog. In fact, conversely, not being a physiologist I would be unhappy about the use of such a large temperature change as 6°C in guinea-pigs.

The avian hearing organ: A status report

Geoffrey A. Manley

Institut für Zoologie, Technische Universität München, Lichtenbergstrasse 4, 85747 Garching, Germany

1 Introduction

The last several years have seen a rapid increase in our understanding of the anatomy and physiology of the hearing epithelium of birds. This paper is a summary of some important new findings. An earlier review can be found in Manley (1990).

Palaeontological and comparative studies suggest that at the time of the divergence of the evolutionary line (Archosauria) leading to both birds and *Crocodilia* about 230M years ago, the auditory papilla was still a relatively unspecialized structure not showing prominent hair-cell specializations along and across the auditory papilla. Nonetheless, the development of specializations must have been rapid at first, as the pattern of hair-cell specialization we see in both archosaur groups is unique. It is, however, to be expected that selection pressures during evolution had similar effects on the large epithelia of mammals and birds (Manley et al., 1989). Study of such organs may thus be instructional in our attempt to understand the mechanisms underlying hair-cell functional specialization in general. For the purposes of this report, only the birds will be considered.

Jahnke et al. (1969) correctly observed that there are no structural grounds for distinguishing discreet hair-cell types in the avian papilla. Nonetheless, the terms "tall" (THC) and "short" (SHC) have been widely used to describe particular structural configurations (e.g. Takasaka and Smith, 1971), THC being taller than they are wide and *vice versa*. More recent detailed anatomical studies verify that avian hair cells form a structural continuum along and across the papilla (Fischer, 1992, 1994; Fischer et al., 1992). Additional terms, such as "intermediate" hair cells, implying the existence of other definable sub-groups should be abandoned. Indeed, because not only hair-cell shape, but other parameters, e.g., of the hair-cell bundle, also change independently along and across the epithelium, a case can be made that every hair cell is unique! In the species we have also studied using TEM (starling, chicken, barn owl and emu), however, cells in an area previously classified as SHC were found to receive no afferent innervation. This finding offers a real structural basis for defining populations of hair cells (which presumably also differ in *function*) and Fischer (1994) has suggested re-defining the terms THC and SHC using the innervation pattern: THC are afferently innervated, SHC receive no afferent innervation. Although there is a rough correspondence between the papillar *areas* defined by this and the earlier definition, not enough species have been studied using the TEM to use the new definition for all species. Thus in this paper, the older definition will be used, except where otherwise specified.

2 Evolutionary trends in papillar structure

2.1 The primitive condition

In order to understand trends over time, we have to know which groups of birds are conservative in their structure and which are considered to be specialized. The most primitive living birds are the flightless *Ratitae* (ostrich, emu, kiwi, etc.), that are, however, not considered to be a monophyletic group (Carroll, 1988). Due to the lack of detailed information on these important species, we (Fischer, Gleich, Köppl, Manley, Yates) have begun a study of the emu. Most hair cells of the emu basilar papilla are remarkably tall and columnar in shape. Although the hair cells generally become smaller and wider towards the abneural side and towards the base of the papilla, it is only on the extreme abneural edge of the basal papillar area that a small area is found whose hair cells fulfil the original criterion for SHC, i.e., they are wider than tall. Even in this primitive papilla, however, an area of SHC, that is, hair cells without afferent innervation, is present (Fischer, pers. comm.). The hair-cell bundles are not all abneurally oriented (bundle long axis parallel to the neural edge), but show rotations of up to 70° towards the apex, the maximum rotation being at about 70% of the papillar length from the basal end and roughly midway across the papilla. From this position, the rotational angle of emu hair-cell bundles decreases to zero rotation in all directions.

Even at this relatively early stage of evolutionary development, the auditory organ thus already shows features regarded as being typical for avian papillae:

✧ The hair cells are taller at the apex and on the neural side and gradually become - generally monotonically - shorter towards the base and the abneural side.

✧ There is a characteristic pattern of rotation of the hair-cell bundles.

✧ The number of stereovilli per bundle is high in the base and falls strongly towards the apex. The height of the bundles shows the reverse trend, with, however, no great differences *across* the papilla at any given position along its length.

✧ The trend in the innervation is similar to that of more advanced species (see below).

2.2 Trends in papillar structure discernable in more modern groups

In general, bird groups show different levels of development and specialization, the primitive ratites being followed by the water birds such as ducks, then primitive land bird groups such as chickens and pigeons and finally advanced land birds such as song birds and owls (Carroll, 1988; Feduccia, 1980). Until recently, substantial information on the structure of the avian ear was only available for the chicken and the pigeon. We have now studied these and a number of other species in detail, including a duck, the barn owl, the budgerigar and several species of song birds, the starling, canary and zebra finch (Fischer, 1992, 1994; Fischer et al., 1988, 1992; Gleich and Manley, 1988; Manley et al., 1993 and Gleich et al., unpublished data). Every species has a unique papillar morphology, with recognizable specializations in most cases. The pigeon and chicken, for example, show (different) specializations for low-frequency reception, the canary and zebra finch for reduced low-frequency sensitivity (Gleich et al., in press) and the barn owl even shows an auditory fovea at high frequencies (Köppl et al., 1993) that has characteristic anatomical features (Fischer et al., 1988; Smith et al., 1985). The trends observed can be regarded as continuations of the following evolutionary developments already manifested in the emu:

✧ The hair cells show an increasing specialization. The cell height, which is related in some way to the response frequency (Fischer et al., 1992), is generally shorter in birds hearing higher frequencies, but these papillae still show a reduction in hair-cell height both towards the base (i.e., towards higher frequencies) and *across* the papilla towards the abneural side. Abneural and basal cells are wider, except in the barn owl. In more advanced species and for higher-frequency responses, the papillae contain increasingly large proportions of areas of SHC. The hair-cell height generally falls steadily across the papilla, although the tallest hair cells are not necessarily at the extreme neural edge. In higher-frequency areas, the hair-cell height falls rapidly across the neural third to half, changing only little across the abneural half. In the barn owl, the auditory foveal area is even more specialized in this respect. Here, only the very first cell on the neural side is higher than wide and has an extremely dense afferent innervation; all others in the transverse section are much shorter (Köppl, 1993; Fischer 1994).

✧ The specialization of the innervation of the hair cells progresses together with the changes in hair-cell shape. In the chicken, starling and barn owl, except at the very apical end, only hair cells over 50-80% of the width of the papilla from the neural side are afferently innervated, depending on the species and the actual papillar position. During evolution, the population of hair cells whose function is confined to the papilla itself - the SHC - became larger; correlated with the acquisition of responses to higher frequencies.

✧ In general, the total number of hair cells falls. This is partly due to a decrease in papillar size with body size (from 5mm down to about 2mm; as so often, the barn owl is an exception, with 11mm). The reduction in hair-cell number is also due to the increase in the number of hair cells with a large surface area. Examples of sensory-cell numbers: 17000 in emus, 10000 in chickens, 4500 in starlings to 3000 in canaries. Interestingly, however, the number of afferent nerve fibres is not proportionately reduced and the ratio of hair cells to nerve fibres falls from about 2 in the emu to 0.5 in the canary (Gleich pers. comm.) and the barn owl (Köppl, 1994). Thus advanced species show a denser afferent innervation, especially on neural hair cells. In the auditory fovea of the barn owl, the most neural hair cell at any one position receives up to 20 afferent fibres (Fischer, 1994).

✧ Additionally, the hair-cell bundles also specialize. Thus, although in any one transverse section of the emu papilla the bundles of neural and abneural hair cells are very similar, they are often different in more advanced species. In the canary and zebra finch, for example, the bundles of abneural cells at a position 50% of the papilla's length have only *half* as many stereovilli as neural cells. An intermediate situation is seen basally in the pigeon, budgerigar and starling. The micromechanics of the papilla's response to sound may thus have become more complex compared to primitive birds.

✧ The pattern of hair-cell bundle rotation is maintained and appears to shift with the presumed frequency map of the cochlea. In the canary and zebra finch, that show a poor low-frequency sensitivity, the maximal rotation is only 30-40 degrees and is found at the extreme apical end of the papilla.

3 Papillar function

3.1 Correlations between cell position and cell function

As the anatomical trends described above in fact differ uniquely between species, any attempt to correlate structure and function across species is difficult and must be undertaken with great care. There is no such thing as "the" avian inner ear.

In the pigeon, chicken and starling, sufficient data are available from traced, characterized afferent fibres to make interesting observations on papillar function and on changes in hair-cell function with the relative position in the epithelial mosaic (Gleich, 1989; Klinke and Smolders, 1993; Manley et al., 1987, 1989; Smolders et al., 1992). The pigeon and chicken on the one hand and the starling on the other belong to relatively primitive and specialized bird groups, respectively. In contrast to the starling, different anatomical (Gleich and Manley, 1988; Lavigne-Rebillard et al., 1985) and physiological (Schermuly and Klinke, 1990a,b; Warchol and Dallos, 1987) specializations for very low frequency responses exist in the apical area of the pigeon's and chicken's papilla. The gradients in hair-cell shape, especially across the papilla's width in the higher-frequency area, are species-specific. Thus, some difference in function is expected between species.

For all three papillae, frequency maps exist (Gleich, 1989; Manley et al., 1987, 1989; Klinke and Smolders, 1993). Whereas in the pigeon, the frequency map is well matched by a linear regression line, the space constants of frequency distribution in the starling and chicken are smaller apically than towards the base. In the starling and chicken, recent anatomical studies have demonstrated that many or most abneural hair cells lack afferent fibres from which recordings can be made. In the pigeon, the area of afferently-innervated hair cells apparently extends further abneurally than in the starling and chicken. In pigeons, afferents in the mid-frequency region were traceable to hair cells at positions up to two-thirds of the distance from neural (Smolders et al., 1992), whereas in starlings and chickens, they were confined to the neural 45% (Gleich, 1989; Manley et al., 1989, Fig. 1). Although the innervation of the pigeon papilla has not been studied in detail, this difference almost certainly reflects differences in innervation patterns. In addition, both starlings and pigeons show changes in response threshold *across* the papilla, the minimal threshold being between 15 and 25% from the neural edge (Fig.1). At the position where the pigeon papilla has its best thresholds, the dimensions of the hair-cell cuticular plate in chickens are such that the plate fills out the hair-cell surface, which is not true in other positions (Brix et al., 1994). This is also the position in the chicken where the efferent innervation is minimal (Fischer, 1992, Fig. 1). Thus morphological correlates of physiological trends exist and need to be studied in more species. In pigeons, but not in starlings, fibre threshold correlated with the frequency selectivity (Gleich, 1989; Klinke and Smolders, 1993). Thus avian afferent fibres fall into one population of varying threshold, tuning etc., correlated with the position of the innervated hair cells across the epithelium.

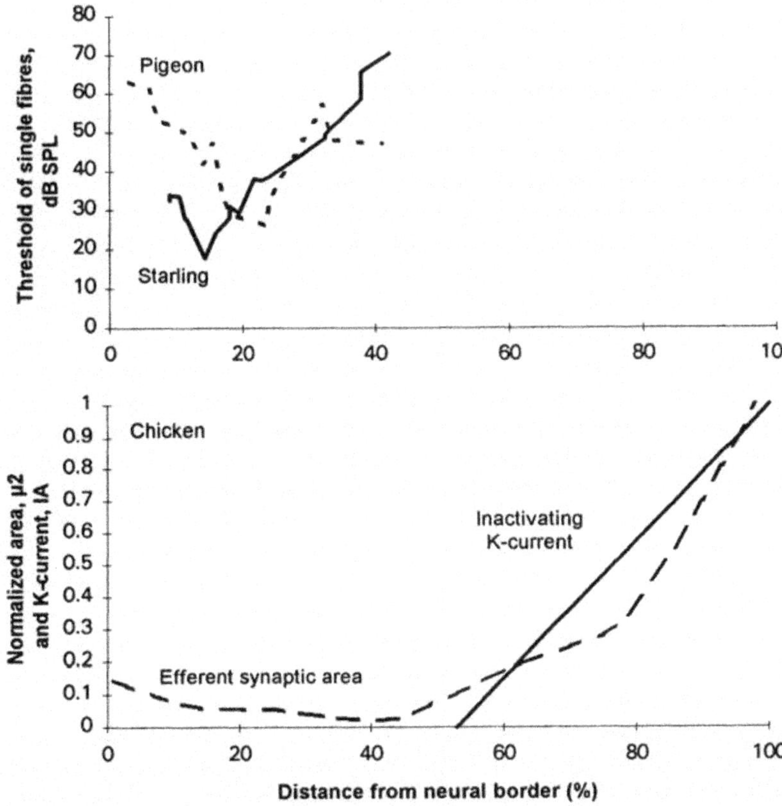

Figure 1. Top: A comparison of the threshold of auditory nerve fibres contacting hair cells as a function of the hair cells' position relative to the neural edge in two avian species, the pigeon (dashed line, after Smolders et al., 1992) and starling (continuous line, after Gleich, 1989 and personal communication). Only five-point weighted averages through the data are shown.

Bottom: A comparison of the normalized area of efferent synapses as a function of hair-cell position across the chicken's papilla at a position 66% from the basal end of the papilla (after Fischer, 1992) and the normalized magnitude of the inactivating potassium current in hair cells from this position (calculated from the data of Murrow and Fuchs, 1990). The values for the current were given for hair cells of different shape ratios (height-width) at the 66% position and have been matched to the probable position of these cells across the papilla according to Fischer's anatomical-positional data.

As yet, no adequate basis for these functional trends has been found, although bundle orientation differences (Gleich, 1989) and differences in ion-channel distributions (Murrow and Fuchs, 1990) are promising leads. Of course, there are other differences in the structure and function of avian and mammalian papillae (for reviews see Klinke and Smolders, 1993; Manley, 1990; Manley et al., 1989), but it is not yet possible to trace functional differences other than those indicated above to specific hair-cell populations. It is nonetheless striking that birds and mammals have independently developed papillae with an obvious similarity in possessing a division of labour between hair-cell areas. Although Klinke and Smolders (1993) claim that "the functional role of avian SHCs is different from that of mammalian OHCs", and that "avian THCs and SHCs are not functionally analogous to mammalian IHCs and OHCs respectively", the available functional data are not yet adequate to judge. As we have suggested (Manley et al., 1989; Manley and Gleich, 1992) a clear functional parallel to mammals does exist, in that in both, an abneural hair-cell area receives an apparently non-transmitting (mammals, Robertson, 1984) or no (birds) afferent innervation and thus has a function confined to the papilla itself. Of course, what exact function SHC, or for that matter, OHC fulfil is still a matter of debate. More data are needed along the lines of the hair-cell membrane channel study of Murrow and Fuchs (1990). The size of the inactivating potassium current in chicken hair cells as found in that study correlates very well with the area of the efferent synapses measured in chicken hair cells from the same papillar position (Fischer, 1992; Fig. 1).

3.2 A possible mechanism by which SHC influence THC

Recent data make it necessary to reconsider some common conceptions of hair-cell function, even in the mammalian cochlea. We have recently demonstrated the presence of high-frequency (up to 11kHz) spontaneous otoacoustic emissions (SOAE) in the barn owl (Manley and Taschenberger, 1993). Together with reports of SOAE in amphibians (e.g. van Dijk et al., 1989) and in lizards (Manley and Köppl, 1993), all with properties resembling those of SOAE in mammals, SOAE are clearly a basic property of tetrapod hair cells (see C. Köppl, this volume). Are the mechanism traditionally considered to be producing SOAE in mammals (active changes in hair-cell length) appropriate for the avian situation? If avian SOAE are a reflection of mechanical activity of SHC, what mechanism(s) could be producing such rapid movements? Avian SHC have no subsurface cisternae and are often extremely short (a few microns high, e.g., Fischer, 1992) with little cytoplasm, suggesting that only stiffness changes or bundle movements could influence papillar micromechanics. In turtles, the hair-cell bundle has been shown to move actively (Crawford and Fettiplace, 1985), but no detailed studies are available. Such a mechanism could feed mechanical energy into the oscillating papilla and it is conceivable that bundle movements are the origin of SOAE in all species, including mammals. Heuristically, it should be assumed that the same mechanism is operational in all groups, before accepting different mechanisms on the basis of compelling evidence. The localization of the active mechanism to the hair-cell bundle in non-mammals at least would laterally couple hair cells in the plane of the tectorial membrane, an important prerequisite for birds (Fig. 2).

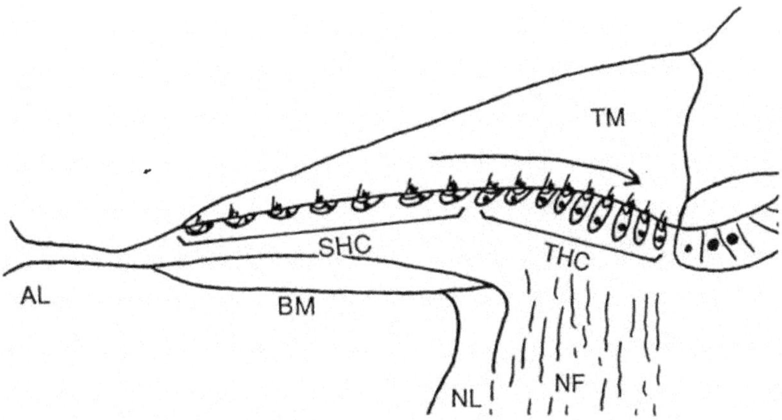

Figure 2. A schematic drawing of a transverse section of the Papilla basilaris of the canary in the apical third. The afferent nerve fibres (NF) mainly innervate the THC. The arrow within the tectorial membrane (TM) is to indicate the plane and direction of the putative mechanical interaction from the SHC over the basilar membrane (BM) to the THC over the neural limbus (NL). AL = abneural limbus.

Perhaps the proposed adaptational motors (Hudspeth and Gillespie, 1994) are fast enough to feed energy into the motion cycle-by-cycle. This mechanism would be appropriate for coupling metabolic energy into the system; would feed back with the appropriate phase and be independent of cell-membrane potential.

The concept of active bundle movements is attractive when applied to birds, where hair cells producing sensitive responses are not found on the free basilar membrane (Gleich, 1989; Klinke and Smolders, 1993; Manley et al., 1987, 1989) and presumably receive their main stimulation via the tectorial membrane. In Fig. 2, it was assumed that SHC exert an effect on THC through active bundle movements. The "division of labour" between hair-cell groups in birds would thus parallel that in mammals, where the OHC are regarded as feeding mechanical energy into the moving organ of Corti at low sound-pressure levels, thus increasing the stimulus to IHC. This hypothesis suggests a degree of functional equivalence of hair-cell populations in these two tetrapod groups. On the other hand, it is possible that SHC affect THC by responding to their large efferent input with a change in stiffness, affecting the response of the hair-cell/tectorial membrane complex. At present, neither the functions of the OHC nor those of the SHC are clearly understood.

3.3 Some physiological differences to mammals

Apart from structural differences between the avian and mammalian hearing organ, a number of differences in peripheral physiology exist (Klinke and Smolders, 1993; Gleich and Manley, 1992; Manley et al., 1989). One of the most interesting is the difference in temperature sensitivity. In common with other non-mammals (Manley, 1990), frequency tuning in the pigeon is temperature sensitive (Schermuly and Klinke, 1985). Whereas in mammals, neural frequency tuning is insensitive to temperature (e.g., Gummer and Klinke, 1983), in non-mammals the centre frequency shifts more than 0.1 octaves for a change in temperature of 1°C. Important in this regard, however, is the finding that not only are avian SOAE temperature sensitive (Manley and Taschenberger, 1993), like those of other non-mammals (e.g. Manley and Köppl, 1994), but that SOAE in guinea pigs also shift frequency with temperature (Ohyama et al., 1992). This suggests that at the level of hair-cell *transduction* in the strict sense, the functional similarities between mammals and birds are greater than at higher processing levels. In the guinea pig, the temperature effect is overridden at a processing stage between hair-cell transduction and the cochlear nucleus, perhaps by the summed tuning characteristics of the basilar-membrane/organ of Corti complex. It is possible that the phenomena described here are related to the fact that transduction in birds is also sensitive to the level of anaesthesia (Kettembeil et al., 1993).

Basilar-membrane motion in birds is probably less sharply tuned than in mammals (Gummer et al., 1987), so that the "tectorial-membrane and hair-cell bundles" complex is also responsible for a significant part of tuning selectivity. How large the role of electrical tuning in frequency selectivity in birds is remains to be clarified (Fuchs et al., 1988; Klinke and Smolders, 1993; Manley, 1979; Manley and Gleich, 1984, 1992). The effect of electrical tuning, that Klinke and Smolders (1993) regard as an "adequate candidate" for "the active contribution to frequency tuning in the avian ear" will diminish towards higher frequencies, making it important when comparing tuning mechanisms to take into account the frequency range in question.

In birds, although primary auditory fibres are at least as sharply tuned as those of mammals in the same frequency ranges (review in Manley, 1990), the tuning curves do not show the mammalian asymmetry (e.g. Gummer et al., 1987; Klinke and Smolders, 1993; Manley et al., 1985). They also show no low-frequency "tails", although in chickens, a break in the low-frequency slope was often observed (Manley et al., 1991). Gleich (1994) used single afferent fibre responses to study the pattern of excitation on the starling's papilla and showed that, like the tuning of primary fibres, it is fairly symmetrical at all sound-pressure levels of the stimuli. This correlates with the lack of spread of excitation to high frequencies in psychoacoustical data for avian species (e.g., Saunders and Pallone, 1980), in clear contrast to findings in mammals.

The ability to regenerate new hair cells (not to be discussed in detail here) is much greater in the hearing organ of birds, which might be interpreted to indicate that avian hair cells are less specialized than those of mammals. However, it is probably the *supporting cells* of birds that are sufficiently unspecialized to be able to respond to damaged hair cells by dividing and producing either new supporting cells or new hair cells (e.g., Corwin et al., 1991). This has yet to be demonstrated in the mammalian cochlea, where the supporting cells are more specialized. Although some studies of hair-cell regeneration in the avian cochlea have suggested that neural thresholds can recover to near-normal in epithelia whose morphology is far from normal, more detailed studies are necessary to determine where nerve-fibres connect to in damaged papillae and to help elucidate whether the phenomenon of regeneration can be used to further understand the functional relationships between THC and SHC in the avian papilla.

4 Acknowledgements

Work in my laboratory was supported by a grant from the Deutsche Forschungsgemeinschaft (SFB 204 "Gehör"). Work on the emu was also supported by a grant from the Australian NH&MRC to B. Johnstone, D. Robertson, R. Patuzzi and G. Yates and an International Reciprocal Exchange Fellowship from the Australian Research Council.

5 References

Brix, J., Fischer, F.P. and Manley, G.A. (1994) The cuticular plate of the hair cell in relation to morphological gradients of the chicken basilar papilla. Hear. Res. in press.

Carroll, R.L. (1988) Vertebrate Palaeontology and Evolution. Freeman, N.Y.

Corwin, J.T., Jones, J.E., Katayama, A., Kelley, M.W. and Warchol, M.E. (1991) Hair cell regeneration: the identities of progenitor cells, potential triggers and instructive cues. In: Regeneration of vertebrate sensory receptor cells, Ciba Foundation Symp. 160, Wiley, Chichester, pp. 103-130.

Crawford, A.C. and Fettiplace, R. (1985) The mechanical properties of ciliary bundles of turtle cochlear hair cells. J Physiol 364, 359-379.

Feduccia, A. (1980) The Age of Birds. Harvard U.P., Cambridge.

Fischer, F.P. (1992) Quantitative analysis of the innervation of the chicken basilar papilla. Hear. Res. 61, 167-178.

Fischer, F.P. (1994) Quantitative TEM analysis of the barn owl basilar papilla. Hear. Res. 73, 1-15.

Fischer, F.P., Köppl, C. and Manley, G. (1988) The basilar papilla of the barn owl *Tyto alba*: A quantitative morphological SEM analysis. Hear. Res. 34, 87-101.

Fischer, F.P., Miltz, C., Singer, I. and Manley, G.A. (1992) Morphological gradients in the starling basilar papilla. J. Morphol. 213, 225-240.

Fuchs, P.A., Nagai, T. and Evans, M.G. (1988) Electrical tuning in hair cells isolated from the chick cochlea. J. Neurosci. 8, 2460-2467.

Gleich, O. (1989) Auditory primary afferents in the starling: Correlation of function and morphology. Hear. Res. 37, 255-268.

Gleich, O. (1994) Excitation patterns in the starling cochlea: A population study of primary auditory afferents. J. Acoust. Soc. Amer. 95, 401-409.

Gleich, O. and Manley, G.A. (1988) Quantitative morphological analysis of the sensory epithelium of the starling and pigeon basilar papilla. Hear. Res. 34, 69-86.

Gummer, A. and Klinke, R. (1983) Influence of temperature on tuning of primary-like units in the guinea pig cochlear nucleus. Hear. Res 12, 367-380.

Gummer, A.W., Smolders, J.W.T. and Klinke, R. (1987) Basilar membrane motion in the pigeon measured with the Mössbauer technique. Hear. Res. 29, 63-92.

Hudspeth, A.J. and Gillespie, P.G. (1994) Pulling strings to tune transduction - adaptation be hair cells. Neuron 12, 1-9.

Jahnke, V., Lundquist, P-G. and Wersäll, J. (1969) Some morphological aspects of sound perception in birds. Acta Otolaryngol. 67, 583-601.

Kettembeil, S., Manley, G.A., Siegl, E. and Oeckinghaus, H. (1993) Time course of the effect of anaesthesia on CAP and $2f_1$-f_2 distortion-product emission in a song bird. 16th Midwinter Res. Mtg. Assoc. Res. Otolaryngol., Abstr. Nr. 411

Klinke, R. and Smolders, J.W.T. (1993) Performance of the avian inner ear. In: J.H.J. Allum, D.J. Allum-Mecklenburg, F.P. Harris and R. Probst (Eds.) Progr. in Brain Res., 97, 31-43.

Köppl, C. (1993) Hair-cell specializations and the auditory fovea in the barn owl cochlea. In: Duifhuis, H., Horst, J.W., van Dijk, P., van Netten, S. (Eds.) Biophysics of hair-cell sensory systems. London, World Scientific Publ. Co., pp. 216-222.

Köppl, C. (1994) Fiber number and diameters in the auditory nerve of the barn owl. 17th Midwinter Res. Mtg. Assoc. Res. Otolaryngol., Abstr. Nr. 381.

Köppl, C., Gleich, O. and Manley, G.A. (1993) An auditory fovea in the barn owl cochlea. J. Comp. Physiol. 171, 695-704.

Lavigne-Rebillard, M., Cousillas, H. and Pujol R. (1985) The very distal part of the basilar papilla in the chicken: A morphological approach. J. Comp. Neurol. 238, 340-347.

Manley, G.A. (1979) Preferred intervals in the spontaneous activity of primary auditory neurones. Naturwiss 66:582

Manley, G.A. (1990) Peripheral Hearing Mechanisms in Reptiles and Birds. Heidelberg, Springer-Verlag.

Manley, G.A. and Gleich, O. (1984) Avian primary auditory neurones: the relationship between characteristic frequency and preferred intervals. Naturwiss. 71:592-594.

Manley, G.A. and Gleich, O. (1992) Evolution and specialization of function in the avian auditory periphery. In: The Evolutionary Biology of Hearing, R.R. Fay, A.N. Popper, D.B. Webster, (Eds.) Springer-Verlag, Heidelberg, N.Y. pp. 561-580.

Manley, G.A. and Köppl, C. (1993) Spontaneous otoacoustic emissions in the bobtail lizard. I: General characteristics. Hear. Res., 71, 157-169.

Manley, G.A. and Köppl, C. (1994) Spontaneous otoacoustic emissions in the bobtail lizard. III. Temperature effects. Hear. Res. 72, 171-180.

Manley, G.A. and Taschenberger, G. (1993) Spontaneous otoacoustic emissions from a bird: a preliminary report. In: H. Duifhuis, J.W. Horst, P. van Dijk, and S. van Netten (Eds.) Biophysics of hair-cell sensory systems. London, World Scientific Publ. Co., pp.33-39.

Manley, G.A., Gleich, O., Leppelsack, H-J. and Oeckinghaus, H. (1985) Activity patterns of cochlear ganglion neurones in the starling. J. Comp. Physiol. A. 157, 161-181.

Manley, G.A., Brix, J. and Kaiser, A. (1987) Developmental stability of the tonotopic organization of the chick's basilar papilla. Science 237, 655-656.

Manley, G.A., Gleich, O., Kaiser, A. and Brix, J. (1989) Functional differentiation of sensory cells in the avian auditory periphery. J. Comp. Physiol. 164, 289-296.

Manley, G.A., Kaiser, A., Brix, J. and Gleich, O. (1991) Activity patterns of primary auditory-nerve fibres in chickens: development of fundamental properties. Hear. Res. 57, 1-15.

Manley, G.A., Schwabedissen, G. and Gleich, O. (1993) Morphology of the basilar papilla of the budgerigar *Melopsittacus undulatus*. J. Morphol. 218, 153-165.

Murrow, B.W. and Fuchs, P.A. (1990) Preferential expression of transient current (I_A) by short hair cells of the chick's cochlea. Proc. Roy. Soc. Lond. (Biol.), 242, 189-195.

Ohyama, K., Sato, T., Wada, H. and Takasaka, T. (1992) Frequency instability of the spontaneous otoacoustic emissions in the guinea pig. Abstr. 15. Mtg, Assoc. Research in Otolaryngol. p. 150.

Robertson, D. (1984) Horseradish peroxidase injection of physiologically characterized afferent and efferent neurones in the guinea pig spiral ganglion. Hear. Res. 15, 113-121.

Saunders, J.C. and Pallone, R.L. (1980) Frequency selectivity in the parakeet studied by isointensity masking contours. J. Exp. Biol. 87, 331-342.

Schermuly, L. and Klinke, R. (1985) Change of characteristic frequencies of pigeon primary auditory afferents with temperature. J. Comp. Physiol. A. 156, 209-211.

Schermuly, L. and Klinke, R (1990a) Infrasound sensitive neurones in the pigeon's cochlear ganglion. J. Comp. Physiol. A. 166, 355-363.

Schermuly, L. and Klinke, R. (1990b) Origin of infrasound sensitive neurones in the papilla basilaris of the pigeon: a HRP study. Hear. Res., 48, 69-78.

Smith, C.A., Konishi, M. and Schull, N. (1985) Structure of the barn owl's (*Tyto alba*) inner ear. Hear. Res 17, 237-247.

Smolders, J.W.T., Ding, D. and Klinke, R. (1992) Normal tuning curves from primary afferent fibres innervating short and intermediate hair cells in the pigeon ear. In: Y. Cazals, L. Demany and K. Horner (Eds.), Auditory Physiology and Perception - Advances in Biosciences, 83, Pergamon, Oxford. pp. 197-204.

Takasaka, T. and Smith, C.A. (1971) The structure and innervation of the pigeon's basilar papilla. J. Ultrastruct. Res. 35, 20-65.

van Dijk, P., Wit, H.P. and Segenhout, J.M. (1989): Spontaneous otoacoustic emissions in the European edible frog (Rana esculenta): Spectral details and temperature dependence. Hear. Res. 42, 273-282.

Warchol, M.E. and Dallos, P. (1987) Single unit response to very low frequency sound in the avian auditory brainstem. Abstracts 10th Mtg. Assoc Res Otolaryngol pp.38-39.

Central neuronal processing

Intensity coding: Dynamic range shifts in cochlear nerve and nucleus

E.F. Evans and W. Zhao

Department of Communication and Neuroscience, Keele University, Keele, Staffs ST5 5BG, UK

1 Introduction

It is well established that the dynamic range of mammalian cochlear nerve and nucleus units can be dramatically extended by background noise or additional tones (Evans, 1974, 1981; Evans and Palmer, 1975; Palmer and Evans, 1982; Costalupes *et al*, 1984; Gibson *et al*, 1985). The addition of these background/additional stimuli shift the rate-level function towards higher levels, as shown diagrammatically in Fig. 1.

In the case of cochlear nerve fibres, the mechanism for this shift is likely to be lateral suppression. It is not clear, however, what the mechanisms are in the case of the cochlear nucleus. As far as the dorsal cochlear nucleus (DCN) is concerned, Evans and Palmer (1975) and Evans and Palmer

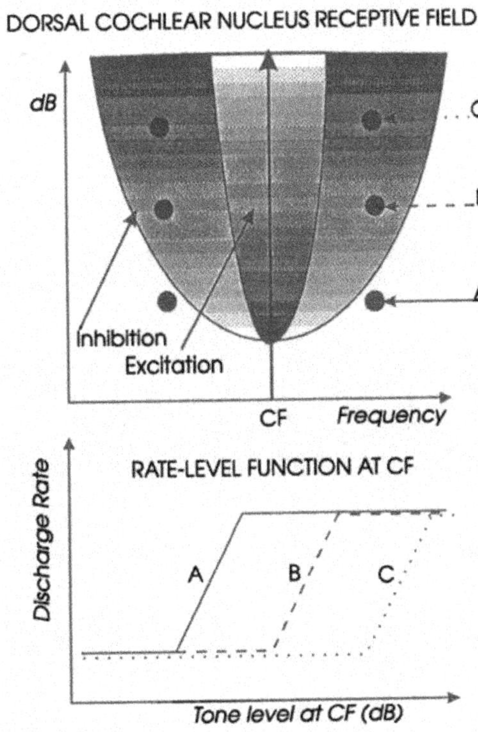

Figure 1. Diagram of relationship between CF (characteristic frequency) tone and side-tones and excitatory and inhibitory receptive fields, and the shift in CF rate-level function with level of side-tones. Upper half: receptive field map defined in terms of tone level and frequency; lower half: rate-level functions at CF with the addition of side-tones A, B, C at the frequencies and levels indicated in the upper half.

(1982) concluded, by comparison with ventral cochlear nucleus and cochlear nerve responses, that the effects must involve synaptic lateral inhibition intrinsic to the cochlear nucleus (Evans and Nelson, 1973 a,b), in addition to any effects of cochlear nerve lateral suppression. This conclusion has been challenged by Gibson *et al* (1985), who maintained that the predominant effects in the cochlear nucleus largely reflected lateral suppression mechanisms at the cochlea/cochlear nerve level.

Following on the demonstration by Caspary *et al* (1987) that on-CF inhibition in the DCN is mediated by glycine, we have recently demonstrated that lateral inhibition in the dorsal cochlear nucleus is glycinergic and can be specifically blocked by micro-iontophoretic application of strychnine, the specific antagonist to glycine (Zhao and Evans, 1990, Evans and Zhao, 1993a,b). The present experiments exploit this finding, by measuring the degree to which the above shifts in dynamic range can be affected by blockade of the lateral inhibitory mechanisms by iontophoretic application of strychnine. In this way, we attempt to fractionate the shifts into components due to synaptic lateral inhibition in the cochlear nucleus, and due to suppression at the cochlear nerve level.

2 Methods

The responses of single units were recorded using 7-barrelled micropipettes in guinea pigs in which anaesthesia was induced with neuroleptanaesthesia (Evans, 1979a) and maintained with alpha-chloralose (40 mg/kg per 2 hours), with monitoring and maintenance of arterial blood pressure, end-tidal CO_2 and gross cochlear action potential to within normal limits (Evans, 1979b). The dorsal cochlear nucleus was exposed by posterior fossa craniotomy and displacement of the cerebellum and electrodes were placed into the dorsal cochlear nucleus under direct vision. The central barrel of the 7-barrelled micro-electrode is NaCl filled for recording; two barrels are used respectively for current balancing (NaCl) and for localisation of the electrode position (Fast Green). The remaining four barrels contained two agonists: GABA and glycine, and two antagonists: strychnine (antagonist to glycine receptors), and bicuculline methylchloride (antagonist to $GABA_A$ receptors). For further details, see Evans and Zhao (1993a,b).

The responses of cochlear nucleus cells recorded extra-cellularly were obtained to pure tone stimuli of 80 ms duration presented 4 times a second, shaped with 5 ms linear rise and fall times. For mapping the excitatory/inhibitory frequency response area, the tones were presented in a pseudo-random sequence of frequencies and intensities so that a range of 60 dB and typically 3 octaves was covered evenly in about 4 minutes of data collection (Evans 1974, 1979b). The resolution in the intensity domain was typically 4 dB; in the frequency dimension: 1/64 of 3 octaves.

Rate-level functions were obtained at the characteristic (best) frequency (CF) of the cell using typically 80 ms tones (at 4 per sec), the levels of which were pseudo-randomly distributed in 16 x 4dB intervals over a 60 dB range, using an algorithm (developed by D.J. MacKay) which ensured an equal number of repeats of each tone level (typically 16) but prevented tones being immediately preceded by tones greater than 16 dB in level or by repeats more than about 10 presentations before. Interleaved with these rate-level

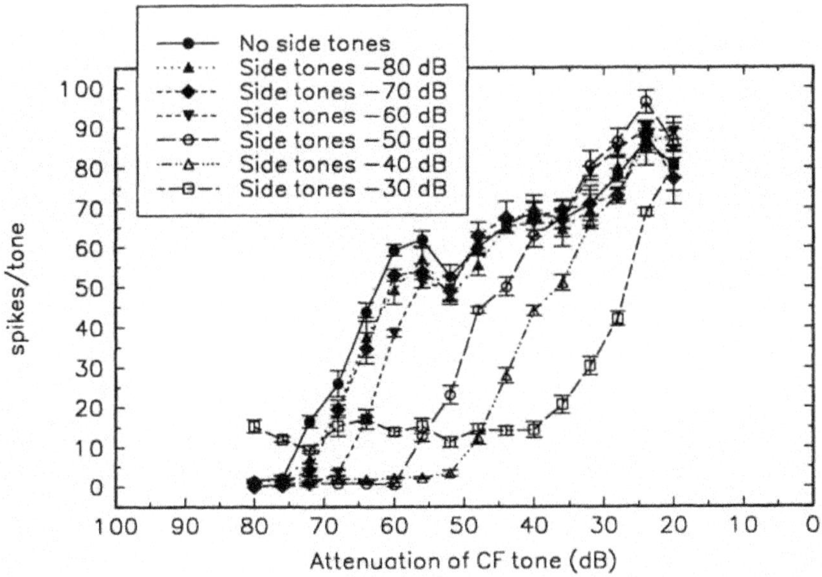

Figure 2. Type I/III unit in DCN. Progressive shift in CF Rate-level functions as levels of side-tones are progressively increased. CF tone at 10.7 kHz; side-tones at 8 and 12 kHz. The dB values in the legend refer to attenuation.

functions at CF, rate-level functions were taken with the addition of one or two 'side-tones' (of identical duration and simultaneously presented with the CF tone), but with fixed levels and frequencies set to produce maximal lateral inhibition of the CF response, as judged from the receptive field map (see Fig. 1). The figures give the means and s.e. of typically 32 presentations (randomized and interleaved as above). The stimulus levels on the figures and in the text are given as dB values of attenuation relative to our maximum (0 dB), approximately equivalent to 110 dB SPL at the frequencies dealt with here (see Fig 15.1 of Evans, 1979b).

In all cases, data were collected before, during and following administration of the antagonist to ensure that the drug effects were fully reversible. The specificity of effects of strychnine blockade of glycinergic lateral inhibition were tested in each case by application of bicuculline, specific for the $GABA_A$ inhibition, unrelated to lateral inhibition (Evans and Zhao, 1993a,b). Also in each case, the specificity of the strychnine application was tested on the same unit by demonstrating that iontophoretically applied strychnine could block inhibition evoked by iontophoretic application of glycine but not by GABA.

Likewise, the specificity of the bicuculline was tested by demonstrating that it blocked inhibition mediated by GABA and not by glycine.

3 Results

Fig. 2 shows the typical effect of changing the levels of the side-tones on the rate-level function of a Type I/III cell having a CF of 10.7 kHz. The left-most curve is the rate-level function for the CF tone alone. The curves progressively to the right are rate-level functions obtained with progressively increasing levels of side-tones (at frequencies of 8 and 12 kHz) as indicated in the legend. The right-most curve represents that obtained with side-tones 30-40 dB above suppression/inhibition threshold, producing a shift of the rate-level function of nearly 40 dB.

Fig. 3 shows the effect of strychnine on another type I/III unit, applied at 80 nA for 5 min. The dashed curve with solid rectangle points is the control CF alone (13 kHz) rate-level function. The corresponding curve with sidetones (at 15 kHz, -20 dB) is the continuous line joining solid circle points. The long dashed (open squares) and dotted (open circles) curves are the CF alone and CF plus side-tone curves respectively, obtained during the application of the strychnine. Thus, the application of strychnine has eliminated

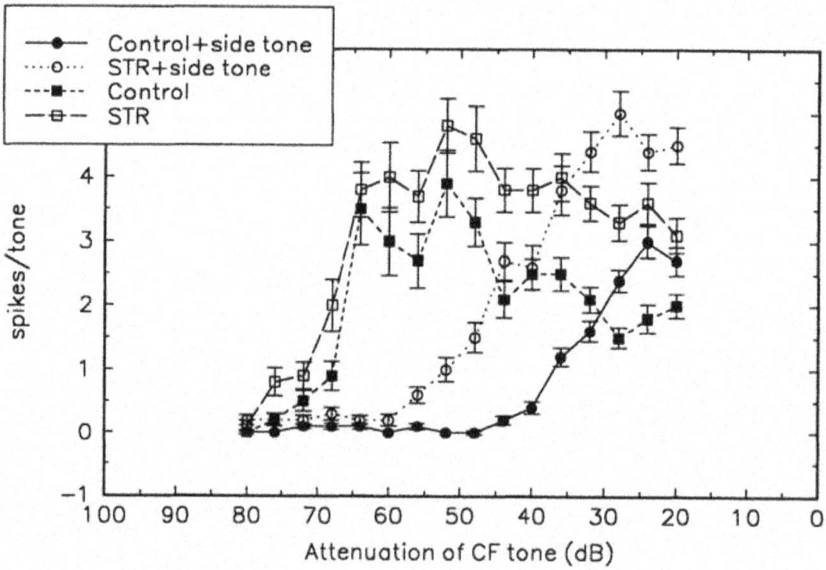

Figure 3. Type I/III unit in DCN. Effect of strychnine producing partial blockade of shift in CF (13 kHz) rate-level function due to addition of side-tones (15 kHz at -20 dB).

about 15 dB of the 30 - 35 dB shift due to the addition of the side-tones.

A more complete blockade of the shift is shown in Fig. 4, in a Type IV unit. The symbols and lines correspond to the conditions in Fig. 3. Thus, the dash-dot curve joining solid squares is the control curve for the CF alone condition, and the continuous line through the solid circle points, the corresponding CF plus side-tone condition, both

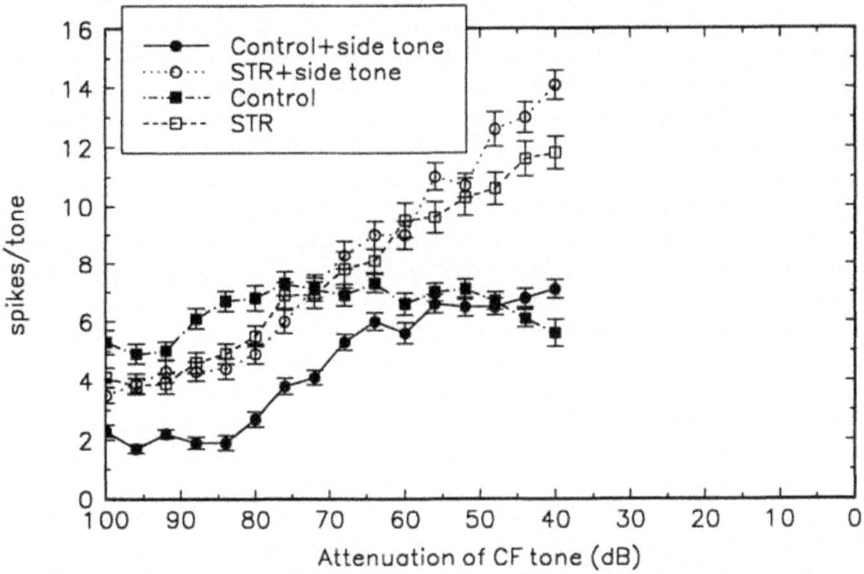

Figure 4. Type IV unit in DCN. Strychnine (open symbols) produces virtually complete blockade of shift in CF (6 kHz) rate-level function due to addition of side-tone (8.5 kHz - 40 dB).

obtained in the 5 min period immediately before application of strychnine. The CF is at 6 kHz (-92 dB threshold) and the side-tone is in the predominant upper frequency inhibitory sideband, at 8.5 kHz (at -40 dB). The dashed and dotted curves through the open squares and circles respectively are the CF alone and CF plus side-tone conditions recorded in the 5 min immediately following application of 80 nA strychnine, (thus during its effect but avoiding possible artefacts due to current passage). During this period, the addition of the side tone has virtually no effect on the CF rate-level function. In other words, the shift due to the presence of the side tone is predominantly due to glycine-mediated lateral inhibition.

To demonstrate that this effect on the shift of the rate-level function is glycine- and not GABA-specific, Fig. 5 shows the same unit, conditions and symbols as Fig. 4, but with bicuculline (antagonist to $GABA_A$ receptors) instead of strychnine. There is no effect on the shift of the rate-level function.

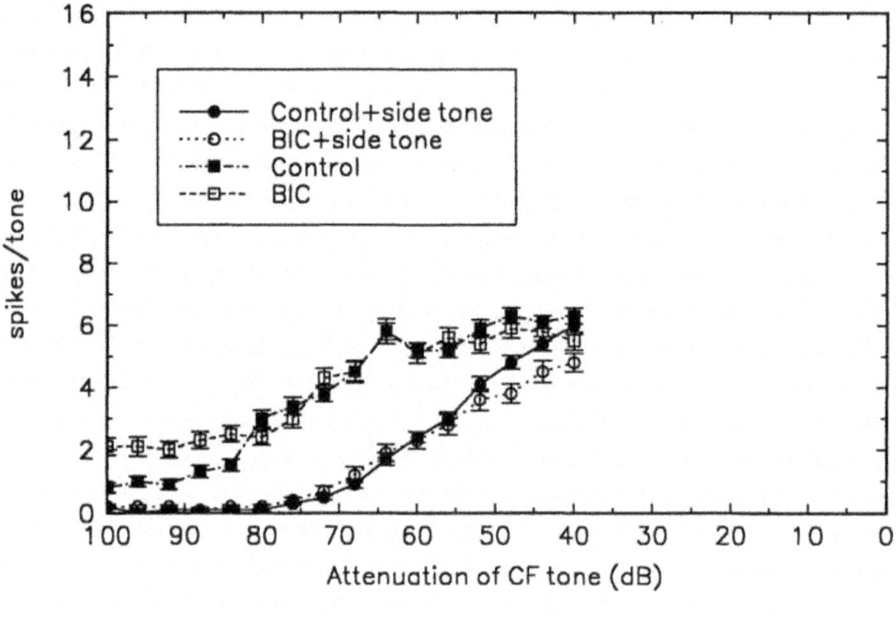

Figure 5. Same unit as Fig. 4. Bicuculline, $GABA_A$ antagonist, has no effect on shift in rate-level function due to side-tone.

4 Discussion

In this small sample of units, it is already clear that in Type IV cells particularly (eg as in Fig. 4), near complete blockade can be obtained of the shift of the rate-level functions due to side-tones in the lateral inhibitory sidebands. In Type I/III units (eg as in Fig. 3), where the spontaneous rates are low, the blockade is so far only partial, suggesting that *both* cochlear nerve suppression and cochlear nucleus inhibition are likely to be involved.

5 Acknowledgments

This work was supported by Grant 032889/Z/90/2 from the Wellcome Trust to EFE.

6 References

Caspary, D. M., Pazara, K. E., Kossl, M., Faingold, C. L., (1987). Strychnine alters the fusiform cell output from the dorsal cochlear nucleus, Brain.Res., 417-273.

Costalupes, J. A., Young, E. D. & Gibson, D. J. (1984). Effects of continuous noise backgrounds on rate response of auditory nerve fibers in cat. J Neurophysiology, 51, 1326-1344.

Evans, E. F. (1974). Auditory frequency selectivity and the cochlear nerve. In: Facts and Models in Hearing: E.Zwicker and E.Terhardt eds., Springer-Verlag, Heidelberg, 118-129.

Evans, E. F. (1979a). Neuroleptanaesthesia for the guinea pig: an ideal anaesthetic procedure for long-term physiological studies of the cochlea. Arch. Otolaryngol., 105, 185-186.

Evans, E. F. (1979b). Single unit studies of the mammalian auditory nerve. In: Auditory Investigations: The Scientific and Technological Basis. H.A. Beagley ed, Oxford University Press, Oxford, 324-367.

Evans, E. F. (1981). The dynamic range problem: place and time coding at the level of cochlear nerve and nucleus. In: Neuronal Mechanisms of Hearing:J Syka and L Aitken ed, Plenum Press, NY, 69-85.

Evans, E. F. & Nelson, P. G. (1973a). The responses of single neurones in the cochlear nucleus of the cat as a function of their location and the anaesthetic state. Experimental Brain Research, 17, 402-427.

Evans, E. F. & Nelson, P. G. (1973b). On the functional relationship between the dorsal and ventral divisions of the cochlear nucleus of the cat. Experimental Brain Research, 17, 428-442.

Evans, E. F. & Palmer, A. R. (1975). Responses of units in the cochlear nerve and nucleus of the cat to signals in the presence of bandstop noise. J. Physiol., 252, 60-62P.

Evans, E. F. & Zhao, W. (1993a). Neuropharmacological and neurophysiological dissection of inhibition in the mammalian dorsal cochlear nucleus. In: The Mammalian Cochlear Nuclei: Organization and Function. Ed by Merchan M. and Juiz J.M., Plenum Press. NY, 253-266.

Evans, E. F. & Zhao, W. (1993b). Varieties of inhibition in the processing and control of processing in the mammalian cochlear nucleus. Progress in Brain Research, 97, 117-126.

Gibson, D. J., Young, E. D. & Costalupes, J. A. (1985). Similarity of dynamic range adjustment in auditory nerve and cochlear nuclei. J.Neurophysiol., 53, 940-958.

Palmer, A. R. & Evans, E. F. (1982). Intensity coding in the auditory periphery of the cat: responses of cochlear nerve and cochlear nucleus neurons to signals in the presence of bandstop masking noise. Hear.Res., 7, 305-323.

Zhao, W. & Evans, E. F. (1990). Pharmacological (microiontophoretic) investigation of receptive-field and temporal properties of units in the cochlear nucleus. British Journal of Audiology, 24, 193.

Comment by R. Klinke

I wonder whether your term "lateral inhibition" applies. What are the arguments that the inhibition you see is brought about by a classical lateral inhibition network?

Reply

The term is used phenomenologically to describe inhibition apparently occuring on the side of a central excitation response area. As our subtraction method shows, the inhibition is actually maximal at the centre of the excitatory region. Thus we have a classical situation as in the retina (the homologue of the cochlear nucleus) where a central excitatory field converges like an iceberg floating in a sea of inhibition, to produce a classical "Mexican hat" profile of cxcitation apparently surrounded by inhibition.

The balance of excitation determines whether the cell in question is a Type III (least), Type IV or Type V (most), but this is an oversimplification.

Comment by A. Rees

You mentioned that $GABA_A$ mediated inhibition is responsible for a tonic background inhibition in the DCN. In our experiments in the IC we find some cells where bicuculline increases the firing rate over the whole of the excitatory response area, but does not change spontaneous firing rate. Do all of the cell types you have studied in the DCN always show an increase in spontaneous acitvity with bicuculline?

Reply

In nearly all our Type IV cells and about half our Types I, I/III and III cells in the guinea pig DCN, we obtained the increase in spontaneous activity with bicuculline as described in Evans and Zhao (1993a,b).

In no units did we observe an increase in evoked activity without increase in spontaneous activity with bicuculline; only with strychnine.

On the neural code for loudness and Its cochlear correlates

Jozef J. Zwislocki and Monita Chatterjee

Institute for Sensory Research and Dpt. of Bioengineering and Neuroscience, Syracuse University, Syracuse NY 13244-5290, U. S. A.

1 Introduction

This paper concerns sensorineural coding of sound intensity culminating in the sensation of loudness. Our investigations have led us to the following conclusions:

1. The whole auditory nerve response in humans, as embodied in the CAP response, roughly parallels the loudness magnitude as a function of sound intensity.
2. The degree of nonlinear compression evident in the CAP I/O function is species dependent.
3. In our animal model, the Mongolian gerbil, IHC I/O functions obtained at single sound frequencies do not parallel the CAP I/O function.
4. The strong compression evident in the IHC I/O functions at CF and higher frequencies is due in part to a shift of maximum excitation toward lower frequencies, as sound intensity is increased. The same shift decreases the apparent compression below CF.
5. The I/O function of the peak IHC response shows a somewhat greater compression than do the areas under the IHC transfer functions.
6. The I/O function of the peak IHC response grows with sound intensity at a slightly slower rate than the CAP.
7. The area under the IHC transfer function, the response area, grows with sound intensity at a slightly faster rate than the CAP.
8. Comparison of single frequency IHC I/O functions to the CAP I/O function indicates that loudness cannot be coded by single cochlear locations.
9. Because the CAP response may under represent the whole nerve response, it is not possible to decide whether loudness depends on the IHC response near the peak of excitation or on the whole population of excited IHCs.

2 CAP Input/output Functions

On the assumptions that the total response of the auditory nerve recorded as a function of sound intensity controls the growth of the human loudness function and that the CAP response reflects the total nerve response with sufficient accuracy, CAP functions are often compared to the loudness function. Since animal CAP functions are frequently used for the purpose, we thought that it would be useful to make an interspecies comparison among them. The task proved to be somewhat more difficult and risky than we had anticipated. A considerable variability is associated with measurement of both the loudness and CAP functions. As a consequence, the hypothesis that the latter parallels the former can be rejected only when the slope difference is substantial. In addition, it must be realized that, because of latency differences among single fiber contributions and their bipolar nature, the CAP response is not an accurate representation of the sum of these contributions. It probably underrepresents the sum, especially at high sound intensities at which the latency differences can be expected to be the greatest. Accordingly, if the whole nerve response parallels the loudness function, the CAP response may exhibit a somewhat greater compression.

For meaningful comparisons between the loudness and CAP functions, the stimulus conditions must be as similar as possible. Whereas such similarity can be found for interspecies comparisons of CAP functions, this is not true for loudness measurements. By contrast to CAP measurements, usually performed with clicks or short sound bursts with steep onsets, sound bursts of moderate duration and relatively gradual onsets are routinely used for loudness measurements. Short sound bursts with steep onsets produce much broader frequency spectra than longer sound bursts with more gradual onsets. Since the CAP response is based on synchronous contributions of individual nerve fibers, which exist only at the stimulus onset, it represents an onset response. By contrast, loudness is believed to be determined by a more extended portion of the sound burst. Fortunately, the loudness function has a rather robust shape and appears to depend little with respect to its slope at moderate and high intensities on the stimulus bandwidth and duration (Scharf, 1978, for review). Also, the slope appears to be fairly frequency independent, except at very low and high frequencies (Scharf, 1978, for review). Comparisons of loudness functions obtained with sinusoids in the midfrequency range and with broad band noise have indicated that the latter produced a somewhat greater slope at low SPLs and a somewhat smaller slope at high SPLs than the sinusoids, but the difference is small enough to have generated a discussion concerning its existence (Scharf, 1978, for review).

Because of the robustness of the loudness function, it does appear meaningful to compare the growth of CAP responses as functions of sound intensity to the corresponding growth of loudness. This is particularly true for sound frequencies above 2 kHz, where the bandwidth produced by the steep stimulus onset becomes less broad relative to the center frequency. However, as a result of the caveats introduced above, detailed comparisons would appear foolish. Therefore, we limit the loudness representation to its logarithmic slope at medium and high SPLs, as established on the basis of numerous studies. This slope is on the order of 0.6 and means that, every time the SPL is increased by 10 dB, the loudness doubles (Scharf, 1978, for review).

CAP functions obtained transtympanically on a human subject and at the round window of a guinea pig with tone bursts in the frequency range between 4 and 8 kHz (Eggermont, Odenthal, Schmidt, and Spoor, 1974) and a CAP function obtained similarly on a Mongolian gerbil at 2 kHz (Hellstrom and Schmiedt, 1990) are compared to the slope of the loudness function in Fig. 1. The slope is indicated by the straight line, the squares indicate the results obtained on the human subject, the circles, those obtained on the guinea pig and the diamonds, those obtained on the gerbil.

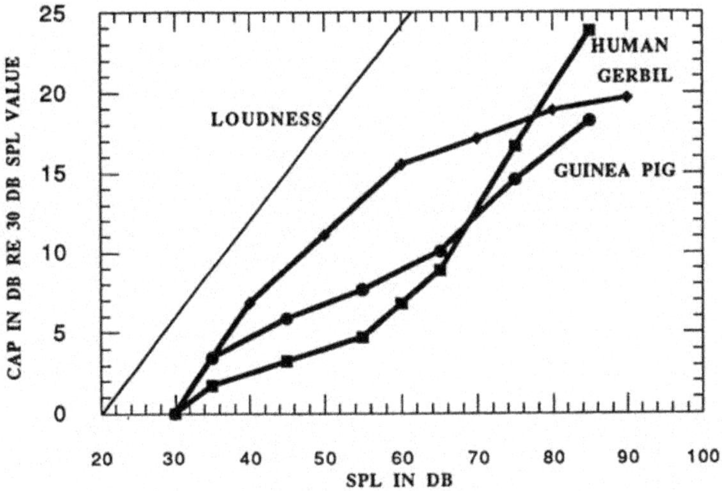

Figure 1. The slope of the loudness function and CAP I/O functions for humans, guinea pigs and Mongolian gerbils.

Several clarifying statements must be made with respect to the empirical curves. Since noise effects make interpretation of the empirical curves at low SPLs uncertain, we have truncated all the curves at 30 dB and normalized them at this SPL. Because of the indirectness of the recordings involved, only slope relationships are significant, anyway. The human and guinea pig curves were obtained by the same authors, presumably, under similar conditions to the limit of feasibility. Both show a flat portion in the medium SPL range which is probably an artifact due to imperfect summation of single fiber contributions. When the human curve is averaged over several subjects (Eggermont, 1978), the plateau nearly disappears but the slope at high SPLs is only slightly reduced. The high SPL slope of the guinea pig curve is supported by very systematic data of Teas, Eldredge and Davis (1962) obtained with a somewhat different method. These data do not show any mid SPL curve flattening. The gerbil data of Fig. 1 are supported by our own measurements and measurements by others at our Institute. In general, good consistency has been obtained.

The slope at high SPLs is of main interest, because the I/O functions of many single fibers saturate at these SPLs, and the lack of a corresponding saturation in the loudness function is the most difficult to explain. Clearly, the human CAP function shown in Fig.1 is nearly parallel to but, rather, somewhat steeper than the loudness function. The slope agreement is even better for the average CAP function. This may be meaningful, since the loudness slope has also been averaged over many subjects. In any event, it is unlikely that the hypothesis according to which the CAP I/O function parallels the loudness I/O function can be rejected, although we do not have sufficient data for a formal statistical test.

The guinea pig curve appears to be clearly flatter than the human curve in the high intensity range. Eggermont et al. thought that both curves were roughly parallel when taken over the entire range of their measurements, but inclusion of low SPLs may have clouded the picture because of uncertain noise effects, as we already mentioned.

Whereas, the human and guinea pig I/O curves do not show any saturation below a SPL of 90 dB, the gerbil curve, which is typical, does. It brings out the most clearly the existing interspecies differences with respect to the CAP. It may be of interest to note in this context that guinea pigs, like cats, have high threshold fibers whose firing rates do not saturate at mid intensity levels (Winter, Robertson and Yates, 1990) but Mongolian gerbils are almost devoid of such fibers (Sokolich, 1977; Schmiedt, 1989; Ohlemiller, Echteler and Siegel, 1991). In addition to the substantive message that the CAP I/O functions differ among animal species with respect to their slopes, we also see here a methodological message that the human loudness function should not be compared to an animal model CAP I/O function unless it is demonstrated that the latter parallels the human CAP function.

3 Direct Cochlear Precursors of the CAP I/O Function

We regard here the I/O functions of IHC receptor potentials as direct precursors of the CAP I/O function. A method for rapid recording of intensity series of IHC and other cochlear transfer functions (Zwislocki, 1986, 1991) has enabled us to construct IHC I/O functions at a large number of sound frequencies and to relate them to features of the transfer functions. The method can be applied to both alternating and direct receptor potentials. The recordings were made intracellularly according to methods described before (Zwislocki and Smith, 1988), which were developed partially from methods described originally by Dallos, Santos-Sacchi and Flock (1982). The data we show here concern alternating potentials since, in the cochlear region of our recordings, they are strongly predominant. The cochlear region corresponds to a CF of about 2 kHz.

Three IHC I/O functions recorded intracellularly are shown in Fig. 2. The one indicated by solid circles has been obtained at CF (2,378 Hz), the one indicated by the triangles at a somewhat higher frequency (2,828 Hz), and the one indicated by the squares at a lower frequency (1,000 Hz). The strong compression evident at CF and the higher frequency, which amounts to almost complete saturation above 60 dB SPL is clearly greater than seen in the gerbil CAP response, as shown in Fig. 1. The I/O function for 1,000 Hz is also nonlinear but in a more complicated way - it shows decompression below 50 dB and increasing compression above. It does not parallel the CAP function. In addition, it could not account for it at low intensities because the sensitivity at 1,000 Hz is much smaller than at CF. We must conclude that, for a given cochlear location, no single frequency I/O function parallels the CAP. Using a mirror image representation, we can infer that, for a given sinusoid, no single cochlear location has an IHC output paralleling the CAP function. Since the CAP I/O function in humans roughly parallels the loudness function,we can infer further that no single cochlear location determines the loudness.

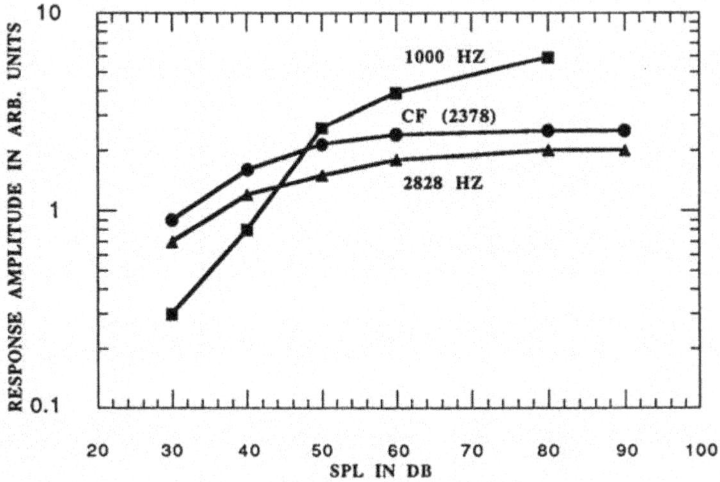

Figure 2. IHC I/O functions determined at CF, a higher and a lower frequency.

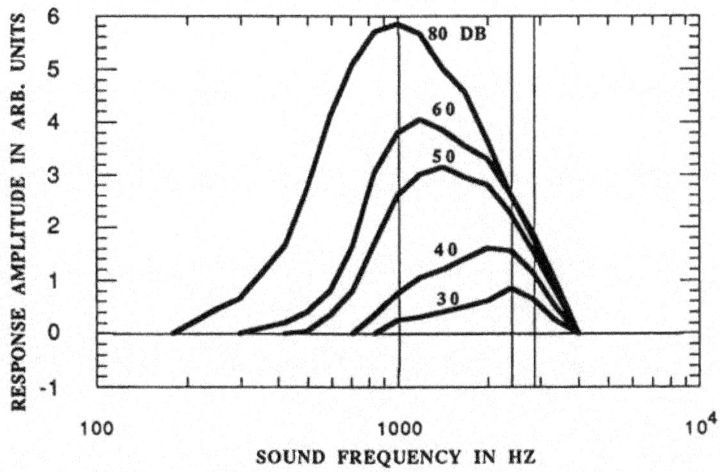

Figure 3. Mongolian gerbil transfer functions taken at 5 SPLs indicated at the curves. The vertical lines indicate cuts that served to construct the I/O function of Fig. 2. Note the peak shift with increasing SPL.

To gain a further insight into the cochlear precursors of the CAP I/O function we show in Fig. 3 an intensity series of IHC transfer functions. The vertical lines indicate the frequencies at which the I/O functions of Fig. 2 have been generated. Note the strong displacement of the peak response toward lower frequencies as SPL is increased. It means that the CF depends on sound intensity. As can be seen in Fig. 3, the shift contributes to the severe compression of the I/O functions at the low intensity CF and higher frequencies and produces the decompression at lower frequencies.

In search of a parameter that would parallel the CAP I/O function, we followed the peak amplitude as a function of SPL and also integrated the areas under the transfer functions. These areas should be roughly directly proportional to the IHC excitation areas in the cochlea. This is so because the transfer functions have been plotted over a log frequency scale, and sound frequency is mapped approximately logarithmically along the cochlea. In other words, the transfer functions can be assumed to be approximate mirror images of excitation distributions along the cochlea. Logically, the CAP function, which represents a global cochlear response, should be related the most directly to these excitation distributions.

The peak and the area I/O functions, together with the gerbil CAP I/O function of Fig. 1 are plotted in Fig. 4. Note that the peak function may be a little flatter than the CAP function, and that the area function is somewhat steeper. Several interpretations of these relationships are possible. First, there is the possibility that the neural response near the peak predominates to the extent that it practically determines the CAP I/O function. In

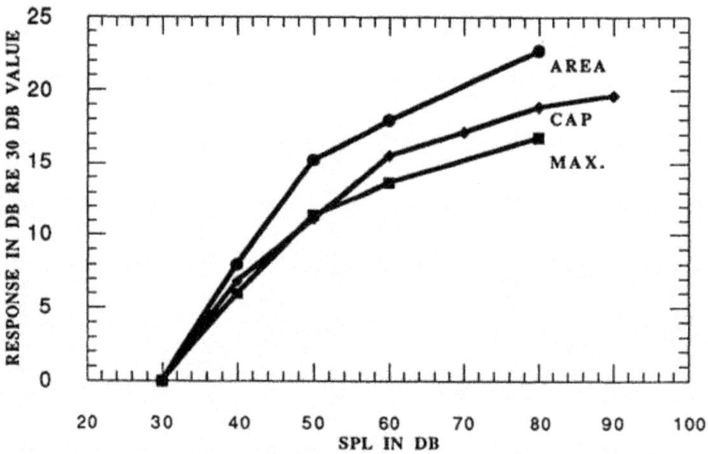

Figure 4. Typical Mongolian gerbil I/O functions for the CAP and for two IHC response parameters - the response maximum and the response area (the area under the transfer function). The IHC curves were determined on one cell that had typical characteristics.

this case, we would infer that maximum cochlear response controls loudness. However, we mentioned at the outset that the CAP probably underrepresents the global nerve response. With this caveat, we could conclude that the whole nerve response linearly reflects the excitation of the whole IHC population, whatever the details may be.

In the end, we can eliminate the possibility of inferred loudness coding by single cochlear locations, but we are left with the dilemma as to the spatial extent of cochlear excitation responsible for the coding - is the extent limited to the region around the excitation maximum or does it include the whole population of excited IHCs?

4 Acknowledgments

We thank Dr. R. L. Smith for the use of gerbil CAP data. This work was supported by NIDCD Grants RO1 DC00074 and PO1 DC00380 and by the DiCarlo Fund.

5 References

Dallos, P., Santos-Sachhi, J. and Flock, A. (1982). Intracellular recordings from cochlear outer hair cells. Science 218, 582 - 584.

Eggermont, J.J. (1978) Stimulus-response relations for promontory-recorded compound action potentials in normal and recruiting ears. In: Naunton and Fernandez (Eds.) Evoked electrical activity in the auditory system. Academic Press, New York.

Eggermont, J.J., Odenthal, D.W., Schmidt, P.H. and Spoor, A. (1974) Electrocochleography. Basic principles and clinical application. Acta Otolaryngol. Suppl. 316, 1-84.

Hellstrom, L.I. and Schmiedt, R.A. (1990) Compound action potential input/output functions in young and quiet-aged gerbils. Hearing Research 50, 163-174.

Ohlemiller, K.K., Echteler, S.M. and Siegel, J.H. (1991) Factors that influence rate-versus-intensity relations in single cochlear nerve fibers of the gerbil. J. Acoust. Soc. Am. 90 (1), 274-287.

Scharf, B. (1978) Loudness. In E.C. Carterette and M.P. Friedman (Eds.) Handbook of Perception. Academic Press, New York.

Schmiedt, R.A. (1989) Spontaneous rates, thresholds and tuning of auditory-nerve fibers in the gerbil: Comparisons to cat data. Hearing Research 42, 23-36.

Sokolich, W.G. (1977) Some electrophysiological evidence for a polarity-opposition mechanism of interaction between inner and outer hair cells in the cochlea. Ph.D. Dissertation, Special Report ISR-S-15. Institute for Sensory Research, Syracuse University, Syracuse, NY.

Teas, D.C., Eldredge, D.H., and Davis, H. (1962) Cochlear responses to acoustic transients: an interpretation of whole-nerve action potentials. J. Acoust. Soc. Am. 34: 1438-1459.

Winter, I.M., Robertson, D., and Yates, G.K. (1990). Diversity of CF rate-intensity functions in guinea pig auditory nerve fibers. Hear. Res. 45, 191-202.

Zwislocki, J.J. (1986) Analysis of cochlear mechanics. Hearing Research 22, 155-169.

Zwislocki, J.J. (1991). What is the cochlear code for pitch? Acta Otolaryngol. (Stockh) 111, 256-262.

Zwislocki, J.J. and Smith, R.L. (1988) Phase reversal in OHC response at high sound intensities. In: J.P. Wilson and D.T. Kemp (Eds.) Cochlear mechanisms: structure, function and models. Plenum Press, London.

Comment by M.A. Cheatham and P. Dallos

Zwislocki and Chatterjee revisit the interesting problem of the representation of peripheral events in the compound action potential (CAP) and the relationship between the latter and loudness growth. One should note, however, that the CAP was extensively studied in the 1970's and a theory for its growth was formulated by Özdamar (1973) and by Özdamar and Dallos (1976). At low sound levels the tone-burst evoked CAP reflects the firing of neurons whose characteristic frequencies (CF) are similar to the frequency of the stimulus. However, as level increases, more and more higher CF fibers, responding on their tail segments, contribute to the response as shown in Fig. 1a. The number of responding fibers is roughly proportional to the size of the CAP which can be obtained from the width of the "across-fiber tuning curve" shown in Fig. 1b. The two segment CAP growth function is, therefore, a natural consequence of the shape of this across-fiber curve. The latter can be obtained directly from populations of nerve fibers (Kiang and Moxon 1974) and is also reflected in the work of Elberling (1976) and Eggermont et al. (1976). The theory described was validated in gerbils by showing that high-pass maskers eliminate the high-level segment of the CAP input-output function (Özdamar and Dallos 1976).

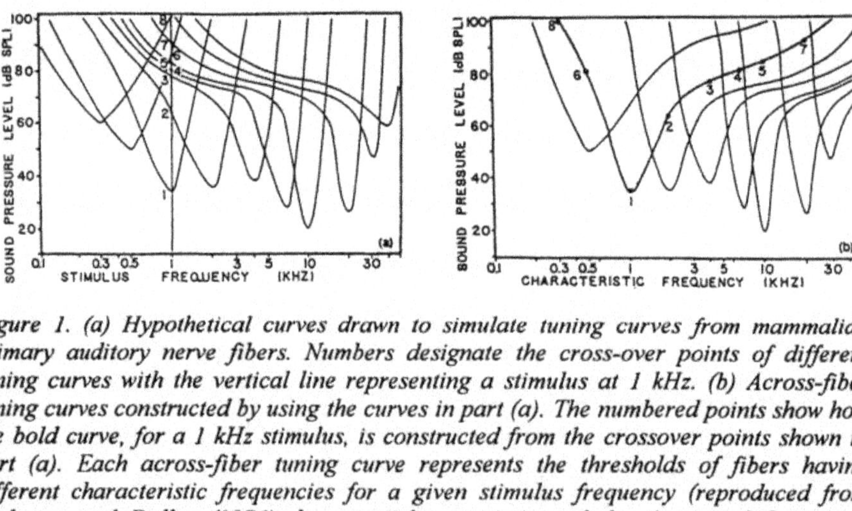

Figure 1. (a) Hypothetical curves drawn to simulate tuning curves from mammalian primary auditory nerve fibers. Numbers designate the cross-over points of different tuning curves with the vertical line representing a stimulus at 1 kHz. (b) Across-fiber tuning curves constructed by using the curves in part (a). The numbered points show how the bold curve, for a 1 kHz stimulus, is constructed from the crossover points shown in part (a). Each across-fiber tuning curve represents the thresholds of fibers having different characteristic frequencies for a given stimulus frequency (reproduced from Özdamar and Dallos (1976), by copyright permission of the Acoustical Society of America).

Eggermont, J.J., Spoor, A. and Odenthal, D.W. (1976). Frequency selectivity of tone-burst electrocochleography. In: R.J. Ruben, C. Elberling and G. Salomon, (Eds.), Electrocochleography, University Park Press, Baltimore MD, pp. 215-256.

Elberling, C. (1976). Simulation of cochlear action potentials recorded from the ear canal in man. Ibid, pp. 151-168.

Kiang, N.Y.S. and Moxon, E.C. (1974). Tails of tuning curves of auditory nerve fibers. J. Acoust. Soc. Am. 55, 620-630.
Özdamar, Ö. (1973). Compound action potentials of the cochlea: Masking experiments and modelling. M.S. Thesis, Northwestern University, Evanston IL.
Özdamar, Ö. and Dallos, P. (1976). Input-output functions of whole nerve action potentials: Interpretation in terms of one population of neurons. J. Acoust. Soc. Am. 59, 143-147.

Reply

We are quite aware of the enormous work performed in the past on the analysis of the whole nerve response. A full discussion of this work would certainly have exceeded the scope of our contribution.

In contradistinction to this work we have been able to avail ourselves of the most recent experimental results. These results indicate, among other things, that tuning curves do not represent accurately the transfer characteristics of the cochlea or the nerve fibers of the auditory nerve. Our reconstructions of the whole nerve response are based on forward transfer functions of the inner hair cells which we have been able to measure. Our observation that the frequency of the IHC peak response at a given cochlear location depends on SPL affects fundamentally our conclusions. This dependence was not known at the time of the Özdamar and Dallos's CAP reconstructions.

With respect to the CAP characteristics, we should state that our work was based on lower sound frequencies than that of Özdamar and Dallos. At these frequencies, the gerbil CAP functions clearly tended toward saturation at high SPLs. The corresponding functions derived from intensity series of IHC transfer functions showed a similar pattern. We should point out parenthetically that our functions are plotted on double log coordinates whereas those of Özdamar and Dallos are plotted on semi log coordinates.

Our approach is similar to that of Özdamar and Dallos, nevertheless, in that we take the total excitation pattern in the cochlea into consideration.

Across-frequency integration by neurones in the ventral cochlear nucleus

A. R. Palmer[1], I.M. Winter[2], D. Jiang[1] and N. James[1]

[1]*MRC Institute of Hearing Research, University Park, University of Nottingham, Nottingham NG7 2RD, U.K. and* [2]*Physiology Laboratory, Downing Street, Cambridge CB2 3EG, U.K.*

1 Introduction

Human listeners demonstrate remarkable abilities in segregating speech from competing sounds such as noise or other speakers (Plomp and Mimpen, 1979; Duquesnoy, 1983). When the interfering sound is speech, the interference cannot be simply removed by filtering, since the target sound and the interference share many spectral and temporal characteristics. Under these circumstances listeners use a range of cues to segregate and attend to a single speaker (Cherry, 1953). One of the most potent of these cues is the fundamental frequency of voicing (F0), which corresponds to the rate of vibration of the vocal folds and varies from 80 to 400 Hz (from adult males to children). Even in the very artificial condition, where listeners are asked to identify pairs of voiced vowels with the same F0, performance is well above chance, suggesting that some kind of template matching process is used (Klatt, 1980; Scheffers, 1983; Assmann & Summerfield, 1989). However, when a pair of vowels is presented with a semitone difference in F0, the identification performance improves significantly and the perception changes: two voices are heard instead of one (Scheffers, 1983; Assmann & Summerfield, 1990). It is difficult to account for these observations soley on the basis of the simple place coding of the sound spectra (Scheffers, 1983; Assmann & Summerfield, 1990).

Several physiological studies have investigated the manner in which the F0 of single vowel sounds, paired vowels sounds on different F0s and of harmonic complexes are signalled by the discharges of fibres in the auditory nerve. The general finding is that low-frequency nerve fibres phase-lock to individual harmonics of the F0, and further, at frequency regions in which more than one harmonic passes through a single neural filter, they beat together and the discharge of the neurone is modulated at the F0 (Smoorenburg & Linschooten, 1977; Delgutte, 1980; Miller and Sachs, 1984; Horst *et al.*, 1985, 1986; Palmer 1990; Delgutte & Cariani, 1991; Palmer and Winter, 1992, 1993). Even for single vowels the F0 seems poorly represented in the distribution of mean discharge rate within the ensemble of auditory nerve fibres (Miller & Sachs, 1983).

Taken together, the psychophysics and the physiology suggest that information concerning the F0 of harmonic complexes (including voiced speech) is likely to be encoded in the timing of impulses in auditory nerve fibres. It is therefore of considerable interest to discover the fate of information encoded in this form in its passage through the cochlear nucleus, which constitutes an obligatory relay in the auditory pathway, and hence the first opportunity for transformation of the temporal code into some other, possibly more robust, representation.

Several studies have measured the capacity of neurones in the cochlear nucleus to signal the modulation in the envelope of tones and have discovered that the different cell types exhibit a hierarchy of sensitivity to modulation. Onset cells respond best to modulation followed by choppers, primarylike-with-a-notch, primarylike and finally by auditory nerve fibres (Frisina *et al.* 1990; see Pfeiffer, 1966 for the basic classification criteria). The role of onset units in the signalling of F0 has also been emphasized more directly in the studies of Kim and his colleagues who demonstrated (based on a very limited sample) that this unit type, better than any other, responded with impulses accurately locked to the pitch period of vowel sounds (Kim *et al*, 1986, Kim & Leonard 1988).

In a series of experiments on units of the ventral cochlear nucleus, we further investigated the representation of the F0 for a range of complex sounds; single and paired vowels in quiet and in noise, harmonic series in sine or alternating phase, and three-tone complexes evoking the "missing fundamental" percept (Palmer & Winter, 1992, 1993). We concluded that the onset cells responded in a manner consistent with the perceived pitch for the range of stimuli that we presented. We hypothesized that the basis for the onset units' ability to respond in this manner was that they responded to coincidences in the times of impulses arriving via auditory nerve fibres representing a wide range of BFs. Since onset units often had response areas which qualitatively appeared to be as sharply tuned as those of auditory nerve fibres, we further hypothesized that many of the off-BF inputs, when activated alone, were only able to generate sub-threshold potentials within the onset cell.

In this paper, we present evidence in support of the hypothesis that onset units, but not chopper or primarylike units, of the ventral cochlear nucleus receive excitatory inputs from auditory nerve fibres with a wide range of best frequencies.

2 Methods

The methods used have been described in detail elsewhere (Palmer *et al* 1986, Palmer 1990) and will only be briefly mentioned here. Responses were measured of units in the ventral cochlear nucleus of pigmented guinea pigs (264-509 g) anaesthetized either with a neuropleptic technique (Evans, 1979) or with 20% Urethane supplemented with phenoperidine as indicated. Recordings were made using tungsten-in-glass microelectrodes inserted into the cochlear nucleus stereotaxically through the intact cerebellum. Sounds were presented, under computer control, in the closed-field via a condenser earphone and calibrated a few millimetres from the tympanic membrane using a probe tube microphone.

3 Results

We have concentrated here on onset units in the ventral cochlear nucleus, but have also analysed units which exhibited chopper and primarylike post-stimulus-time histograms to BF tones at 20 and 50 dB above threshold (Pfeiffer 1966).

3.1 Rate versus level functions to BF tones and to wideband noise

Assuming that auditory nerve fibres operate as simple linear filters, it is possible to estimate their effective bandwidth from measurements of their relative thresholds to tones and to wideband noise of known spectral density (see Evans, 1975a). An example of such a measurement for an auditory nerve fibre, a chopper unit and for an onset unit is shown in Fig.1 A-C respectively. For both the auditory nerve fibre and for the chopper unit the difference in threshold is of the order of 20 dB (as indicated in the figures by the arrows), a value consistent with the effective bandwidth of their response areas measured in the usual way with single tones. For the onset unit, however, the difference in thresholds to the tone and noise is very small and the noise is more effective in driving the unit than the BF tone. The histograms shown in Fig. 1 D-F indicate the values of threshold differences

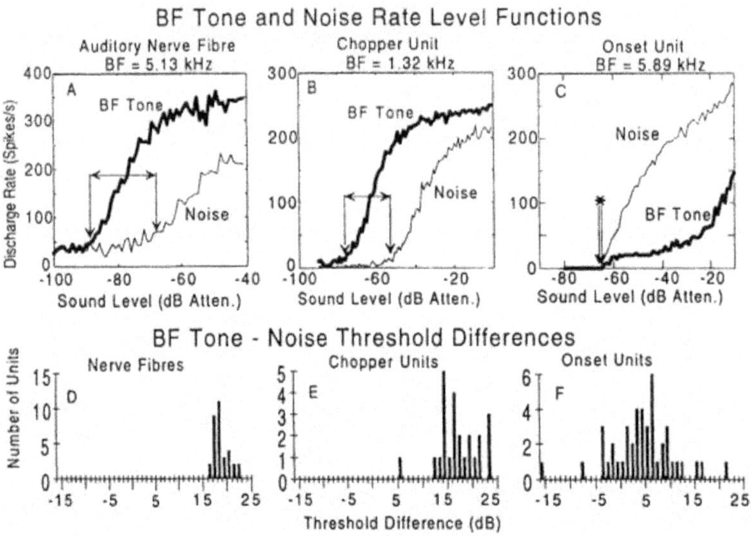

Figure 1. A,B,C show discharge rate versus level functions for 50-ms bursts of BF tones (thick lines) and noise (thin lines) for an auditory nerve fibre, a chopper unit and for an onset unit respectively. The noise was 20 kHz wide and its overall RMS level was approximately matched to that of the BF tone. D,E,F show histograms of the differences in threshold to BF tones and to noise (see text).

found in our samples of fibres, choppers and onset units (mean values are 19.4, 17.7, and 5.5 dB respectively). If onset units are acting as coincidence detectors, as we hypothesize, it is probably incorrect to treat them as simple energy detectors and we have therefore not calculated the putative effective bandwidths from the threshold differences. If such a bandwidth calculation were appropriate for wideband signals the bandwidth derived from the threshold difference would have been of the order of 20 kHz for many onset units (consistent with data in section 3.4). At the very least, this analysis indicates that the onset unit is performing some kind of integration over a wide band of noise energy.

3.2 Facilitation of the responses to BF tones by non-excitatory tones

Many onset units, while having similar thresholds for the noise and BF tones, had response areas that appeared as narrowly tuned as auditory nerve fibres. One explanation for this is that they receive sub-threshold inputs at off-BF frequencies. To test this hypothesis we measured the rate-versus-level functions of onset units in the presence of tones outside the response area which themselves did not activate the unit. We typically chose a frequency half an octave below the BF and a sound level 10-15 dB below the single tone threshold at that frequency. An example of this type of analysis is shown in detail in Figure 2. The response area of the onset unit is shown in Figure 2A (after the method of Evans, 1975b), in which the length of the lines represent the number of spikes evoked by a 50-ms tone burst plotted at the appropriate frequency and sound levels. The peri-stimulus-time histograms of responses for frequencies and levels indicated by the arrows (Fig. 2B) illustrate the basis for the onset unit classification. The two rate-versus-level functions to the BF tones taken at the start and end of the analysis (Fig. 2D) show that the threshold to the BF tone did not change throughout, while the arrow on the 4.18 kHz rate-versus-level function (Fig. 2C) shows the level at which it was set to obtain the two-tone rate level functions shown in Fig. 2E. The major result to note from these analyses is that when the rate-versus-level function was determined in the presence of a simultaneously gated tone, which itself did not evoke activity, the threshold to the BF tone was reduced by a significant margin (16 dB in this instance, but up to 20 dB in some cases) as indicated in Fig. 2E by the arrows marked "facilitation". Note also that, for this onset unit, the second tone was required to be gated and no facilitation was seen when a continuous second tone was presented at the same frequency and level. Using this analysis, we have also seen occasional examples of inhibition or suppression in onset units, due to the off-BF tone.

3.3 Frequency Threshold Curves (FTC) with a fixed BF tone present

The facilitation of the threshold at BF by a second tone, while indicating the presence of sub-threshold inputs which can sum with the BF input, provides no indication of the extent of the frequency region over which the onset unit receives sub-threshold inputs. We have therefore mapped out the range of frequencies capable of producing BF facilitation by using a threshold tracking algorithm (after Rose and Weiss, 1988) in the

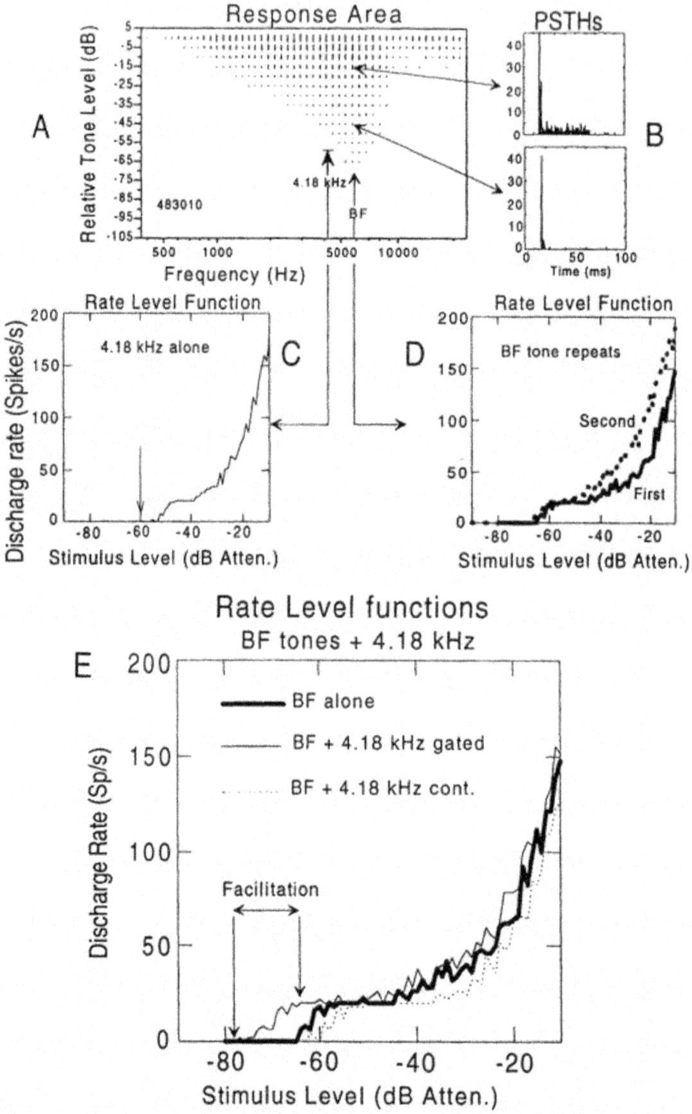

Figure 2. A. The response area of the onset unit determined by presentation of 50-ms tones at randomized levels and frequencies. B. Post stimulus time histograms to BF tones 20 and 50 dB suprathreshold. C, D and E show rate-versus-level functions to combinations of BF tones with 4.18 kHz tones as indicated.

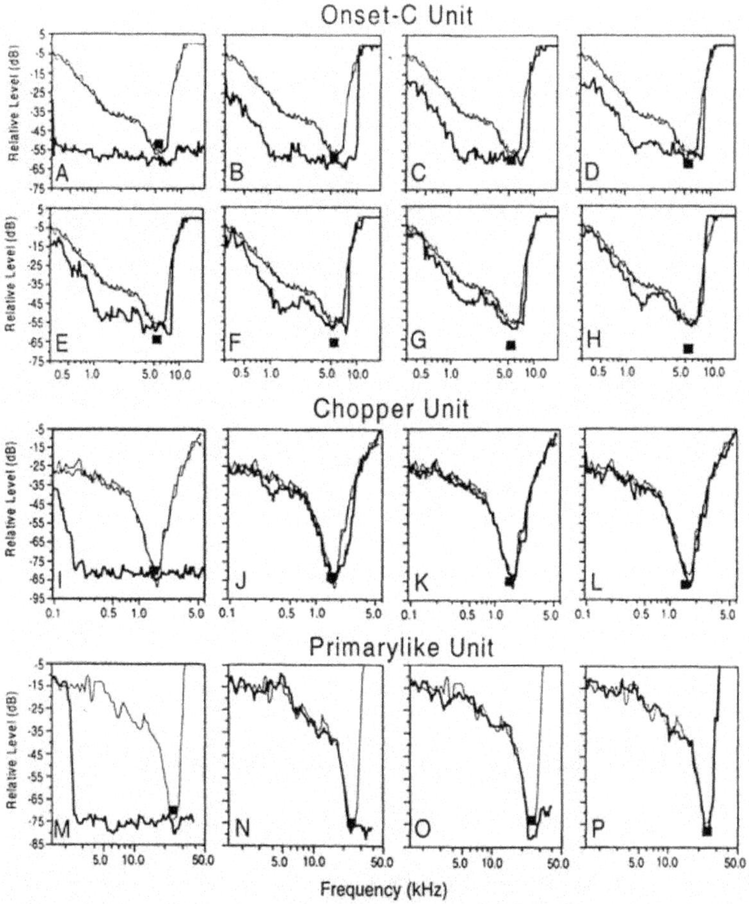

Figure 3. A-H FTCs of an onset-C unit. The thin curves are FTCs to single tones taken at the beginning and the end of the analysis. The filled squares indicate the level and frequency of a second tone present when the FTC shown by the thicker line in each panel was measured. I-L FTCs of a sustained chopper unit in the same format as A-H. M-P FTCs of a primarylike unit in the same format as A-H except that the tone alone FTC was only available for the start of the analysis as the unit was lost.

presence of BF tones at fixed levels above and below the threshold for the BF tone alone. The curves so obtained can be considered as iso-facilitation curves, with a facilitation value corresponding to the number of decibels which the fixed BF tone is below its threshold when presented alone. Examples of such measurements for an onset unit, a chopper unit and for a primarylike unit are shown in Figure 3. The thin lines in Fig. 3

indicate the FTC determined using only a single tone while the thicker line in each panel indicates the FTC measured in the presence of the BF tone at the level indicated by the filled square. When the tracking tone level exceeded the BF tone level both tracked together so that when the BF tone level was suprathreshold the analysis simply tracked the threshold at the BF and a horizontal line results, as seen in Figs. 3A, I and M. For the onset unit, the FTC measured in the presence of sub-threshold BF tones is substantially wider than that to a single tone. Thus for example in Fig. 3E, the combination of a BF tone of about 5 dB below threshold with a 1 kHz tone 20 dB below its own threshold is sufficient to exceed the unit's firing threshold. Even when the BF tone is more than 10 dB sub-threshold as in Fig. 3H there is still a range of frequencies centred at 1.5 kHz where facilitation can be observed. While the facilitation might be thought of as either the BF facilitating the other frequencies or the other frequencies facilitating the BF, we believe, from measurements of firing latency, that the correct interpretation is the facilitation of the activity at BF by the off-BF tones. In the onset unit depicted in Fig. 3 the facilitation was more pronounced at frequencies below BF, but we have observed above BF and below BF facilitation alone or together. We have also revealed strong inhibitory side band inhibition in some onset units using this technique and in some instances we have been unable to demonstrate any facilitation in onset units apparently no different in their characteristics from that in Fig. 3. The picture is somewhat different for chopper units. For this unit type, we frequently saw evidence of inhibitory side bands. We also saw some facilitatory effects, but only when the BF tone was within a few decibels of threshold as can be seen on the high frequency side of the FTC in Fig. 3J. The facilitatory effects we observed did not span as wide a frequency range, nor were they as pronounced as those in onset units, and the range of BF tone levels which showed effects was more restricted.

We have obtained FTC data of this kind in only a limited sample of primarylike units. An example is shown in Figs. 3M-P. Like the chopper units, the effects which we observed in this unit class were more restricted in terms of the strength, range of frequency and the range of BF tone levels which elicited any facilitation.

3.4 Response as a function of the width of bands of noise

The limitation of the two-tone analysis described above is that, when complex or wideband sounds are presented, many of the facilitatory inputs will be simultaneously activated and each may contribute to raising the intracellular potential to the firing threshold: inputs too weak to produce significant BF facilitation when presented alone may be effective in concert with other weak inputs. The two-tone paradigms would fail to demonstrate such interactions. Thus, in order to provide a better estimate of the bandwidth over which neurones in the ventral cochlear nucleus integrate across frequency when presented with wideband sounds, it is necessary to measure their output as a function of the stimulus bandwidth. Such an analysis for the onset unit shown in Fig. 3A-H and for a chopper unit are shown in Figure 4. The paradigm consisted of fixing the frequency of one edge of a noise at the unit BF and progressively widening the band either upwards or downwards in frequency. The abscissa scale indicates the upper or lower

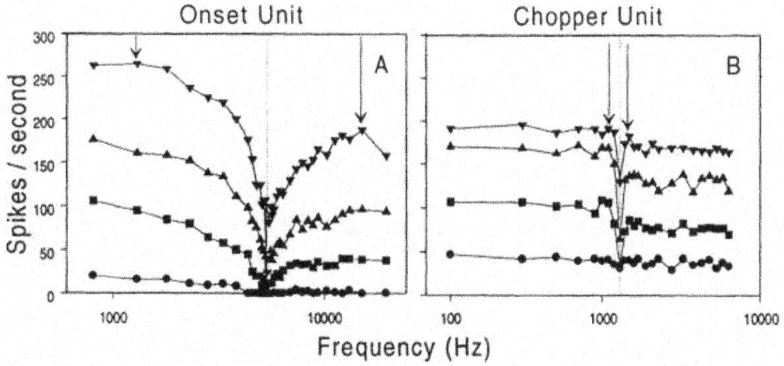

Figure 4. A. Discharge rate as a function of the bandwidth and level of a noise and of the level of a BF tone for a chopper unit. The ordinate indicates either the upper or lower frequency cut-off of the noise. The other cut-off was always at BF. The dotted line passes through the BF and those points determined using a single BF tone. B. The same analysis as in A for the onset unit also shown in Fig. 3A-H. The spectral density of the noise bands was 54 dB SPL for the inverted triangles, 38 dB SPL for the triangles, 22 dB SPL for the squares and 6 dB SPL for the circles.

cut-off frequency of the noise band. The dotted line passes through the points determined using a single tone at the BF. The BF tone was less effective in driving either unit than the narrowest bands of noise (100 Hz) due to the integration of the noise energy which all fell within the unit's response area (100 Hz represents an increase over the spectral density of 20 dB). The discharge rate of this onset unit to the BF tone increased from 24 to 84 spikes per second as the level was increased from 54 to 74 dB SPL which is consistent with the difference in discharge rate between the BF tone and 100 Hz noise bands in Fig. 4A. Similarly at the highest level in Fig. 4B the discharge rate to the BF tone is 130 spikes per second while the discharge to the 100 Hz noise bands is of the order of 190 spikes per second which is consistent with the discharge to the BF tone at 20 dB higher level (187 spikes per second). The arrows in Fig. 4 indicate the cut-offs of the noises at which no further increase in the discharge rate of the unit was observed. Note that the onset unit continues to increase its discharge rate as the low-frequency cut off of the noise is decreased to 1300 Hz and the high-frequency cut off increases to 15300 Hz. Thus components of the noise spanning 14000 Hz are affecting the output of this neurone. In contrast, for the chopper unit, increases in bandwidth from the single tone to 100 Hz in the high-frequency direction produce an increase in output, but no further changes in discharge occur as the noise bandwidth is further increased in this direction. In the low-frequency direction the output discharge rate increases as the noise is increased in bandwidth only over a very limited range of frequency unlike the case for the onset unit. We do not have data of this type for primarylike units.

4 Discussion

The facilitation of the responses to BF tones by a second tone demonstrates inputs off-BF which alone are insufficient to cause onset units to respond. Using two-tone FTCs, we have mapped out the combinations of BF tones and off-BF tones which together cause the unit to fire. Both the rate-versus-level analyses with single fixed tones and the two-tone FTC analyses on a single unit reveal the same facilitation of the BF threshold. While we deliberately concentrated on onset units we have obtained data on chopper and primarylike units, which appear to present a different picture. As yet we have no evidence for strong excitatory inputs to choppers and primarylike units which span wide ranges of auditory nerve fibre BFs.

The onset units of the ventral cochlear nucleus are able to extract the F0 of various harmonic complex sounds (Palmer & Winter, 1992,1993) and, because their output is more precisely timed at the F0 than that of other cells types, it has been described as a "pitch period following response" (Kim & Leonard, 1988). The output of onset units is not, however, unique in representing F0 since responses modulated at the F0 have been reported in virtually all cell types of the cochlear nucleus (Kim *et al*, 1986), a result consistent with the sensitivity of the different cell types to amplitude modulated stimuli (Frisina *et al*, 1990; Rhode, 1991). However, reducing or removing the modulation of the input at the BF of many onset units did not abolish their response to the F0 (Palmer & Winter, 1993), suggesting that while their non-linear responses to modulation may explain much of the precision of their time locked output (see Wang and Sachs 1994) this cannot be the full explanation. It was results such as these that led us to propose (as have others), that the onset cells were acting as coincidence detectors and that they received as input discharges from auditory nerve fibres spanning a wide range of BFs, thus allowing for the possibility that responses phase-locked to low-frequency harmonics, as well as responses at higher frequency to F0 modulation, could contribute to the activation of the onset unit. Leaving aside the nature of the coincidence detection, for which we have other supporting evidence, the experiments reported here sought only to measure the integration of input from auditory nerve fibres spanning a wide range of BFs.

How then do the various measures which we have obtained using these different analyses on the same unit interrelate? The width of the two-tone FTC in Fig. 3B at a level equal to the spectral density of the most intense noise used in Fig. 4B (-51dB of attenuation in Fig. 3 corresponds to the 54 dB SPL spectral density in Fig. 4), has a width approximately equal to the 14000 Hz spacing of the arrows in Fig. 4B (i.e. the range of frequencies contributing to increase in the discharge rate). Since the width of the two-tone FTC is dependent on the BF tone level this comparison is arbitrary and perhaps coincidental. Computation of the filter bandwidth based on the threshold difference between the BF tone and a matched broadband noise gives a value of 10000 Hz, which, given the difficulties in determination of threshold, is of the same order as the 14000 Hz revealed by the bandwidth analysis. However, we suggested that computations of the bandwidth from the threshold differences may be inappropriate for a coincidence detector. Comparison of the responses to 100 Hz bands of noise with the BF tone rate-versus-level function suggested that the output varied in a wav which *was* consistent with the extra energy in the noise (see section 3.4). For wider bands of noise, however, the discharge to the noise was considerably greater than predicted from the BF rate-versus-level function, a result which reinforces our reservation concerning estimation of the effective bandwidth from the tone/noise threshold difference.

Taken together all the analyses point to the fact that onset units receive input from auditory nerve fibres with a wide range of BFs. They are, however, not to be thought of as simply wide band detectors as the effectiveness of the various off-BF inputs varied over a wide range. Every onset cell showed a definable BF and the inputs were weighted, decreasing in effectiveness at higher and lower frequencies. Chopper or primarylike units either showed little evidence of off-BF inputs or evidence of inhibition at these frequencies.

What are the possible functions of the onset units in the ventral cochlear nucleus? First, we should point out that, in common with all other studies of the ventral cochlear nucleus, we identify different onset unit types (Onset-L, Onset-C, Onset-I; Rhode, 1991). Certainly, some of the onset units project out of the cochlear nucleus (Adams 1979) and could constitute a pathway for information concerning the F0 of complex sounds. Another suggestion, based on the fact that onset units often have wide dynamic ranges as a result of non-saturating rate-versus-level functions (like those shown in Figs. 1C, 2C,D,E), is that onset units may contribute a pathway concerned with sound intensity (see Fig. 12A, Rhode, 1991). None of the data presented here can gainsay either possibility. However, at least two other options, which are not mutually exclusive, exist for the function of onset units. The onset unit responses are probably measured from cells with large multipolar or stellate type morphologies (Smith & Rhode, 1989). In the slice preparation, one such group of stellate cells has a dorsally directed axon headed in the direction of the dorsal cochlear nucleus (Oertel *et al* 1990). It may be, therefore, that some of the onset cells constitute an interneuronal pathway to the cells of the dorsal cochlear nucleus. Certainly, some of the properties of the onset cells match those required for an interneurone providing the inhibitory input to the type II cells (see Spirou & Young, 1991). In other studies, large stellate cells in the ventral cochlear nucleus have been identified as the source of an inhibitory commisural pathway to the opposite cochlear nucleus (Cant & Gaston, 1982; Wenthold 1987), the function of which is yet to be determined.

5 Acknowledgements

We thank P. Moorjani for technical assistance and Professor A.Q. Summerfield and Dr. A. Rees for helpful comments on the manuscript.

6 References

Adams, J.C. (1979) Ascending projections to the inferior colliculus. J. Comp. Neurol., 183, 519-538.

Assmann, P. and Summerfield, A.Q. (1989) Modeling the perception of concurrent vowels: vowels with the same fundamental frequency. J. Acoust. Soc. Amer., 85, 327-338.

Assmann, P. and Summerfield, A.Q. (1990) Modeling the perception of concurrent vowels: Vowels with different fundamental frequencies. J. Acoust. Soc. Amer., 88, 680-697.

Blackburn, C.C. and Sachs, M.B. (1990) The representation of the steady-state vowel /ε/ in the discharge patterns of cat anteroventral cochlear nucleus neurons. J. Neurophysiol., 63, 1191-1212.

Cant, N.B. and Gaston, K.C. (1982) Pathways connecting the right and left cochlear nuclei. J. Comp. Neurol., 212, 313-326.

Cherry, E.C. (1953) Some experiments on the recognition of speech with one and with two ears. J. Acoust. Soc. Amer., 25, 975-979.

Delgutte, B. (1980) Representation of speech-like sounds in the discharge patterns of auditory nerve fibers. J. Acoust. Soc. Amer, 68, 843-857.

Delgutte, B. and Cariani, P. (1992) Coding of fundamental frequency in the auditory nerve: A challenge to rate-place models. In: The Auditory Processing of Speech. (M.E.H. Schouten ed.), p. 37-46.

Delgutte, B. and N. Y. S. Kiang. (1984) Speech coding in the auditory nerve: I. Vowel-like sounds. J. Acoust. Soc. Am., 75, 866-878.

Duquesnoy, A.J. (1983) Effect of a single interfering noise or speech sources upon the binaural sentence intelligibility of aged persons. J. Acoust. Soc. Amer., 74, 739-743.

Evans, E.F. (1979) Neuroleptanaesthsia for the guinea pig. Arch. Otolaryngol., 105, 185-186.

Evans, E.F. (1975a) Cochlear nerve and cochlear nucleus. In: Handbook of Sensory Physiology V/2. (W.D. Keidel and W.D. Neff, Eds.), Springer-Verlag, New York, pp. 1-108.

Evans, E.F. (1975b) Normal and abnormal functioning of the cochlear nerve. In: Sound Reception in Mammals. (R.J. Bench and J.D. Pye, Eds.) Academic press, London.

Frisina, R.D., Smith, R.L. and Chamberlain, S.C. (1990) Encoding of amplitude modulation in the gerbil cochlear nucleus. Hearing Res., 44, 99-122.

Horst, J. W., E. Javel and G. R. Farley. (1985) Extraction and enhancement of spectral structure by the cochlea. J. Acoust. Soc. Amer., 78, 1898-1901.

Horst, J. W., E. Javel and G. R. Farley. (1986) Coding of spectral fine structure in the auditory nerve: I. Fourier analysis of period and interspike interval histograms. J. Acoust. Soc. Amer., 79, 398-416.

Kim, D. O., W. S. Rhode and S. R. Greenberg. (1986) Responses of cochlear nucleus neurons to speech signals: Neural encoding of pitch, intensity and other parameters. In: Auditory Frequency Selectivity; (B.C.J. Moore & R.D. Patterson eds.), Plenum Press, New York, pp. 281-288.

Kim, D.O. and Leonard, G. (1988) Pitch-period following response of cat cochlear nucleus neurones to speech sounds". In: Basic Issues in Hearing (H. Duifhuis, J.W. Horst and H.P. Wit, Eds.), Academic Press, London, pp. 252-260.

Klatt, D.H. (1980) Speech perception: a model of acoustic-phonetic analysis and lexical access. In: Perception and Production of Fluent Speech. (R. Cole, Ed.), Erlbaum, New York, pp. 243-288.

Miller, M. I. and M. B. Sachs. (1983) Representation of stop consonants in the discharge patterns of auditory-nerve fibers. J. Acoust. Soc. Amer., 74, 502-517.

Miller, M. I. and M. B. Sachs. (1983) Representation of voice pitch in the discharge patterns of auditory-nerve fibers. Hearing Res., 14, 257-279.

Oertel, D., Wu, S.H. and Dizack, C. (1990) Morphology and physiology of cells in slice preparation of posteroventral cochlear nucleus of mice. J. Comp. Neurol., 295, 136-154.

Palmer, A.R. (1990) The representation of the spectra and fundamental frequencies of steady-state single- and double-vowel sounds in the temporal discharge patterns of guinea pig cochlear-nerve fibers. J. Acoust. Soc. Amer., 88, 1412-1426.

Palmer, A.R. and Winter, I.M. (1992) Cochlear nerve and cochlear nucleus responses to the fundamental frequency of voiced speech sounds and harmonic complex tones. In: Auditory Physiology and Perception (Y. Cazals, L. Demany and K. Horner, Eds.), pp. 231-239.

Palmer, A.R. and Winter, I.M. (1993) Coding of the fundamental frequency of voiced speech sounds and harmonic complex tones in the ventral cochlear nucleus. In: The Mammalian Cochlear Nuclei: Organization and Function. (M.A. Merchan, J. Juiz, D.A. Godfrey and E. Mugnaini, Eds.), Plenum Press, New York, pp. 373-384.

Palmer, A.R., Winter, I.M. and Darwin, C.J. (1986) The representation of steady-state vowel sounds in the temporal discharge patterns of guinea pig cochlear nerve and primarylike cochlear nucleus neurons. J. Acoust. Soc. Amer., 79, 100-113.

Pfeiffer, R.R. (1966) Classification of response patterns of spike discharges for units in the cochlear nucleus: tone-burst stimulation. Exp. Brain. Res., 1, 220-235.

Plomp, R. and Mimpen, A.M. (1979) Speech reception threshold for sentences as a function of age and noise level. J. Acoust. Soc. Amer., 66, 1333-1342.

Rose, C. and Weiss, T.F. (1988) Frequency dependence of synchronization of cochlear nerve fibers in the alligator lizard: evidence for a cochlear origin of timing and non-timing neural pathways. Hearing Res., 33, 151-166.

Scheffers, M.T.M. (1983) Sifting vowels: Auditory pitch analysis and sound segregation. Doctoral Thesis, University of Groningen.

Smith, P.H. and Rhode, W.S. (1989) Structural and functional properties distinguish two types of multipolar cells in the cat ventral cochlear nucleus. J. Comp. Neurol., 282, 595-616.

Smoorenburg, G. F. and Linschoten D. H. (1977) A neurophysiological study on auditory frequency analysis of complex tones. In Psychophysics and Physiology of Hearing, (E.F. Evans and J.P. Wilson, Eds), Academic Press, London, pp. 175-183.

Spirou , G.A. and Young, E.D. (1991) Organization of dorsal cochlear nucleus type IV unit response maps and their relationship to activation by bandlimited noise. J. Neurophysiol., 66, 1750-1768.

Wang, X. and Sachs, M.B. (1994) Neural encoding of sungle-formant stimuli in the cat. II. Responses of anteroventral cochlear nucleus units. J. Neurophysiol., 71, 59-78.

Wenthold, R.J. (1987) Evidence for a glycinergic pathway connecting the two cochlear nuclei: an immunohistochemical and retrograde transport study. Brain Res., 415, 183-187.

Comment by A.J.M. Houtsma

With respect to the relevance of phase-locking to F_0 in 8th-nerve fibers and onset units of the VCN for pitch perception of complex tones, there appears to be an interesting paradox. On the one hand there is, as you have shown, plenty of evidence for information of F_0 up to the level of the VCN. This is also true for complex-tone stimuli that have many high-order harmonics (e.g. from the 15th through the 25th), without the fundamental being present (Horst, Javel and Farley, 1986; Kim and Leonard, 1988). On the other hand, psychophysical experiments on pitch discrimination or identification for harmonic complexes with many partials (Hoekstra, 1979; Houtsma and Smurzynski, 1990) have shown that, if all harmonics are higher than order 11 or 12 and therefore unresolved by the cochlea, pitch discrimination or identification performance becomes

(a) phase dependent and

(b) very poor compared with performance for low-order resolved harmonics. This supports your suggestion that information concerning F_0 is likely to be encoded in the timing of impulses in auditory-nerve fibers and VCN onset units, at least for high-order unresolved harmonics. But it also shows that the central auditory nervous system can use this information only very inefficiently compared with the information contained in the low-order resolved harmonics.

Kim, D.O. and Leonard, G. (1988). Pitch-period following response of cat cochlear nucleus neurones to speech sounds. In: Basic Issues in Hearing, (H. Duifhuis, J.W. Horst, and H.P. Wit, Eds), Acad. Press, London, pp. 252-260

Hoekstra, A. (1979). Frequency discrimination and frequency analysis in hearing. Ph.D. Dissertation, University of Groningen.

Horst, J.W., Javel, E., and Farley, G.R. (1986). Coding of spectral fine structure in the auditory nerve I. Fourier analysis of period and interspike interval histograms. J. Acoust. Soc. Am. 79, 398-416.

Houtsma, A.J.M. and Smurzynski, J. (1990). Pitch identification and discrimination for complex tones with many harmonics. J. Acoust. Soc. Am. 87, 304-310.

Reply

We agree entirely with Professor Houtsma who correctly states that there is good psychophysical evidence that information concerning the F_0 of complex sounds may be carried both by resolved and by unresolved harmonics (see in addition the elegant demonstration by Carlyon et al, 1992). Consistent with this, we have previously shown that the responses of high-frequency onset cells in the cochlear nucleus are dependant on the phase relationships of harmonic complexes (Palmer and Winter 1992, 1993). Our physiological data demonstrate that the activity of peripheral auditory neurones carries information concerning F0, but obviously say nothing about the efficiency with which such information is analysed more centrally.

Carlyon, R.P., Demany, L. and Semal, C. (1992). Detection of across-frequency differences in fundamental frequency, J. Acoust. Soc. Amer., 91, 279-292.

Comment by D.R.F. Irvine

I have a comment and a question. They concern the implications of the data for the site and mechanisms of injury-induced reorganization of frequency maps.

I mentioned in my paper that we have evidence for reorganization in some regions of the central nucleus of the inferior colliculus (ICC) after restricted cochlear lesions in adult cats. What I did not have time to mention was that reorganization is always associated with the appearance of simple onset responses in the high-frequency region of ICC deprived of its normal input by the lesion. In penetrations through ICC in which sustained responses were seen throughout the deprived regions, there was no evidence of reorganization (i.e. in these regions, the changes in the frequency maps can be explained in terms of the residue of pre-lesion responses). (Irvine and Rajan, 1994).

In this context, I wonder whether you have any evidence on whether the onset cells in VCN that exhibit subthreshold (or perhaps unexpressed for some other reason) frequency convergent input include cell types that send their axon out of the CN?

Octopus cells, a group of cells associated with onset type responses, project out of the cochlear nucleus to the contralateral ventral nucleus of the lateral lemniscus which in turn projects to the inferior colliculus (Warr, 1982). While we deliberately targetted our electrodes at the octopus cell area and therefore our sample should contain the responses of octopus cells they are probably a very small minority. Most of our onset responses are likely to derive from multipolar cells, a cell type which also sustains chopper type temporal response patterns. Thus while it is known that multipolar cells in the ventral cochlear nucleus do project to the inferior colliculus (Adams, 1979) we have no way of knowing whether those cells supporting onset type response patterns are amongst them. The only unequivocal data which demonstrate both physiological response type and morphological substrate are from physiological studies combined with intracellular labelling. Such data have been obtained for onset responding units in the ventral cochlear nucleus and suggest that the cells project out, but the stains often fade before reaching their final termination site (e.g. Rhode et al., 1983). Injection into fibres of the intermediate acoustic stria allow axon projections to be traced, but often at the expense of the location of the soma (see Smith et al., 1991). Thus we do not yet know whether the onset cells showing facilitation project to the inferior colliculus.

Adams, J.C. (1979) Ascending projections to the inferior colliculus. J. Comp. Neurol. 183, 519-538.

Rhode, W.S., Oertel, D. and Smith, P.H. (1983) Physiological response properties of cells labelled intracellularly with horseradish peroxidase in the cat ventral cochlear nucleus. J. Comp. Neurol. 213, 448-463.

Smith, P.H., Joris, P.X., Banks, M.I. and Yin, T.C.T. (1991) Responses of cochlear nucleus cells and projections of their axons. In: The mammalian cochlear nuclei. Eds. M.A. Merchan, J.M. Juiz, D.A. Godfrey and E.Mugnaini, Plenum Press, New York, 349-360.

Warr, W.B. (1982) Parallel ascending pathways from the cochlear nucleus: Neuroanatomical evidence of functional specialization. In: Contributions to sensory physiology, Academic Press, Vol. 7, 1-38.

The dorsal cochlear nucleus (DCN): Mechanisms and function

I. Nelken and E. D. Young

Center for Hearing Sciences, Department of Biomedical Engineering, the Johns Hopkins University, 720 Rutland Av., Batimore MD 21205, USA

1 Introduction

The dorsal cochlear nucleus (DCN) of the cat is a layered structure, with some similarities to the cerebellum (Berrebi and Mungaini 1991, Mugnaini and Morgan 1987). It has an intricate internal circuitry, with many interneuron types, most of which are inhibitory. Although the DCN receives auditory nerve fiber input (Ryugo 1992) it also receives input from other sources, including other divisions of the cochlear nucleus (Adams 1983, Smith and Rhode 1989, Snyder and Leake 1988), higher stations of the auditory pathways (Conlee and Kane 1982, Kane 1977, Kane and Finn 1977), and non-auditory sources. One non-auditory source is a projection from the somatosensory dorsal column nuclei which reaches the granule cell domains of the DCN (Itoh et al. 1987, Weinberg and Rustioni 1987, Wright and Ryugo 1994).

We recorded single-unit activity using extracellular electrodes in the DCN of unanesthetized, decerebrate cats. We used a large set of sounds, including single-tone sounds, two-tone sounds, BBN, narrow noise bands and noise notches, to characterize the responses of each unit. We compared quantitatively the responses to the various stimuli in order to dissect the mechanisms which shape the responses of DCN units to complex sounds.

2 Properties of DCN type II and type IV units

DCN principal cells display the so-called type IV response characteristic (Evans and Nelson 1973, Young and Brownell 1976), which is dramatically different from auditory nerve responses to sound. The defining property of type IV units is their inhibition by BF tones at high levels. Fig. 1A shows the responses of a type IV unit to BF tones and broad-band noise (BBN). At low levels, both stimuli are excitatory; at high levels, BF tones strongly inhibit the unit whereas BBN remains weakly excitatory. Spirou and Young (1991) studied the responses of type IV units to tones across a range of frequencies and sound levels (tone response map). Fig. 1C shows a type IV response map. Note the predominance of inhibitory responses. Type IV response maps show a large variability in the arrangement of excitatory and inhibitory regions, but they have some common features. The area outlined by dashed lines in Fig. 1C is called the central inhibitory area (CIA); CIA is commonly found in type IV response maps. It can be accounted for by

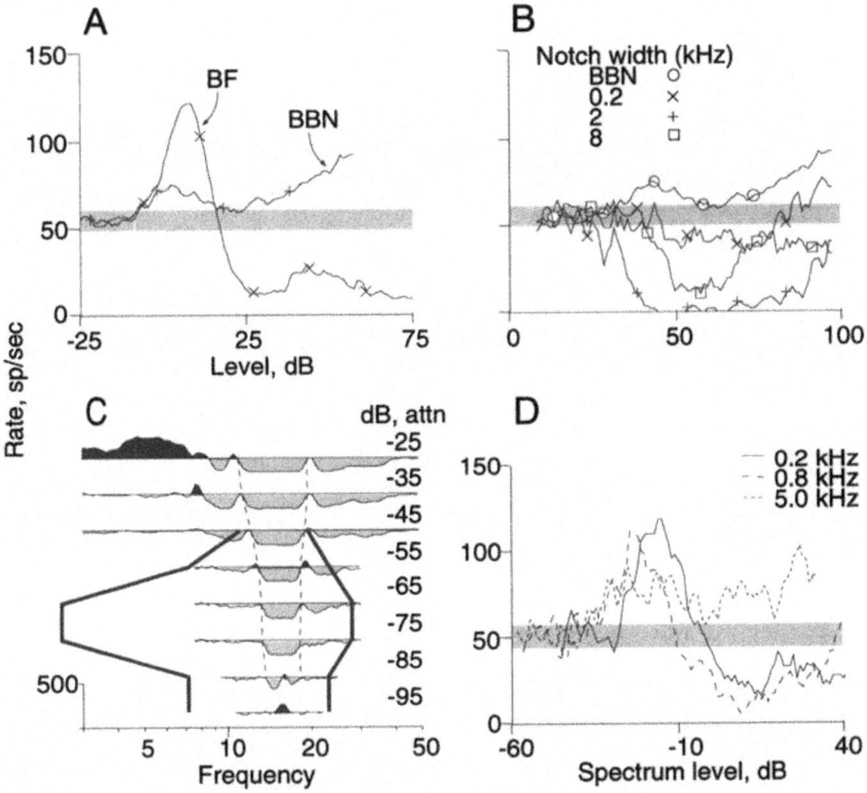

Figure 1. General characteristics of type IV responses. A: Rate-level functions of a type IV unit to BF tones and BBN. Shaded bar is spontaneous rate. B: Rate-level functions of the same type IV unit to BBN and notch stimuli. C: A response map (rate vs. frequency at 8 levels; horizontal lines in each plot are spontaneous rate) of a type IV unit. The dashed lines outline the central inhibitory area (CIA); the bold lines show the width of the widest inhibitory notch at each level. D: Response of a type IV unit to noise bands of increasing bandwidth, arithmetically centered at BF.

assuming that type IV units receive excitatory auditory nerve input and inhibitory input from a DCN inhibitory interneuron. The interneuron in this model is the type II unit which is most likely recorded from vertical or tuberculoventral cells (Young 1980), a class of glycinergic DCN interneuron (Lorente de Nó 1981, Osen et al. 1990, Saint Marie et al. 1991, Wickesberg and Oertel 1988). Type II units do not show spontaneous activity and are activated strongly by tones (Fig. 2A) (Young and Brownell 1976). The hypothesis of an inhibitory type II-type IV synapse is supported by cross-correlation analysis of DCN type II and type IV units (Voigt and Young 1980, Voigt and Young 1990). However, other parts of the tone response maps, mostly above-BF inhibitory regions, cannot be explained by this mechanism.

Responses to BBN stimuli have been important in studying DCN unit properties. Despite the predominance of inhibition in their tone response maps, type IV units usually give excitatory responses to BBN (Fig. 1A). Consistent with the model in which type II units inhibit type IV units, type II units give little or no response to BBN (Fig. 2A).

To study the transition between narrow-band (inhibitory) and wide-band (excitatory) stimuli, we used a band-widening paradigm in which we measured the rate-level functions of type IV units in response to a sequence of noise bands of increasing bandwidth. The responses of a type IV unit to such stimuli is shown in Fig. 1D. This unit, like all other type IV units in our sample, is disinhibited at higher levels when the noise bandwidth is increased. We used the firing rate at 50 dB re threshold as a measure of the disinhibition of type IV units with increase in bandwidth. The disinhibition bandwidth, at which the firing rate of the unit starts to increase rapidly, is only weakly correlated with BF (Nelken and Young 1994). In contrast with the uniform disinhibition at high levels, at low levels the behaviour of the responses is much more variable. Some units, like the one shown here, show a reduction in firing rate with increase in bandwidth at low levels; other units show an increase in firing rate with increase in bandwidth, or a non-monotonic relationships between the two variables. Fig. 2D shows the responses of a type II unit to a band-widening experiment. The responses of this unit, and all other type II units which were tested, are a monotonic decreasing function of the stimulus bandwidth at all levels.

3 Responses of DCN type II and type IV units to notch noise

Spirou and Young (1991) discovered another intriguing property of type IV units: many of them are inhibited by band-reject (notch noise) stimuli, in which a narrow band of frequencies around the unit's BF is filtered out from a BBN. This result is surprising since the tone response map suggests that a narrow band of energy overlying the type IV unit BF is inhibitory by itself; therefore, subtracting such a band from a wide-band stimulus should not make the wide-band stimulus more inhibitory, which is the experimental result.

Fig. 1B is an example of the responses of a type IV unit to notch noise. It can be seen that the unit is already weakly inhibited at the narrowest notch width tested (0.2 kHz); at larger notch widths, the unit is more strongly inhibited. We defined the minimum inhibitory notch width as the narrowest notch width which is inhibitory at threshold. For the unit in Fig. 1, this width would be 0.2 kHz. We found that the minimum inhibitory notch width is only weakly correlated with BF. It is however significantly correlated with the strength of responses to BBN: units which are only weakly excited by BBN, like the unit in Figs. 1A and 1B, tend to be inhibited by narrow notches; units which are more strongly excited by BBN tend to be inhibited only by wider notches (Nelken and Young 1994).

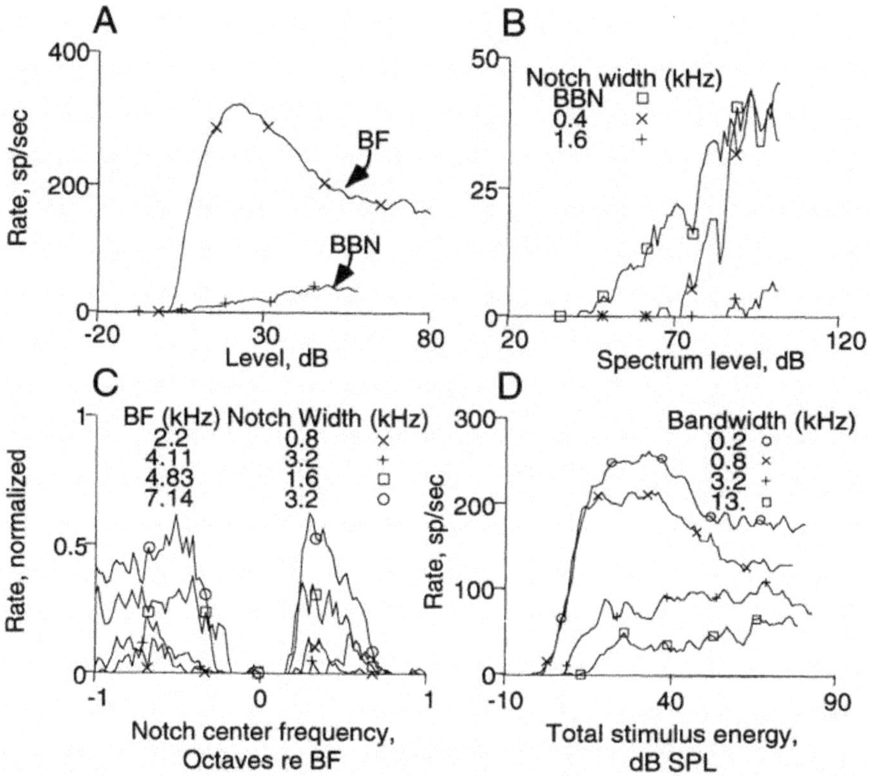

Figure 2. General characteristics of type II responses. A: Rate-level functions of a type II unit to BF tones and BBN. B: Rate-level functions of the same type II unit to BBN and notch stimuli. Note change in ordinate scale. C: Responses of four type II units to notch stimuli with varying center frequency (abscissa). The rate is normalized by the maximal firing rate of each unit to BF tones. D: Response of a type II unit to noise bands of increasing bandwidth, arithmetically centered at BF.

Responses to pure tones are usually inconsistent with the responses of type IV units to wideband stimuli such as BBN and notches. A demonstration of this fact is shown in Fig. 1C. A response map of a type IV unit is shown. On this map, we superimposed the borders of the central inhibitory area (in dashed lines). The central inhibitory area is believed to be the effect of type II units (Spirou and Young 1991). Also superimposed on the response map is the widest inhibitory notch at each level (in thick continuous lines). Note that inhibitory notches may be wider than any single-tone measure of the inhibitory responses of the type IV unit, showing a significant amount of spectral integration outside the response map of the unit. This non-linearity is addressed below in our model of type IV responses.

Fig. 2B shows the responses of a type II unit to notch stimuli, centered at the BF of the unit. Note that the unit is completely shut off when presented with wide enough notches. However, the unit may still be excited by notches when their center frequency is off the BF of the unit; this is shown in Fig. 2C, where the responses of four type II units to notches of varying center frequency are shown. It can be seen that the units are silent as long as the unit's BF lies within the notch.

4 Model of DCN type II and type IV responses

As mentioned before, type II units are thought to be responsible for the inhibition of type IV units by BF tones. Spirou and Young (1991) tried to explain the notch inhibition using the type II - type IV inhibitory circuit. Subsequent results suggest that this explanation is insufficient (Nelken and Young 1994), that is the responses of type II units are inappropriate for explaining the inhibition of type IV units by notch noise. In this section, we present the case for the existence of a second source of inhibition to type IV units, which shapes their responses to wide-band stimuli. Fig. 3 shows a hypothesis for a circuit which can explain the responses of type IV units to both narrow-band and wide-band stimuli. It consists of a tonotopically organized input represented by the horizontal line at the bottom, type II and type IV units, and a wide-band inhibitor (WBI). The WBI inhibits both type II units and type IV units. It is assumed to be weakly excited by tones and strongly excited by noise. The WBI strongly inhibits type II units, producing their weak BBN responses. The WBI's effects on type IV units, on the other hand, is postulated to be weaker, for reasons explained below.

Narrow-band stimuli are assumed to excite the WBI only weakly, and the major interactions are between the excitatory input, the type II and the type IV unit. Type II units are known to have a somewhat higher threshold to tones than type IV units (Young, et al. 1976); this fact is not explicitly accounted for by the model, but could arise through specific input connections to type II units from high-threshold excitatory inputs or from spontaneously active inhibitory inputs. At low levels the type IV units are excited by the tonotopic input and the type II units are silent; once the type II units are activated, their strong inhibitory effect on the type IV units causes the type IV units to decrease their firing rate, and eventually to be shut off. This produces the central inhibitory area of type IV units, as previously described (Spirou and Young 1991).

When the circuit is excited by wide-band stimuli, on the other hand, the WBI is strongly active and suppresses the type II unit. As a result, the excitatory drive on the type IV units is uncovered. The WBI is assumed to affect type IV units only weakly, not enough to reverse the excitatory drive, and therefore type IV units are excited by BBN. However, when the excitatory drive is weakened, as is the case with notch noise, the WBI is strong enough to suppress the spontaneous activity of the type IV units, producing the inhibitory responses to notch noise.

Properties of the type II-type IV circuit have been described in the past (Voigt and Young 1980, 1990; Spirou and Young 1991). The reasons for postulating the existence of a separate WBI are described in detail in Nelken and Young (1994). The argument has two parts:

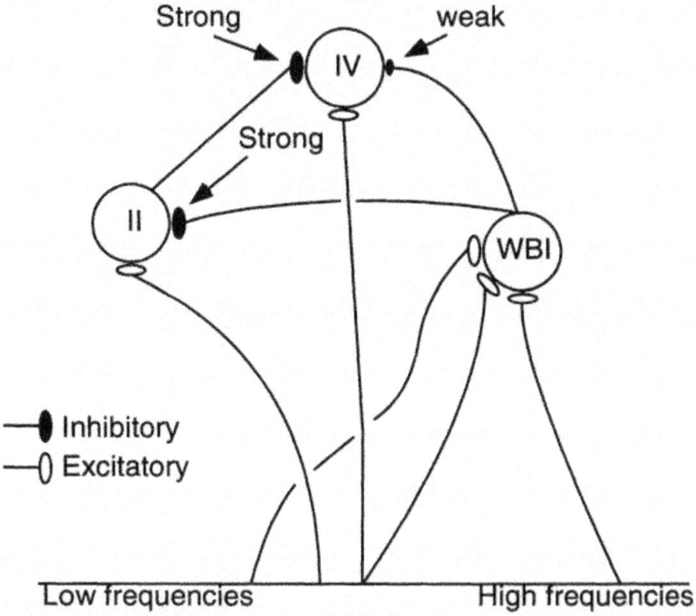

Figure 3. A qualitative model for DCN responses to complex sounds. Details in the text.

- First, we present evidence for a low-threshold wideband inhibitory input to type IV units by analyzing rate-level functions at sound levels just above threshold. Notch noise stimuli of the appropriate notch width produce inhibition at threshold in this regime (Fig. 1B). When BBN is presented, this inhibition appears to summate with excitation produced by energy in the band of noise centered on BF, resulting in BBN rate-level functions with decreased slope and maximum firing rate (Nelken and Young 1994). A range of slopes and maximal firing rates is observed, but these variables are strongly correlated and they are also correlated with the minimum inhibitory notch width; these correlations support the conclusion that a single inhibitory source is responsible for the effects of BBN and notch noise.

- Second, we present evidence that properties of the low-threshold inhibition are inconsistent with properties of type II units. We show that type IV units may be inhibited by notch stimuli with no energy within the central inhibitory area of the type IV unit (Fig. 1C); such stimuli wouldn't excite at all the type II units which inhibit the type IV unit (Fig. 2C). There is also a tendency of the low-threshold inhibitory source to have lower thresholds to BBN than the typical type II unit (Nelken and Young 1994). More evidence is based on the behaviour of type II and type IV units to noise bands of increasing bandwidth. Type II units lower their firing rate monotonically with increase in bandwidth at all levels (Fig. 2D). Therefore, type IV units are expected to increase their firing rate monotonically with bandwidth. Most type IV units in our sample show a more complicated dependence of firing rate on bandwidth, including some units with monotonically decreasing firing rate at low levels (Fig. 1D); this finding is inconsistent with a model in which type II units are the only inhibitory source on type IV units.

There is one class of units which is a possible candidate for being the WBI: these are the onset-C units described by Palmer and Winter (1993). These may be the same as the onset-C units of Rhode and Smith (1986) and stellate-D units of Oertel et al. (1990) although definitive evidence for this is lacking. Palmer and Winter's onset-C units are weakly activated by tones, strongly activated by noise, and show two-tone facilitation. They may well be both the WBI of type IV units, as we suggest here, and the WBI of the type II units, as originally suggested by Palmer and Winter (1993). As long as there is no evidence to the contrary, this is the most parsimonious model. However, it may be that different populations act as WBI on type II units and on type IV units. Further work is needed to clarify this issue.

An interesting feature of this model is that it cannot be identified by pure tones or other narrow-band stimuli, since these stimuli wouldn't excite the WBI; nor can it be identified by second-order white-noise methods alone (e.g. second-order Wiener-Volterra kernels or the STRF, see the review by Eggermont (1993)), since white noise excites type II units only weakly. Theoretically, computing Wiener-Volterra kernels of high enough order would be enough to completely characterize type IV units; however, this order seems to be much too high for any practical purposes. The ad-hoc approach presented here, using a large class of narrow-band and wide-band stimuli to characterize a unit, is clearly better at dissecting the mechanisms underlying type IV responses. At present, however, it doesn't have any theoretical foundation, and therefore has to be implemented on a case-by-case basis.

5 Function of DCN type II and type IV units

The function of the DCN in hearing is unclear at present. It has been proposed in the past (Young et al. 1992) that the sensitivity of DCN type IV units to notch stimuli may be used for the detection of spectral cues for sound localization. It has been shown (Rice et al. 1992) that the first notch of the head-related transfer function (HRTF - the transfer function from free field to the eardrum, which is direction-dependent) can be used as a cue for both azimuth and elevation of a broadband sound source; this notch can be detected by some type IV units. However, recent behavioural studies show that cats can discriminate between sources at different elevations with small deficits, if at all, when their dorsal acoustic stria (the output pathway of the DCN) is lesioned (Masterton and Sutherland 1994). The only behavioural problem in such cats is a serious deficit in their unconditioned head turning reflex to elevated speakers (Sutherland 1991). Although the interpretation of lesion experiments is complicated, it seems that the DCN is neither necessary nor sufficient for elevation discrimination.

We suggest here a different role for DCN type IV units. This function is a rewording of the fact that type IV units tend to be inhibited both by narrow-band stimuli, or spectral maxima, and by notch noise, or spectral minima. In other words, they are inhibited by sharp features in the spectrum, depending on their frequency location. Therefore we suggest that type IV units are detectors of interesting features in the stimulus spectrum, features which may carry important information about the external world. For example, many natural sounds are defined by their spectral peaks (human speech as well as many animal communication sounds (Suga 1992)). As mentioned above, spectral notches are thought to be important in sound source direction estimation (Blauert 1983, Rice et al. 1992). In this interpretation, the information carried by type IV units is not specifically or exclusively used for direction estimation; rather, it may be that type IV units became sensitive to notches because of the importance of notches in direction estimation, which made them "interesting features" in the spectrum.

In the model presented above, the strength and threshold of the type II inhibition determine what is a narrow spectral peak by determining the bandwidth at which the type IV unit's responses are disinhibited at high stimulus levels. As mentioned above, the disinhibition bandwidth is variable and is uncorrelated with BF. Therefore, the type IV units present an array of sensitivities to spectral peaks. The same is true for their notch sensitivity: it is only weakly correlated with BF, so that at the same BF, different type IV units show different notch sensitivity. Finally, the disinhibition bandwidth and the notch sensitivity (as measured by the minimal inhibitory notch width) are uncorrelated or only weakly correlated. Therefore, type IV units present an array of sensitivities to spectral maxima of varying widths and spectral minima of varying widths. In this way, type IV units can support a multi-resolution analysis of the information-bearing regions (Suga 1992) in the spectral envelope.

In addition to their function in shaping the responses of type IV units to narrow-band stimuli, type II units also participate in additional circuits. It is known that vertical cells project tonotpically to the ventral cochlear nucleus (Wickesberg and Oertel 1988), and they seem to have inhibitory effects in the VCN. This projection was implicated in monaural echo suppression (Wickesberg and Oertel 1990). We propose here another possible role for this circuit: that of a whitening filter. It is easiest to understand this idea by considering the responses of type II units to notch stimuli of varying center frequency (Fig. 2C). Type II units are weakly excited by such stimuli, as long as their BF is outside the notch. When a type II unit's BF is in the notch, that unit would stop firing altogether. Therefore type II input to the VCN would tend to inhibit more strongly frequency regions outside the notch than inside the notch. As a result, the difference in the activity within and outside the notch region would be less pronounced in the VCN than the expected without type II input; in other words, the representation of the spectrum would be whiter than the input spectrum itself.

This mechanism may be important in the identification of sound sources, since the notch which is introduced by the HRTF distorts the actual spectrum on the sound source. DCN type II units may help in identifying these notches and in reducing their effects at the level of the VCN.

To summarize, we propose here that DCN units participate in relatively high-level mechanisms of sound processing. We hypothesize that this is the reason it is hard to find behavioural deficits in DCN-lesioned cats. Since the information which is coded in the activity of DCN type II and type IV units is also available in the VCN, it is possible to extract it also at higher auditory stations, such as the inferior colliculus, the medial geniculate body, or the auditory cortex. In this view, the DCN may be a useful, but not necessary, to the higher stations in that it directs the "attention" of the system to important features. When it is absent, processing in the auditory system may be less efficient but is certainly still possible. We therefore need much more sophisticated behavioural tasks in order to show actual deficits in DCN-lesioned animals.

One serious drawback of the description given above is in that it does not take into account the multisensory integration which takes place at the external layer of the cat DCN. For example, we documented somatosensory effects on DCN units (Young et al. 1993). Probably the hardest question about the DCN at present is what information is sent to the DCN via its external layer, and how is this information integrated with the auditory inputs to the DCN. Better understanding of these issues will be probably essential in forming a satisfactory model of DCN function within the auditory system.

6 Acknowledgements

Supported by grant DC00115 from NIDCD and by the W.M. Keck and Fulbright foundations.

7 References

Adams, J.C. (1983) Multipolar cells in the ventral cochlear nucleus project to the dorsal cochlear nucleus and the inferior colliculus. Neurosci. Lett. 37, 205-208.

Berrebi, A.S., and Mungaini, E. (1991) Distribution and targets of the cartwheel cell axon in the dorsal cochlear nucleus of the guinea pig. Anat. Embryol. 183, 427-454.

Blauert, J. (1983) Spatial Hearing Cambridge, Massachusetts: The MIT Press.

Conlee, J.W., and Kane, E.S. (1982) Descending projections from the inferior colliculus to the dorsal cochlear nucleus in the cat: an autoradiographic study. Neuroscience. 161-178.

Eggermont, J.J. (1993) Wiener and Volterra analyses applied to the auditory system. Hear. Res. 66, 177-201.

Evans, E.F., and Nelson, P.G. (1973) The responses of single neurons in the cochlear nucleus of the cat as a function of their location and the anaesthetic state. Exp. Brain Res. 17, 402-427.

Itoh, K., Kamiya, H., Mitani, A., Yasui, Y., Takada, M., and Mizuno, N. (1987) Direct projection from the dorsal column nuclei and the spinal trigeminal nuclei to the cochlear nuclei in the cat. Brain Res. 400, 145-150.

Kane, E.S. (1977) Descending inputs to the cat to the cat dorsal cochlear nucleus: An electron microscopic study. J. Neurocytol. 6, 583-605.

Kane, E.S., and Finn, R.C. (1977) Descending and intrinsic inputs to dorsal cochlear nucleus of cats: A horseradish peroxidase study. Neuroscience. 2, 897-912.

Lorente de Nó, R. (1981) The Primary Acoustic Nuclei New York: Raven Press.

Masterton, R.B., and Sutherland, D.P. (1994) Discrimination of sound source elevation in cats: I. Role of dosral/intermediate and ventral acoustic striae. Abst. of the Assoc. for Res. in Otolaryngol. 17

Mugnaini, E., and Morgan, J.I. (1987) The neuropeptide cerebellin is a marker for two similar neuronal circuits in rat brain. Proc. Natl. Acad. Sci. USA. 84, 8692-8696.

Nelken, I., and Young, E.D. (1994) Two separate inhibitory mechanisms shape the responses of Dorsal Cochlear Nucleus type IV units to narrow-band and wide-band stimuli. J. Neurophysiol. in press

Oertel, D., Wu, S.H., Garb, M.W., and Dizack, C. (1990) Morphology and physiology of cells in slice preparations of the posteroventral cochlear nucleus of mice. J. Comp. Neurol. 295, 136-154.

Osen, K.K., Ottersen, O.P., and Storm-Mathisen, J. (1990) Colocalization of glycine-like and GABA-like immunoreactivities. A semiquantitative study of individual neurons in the dorsal cochlear nucleus of cat. In O.P. Ottersen, and J. Storm-Mathisen (Ed.), Glycine Neurotransmission . New York: John Wiley & Sons, pp. 417-451.

Palmer, A.R., and Winter, I.M. (1993) Best-frequency (BF) threshold reductions caused by off-BF non-excitatory tones in onset units of the cochlear nucleus. Abst. of the Assoc. for Res. in Otolaryngol. 16

Rhode, W.S., and Smith, P.H. (1986) Encoding timing and intensity in the ventral cochlear nucleus of the cat. J. Neurophysiol. 56, 261-286.

Rice, J.J., May, B.J., Spirou, G.A., and Young, E.D. (1992) Pinna-based spectral cues for sound localization in cat. Hearing Res. 58, 132-152.

Ryugo, D.K. (1992) The Auditory Nerve: Peripheral Innervation, Cell Body Morphology, and Central Projections. In D.B. Webster, A.N. Popper, and R.R. Fay (Ed.), The Mammalian Auditory Pathway: Neuroanatomy . New York: Springer-Verlag, pp. 23-65.

Saint Marie, R.L., Benson, C.G., Ostapoff, E.M., and Morest, D.K. (1991) Glycine immunoreactive projections from the dorsal to the anteroventral cochlear nucleus. Hearing Res. 51, 11-28.

Smith, P.H., and Rhode, W.S. (1989) Structural and functional properties distinguish two types of multipolar cells in the ventral cochlear nucleus. J. Comp. Neurol. 282, 595-616.

Snyder, R.L., and Leake, P.A. (1988) Intrinsic connections within and between cochlear nucleus subdivisions in cat. J. Comp. Neurol. 278, 209-225.

Spirou, G.A., and Young, E.D. (1991) Organization of dorsal cochlear nucleus type IV unit response maps and their relationship to activation by bandlimited noise. J. Neurophysiol. 66, 1750-1768.

Suga, N. (1992) Philosophy and stimulus design for neuroethology of complex-sound processing. Phil. Trans. R. Soc. Lond. B. 336, 423-428.

Sutherland, D.P. (1991) A role of the dorsal cochlear nucleus in the localization of elevated sound sources. Abst. of the Assoc. for Res. in Otolaryngol. 14, 33.

Voigt, H.F., and Young, E.D. (1980) Evidence of inhibitory interactions between neurons in the dorsal cochlear nucleus. J. Neurophysiol. 44, 76-96.

Voigt, H.F., and Young, E.D. (1990) Cross-correlation analysis of inhibitory interactions in dorsal cochlear nucleus. J. Neurophysiol. 64, 1590-1610.

Weinberg, R.J., and Rustioni, A. (1987) A cuneocochlear pathway in the rat. Neuroscience. 20, 209-219.

Wickesberg, R.E., and Oertel, D. (1988) Tonotopic projection from the dorsal to the anteroventral cochlear nucleus of mice. J. Comp. Neurol. 268, 389-399.

Wickesberg, R.E., and Oertel, D. (1990) Delayed, frequency-specific inhibition in the cochlear nuclei of mice: a mechanism for monaural echo suppression. J. Neurosci. 10, 1762-1768.

Wright, D.D., and Ryugo, D.K. (1994) Projections from dorsal column nuclei neurons form mossy fiber-like terminals in the dorsal cochlear nucleus of the rat. Abst. of the Assoc. for Res. in Otolaryngol. 17.

Young, E.D., and Brownell, W.E. (1976) Responses to tones and noise of single cells in dorsal cochlear nucleus of unanesthetized cats. J. Neurophysiol. 39, 282-300.

Young, E.D., Nelken, I., and Conley, R.A. (1993) Somatosensory inputs to dorsal cochlear nucleus (DCN). Soc. Neurosci. Abstr. 19, 532.

Young, E.D., Spirou, G.A., Rice, J.J., and Voigt, H.F. (1992) Neural organization and responses to complex stimuli in the dorsal cochlear nucleus. Phil. Trans. R. Soc. Lond. B. 336, 407-413.

Comment by E.F. Evans

1) I like your conclusion if only for the fact that the feature sensitivity to spectral profiles (e.g., tone in notch noise) would be expected to be maintained over a very wide dynamic range by the inhibititory mechanisms as explored in my paper.

2) Where do the wide-band inhibitors originate? Could they represent the intranuclear pathway from the ventral cochlear nucleus to the dorsal cochlear nucleus, capable of mediating fast inhibition as shown by us (Evans and Nelson, 1973) and later by Shofner and Young (1987)?

Evans, E.F., and Nelson, P.G. (1973) The responses of single neurons in the cochlear nucleus of the cat as a function of their location and the anaesthetic state. Exp. Brain Res. 17, 402-427.

Shofner, W.P. and Young, E.D. (1987) Inhibitory connections between AVCN and DCN: Evidence from lidocaine injection in AVCN. Hearing Res. 29, 45-53

Reply

At present we don't have any data about the source of the wide-band inhibitor. We have some data about its properties (e.g. bandwidth and thresholds) which can be used to rule out same sources (e.g. type II units of the DCN). Our current working hypothesis is that the WBI is indeed the VCN onset units that A. Palmer and his co-workers study but we must test those units with the kind of stimuli we used in the DCN.

Anatomical basis for fast feedback from the lateral nucleus of the trapezoid body to the cochlear nuclei

George A. Spirou and Albert S. Berrebi

West Virginia University School of Medicine
Department of Otolaryngology, PO Box 9200 Health Sciences Center
Morgantown, WV 26506 USA

1 Introduction

Current concepts of sensory coding by the auditory brainstem emphasize the roles of the principal cell groups of the superior olivary complex yet generally exclude consideraton of periolivary nuclei (PON), except for the neurons of the olivo-cochlear system, despite the fact that individual PON can rival or exceed the principal cell groups in size and number of constituent neurons. Lack of consideration of the PON stems from the scant amount of information about their internal organization, physiology, and connections with other auditory cell groups. Reflecting this lack of information, various schemes have been used for parcelling periolivary neurons into groups with the result that nomenclature is not consistent, especially when authors describe on the order of ten separate nuclei (Boudreau and Tsuchitani, 1967; Morest, 1968; Warr, 1969; Guinan et al., 1972; Schofield and Cant, 1991). The ventrolateral periolivary region, located ventral, anterior and posterior to the lateral superior olive (LSO) and lateral to the medial superior olive (MSO), is the focus of this report. This region has been subdivided into as many as five separate nuclei. However, one nucleus that is consistently identified is the lateral nucleus of the trapezoid body (LNTB), although its exact borders are a source of debate (Cajal, 1911; Stotler, 1953; Taber, 1961; see discussion in Schofield and Cant, 1991).

The ventrolateral periolivary region receives ascending input through collaterals of bushy cells (Stotler, 1953; Tolbert et al., 1982; Rouiller and Ryugo, 1984; Friauf and Ostwald, 1988; Spirou et al., 1990; Smith et al., 1991), and perhaps contributes more descending input to the cochlear nuclei (CoN) than any other PON (Adams and Warr, 1976; Elverland, 1977; Winter et al., 1989). In general, the lateral PON receive a lesser descending projection from the inferior colliculus than the medial PON (Spangler and Warr, 1991). Therefore, those ventrolateral periolivary neurons projecting to the CoN participate in a direct feedback loop perhaps under little descending influence. Lateral portions of the superior olive, when activated electrically, can exert significant excitatory effects on individual cochlear nucleus units (Comis and Whitfield, 1968; Pickles, 1976). These effects may be mediated in part by the ventrolateral periolivary neurons, but more detailed description of their structure and physiology is required to assess this possibility. We present here analysis of the internal organization of the ventrolateral periolivary region of the cat and visualization of its 3-dimensional structure in relationship to other auditory nuclei. Light microscopic immunocytochemistry is used to identify PEP-19-positive cell bodies, fibers and puncta within the ventrolateral periolivary region and suggests that the CoN give rise to projections to this region which terminate in large, secure axosomatic synaptic junctions. PEP-19 immunolabeling patterns, Nïssl staining patterns and 3-dimensional reconstructions support a simplified categorization scheme for ventrolateral periolivary nuclei in which nearly all of this region is called the LNTB. Finally, tract tracing studies are employed to describe connections between the LNTB and the CoN. These anatomical data form a basis for proposing a fast feedback pathway from LNTB to the ipsilateral CoN.

2 Methods

Five adult cats (2-4 kg) were used for these experiments. Two animals were prepared for Nïssl staining, PEP-19 immunocytochemistry and 3-dimensional reconstructions; one animal for immuno-electron microscopy; and two animals for tract tracing. All animals were deeply anesthetized and tissues fixed by vascular perfusion of mixed aldehydes. Immunocytochemical protocols for use of antiserum directed against the putative calcium binding protein PEP-19 (Ziai et al., 1986; Mugnaini et al., 1987) were identical to those described in Berrebi and Mugnaini (1991). Three dimensional reconstructions were performed on tissue sectioned in the coronal plane and processed for Nïssl. Fiducial marks were created in the tissue for proper alignment of sections by placing register pins and blocking the brain while the skull was held in a stereotaxic frame. The CoN, principal superior olivary complex (SOC) nuclei, lateral PON, tissue edges and register pins were drawn using a camera lucida. The drawings were captured using a video camera, edited to clarify nuclear boundaries using image processing software (BDS Images) and imported into CAD/CAM software for 3-dimensional rendering and viewing.

Tract tracing was performed with biotinylated dextran-amine (BDA, low molecular weight form, Molecular Probes). For these experiments, cats were decerebrated using previously described techniques (Spirou and Young, 1991). BDA was iontophoresed into the LNTB (one animal) or CoN (one animal); after 40 hours the animals were sacrificed and their brainstems sectioned and processed using the Elite-ABC kit (Vector Laboratories).

3 Results

Nïssl. The ventrolateral periolivary region is situated lateral to the MSO and ventral, anterior and posterior to the LSO. Analysis of this region in Nïssl-stained material reveals cells of various shapes, sizes and staining patterns. One easily identifiable cell type has a diffuse staining pattern similar to that of CoN globular bushy cells (gbc-like) (Taber, 1961; Adams, 1983). These cells cluster in the posterior part of the ventrolateral periolivary region, although they are found ventrally throughout the rostro-caudal extent of the region. Quantitative analysis of gbc-like cell body size and shape reveals a homogeneous population of medium sized (mean = 175 μm^2, S.D = 50 μm^2) round or oval cells (Spirou et al., in preparation). The posterior region where these cells cluster has been termed the posteroventral periolivary cell group (pvPO) by other authors (Warr, 1969; Schofield and Cant, 1991).

PEP-19 immunocytochemistry. Further clarification of the anatomical features of the ventrolateral periolivary region and its parcellation into distinct nuclei is made in material processed for PEP-19 immunocytochemistry (Figures 1, 2). This antigen is distributed in fibers and puncta and a subpopulation of cell bodies in the SOC. The LSO and MSO are diffusely immunostained (Figure 1A), providing clear landmarks for identifying the ventrolateral periolivary region. PEP-19-immunoreactive (-IR) axons within the trapezoid body branch and enter the ventrolateral periolivary region in large fascicles. Once the axons enter this region, they further branch into many smaller fascicles that run both within and transverse to the coronal plane of section. Work in progress suggests that the main, if not the only, source of PEP-19 labeled fibers reaching the cat SOC are bushy cells of the CoN (Berrebi and Spirou, unpublished). The absence of PEP-19-IR axons and puncta medial to the MSO clearly defines the border between the ventrolateral periolivary region and the other prominent ventral periolivary cell group, the ventral nucleus of the trapezoid body.

Three zones of the ventrolateral periolivary region can be identified based on their PEP-19 immunolabeling pattern. The first zone, that coinciding with the areas containing gbc-like cells and referred to in the literature as pvPO, is devoid of PEP-19-IR cell bodies; however, this region contains a substantial plexus of immunolabeled axons and numerous punctate profiles. The puncta tend to be rather large, on the order of 6-8 μm^2, and in some cases occur in distinct rings which appear to encircle and define the perimeters of unlabeled cell bodies (Figure 1B). This region is located ventrally and medially and marked with asterisks in Figures 1A and 2.

The second zone constitutes most of the volume of the ventrolateral periolivary region. This zone is distinguished by having the highest density of immunolabeled puncta and fiber bundles. Large punctate profiles are found throughout this region, although on average profiles are smaller than in the first zone and usually do not form rings of synapses (Figure 1C). Occasional PEP-19-IR cell bodies are also distributed in this region, usually located dorsally near the LSO.

The third zone is situated caudal to the LSO, and contains the greatest density of immunolabeled cell bodies, which in general are not contacted by PEP-19-positive puncta (Figure 2). Therefore, the density of terminals in this region is much less than that found in the first two regions. Based on experimentally induced degeneration studies, Warr (1969) called the territory posterior to the LSO the posterior periolivary nucleus (pPO) and reported that its inputs were distinguishable from those of the remainder of the ventrolateral periolivary region. The zone containing abundant PEP-19-labeled cell bodies appears coextensive with the pPO.

Based on the PEP-19 immunolabeling pattern, the first two zones that we describe are distinct from the third zone but similar to each other in that they contain numerous and large immunolabeled puncta and mostly unlabeled cell bodies. Based on the common PEP19-IR innervation of the two zones, we propose a simplified classification scheme in which these zones together comprise the LNTB. Since the first zone, referred to by others as pvPO, is easily distinguished by the presence of gbc-like cells and pericellular rings, we

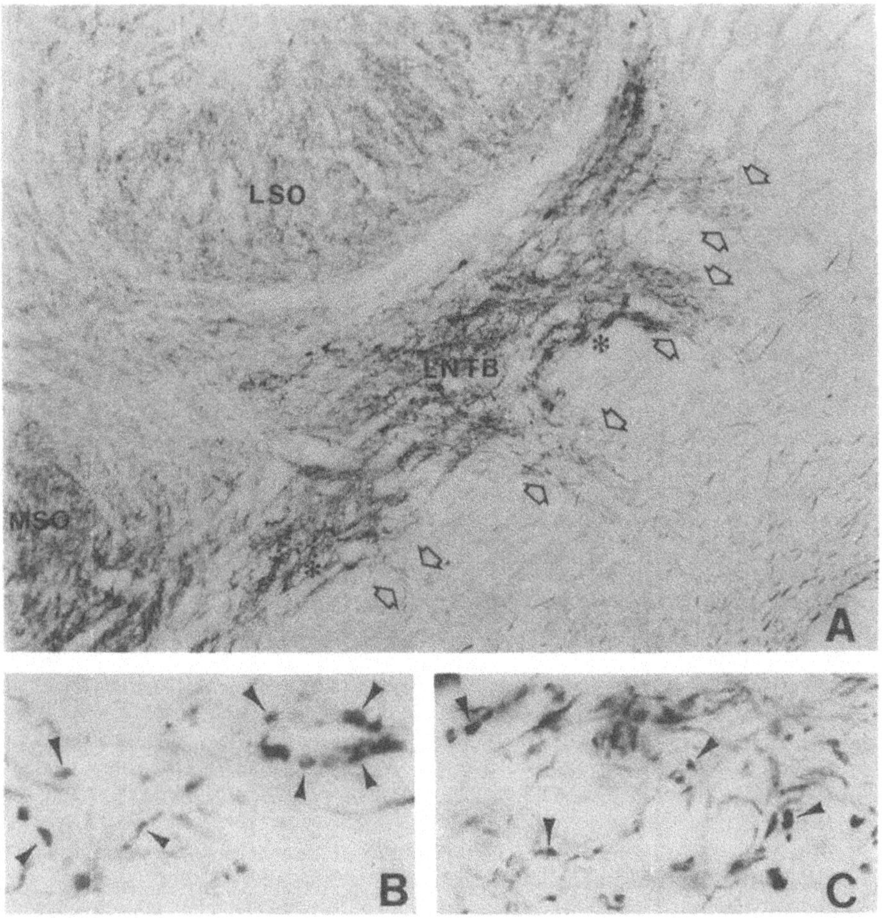

Figure 1. PEP-19 immunolabeling in the ventrolateral SOC. (A) Coronal view of the ventrolateral brainstem at a mid rostro-caudal location, showing the LSO and MSO and features of the innervation and labeling of the ventrolateral PON. Open arrows enclose labeled branches of trapezoid body fibers [X160]. (B) Higher magnification view of immunolabeled puncta apposed to PEP-19-negative periolivary neurons located medially and ventrally (asterisks in A). Puncta, which represent terminal boutons, are large and form pericellular rings (arrowheads) [X800]. (C) Higher magnification view of denser terminal (arrowheads) and axonal labeling found laterally in the LNTB [X800].

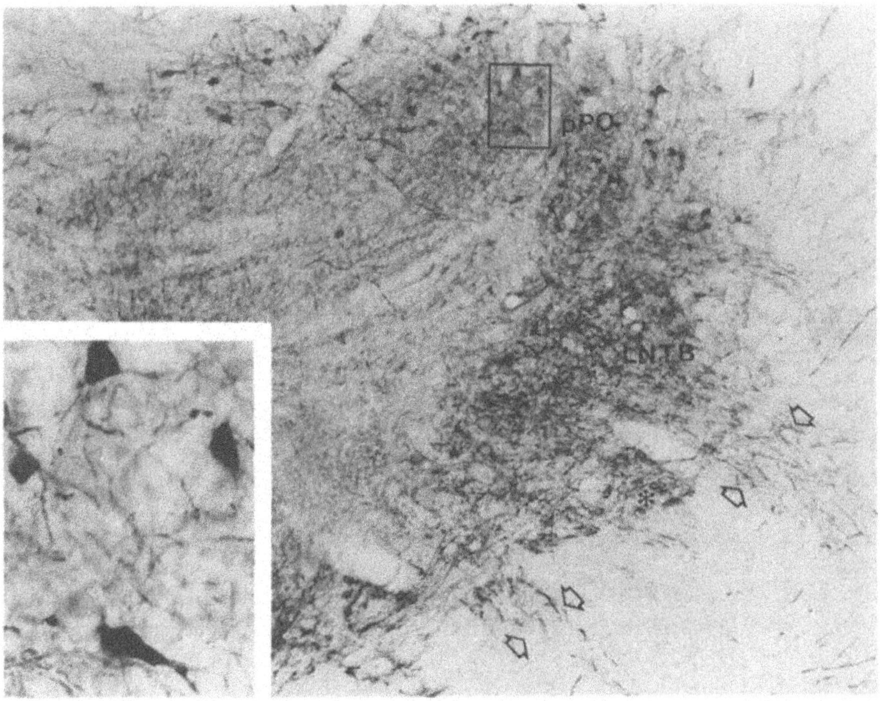

Figure 2. Same orientation as in Figure 1. This section is located caudal to the LSO. The highest density of PEP-19 positive cell bodies is found in the region labeled pPO (see text). Fiber fascicles are marked with open arrows [X160]. Asterisk has same meaning as in figure 1. ***Inset:*** *Higher power view of labeled cell bodies (boxed in the main figure) are free of labeled axosomatic puncta [X700].*

propose that it be referred to as the posteroventral portion of the LNTB, or pvLNTB. The PEP-19 labeling patterns in the third zone support Warr's (1969) designation of the pPO as a periolivary nucleus distinct from the LNTB.

To confirm that PEP-19-IR puncta represent presynaptic boutons within the LNTB, and to determine the post synaptic targets of these boutons, we performed pre-embedding electron microscopic immunocytochemistry (not shown). Numerous immunolabeled axons and synaptic terminals were observed throughout the LNTB. The largest PEP-19-IR synaptic terminals measured up to $8 \mu m^2$ and were exclusively found in apposition to immunonegative cell bodies and dendrites. The boutons contained round synaptic vesicles and formed asymmetric synaptic junctions. Thus, according to well established

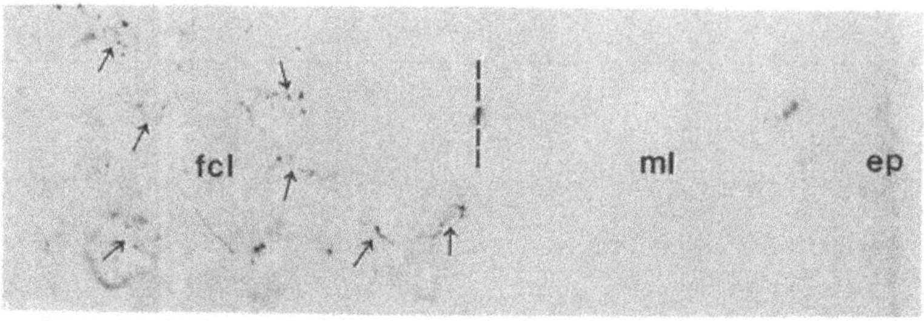

Figure 3. Labeled fibers and boutons (arrows) anterogradely labeled from the LNTB. In the DCoN labeled terminals are found in the deep layers but absent from the molecular layer. ep, ependyma; ml, molecular layer; fcl, fusiform cell layer. Dashed line indicates border between ml and fcl [X320].

ultrastructural criteria (Peters et al., 1991), the PEP-19-IR terminals within LNTB represent excitatory synaptic boutons.

Tract Tracing. The feedback connections between the LNTB and the CoN are currrently being investigated using iontophoretic injections of the tract tracing molecule BDA. In the case presented here, the injection site extended throughout the medio-lateral extent of the LNTB and was centered at a mid LSO location. The majority of retrogradely labeled cells in the ipsilateral CoN were bushy cells, but multipolar cells of the PVCoN and auditory nerve root region were also observed. Labeled cell bodies were not found in the DCoN. Labeled axons were found in the dorsal, intermediate and ventral acoustic striae. Labeled fibers and puncta were found in all subdivisions and throughout the rostral-caudal extent of the ipsilateral DCoN and VCoN and were evident throughout the entire dorso-ventral extent of the DCoN. Fibers gave rise to a fine axonal plexus with a moderate amount of branching and small boutons. One notable feature of labeling in the DCoN was the absence of terminals in the molecular layer (Figure 3). This case illustrates that a relatively restricted portion of the rostro-caudal dimension of the LNTB can innervate a large rostro-caudal extent in the CoN. Confirmation that fibers terminating in the DCoN originate in the LNTB was made by applying a small iontophoretic injection of BDA into the DCoN and identifying retrogradely labeled neurons in the LNTB. Precise descriptions of the topography of LNTB-CoN connections will have to await further analysis and additional cases using systematically placed, restricted injection sites.

3-Dimensional Reconstructions. The SOC is composed of many cell groups whose geometry is difficult to appreciate in any single plane of section. To better understand the relationships among brainstem auditory nuclei, we have developed techniques for 3-dimensional visualization of their nuclear boundaries.

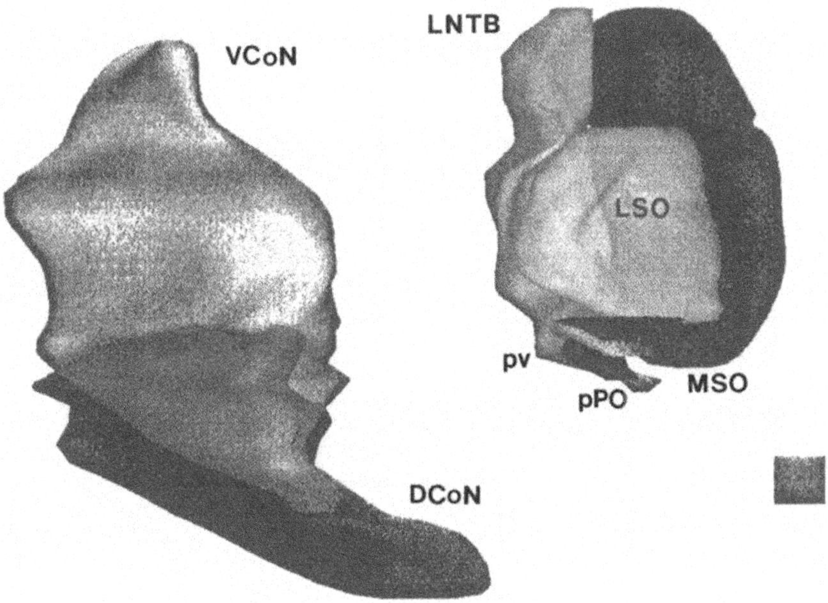

Figure 4. Three-dimensional reconstruction of selected SOC nuclei and the CoN. Dorsal view, rostral is to the top, lateral to the left. Nuclei shown are the LNTB, pvLNTB, pPO, LSO, MSO and the DCoN and VCoN. The calibration square is 0.5mm on each side.

Figure 4 is a dorsal view of such a 3-dimensional reconstruction. Our current scheme for parceling the ventrolateral periolivary region is shown in this figure. We identify two nuclei in this region, the LNTB and pPO. The LNTB and MSO span the entire rostro-caudal extent of the SOC. The pvLNTB defines the caudal limit of the LNTB and extends rostrally through the ventromedial portion of the LNTB. The pPO is located caudal to the LSO.

The relationship of the LNTB and pPO to other SOC nuclei and the CoN is also shown in the figure. The LSO is partially surrounded by the LNTB and pPO. One can appreciate the rostro-caudal position of the LSO, situated slightly caudal within the SOC yet not extending to the caudal border of the complex. The MSO spans nearly the entire rostro-caudal extent of the complex, shifting closer to the LNTB at its rostral end. The larger volume of tissue occupied by the CoN relative to the SOC principal nuclei is apparent. The CoN extends much further caudally than the LNTB, mostly due to the position of the DCoN. The LNTB is closest to the CoN, with which it is reciprocally connected.

4 Discussion

Viewing the ventrolateral PON in 3-dimensional reconstructions simplifies understanding of the complex geometrical arrangements of this brainstem territory. The resulting 3-D structure can be used to plot characteristics of individual neurons and to investigate topographical relationships between specific subregions and other auditory nuclei. For example, the connectivity of the pvLNTB is an unresolved issue, since these neurons reportedly do not project to either the CoN or inferior colliculus (Adams, 1983; Schofield and Cant, 1991). The 3-D templates can be used to guide the injection of tract tracing molecules into the pvLNTB and plotting of the subsequent labeling patterns. Also, recent descriptions of projections from the LNTB to the MSO, two structures running in parallel through the length of the SOC, make visualization of the relationship of these structures useful for plotting their connectivity following more detailed tract tracing studies.

Previous studies report significant effects of electrical activation of the lateral SOC and pharmacological manipulation of the CoN on behavioral and CoN single unit measures (Comis and Whitfield, 1968; Pickles and Comis, 1973; Pickles, 1976). Electrical stimulation results in excitation of many CoN neurons, due at least in part to cholinergic innervation. These effects are correlated with substantial widening of critical bandwidths and lowering of detection thresholds following atropine application to the CoN (Pickles and Comis, 1973; Pickles, 1976). Immunocytochemical and histochemical studies reveal the presence of glycinergic, GABAergic and cholinergic neurons in the LNTB, although the numbers and precise distribution of these neurons have not been determined (Osen et al., 1984; Thompson et al., 1985; Peyret et al., 1986; Helfert et al., 1989).

Preliminary arguments can be made that the PEP-19 immunolabelled fibers and terminals originate from bushy cells of the VCoN. Previous authors, using the degeneration technique or intracellular labelling of globular bushy cells, have described the presence of large terminals in the LNTB originating in the VCoN (Stotler, 1953; Harrison and Warr, 1962; Smith et al., 1991). In our own material, the large and medium sized fibers of the trapezoid body, which arise from bushy cells of the VCoN (van Noort, 1969; Brownell, 1975; Warr, 1982; Tolbert et al., 1982; Friauf and Ostwald, 1988; Rouiller and Ryugo, 1985; Spirou et al., 1990; Smith et al., 1991) were well labeled, so it is likely that they contribute a significant percentage of PEP-19 labeled terminals to the LNTB. PEP-19 positive cell bodies were found in highest density in the pPO, scattered within the LNTB and dorsolateral periolivary regions and absent from other SOC nuclei. Thus, it is possible that some proportion of PEP-19 labeling in the LNTB may arise from intrinsic neurons. Iontophorectic injections of BDA into the LNTB retrogradely labeled cells in the CoN, and very few cells in the pPO or other SOC nuclei. The short survival times necessitated by the decerebrate preparation is not sufficient to assess retrograde labeling from the lateral lemniscal nuclei or inferior colliculus, although other studies have indicated a relatively sparse projection to the LNTB from these territories (Spangler and Warr, 1991).

The presence of large synaptic terminals on the cell bodies and dendrites of LNTB neurons suggests that they are strongly influenced by the source or sources of these inputs. In some cases the large terminals appear to encircle the cell body, resulting in a synaptic complex that rivals in size the modified endbulbs found on globular bushy cells of the cochlear nucleus (Cajal, 1911; Lorente de Nó, 1981; Fekete et al., 1984). These considerations indicate that the strongest input to LNTB neurons occurs via bushy cells of the VCoN, and may represent a very fast activation of the LNTB. In fact, the time course of activation of the LNTB may occur prior to auditory nerve activation of DCoN neurons, which can have first spike latencies 2-3 msec longer than bushy cells (Shofner and Young, 1985; Blackburn and Sachs, 1989).

Descending projections from the SOC are substantial and support the notion that the LNTB contributes a major descending input to the CoN (Adams and Warr, 1976; Elverland, 1977; Winter et al., 1989). We observed anterogradely labeled terminals in all subdivisions of the CoN following a relatively restricted tracer injection at one rostro-caudal level of the LNTB but incorporating the entire medial-lateral extent of the nucleus. A salient feature of the termination patterns in the DCoN is that the molecular layer is clear of inputs, indicating that cartwheel cells and apical dendrites of pyramidal cells are probably not contacted. Since the DCoN was free of retrogradely labeled cell bodies, these terminals cannot originate from local neurons. Qualitatively, terminal densities in the VCoN were similar to the DCoN. Quantitative descriptions of the patterns of termination relative to VCoN subdivisions (as described by Osen, 1969; Brawer et al., 1974; Lorente de Nó, 1981) requires further analysis.

Anterogradely labeled terminals were found in the cochlear nerve root region, anterior PVCoN and AVCoN, which are all locations where bushy cells are found (Osen 1969, Brawer et al. 1974, Lorente de Nó 1981). The possibility exists, therefore, that LNTB neurons feedback onto neurons putatively responsible for their ascending input (see also Figure 7 of Winter et al. 1989). In addition, regions of the CoN that clearly do not contribute ascending inputs to the LNTB, such as the DCoN, receive descending inputs. Thus, the anatomical substrates exist for widespread effects on CoN physiology following activation of the LNTB. Since the LNTB neurons are located proximal to and take direct routes to the CoN, and receive short latency, potentially strong (secure) input from the CoN, their input may precede all other descending activity entering the CoN and may even precede the arrival of auditory nerve fiber input to the DCoN. These hypotheses are currently being investigated in ongoing physiological experiments.

5 Acknowledgements

We gratefully appreciate the assistance of Sarathy Sribyasham and Stephanie Kessinger in the preparation of this manuscript. Dr. James I. Morgan of the Roche Institute of Molecular Biology kindly provided the PEP-19 antiserum. This work was supported by NIH grant DC01387.

6 References

Adams, J.C. (1983) Cytology of periolivary cells and the organization of their projections in the cat. J. Comp. Neurol. 215, 275-289.

Adams, J. C., and Warr, W. B. (1976) Origins of axons in the cat's acoustic striae determined by injection of horseradish peroxidase into severed tracts. J. Comp. Neurol., 170, 107-122.

Berrebi, A. S., and Mugnaini, E. (1991) Distribution and targets of the cartwheel cell axon in the dorsal cochlear nucleus of the guinea pig. Anat. Embryol., 183, 427-454.

Blackburn, C. C., and Sachs, M. B. (1989) Classification of unit types in the anteroventral cochlear nucleus: PST histograms and regularity analysis. J. Neurophysiol., 62, 1303-1329.

Boudreau, J.C. and Tsuchitani, C. (1970) Cat superior olive S-segment cell discharge to tonal stimulation. Contr. Sens. Physiol. 4, 143-213.

Brawer, J.R., Morest, D.K. and Kane, E.C. (1974) The neuronal architecture of the cochlear nucleus of the cat. J. Comp. Neurol. 155, 251-300.

Brownell, W. E. (1975) Organization of the cat trapezoid body and the discharge characteristics of its fibers. Brain Res., 94, 413-433.

Cajal, S. Ramon y. (1911) Histologie du Système Nerveux de l'Homme et des Vertébrés. Maloine, Paris.

Comis, S. D., and Whitfield, I. C. (1968) Influence of centrifugal pathways on unit activity in the cochlear nucleus. J. Neurophysiol., 31, 62-68.

Elverland, H. H. (1977) Descending connections between the superiro olivary and cochlear nulcear complexes in the cat studied by autoradiographic and horseradish peroxidase methods. Exp. Br. Res., 27, 397-412.

Fekete, D. M., Rouiller, E. M., Liberman, M. C., and Ryugo, D. K. (1984) The central projections of intracellularly labeled auditory nerve fibers in cats. J. Comp. Neurol., 229, 432-450.

Friauf, E., and Ostwald, J. (1988) Divergent projections of physiologically characterized rat ventral cochlear nucleus neurons as shown by intra-axonal injection of horseradish peroxidase. Exp. Brain Res., 73, 263-284.

Guinan, J.J., Norris, B.E. and Guinan, S.S. (1972) Single auditory units in the superior olivary complex II: Locations of unit categories and tonotopic organization. Intern. J. Neuroscience 4, 147-166.

Harrison, J. M., and Warr, W. B. (1962). A study of the cochlear nuclei and ascending auditory pathways of the medulla. J. Comp. Neurol., 126, 51-63.

Helfert, R.H., Bonneau, J.M., Wenthold, R.J. and Altschuler, R.A. (1989) GABA and glycine immunoreactivity in the guinea pig superior olivary complex. Brain Research 501, 269-286.

Lorente de Nó, R. (1981) The Primary Acoustic Nuclei. New York: Raven Press.

Morest, D.K. (1968) The collateral system of the medial nucleus of the trapezoid body of the cat, its neuronal architecture and relation to the olivo-cochlear bundle. Brain Research 9, 288-311.

Mugnaini, E., Berrebi, A. S., Dahl, A.-L., and Morgan, J. I. (1987) The polypeptide PEP-19 is a marker for Purkinje neurons in cerebellar cortex and cartwheel neurons in dorsal cochlear nucleus. Archives Italiennes de Biologie. 126, 41-67.

Noort, J. v. (1969) The structure and connections of the inferior colliculus. The Netherlands: Van Gorcum and Comp.

Osen, K.K. (1969) Cytoarchitecture of the cochlear nuclei in the cat. J. Comp. Neurol. 136, 453-484.

Osen, K.K., Mugnaini, E., Dahl, A.-L. and Christiansen, A.H. (1984) Histochemical localization of acetylcholinesterase in the cochlear and superior olivary nuclei. A reappraisal with emphasis on the cochlear granule cell system. Archives Italiennes de Biologie 122, 169-212.

Peters. A., Palay, S.L. and Webster, H.deF. (1991) The Fine Structure of the Nervous System. Oxford University Press.

Peyret, D., Geffard, M., and Aran, J.-M. (1986) GABA immunoreactivity in the primary nuclei of the auditory central nervous system. Hearing Res. 23, 115-121.

Pickles, J. O. (1976) Role of centrifugal pathways to cochlear nucleus in determination of critical bandwidth. J. Neurophysiol. 39, 394-400.

Pickles, J. O., and Comis, S. D. (1973) Role of centrifugal pathways to cochlear nucleus in detection of signals in noise. J. Neurophysiol., 36 1131-1137.

Rouiller, E. M., and Ryugo, D. K. (1984) Intracellular marking of physiologically characterized cells in the ventral cochlear nucleus of the cat. J. Comp. Neurol., 225 167-186.

Schofield, B. R., and Cant, N. B. (1991) Organization of the superior olivary complex in the guinea pig. I. Cytoarchitecture, cytochrome oxidase histochemistry, and dendritic morphology. J. Comp. Neurol. 314, 645-670.

Shofner, W. S., and Young, E. D. (1985) Excitatory/Inhibitory response types in the cochlear nulceus: relationships to discharge patterns and responses to electrical stimulation of the auditory nerve. J. Neurophysiol. 54, 917-939.

Smith, P.H., Joris, P.X., Carney, L.H. and Yin, T.C.T. (1991) Projections of physiologically characterized globular bushy cell axons from the cochlear nucleus of the cat. Journal of Comparative Neurology 304, 387-407.

Spangler, K.M. and Warr, W.B. (1991) The descending auditory system, in Neurobiology of Hearing: The Central Auditory System. Altschuler, R.A., Bobbin, R.P., Clopton, B.M. and Hoffman, D.W., eds. Raven Press, New York.

Spirou, G. A., Brownell, W. E., and Zidanic, M. (1990) Single fiber recordings from the cat trapezoid body and HRP labeling of globular cell axons. J. Neurophysiol., 63 1169-1190.

Spirou, G. A., and Young, E. D. (1991) Organization of dorsal cochlear nucleus type IV unit response maps and their relationship to activation by bandlimited noise. J. Neurophysiol., 66 1750-1768.

Stotler, W. A. (1953) An experimental study of the cells and connections of the superior olivary complex of the cat. J. Comp. Neurol. 98, 401-432.

Taber, E. (1961) The cytoarchitecture of the brain stem of the cat. I. Brain stem nuclei of cat. J. Comp. Neurol., 116 27-70.

Thompson, G. C., Cortez, A. M., and Lam, D. M.-K. (1985) Localization of GABA immunoreactivity in the auditory brainstem of guinea pigs. Br. Res. 339, 119-122.

Tolbert, L. P., and Morest, D. K. (1982) The neuronal architecture of the anteroventral cochlear nucleus of the cat in the region of the cochlear nerve root: Electron microscopy. Neurosci. 7, 3053-3068.

Warr, W. B. (1982) Parallel ascending pathways from the cochela nucleus: neuroanatomical evidence of functional specialization. Contr. Sens. Physiol. 7, 1-38.

Winter, I. M., Robertson, D., and Cole, K. S. (1989) Descending Projections from Auditory Brainstem Nuclei to the Cochlea and Cochlear Nucleus of the Guinea Pig. J. Comp. Neurol. 280(1), 143-157.

Ziai, R., Pan, Y.-C., Hulmes, J. D., Sangameswaran, L., and Morgan, J. I. (1986) Isolation, sequence, and developmental profile of a brain-specific polypeptide, PEP-19. Proc. Nat. Acad. Sci. 8420-8423.

Comment by E.F. Evans

Can you say more about the "fast feedback" connections to the cochlear nucleus from the LNTB? In particular can you say whether the feedback is excitatory or inhibitory, e.g. from the shape of the synaptic vesicles?

Reply

At present our efforts have been dedicated to understanding the topography of the connections between these two cell groups. Of course, understanding the nature of the projection in terms of its excitatory or inhibitory nature and the identity of the neurotransmitters involved are crucial to providing an appropriately detailed description of this projection. Our next efforts will be dedicated to viewing in the electron microscope labeled terminals found in the different regions of the cochlear nuclei and the particular cell types innervated. We expect to find multiple transmitter types and morphologies indicative of both excitatory and inhibitory synaptic transmission. These results would correspond to results of histochemical and immunocytochemical studies of the superior olivary complex.

Comment by A. Rees

Did you find any evidence for connections between the LNTB and more central nuclei in the pathway?

Reply

We see evidence for a projection from LNTB to MSO in agreement with the report of Cant and Hyson (1992), however, these projections are difficult to distinguish from the projection of bushy cells into the same nucleus when using the tracer BDA. Some neurones of the pPO are retrogradely labeled from the LNTB, and we see some evidence in the electron microscope of immunolabeled terminals in the LNTB having flattened vesicles which may originate from pPO neurones. The presence of connections rostral to the ventral nucleus of the lateral lemniscus is difficult to assess due to the short length of survival of the animal post BDA injection (40-48 hours). However, we do find a few labeled axons dorsal in the lateral lemniscus indicating that connections with more rostral nuclei do exist.

Cant, N.B. and Hyson, R.L. (1992) Projections from the lateral nucleus of the trapezoid body to the medial superior olivary nucleus in the gerbil. Hear. research 58, 26-34.

Comment by T. Yin

Since the designation of globular bushy cells in the cochlear nuleus is based on both Nïssl and Golgi stains, I am surprised by your use of the term "globular-bushy cell-like" from Nïssl staining only. Do you have other evidence for suggesting that these cells are gbc-like?

Reply

Besides the similarity in Nïssl staining patterns we have quantified the morphology of these cells and find them to be round or oval in shape. In addition, we have described a pattern of afferent innervation of "gbc-like" cells via large synaptic terminals that may resemble modified end bulbs, which is another similarity to globular bushy cells. In the absence of descriptions of dendritic patterns perhaps we should more accurately refer to these cells as globular cell-like, or "gc-like". However, reference to the cochlear nucleus cells as globular bushy cells is now common in the literature, and we have simply adopted this accepted terminology. Included in our hypothesis that gbc-like cells are a kind of bushy cell is the suggestion that these cells would show similar physiological characteristics such as non-linear i-v curves, irregular spike intervals and primary-like or primary-like with notch PSTHs.

We would find physiological similarities more compelling in drawing the parallel between the two cell types than the particulars of dendritic tree morphology.

Relative importance of different acoustic cues to the directional sensitivity of inferior-colliculus neurons

B. Delgutte[1,2], P.X. Joris[3], R.Y. Litovsky[3], and T.C.T. Yin[3]

[1]*Eaton-Peabody Laboratory, Massachusetts Eye and Ear Infirmary, Boston, MA 02114, USA;* [2]*Research Laboratory of Electronics, Massachusetts Institute of Technology, Cambridge, MA 02139, USA;* [3]*Department of Neurophysiology, University of Wisconsin, Madison, WI 53706, USA.*

1 Introduction

Sound localization is based on multiple acoustic cues such as interaural differences in time and level, spectral cues, and changes in these cues resulting from head movements (Blauert, 1983; Searle et al., 1976). Physiological studies done in the free field have shown that many cells in the inferior colliculus (IC) are sensitive to the direction of sound sources (Aitkin et al., 1985; Calford et al., 1986; Aitkin and Martin, 1987, 1990). These directionally-sensitive cells are likely to play an important role in sound localization. However, free-field studies cannot determine which of the many possible acoustic cues are responsible for this directional sensitivity because they do not allow independent control over each cue.

Control over individual acoustic cues is achieved in dichotic studies that deliver stimuli through closed acoustic systems. Many studies have demonstrated that cells in the IC and the superior olive are sensitive to interaural time (ITD) and level (ILD) differences (Rose et al., 1966; Goldberg and Brown, 1969; reviewed by Irvine, 1986). However, with few exceptions (e.g. Caird and Klinke, 1987), most of these studies varied a single cue without consideration of possible interactions between cues. Furthermore, most studies have focused on pure tone stimuli, which do not include the spectral cues provided by directionally-dependent filtering of acoustic stimuli by the head and the pinnae.

Recent advances in digital technology have made it possible to simulate the sound pressure waveforms produced in the ear canals by free-field sound sources through closed acoustic systems (Blauert, 1983; Wightman and Kistler, 1989; Poon and Brugge, 1993). Such "virtual-space" (VS) techniques provide stimuli with multiple, realistic localization cues, and also give precise control over individual localization cues. They are beginning to provide information about which cues are most important for sound localization by human listeners (Wightman and Kistler, 1992). In this paper, we used VS techniques for identifying which acoustic cues are most important for the directional sensitivity of single units in the central nucleus of the IC of anesthetized cats. We used head-related transfer functions (HRTF's) measured in the cat by Musicant et al. (1990) to synthesize VS stimuli possessing realistic ITD's, ILD's, and spectral shape. Although this approach ignores other important cues such as echoes and head and pinna movements, it provides a first important cues such as echoes and head and pinna movements, it provides a first approximation applicable to an animal at rest in an anechoic environment. This brief report focuses on VS stimuli located in the horizontal plane, although our experiments were also concerned with stimuli in the median vertical plane.

2 Method

Methods for recording from single units in the IC of barbiturate-anesthetized cats are essentially the same as described by Yin et al. (1986). The only significant difference with the earlier studies is that we focused on units with high characteristic frequencies (CF > 2-4 kHz), for which spectral cues might be important.

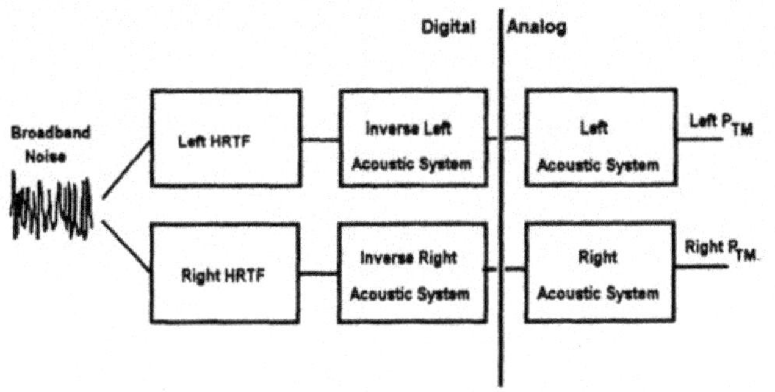

Figure 1. Block diagram of the signal processing used for synthesizing virtual-space stimuli.

The method for synthesizing virtual-space stimuli (Fig. 1) is similar to that used in the human psychophysical experiments of Wightman and Kistler (1989) and the physiological study of Poon and Brugge (1993). The input signal is a sample of pseudo-random broadband noise, 200 msec in duration, with significant energy between 2 and 35 kHz, the range in which the measurements of Musicant et al. (1990) were most reliable. This signal is first processed through digital filters constructed from acoustic measurements made in one "standard" cat by Musicant et al. (1990). These filters (one for each ear) represent the directionally-dependent transformation of sound pressure from the free field to the ear canal. Stimuli in each ear were then processed through another digital filter that compensated for the transfer function of the closed acoustic system measured with a calibrated probe-tube microphone. With compensation, the sound pressures (magnitude and phase) produced in both ear canals by our closed systems are the same as those that would occur for free-field stimuli originating from a particular direction in the standard cat.

The VS stimuli described above include three cues to sound localization (ITD, ILD, and spectral shape), and referred to as "full-cue". We have also generated modified VS stimuli in which one or more of these cues was set to a constant for every azimuth. Table I lists some of these "partial-cue" stimuli. "0-ITD" stimuli were generated by delaying the waveforms of the full-cue stimuli at the two ears so as bring the ITD to zero for every azimuth. ITD was measured by picking the maximum of the crosscorrelation function between the waveforms in the left and right ear. "Δ-ITD" stimuli were generated by taking the full-cue waveforms for zero azimuth, where the ITD is 0, then introducing the appropriate ITD for each azimuth. These stimuli are similar to those used by Yin et al. (1986) for studying ITD sensitivity for broadband noise, except that there is a known mapping between ITD and azimuth. The manipulation of ILD cues was necessarily more complicated because of the difficulty in defining ILD for a broadband stimulus. The sound pressure level (SPL) was measured for each ear and each azimuth in either of two ways: broadband, or narrowband. The broadband SPL is the r.m.s. amplitude of the stimulus waveform. The narrowband SPL was measured using a third-octave Gaussian bandpass filter whose center frequency was at the CF of the neuron. After measuring SPL's, "0-ILD" stimuli were generated by adjusting the gains of the full-cue stimuli so as to make their SPL's at both ears coincide with those of the stimulus at zero azimuth. Thus, SPL's in both ears did not vary with azimuth for these stimuli, and the ILD was always equal to the ILD at zero azimuth, which is approximately zero. Finally, we generated "Δ-ILD" stimuli by taking the full-cue waveforms for zero azimuth, and then introducing gains so as create the appropriate SPL in each ear for each azimuth, and therefore the appropriate ILD.

Table 1: Cue manipulations for the virtual-space stimuli.

	ITD	ILD	Spectral Shape
Full Cue	+	+	+
0-ITD	-	+	+
Δ-ITD	+	-	-
0-ILD	+	-	+
Δ-ILD	-	+	-

3 Results

Our results are based on data from 60 well-characterized single units in 10 cats. Two questions are of particular interest: how binaural interactions shape the directional responses to VS stimuli, and which localization cues are most important for this directional sensitivity.

3.1 Binaural interactions in responses to VS stimuli

A majority of units in our sample showed directional sensitivity for VS stimuli at moderate stimulus levels. Figure 2 shows data for a single unit with a CF of 9 kHz. The top panel shows the average discharge rate in response to the VS stimuli as a function of azimuth. The stimulus level was approximately 20 dB above threshold for 0 azimuth. In this figure as in all others, positive azimuths correspond to VS stimuli located contralaterally to the recording site. When the VS stimuli were presented binaurally (as would naturally occur in the free-field), the response was clearly directional: there was little response for azimuths on the ipsilateral side, a steep rise in response for azimuths near zero, and a broad maximum on the contralateral side. In order to examine the role of binaural interactions, VS stimuli were also presented to the contralateral ear only. This condition corresponds to plugging one ear in free-field experiments. The monaural response was much less directional than the binaural response. Thus, binaural interactions are important for the directional sensitivity of this unit.

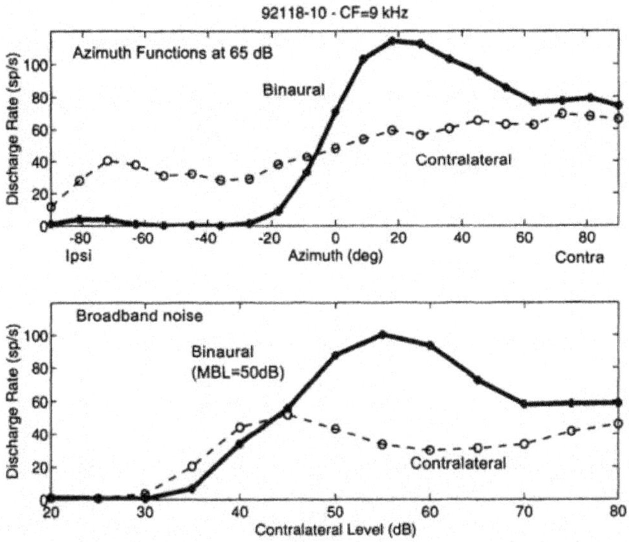

Figure 2. Binaural interactions in the response of a single IC unit for VS stimuli (Top) and broadband noise (Bottom).

An advantage of VS techniques over free-field stimulation is that they provide independent control over the inputs to each ear, making it possible to study binaural interactions. The dashed line in the bottom panel of Fig. 2 shows the response to a 200-msec broadband noise presented to the contralateral ear as a function of stimulus level. The solid line shows responses for a binaural condition used for studying ILD sensitivity (Irvine and Gago, 1990): As the stimulus level was increased in the contralateral ear, the level in the ipsilateral ear was correspondingly decreased so as to keep the mean binaural level (MBL) constant at 50 dB. This condition crudely mimics the changes in level that occur when a free-field stimulus moves from the ipsilateral to the contralateral side. For ILD's favoring the contralateral ear (contra levels > 50 dB), the binaural response is greater than the monaural response obtained with contralateral stimulation, meaning that the ipsilateral ear has a facilitatory influence. On the other hand, for ILD's favoring the ipsilateral side, the binaural response is smaller than the contralateral response, meaning that the ipsilateral ear is inhibitory. Such mixed facilitatory and inhibitory binaural interactions, which are commonly seen in the IC (Semple and Kitzes, 1987; Irvine and Gago, 1990), are also apparent for the VS stimuli in the top panel. The binaural response is greater than the monaural response for contralateral azimuths, but smaller than the monaural response for ipsilateral azimuths. Thus, the binaural interactions found with VS stimuli are consistent with those found for broadband noise using the stimulus paradigms of traditional dichotic studies.

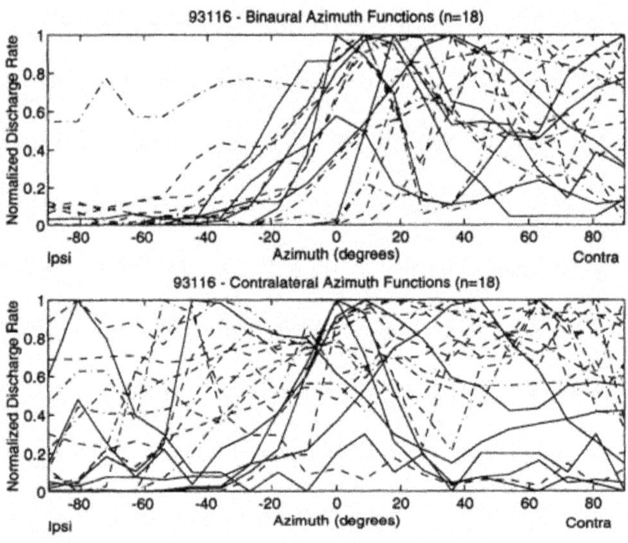

Figure 3. Azimuth functions for 18 units from the same cat measured with VS stimuli presented binaurally (Top) and contralaterally (Bottom).

The importance of binaural interactions for the directional sensitivity of IC neurons is a general finding. The top panel of Fig. 3 shows binaural azimuth functions for 18 units from one cat. Unit CF's ranged between 4 and 30 kHz. With one exception, all units show little response for ipsilateral azimuths, and strong response for a range of contralateral azimuths. Most units also show a steep rise in response which occurs at different azimuths for different units. The bottom panel shows responses of the same units to VS stimuli presented to the contralateral ear alone. Again, this condition corresponds to plugging one ear in the free field. The contralateral azimuth functions do not show the orderly pattern seen for the binaural condition, and many of them are less directional. Thus, binaural interactions are important for the directional sensitivity of this population of units.

3.2 Effect of selective cue manipulations on responses to VS stimuli

All the binaural data shown so far were for "full-cue" VS stimuli, which include all 3 localization cues. A major advantage of VS techniques is their ability to selectively manipulate each cue. Fig. 4 shows results for a contralaterally-excited, ipsilaterally-inhibited unit with a CF of 14 kHz. The top panel shows the effects of manipulating ITD. The azimuth function for the full-cue condition showed a typical directional sensitivity for our sample of units. When ITD was set to zero for every azimuth (dashed line), the response was largely similar to the full-cue response. This suggests that ITD is not the primary determinant of the directional sensitivity of this unit. When ITD only was varied with azimuth (dot-dash line), the response was not very directional, confirming that this unit is not very sensitive to ITD.

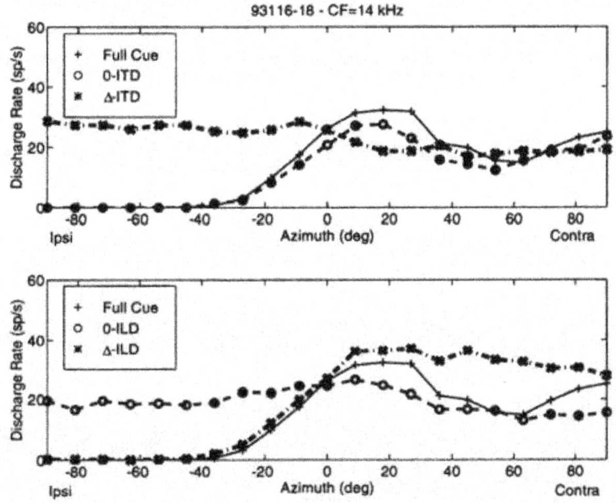

Figure 4. Azimuth functions for a single unit in response to modified VS stimuli. Top: Cue manipulations involving ITD. Bottom: Manipulations involving ILD. The stimulus level was 15 dB above threshold for zero azimuth for all conditions.

The bottom panel of Fig. 4 illustrates the effect of manipulating ILD. In this case, the ILD was measured in a 1/3-octave band centered at the unit CF. The solid line is the same full-cue response as on top. When ILD was fixed to its value at 0 azimuth, the response became almost flat, suggesting that ILD is very important for the directional sensitivity of this unit. The response for the Δ-ILD condition showed the same rapid rise in response seen for the full-cue condition for azimuths near zero, but failed to show the broad dip seen for azimuths near 40-60 degrees. Thus, while ILD is important, level cues alone do not fully predict the directional response of this unit, suggesting that there may also be sensitivity to spectral cues. In fact, for the full-cue and Δ-ILD conditions, the SPL's in a third octave band centered are the CF are the same in each ear, yet the responses are different. This behavior suggests that this unit performs a more complex form of spectral integration than a third-octave filter.

Figure 5 summarizes the effects of cue manipulations for a population of IC units from 10 cats. For each partial-cue condition, we computed the correlation coefficient between the azimuth function for that condition and the function for the full-cue condition. This gives a measure of similarity between the shapes of the two curves. For the 0-ITD condition, the correlation coefficients are near one for the vast majority of units. Thus, setting ITD to zero has little effect on the directional response of this population of units. For the Δ-ITD condition, correlation coefficients never approach one, and are even negative in some cases, confirming that ITD is not the major determinant of directional sensitivity for these high-CF units. Results of ILD manipulations are clearly

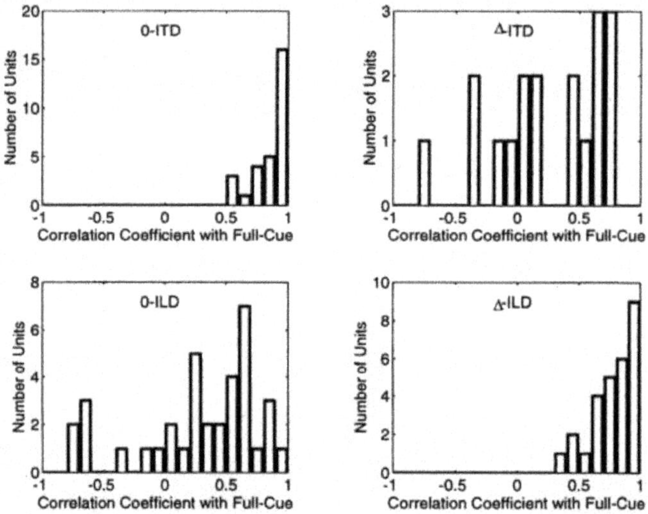

Figure 5. Histograms of the correlation coefficients between the azimuth functions for each partial-cue condition and the function for the full-cue VS stimuli.

different. For the 0-ILD condition, the vast majority of correlation coefficients are well below one, suggesting that ILD is important for the directional sensitivity of this population. For the Δ-ILD condition, some of the correlation coefficients are near one, while others are significantly smaller. Thus, while level cues are important, they do not entirely determine the directional sensitivity of these units. Again, this suggests that spectral cues may be important for some units.

4 Discussion

Our results demonstrate how virtual-space techniques can address questions about neural mechanisms for sound localization that cannot be directly answered through either free-field or traditional dichotic studies alone. Our principal finding is that ILD is the most potent cue for the directional sensitivity of high-CF inferior-colliculus neurons. Another important finding is that binaural interactions studied with VS stimuli are consistent with those found using traditional dichotic paradigms. This result confirms that information obtained in detailed parametric studies of binaural interactions can be applied to the more complex situation found in the free field.

A limitation of our study is that we used acoustic data from one standard cat of Musicant et al. (1990) for generating VS stimuli in all of our experiments. Thus, the sound pressure waveforms of VS stimuli in the ear canal did not exactly match those that would occur in the free field for each individual animal. Several arguments suggest that this limitation may not be severe for the questions that we are addressing in this paper. The most prominent features of HRTF's, and in particular the spectral notches in the 8-20 kHz region appear to be stable across animals (Musicant et al., 1990; Rice et al., 1992). Psychophysical data from human listeners show that localization, particularly in the horizontal plane, can be quite accurate and comparable to free-field localization for naive subjects listening to VS stimuli synthesized using someone else's HRTF's. The general shapes of azimuth functions measured with VS stimuli are similar to those obtained in free-field studies for IC units in the same range of CF's (Aitkin and Martin, 1986; Calford et al., 1985), suggesting that the most important cues for directional sensitivity were present in our VS stimuli. Further, binaural interactions for VS stimuli were generally consistent with those for broadband noise, suggesting that the underlying neural mechanisms may not depend on the exact shape of the stimulus spectrum.

As a whole, our sample of high-CF units showed little sensitivity to ITD for VS stimuli. This result contrasts with physiological studies demonstrating that many high-CF neurons in the IC and the lateral superior olive are sensitive to the ITD of amplitude modulated (AM) tones (Yin et al., 1984; Joris and Yin, 1992; Batra et al., 1993). ITD sensitivity of high-CF units has not been studied for long-duration broadband stimuli such as our VS stimuli. For such stimuli, effective AM frequencies are primarily determined by the bandwidths of the cochlear filters, and are likely to be higher than the low modulation frequencies (< 600 Hz) of the AM tones used in studies of ITD sensitivity. Many natural stimuli such as speech, animal vocalizations, and sounds produced by animals in motion show more pronounced low-frequency AM than do our VS stimuli. Thus, our results may somewhat underestimate the importance of ITD cues for the directional sensitivity of IC units with natural stimuli. This issue could be investigated using VS techniques by replacing the broadband noise input in Fig. 1 by waveforms showing more pronounced AM.

It is difficult to make a firm distinction between ILD and spectral cues because ILD depends on frequency (Musicant et al., 1990). Nevertheless we feel that such a distinction is useful for relating our results with those of studies of binaural interactions which manipulate ILD without changing the spectrum (Rose et al., 1966; Semple and Kitzes, 1987; Irvine and Gago, 1990). In our experiments, ILD was defined either by integrating intensity over the entire 40 kHz bandwidth of our stimuli, or by measuring intensity in a 1/3-octave band centered at the CF of each unit. The latter definition seems to be the most appropriate because most units in the central nucleus of the IC are sharply tuned, and the effective bandwidths of auditory-nerve fibers are approximately 1/3-octave (Evans and Wilson, 1973). Some units such as that of Fig. 4 had clearly different directional responses for the full-cue and Δ-ILD conditions, although these stimuli have the same intensities in the 1/3-octave band centered at the CF. These units behave very differently from auditory-nerve fibers, for which the response to broadband stimuli is primarily determined by the intensity in a 1/3-octave band centered at the CF (Evans and Wilson, 1973). Thus, these units may perform a more complex form of spectral integration than that of auditory-nerve fibers. This conclusion is consistent with findings of complex response areas with prominent lateral inhibition for many IC neurons (Ehret and Merzenich, 1988). Complex spectral integration may also arise at more peripheral levels of the auditory system: for example it has been demonstrated for Type IV neurons in the dorsal cochlear nucleus using stimuli with sharp spectral notches similar to those occurring with free-field stimulation (Young et al., 1992). The IC may differ from more peripheral levels in that many neurons show both powerful binaural interactions and complex spectral integration. Understanding neural mechanisms of spectral integration is important not only for sound localization, but also for the recognition of speech and animal vocalizations.

Our physiological results are generally in harmony with psychophysical data on sound localization. The most directly comparable psychophysical experiments are those of Wightman and Kistler (1992), who used VS stimuli very similar to our broadband noise. Wightman and Kistler showed that ITD is the dominant cue for localizing noise possessing frequency components below 1-2 kHz. However, when their stimuli were highpass-filtered at 2 kHz, ILD cues became dominant. Because localization of highpass noise is likely to be based primarily on high-CF neurons such as those we studied, the Wightman and Kistler results are consistent with our finding that ILD is the most potent cue for the directionality of high-CF neurons.

Our results may also be related to psychophysical experiments conducted in the free field. In both cats and humans, the minimum audible angle (MAA) is smaller for azimuths near zero than for more lateral azimuths (Mills, 1958; Heffner and Heffner, 1988). Figure 3 shows that a majority of our directional neurons show a steep rise in response for azimuths near zero. If sound localization were based on the pattern of activity in a neural population such as that of Fig. 3, one would expect changes in this pattern resulting from a small change in azimuth to be most pronounced for azimuths near the midline, consistent with the MAA data.

5 Acknowledgments

We thank Mr. Ravi Kochhar for invaluable assistance with software for synthesizing VS stimuli. This research was supported by NIH Grants DC00119 and DC00116.

6 References

Aitkin, L.M., and Martin, R.L. (1987) The representation of stimulus azimuth by high best-frequency azimuth-selective neurons in the inferior colliculus of the cat. J. Neurophysiol. 57:1185-1200.

Aitkin, L.M., and Martin, R.L. (1990) Neurons in the inferior colliculus of cats sensitive to sound-source elevation. J. Neurophysiol. 50:97-106.

Aitkin, L.M., Pettigrew, J.D., Calford, M.B., Philips, S.C., and Wise, L.Z. (1985) Representation of stimulus azimuth by low-frequency neurons in inferior colliculus of the cat. J. Neurophysiol. 53:43-59.

Batra, R., Kuwada, S., and Stanford, T.R. (1993) High-frequency neurons in the inferior colliculus that are sensitive to interaural delays of amplitude-modulated tones: Evidence for dual binaural influences. J. Neurophysiol. 70:64-80.

Blauert, J. (1983) Spatial Hearing. The Psychophysics of Human Sound Localization. MIT Press, Cambridge, MA.

Caird, D., and Klinke, R. (1987) Processing of interaural time and intensity differences in the cat inferior colliculus. Exp. Brain Res. 68:379-392.

Calford, M.B., Moore, D.R., and Hutchings, M.E. (1986) Central and peripheral contributions to coding of acoustic space by neurons in inferior colliculus of cat. Hear. Res. 55:587-603.

Ehret, G., and Merzenich, M.M. (1988) Complex sound analysis (frequency resolution, filtering and spectral integration) by single units of the inferior colliculus of the cat. Brain Res. Rev. 13:139-163.

Evans, E.F., and Wilson, J.P. (1973) The frequency selectivity of the cochlea. In: Basic Mechanisms in Hearing, A.R. Møller, ed, New York: Academic, pp. 519-553.

Goldberg, J.M., and Brown, P.B. (1969) Response of binaural neurons of dog superior olivary complex to dichotic tonal stimuli: some physiological mechanisms of sound localization. J. Neurophysiol. 31:639-656.

Heffner, R.S., and Heffner, H.E. (1988) Sound localization acuity in the cat: Effect of azimuth, signal duration and test procedure. Hear. Res. 36:221-232.

Irvine, D.R.F. (1986) The auditory Brainstem. Berlin: Springer-Verlag.

Irvine, D.R.F., and Gago, G. (1990) Binaural interaction in high-frequency neurons in inferior colliculus of the cat: Effects of variations in sound pressure level on sensitivity to interaural level differences. J. Neurophysiol. 63:570-591.

Joris, P.X., and Yin, T.C.T. (1992) Responses of single units in the LSO circuit to amplitude-modulated sounds. Soc. Neurosci. 18:149.

Mills, A.W. (1958) On the minimum audible angle. J. Acoust. Soc. Am. 30:237-246.

Musicant, A.D., Chan, J.C.K., and Hind, J.E. (1990) Direction-dependent spectral properties of cat external ear: New data and cross-species comparisons. J. Acoust. Soc. Am. 87:757-781.

Poon, P.W.F., and Brugge, J.F. (1993) Virtual-space receptive fields of single auditory-nerve fibers. J. Neurophysiol. 70:667-677.

Rice, J.J., May, B.J., Spirou, G.A., and Young, E.D. (1992) Pinna-based spectral cues for sound localization in cat. Hear. Res. 58:132-152.

Rose, J.E., Gross, N.B., Geisler, C.D., and Hind, J.E. (1966) Some neural mechanisms in the inferior colliculus of the cat which may be relevant to localization of a sound source. J. Neurophysiol. 29:288-314.

Searle, C.L., Braida, L.D., Davis, M.F., and Colburn, H.S. (1976) Model for auditory localization. J. Acoust. Soc. Am. 60:1164-1175.
Semple, M.N., and Kitzes, L.M. (1987) Binaural processing of sound pressure level in the inferior colliculus. J. Neurophysiol. 57:1130-1147.
Wenzel, E.M., Arruda, M., Kistler, D.J., and Wightman, F.L. (1993) Localization using nonindividualized head-related transfer functions. J. Acoust. Soc. Am. 94:111-123.
Wightman, F.L., and Kistler, D.J. (1989) Headphone simulation of free-field listening. I: Stimulus synthesis. J. Acoust. Soc. Am. 85:858-867.
Wightman, F.L., and Kistler, D.J. (1992) The dominant role of low-frequency interaural time differences in sound localization. J. Acoust. Soc. Am. 91:1648-1661.
Yin, T.C.T., Chan, J.C.K., and Irvine, D.R.F. (1986) Effects of interaural time delays of noise stimuli on low-frequency cells in the cat's inferior colliculus. I. Responses to wideband noise. J. Neurophysiol. 55:280-300.
Yin, T.C.T., Kuwada, S., and Sujaku, Y. (1984) Interaural time sensitivity of high-frequency neurons in the inferior colliculus. J. Acoust. Soc. Am. 76:1401-1410.
Young, E.D., Spirou, G., Rice, J.J., and Voigt, H.F. (1992) Neural organization and responses to complex stimuli in the dorsal cochlear nucleus. Phil. Trans. R. Soc. Lond. 336:407-413.

Comment by D. Green

First let me congratulate the authors on a very interesting paper. The use of head-related transfer functions (HRTF) has provided new information for the study of sound location.

I am concerned about one point. As I understand it, the HRTF used in the experiments were obtained from cat, measured in other experiments. Thus, we may assume that the HRTFs used for the animals in this experiment have at least some error component in the spectra used to represent the different sound locations. First, how large do you think this error component is? Second, will this error, whatever its size, degrade some cues more than others? For example, perhaps the interaural level cue is less affected by the exact shape of the HRTF than is the interaural time cue and hence the level appears to be more robust when you modify the cues as you did in table I?

Reply

The issue you raise has been of concern to us, and some general arguments suggesting that variability in HRTF may not be a severe limitation are in the written discussion. Concerning specifically your point that different localization cues (e.g. ITD and ILD) might be differentially affected by inaccuracies in the HRTF, both ITD and ILD, when measured over a 1/3 octave band, are smooth functions of azimuth and frequency, so that they are likely to be stable across animals. The major irregularity in these functions are due to a prominent spectral notch in the 8 - 18 kHz region, which is also stable across animals (Musicant et al., 1990; Rice et al., 1992). A possible direction for future studies that would settle the issue would be to examine how cats trained to localize sounds respond to VS stimuli.

At a more general level, the neural mechanisms that we are studying appear to be similar for VS stimuli and broad band noise, so that models for the behaviour of IC cells constructed from responses to VS stimuli are likely to be generally applicable, including the free-field situation.

The role of inhibition In determining neuronal response properties in the inferior colliculus

F. E. N. Le Beau, M. S. Malmierca and A. Rees

University of Newcastle upon Tyne, Department of Physiological Sciences, Framlington Place, Newcastle upon Tyne, NE2 4HH, UK

1 Introduction

Neuronal responses in the inferior colliculus (IC) depend on inhibitory as well as excitatory interactions. Indeed, it has been suggested that the central nucleus of the inferior colliculus contains as many inhibitory as excitatory synapses (Oliver *et al.*, 1994). Immunocytochemical studies show that this inhibition is mediated by the neurotransmitters γ-aminobutyric acid (GABA) and glycine. GABA is found in both terminals and somata (Oliver and Beckius, 1992; Oliver *et al.*, 1994), while glycine is restricted to terminals only (Saint Marie *et al.*, 1989). These findings imply that GABAergic inhibition in the IC originates from both extrinsic and intrinsic sources, but all the glycinergic inputs originate outside the IC. The extrinsic sources of GABA terminals are the lateral superior olive (Saint Marie *et al.*, 1989) and the dorsal nucleus of the lateral lemniscus (Adams and Mugnaini, 1984), while glycinergic projections arise in the lateral superior olive and the ventral nucleus of the lateral lemniscus (Saint Marie and Baker, 1990).

Evidence for inhibitory interactions within the IC has also accumulated from physiological studies. The first report of stimulus-dependent IPSPs in intracellular records was made by Nelson and Erulkar (1963), but many features of extracellularly recorded responses are also indicative of inhibitory activity. Nonmonotonic functions of firing rate versus level (intensity) have been reported for between 24-50% of neurones in the IC (Rose *et al.*, 1963; Semple and Kitzes, 1985; Rees and Palmer, 1988), and many IC neurones show level-dependent changes in their temporal firing patterns. The frequency response areas of IC neurones are diverse with many suggesting the operation of frequency-dependent inhibitory inputs (for review see Ehret and Merzenich, 1988).

With extracellular recordings alone it is not possible to be certain about the nature or origins of such responses; if they are due to inhibition, is this mediated by inhibitory synapses within the IC, or is it the consequence of inhibition operating at a more peripheral level? One method that can help to discriminate between these possibilities is microiontophoresis. Recently, several studies have used it to study inhibition in the IC (Faingold *et al.*, 1989, 1991; Vater *et al.*, 1992; Yang *et al.*, 1992). These studies showed that GABA and glycine are responsible for several features of the responses of IC neurones to sounds. Faingold *et al.* (1989, 1991) showed that the effects of blocking $GABA_A$ receptors with the antagonist bicuculline included: i) transformation of an onset into sustained response, ii) elimination of level-dependent nonmonotonicity, and iii) abolition of binaural inhibition. In chinchilla, Caspary and Palombi (1993) measured the effects of bicuculline on frequency tuning curves. They reported that although the firing rate of the cells increased with bicuculline, their frequency tuning curves did not broaden. In contrast, tuning curves for the majority of IC units recorded in the horseshoe bat (Vater *et al.*, 1992), and 47% of those in the mustache bat (Yang *et al.*, 1992) broadened in the presence of bicuculline.

Another feature of neuronal responses in the IC that might be sensitive to inhibition is the regularity of their spike discharge. Regularity analysis has been used extensively in both the ventral (e.g. Bourk, 1976; Young *et al.*, 1988) and dorsal (Parham and Kim, 1992) cochlear nuclei to quantify spike discharge regularity (evident as chopping in the PSTHs of some neurones) and classify neuronal sub-types. Regularly discharging neurones have been noted in the inferior colliculus (Willot, 1978; Langner and Schreiner, 1988), but their regularity has not been analysed quantitatively. In the ventral cochlear nucleus iontophoresis of GABA decreases the regularity of chopper cells converting a sustained into a transient chopper (Ebert and Ostwald, 1992).

The first aim of our iontophoretic experiments was to define the contribution of GABA to the frequency response areas of neurones in the guinea-pig IC. To measure response areas we have adopted the method developed by Evans (1979) which provides an estimate of the excitatory and inhibitory response areas. Our second aim was to study the effects of inhibitory transmitter antagonists on the regularity of firing of IC neurones.

2 Methods

The experiments were performed on 17 pigmented guinea-pigs (300-650 g) anaesthetised with urethane (1.5g/kg i.p.). Electrode penetrations were made stereotaxically into the IC and calibrated sound stimuli were presented monaurally and binaurally through a closed acoustic system (Rees, 1990).

Recording and iontophoresis were performed with a glass recording electrode combined with a multibarrelled micropipette (after Stone, 1985). The barrels were filled with bicuculline methiodide (5 mM, pH 3-4) and strychnine (10 mM, pH 3-4). A further barrel filled with 0.5 mM NaCl (pH 3-4) was used to balance current and test for current and pH effects. Retaining and ejection currents were applied using a Medical Instruments Neurophore System. The times of recorded action potentials were logged by computer. In all experiments the unit's firing rate was allowed to stabilise prior to collecting data during the application of each drug and the subsequent recovery period.

Frequency response areas were mapped by presenting 960 tone bursts (25 ms duration, repetition rate 5/s) varying in a pseudorandom sequence of frequency and attenuation over several octaves around a neurone's best frequency (BF). The number of spikes elicited by each tone was counted, and the value plotted as a bar centred on the appropriate frequency and attenuation coordinate on the response area diagram with bar length proportional to the number of spikes fired (Evans 1979). An estimate of the inhibitory response area can be derived by subtracting the control response area from that obtained during application of the inhibitory transmitter antagonist (Evans and Zhao,

1993). In addition, to emphasise the expansion that occurs with the antagonist, a second type of subtraction plot shows only the responses to stimuli that activated the cell in the presence of bicuculline, but not in the control.

Regularity analysis was applied to responses to BF tones (5 ms rise/fall time, 75 ms duration, repetition rate 4/s). Several hundred repetitions of the stimulus were presented and the spike times used to compute a PSTH, the mean interspike interval (ISI) and its standard deviation (SD) in 100-μs bins over the course of the response. Regularity was measured by calculating the coefficient of variation (CV = SD/mean ISI); regularity is inversely proportional to CV. Units were classified as regular if their mean CV was equal or less than 0.5 (Young *et al.*, 1988).

Following the experiment the animal was perfused, and Nissl stained sections of the midbrain were prepared to locate the recording sites. Based on our own cytoarchitectural map in the guinea-pig (Malmierca *et al.*, 1994), the units described were in the central nucleus of the inferior colliculus or close to its border with the dorsal cortex.

3 Results

The results are based on a sample of 42 units for which we have studied the effects of the inhibitory antagonists on frequency response area and spike discharge regularity.

3.1 Frequency response areas

We have divided the neurones in our sample into two groups, I and II, according to the shape of their frequency response areas in control conditions. Group I (60%, 21/35) units are characterised by a V-shaped response area (Fig. 1a), which may or may not include a low-frequency tail. Group II units (40%, 14/35) are characterised by excitatory response areas that have one of several complex patterns. These include i) *closed* response areas (Fig. 2a), which contain an island of excitation for frequencies around BF at low intensities, but have little response to the same frequencies at high intensities, ii) *tilting* response areas, where the response is weak or absent at the high- or low-frequency edges of the area, and iii) *narrow* response areas in which excitation is restricted to frequencies close to BF with an isolated region of excitation at frequencies below BF (Fig. 3a).

Effects of bicuculline: For 35 units in our sample we obtained frequency response areas during the application of bicuculline. We were able to make a complete sequence of post-bicuculline recordings for 60% (21/35) of these units. In only one case did the unit's response fail to recover to its control level. The remaining units were lost before the collection of post-drug data could be completed.

The effect of bicuculline on a group I neurone is shown in Fig. 1. During application of bicuculline (Fig. 1b) the discharge rate at all driven frequencies was greater than in the control (Fig. 1a) but there was little or no increase in spontaneous activity. The range of frequencies and intensities that activate the unit was not changed by bicuculline as evidenced in the subtraction plot (Fig. 1c). This shows the inhibitory response area, and demonstrates that the inhibition was operating across the whole of the excitatory response area. Horizontal bars denote points for which the control response exceeded that with bicuculline. In Fig. 1d a response is only plotted if it was elicited by a stimulus that excited the cell with bicuculline but not in the control. The absence of any driven responses in this plot confirms that the response area of the unit did not expand with bicuculline.

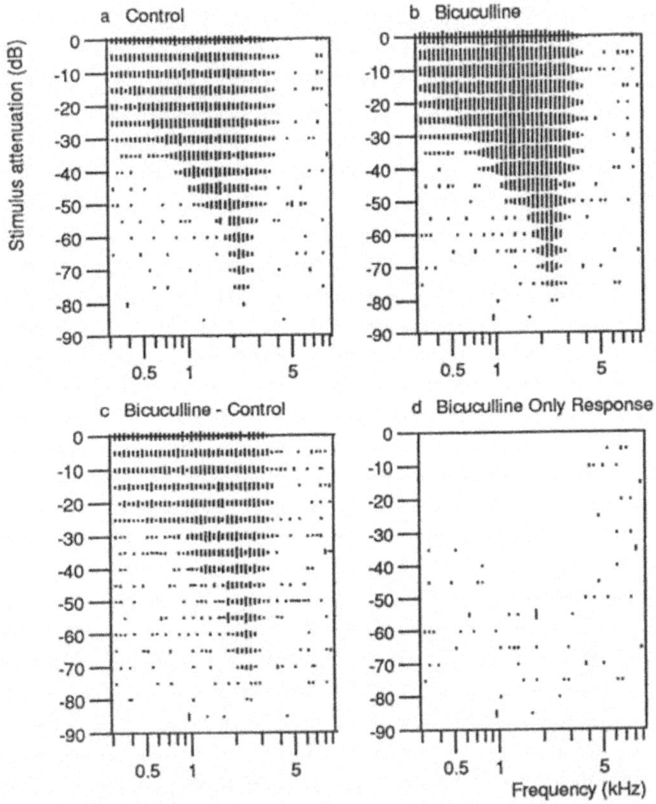

Figure 1. Effects of bicuculline on the frequency response area of a group I neuron. BF = 2.3 kHz, contralateral monaural stimulation. Discharge rate increased in the presence of bicuculline but there was no expansion of the excitatory response area.

An example of a group II, closed-response, neurone is depicted in Fig. 2. In the control response (Fig. 2a) this neurone was excited most by a range frequencies around BF from 5-30 dB above threshold, but the response became progressively weaker with higher intensity stimuli in the same frequency range. When bicuculline was applied, the unit was strongly activated by these higher intensity stimuli, and the range of frequencies to which the unit responded increased (Fig. 2b). The subtraction plot (Fig. 2c) shows that the GABAergic inhibition blocked by bicuculline was operating over the entire control response area as well as extending above and lateral to it. The bicuculline only plot (Fig. 2d) demonstrates the extent of the expansion.

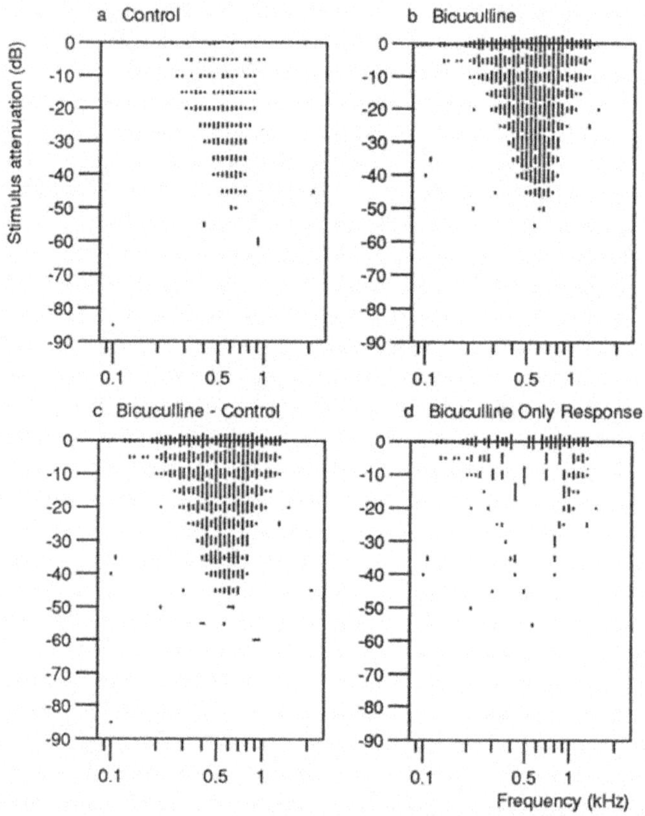

Figure 2. Effects of bicuculline on the frequency response area of a group II neuron. BF = 0.65 kHz, contralateral monaural stimulation. Discharge rate increased with bicuculline and the excitatory response area expanded.

The responses of another type of group II unit are shown in Fig. 3. This unit was sharply tuned with a BF of 5 kHz. In addition to the response around BF there was a second, isolated, region of excitation around 0.7 kHz that was only activated at the highest intensities (Fig. 3a). Application of bicuculline (Fig. 3b) not only increased the firing rates in these regions of the response area, it also revealed an excitatory input at all frequencies in between. As well as increasing the stimulus-driven response of this unit, blockade of GABA also resulted in an increase in the neurone's spontaneous activity. This unit was lost a few seconds prior to the completion of the bicuculline response. The

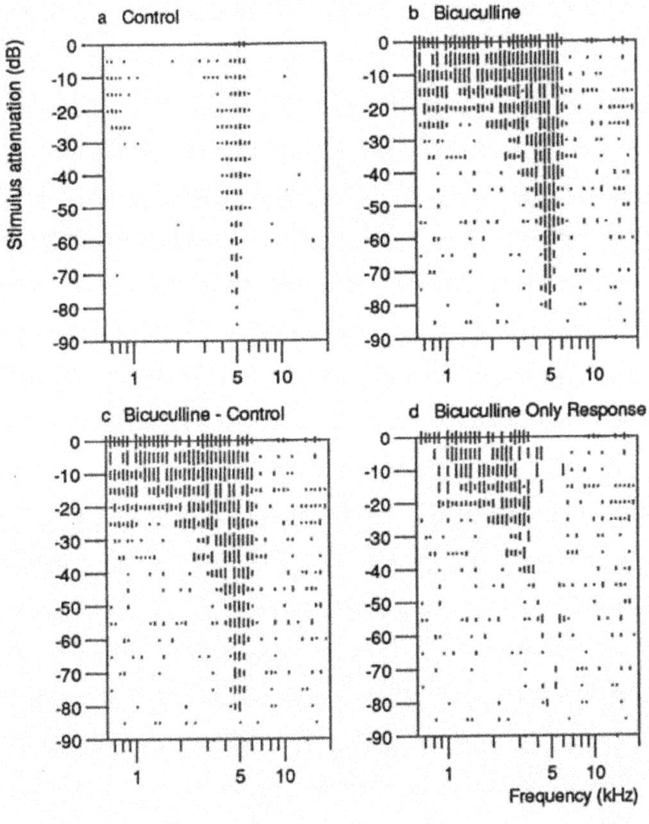

Figure 3. Effects of bicuculline on the frequency response area for a group II neuron. BF = 5 kHz, contralateral monaural stimulation. Discharge rate increased in the presence of bicuculline and removal of inhibition revealed an additional region of excitation.

isolated spaces within the otherwise vigorous excitatory response area elicited with bicuculline correspond to stimulus combinations that were presented after the unit was lost. The subtraction plot (Fig. 3c) emphasises the extent to which the excitation present in the control was subject to inhibition, while Fig. 3d highlights the areas in which the cell's excitatory input was completely inhibited in the control.

To compare the changes in response areas after blocking the GABAergic inhibition we have measured the percentage increase in bandwidth at 10- and 30-dB above threshold for both monaural and binaural stimulation. (In the binaural condition, the stimuli were presented at equal level to the left and right ears.) With contralateral monaural stimulation half of the group I units showed little (< 10%) or no change in either 10 or 30 dB bandwidth. The greatest change for a group I unit was an increase of 64 % at 10 dB. In contrast, the bandwidth of all except one of the group II units increased by more than 10%, and half increased their 10 dB bandwidth by over 50%. The largest change at 10 dB for group II was an increase of 560%. Similar changes occurred with binaural stimulation, although fewer cells were studied with binaural stimulation (16 group I and 6 group II).

In addition to the changes bicuculline induced on response area size and shape, it also produced a change in the BF threshold of 38% (8/21) group I and 28.5% (4/14) of group II units. The magnitude of this shift in sensitivity was similar for both groups with an average threshold reduction of 4.4 dB and 6.8 dB for groups I and II, respectively. We never observed a change in BF during the application of bicuculline.

Effects of strychnine: In ten units we were able to test the effects of the glycine antagonist strychnine following completion of the bicuculline measurements. In 8 of these units (6 group I, 2 group II), strychnine caused an increase in discharge rate and an increase (>10%) in the 30-dB bandwidth. The sample is too small, however, to make any quantitative comparison with the results obtained with bicuculline, but the data demonstrate that glycinergic inhibition is also, in part, responsible for shaping the frequency response areas of IC neurones.

3.2 Regularity Analysis

We have studied the effects of bicuculline on the discharge regularity of 15 units that had control CV below 0.5. In 12 cells there was an increase in regularity over the first 10 ms of the response and 6 of these also showed an increase in regularity in the later part of their response to a tone burst.

An example of the effect of bicuculline on discharge regularity is shown in Fig 4. The neurone's control PSTH (Fig. 4a) has a pronounced onset peak followed by a period of activity at a lower firing rate. The mean ISI increased from 6 ms to about 14 ms over

Figure 4. Effects of bicuculline on regularity of firing. BF = 0.6 kHz, contralateral monaural stimulation. Bicuculline increased discharge rate, changed PSTH shape (a chopping pattern appears), and increased regularity of discharge. Main panel: PSTH, lower inset: mean interstiulus interval (ISI) and standard deviation (SD), upper inset: coefficient of variation (CV).

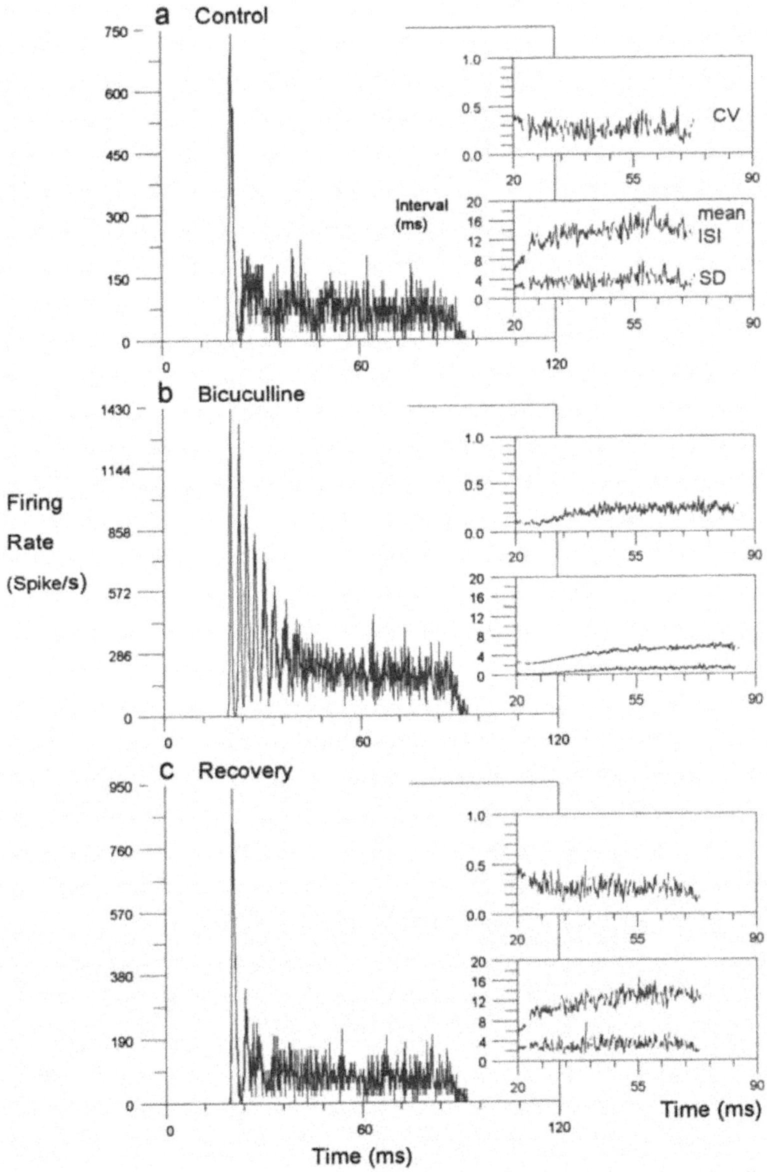

a Control
b Bicuculline
c Recovery
Firing
Rate
(Spike/s)
Interval
(ms)
CV
mean
ISI
SD
Time (ms)
Time (ms)

the course of the response, with the most rapid change occurring near the onset. The cell fired regularly with a CV of 0.4 at the onset that declined 25 ms after the beginning of the response to a mean value of 0.26. During application of bicuculline (Fig. 4b) a transient chopping pattern appeared in the first 20 ms of the PSTH. The mean ISI of the response is lower than in the control, commensurate with the approximate doubling in firing rate in the absence of GABA inhibition. The increase in the regularity of the neurone during the early part of the response, is evidenced by a reduction in the CV from 0.4 in the control to 0.1 with bicuculline. In the later part of the response the CV is virtually the same as in the control. Fig. 4c demonstrates that the response almost reverts to that seen in the control after the application of bicuculline was stopped.

We were also able to test the effect of strychnine in this cell. The neurone's discharge rate increased substantially, but the distinctive chopping that appeared during the application of bicuculline was not present during glycine blockade.

4 Discussion

All the neurones studied here received a GABAergic inhibitory input mediated by $GABA_A$ receptors, since bicuculline altered at least one aspect of each unit's response. Removal of this inhibition produced several distinct effects in different units including increases in discharge rate, changes in the size and shape of the frequency response areas, and increases in discharge regularity. By combining the detailed mapping of frequency response areas with iontophoresis we have been able to reveal some of the patterns of excitation and inhibition that operate to shape the responses of neurones in the IC of the guinea-pig.

In half the units classified as group I, the shape and size of the response area is not changed by bicuculline, despite the significant increase in firing rate seen at all frequencies that drove the cell. Similar observations were made in the mustache bat (Yang *et al.*, 1992) where tuning curve width was unaffected with bicuculline in 53% of neurones. In chinchilla, Caspary and Palombi (1993) found that in 95% of their sample bicuculline caused a substantial increase in discharge rate but no expansion of the excitatory response area. A finding that lead the authors to conclude that GABA does not mediate lateral inhibition in these neurones. In contrast, our group II units showed more dramatic changes in the size and shape of their response areas. Similarly in the horseshoe bat, the tuning curves of almost all neurones in the IC expanded in the presence of bicuculline (Vater *et al.*, 1992) as did the remainder of the units recorded by Yang *et al.* (1992). The bat studies focused mainly on cells from the 60 kHz region of the colliculus, but both groups noted changes at other BFs as well. Several different inhibitory interactions may be responsible for generating the response areas of group II neurones, including level- and frequency-dependent inhibition. The expansion of frequency response areas in the guinea-pig suggests that frequency-dependent GABAergic inhibition is not solely a feature of the specialised auditory system in the bat. In addition, whilst we do not know how anaesthesia may have affected the balance of excitation and inhibition in our experiments, the qualitative similarity between our results and those in unanaesthetised bat suggests that they reflect physiological mechanisms.

Despite the lack of expansion in the responses areas of half of group I units with blockade of $GABA_A$ receptors, the marked increase in firing rate seen in all these units demonstrates the presence of GABAergic inhibition. The subtraction plots (Figs. 1c, 2c and 3c) reveal that this inhibition operates at all frequencies that excite the cell and is by no means confined to lateral side-bands. This result could arise if the distribution of a frequency specific inhibitory input coincides with the excitatory input. On the other hand, the inhibition might be a non-stimulus dependent, tonic input that reduces the effectiveness of the frequency-dependent excitation, similar to the $GABA_A$-meditated background inhibition described in the dorsal cochlear nucleus (Evans and Zhao, 1993). This seems unlikely because, in contrast to cells in the dorsal cochlear nucleus, many units in our sample showed no increase in spontaneous activity with bicuculline (Figs. 1, 2). The absence of significant spontaneous firing also prompts a caution that the subtraction plots derived in these experiments may not reveal the full extent of the inhibitory receptive fields of these units. Because many units have little or no spontaneous activity stimuli that activate a purely inhibitory input will not evoke a detectable response.

We have also demonstrated that GABA inhibition influences the discharge regularity of neurones in the IC. In most units the changes in regularity seen with bicuculline are greatest over the first 20 ms of the response. The regularity of stellate neurones in the ventral cochlear nucleus is a characteristic of their intrinsic membrane properties activated when they are driven by a steady depolarising current (Oertel, 1983). If regularity in the IC depends on a similar mechanism, one might anticipate that the level of inhibition would be an important determinant of a cell's response since any hyperpolarising input that reduced the strength of the depolarisation might reduce the regularity of discharge. There are, however, no equivalent data on the membrane properties of IC neurones. In addition, the explanation may not be so simple, since elimination of glycinergic inhibition provoked a significant increase in discharge rate, without a comparable change in regularity.

These experiments, together with the results of previous studies (Faingold *et al.*, 1991) demonstrate that the effects of inhibition in the inferior colliculus are many and varied, a finding that is perhaps not surprising given the several sources of inhibitory innervation to the IC, and the finding that cells within the IC containing GABA belong to more than one morphological class (Oliver *et al.*, 1994). Further experiments combining iontophoresis with the selective block or destruction of the brainstem nuclei that are the sources of the different inhibitory inputs, will be necessary to disentangle the contributions of these different connections (*cf.* Liang and Kelly, 1992).

5 Acknowledgements

We thank Alan Palmer for helpful comments on the manuscript. Supported by the Royal Society, the Wellcome Trust and the Nuffield Foundation. F.E.N.LB was supported by a University Junior Research Fellowship. M.S.M. was supported by Fellowships from the Spanish MEC and the EU.

6 References

Adams J. and Mugnaini, E. (1984) Dorsal nucleus of the lateral lemniscus: A nucleus of GABAergic projection neurones. Brain Res. Bull. 13, 585-590.

Bourk, T.R. (1976) Electrical responses of neural units in the anteroventral cochlear nucleus of the cat. Ph.D. Dissertation, MIT, Cambridge, Massachusetts

Caspary, D.M. and Palombi, P.S. (1993) GABA inputs control discharge rate within the excitatory response area of chinchilla inferior collicular neurones. Ass. Res. Oto. Abs. 16: 109

Ebert, U and Ostwald, J. (1992) GABA alters the temporal discharge pattern of chopper neurones in the ventral cochlear nucleus. Europ. J. Neurosci. Suppl. 5, 144.

Ehret, G. and Merzenich, M.M. (1988) Complex sound analysis (frequency resolution, filtering and spectral integration) by single units of the inferior colliculus of the cat. Brain Res. Reviews 13, 139- 163.

Evans, E.F. (1979) Single unit studies of the mammalian auditory nerve. In: Auditory Investigations: The Scientific and Technological Basis" (H.A. Beagley, Ed.), Oxford University Press, Oxford, pp 324-367.

Evans, E.F. and Zhao, W. (1993) Neuropharmacological and neurophysiological dissection of inhibition in the mammalian dorsal cochlear nucleus. In: "The Mammalian Cochlear Nuclei: Organization and Function", (M.A. Merchán, J. Juiz, D.A. Godfrey and E. Mugnaini, Eds.), Plenum Press, New York, pp 373-384

Faingold, C.L., Gehlbach, G. and Caspary, D.M. (1989) On the role of GABA as an inhibitory neurotransmitter in inferior colliculus neurons: iontophoretic studies. Brain Res. 500, 302-312.

Faingold, C.L., Gehlbach, G. and Caspary D.M. (1991) Functional pharmacology of inferior colliculus neurons. In: Neurobiology of Hearing: Vol. 2: The Central Auditory System (R.A. Altschuler, R.P. Bobin, B.M. Clopton, and D.W. Hoffman, Eds), Raven Press, New York, pp 223-251.

Langner, G. and Schreiner, C.E. (1988) Periodicity coding in the inferior colliculus of the cat. I. Neuronal mechanisms. J. Neurophysiol. 60, 1799-1829

Liang, L. and Kelly J.B. (1992) Inhibitory influence of the dorsal nucleus of the lateral lemniscus on binaural responses in the rat's inferior colliculus. J. Neurosci. 12, 4530-4539

Malmierca, M.S., Rees, A., Le Beau, F.E.N., Bjaalie, J.G. (1994) The laminar organization of frequency-specific local axons within and between the inferior colliculus of the guinea-pig. J. Comp. Neurol. *submitted.*

Nelson, P.G. and Erulkar, S.D. (1963) Synaptic mechanisms of exitation and inhibition in the central auditory pathway. J. Neurophysiol. 26, 908-923

Oertel, D. (1983) Synaptic responses and electrical properties of cells in brain slices of the mouse anteroventeral cochlear nucleus. J. Neurosci. 3, 2043-2053.

Oliver, D.L. and Beckius, G.E. (1992) Fine structure of GABA-labelled axonal endings in the inferior colliculus of the cat: immunocytochemistry on deplasticized ultrathin sections. Neurosci. 46, 455-463.

Oliver, D.L., Winer, J.A., Beckius, G.E. and Saint Marie, R.L. (1994) Morphology of GABAergic neurons in the inferior colliculus of the cat. J. Comp. Neurol. 340, 27-42.

Parham, K. and Kim, D.O. (1992) Analysis of temporal discharge characteristics of dorsal cochlear nucleus neurons of unanaesthetized decerebrate cats. J. Neurophsiol. 67, 1247-1263.

Rees, A. (1990) a closed-field sound system for auditory neurophysiology. J. Physiol. 430, 6P.

Rees, A., and Palmer, A.R. (1988) Rate-intensity function and their modification by broadband noise for neurons in the guinea-pig inferior colliculus. J. Acoust. Soc. Am. 83, 1488-1498.

Rose, J.E., Greenwood, D.D., Goldberg, J.M. and Hind J.E. (1963) Some discharge characteristics of single neurons in the inferior colliculus of the cat. I. Tonotopical organization, relation of spike counts to tone intensity, and firing patterns of single elements. J. Neurophysiol. 26, 294-320.

Saint Marie, R.L., and Baker, R.A. (1990) Neurotransmitter specific uptake and retrograde transport of (^{3}H)-glycine from the inferior colliculus by ipsilateral projections of the superior olivary complex and nuclei of the lateral lemniscus. Brain Res. 524, 244-253.

Saint Marie, R.L., Ostapoff, E.-M., Morest, D.K., and Wenthold, R.J. (1989) Glycine-immunoreactive projections of the cat lateral superior olive: possible role in midbrain ear dominance. J. Comp. Neurol. 279, 382-396.

Semple, M.N. and Kitzes, L.M. (1985) Single unit responses in the inferior colliculus: different consequences of contralateral and ipsilateral auditory stimulation. J. Neurophysiol. 53, 1467-1482.

Stone, T.W. (1985) Microiontophoresis and pressure ejection. John Wiley & Sons, Chichester.

Vater, M., Habbicht, H., Kössl, M., and Groethe, B. (1992) The functional role of GABA and glycine in monaural and binaural processing in the inferior colliculus of horseshoe bats. J. Comp. Physiol. A 171, 541-553.

Willot, J.F. (1983) Central Nervous System Physiology. In: The Auditory Psychobiology Of The Mouse (J.F. Willot, Ed.) Thomas, Springfield, pp 305-338.

Yang, L., Pollak, G. D., and Resler, C. (1992) GABAergic circuits sharpen tuning curves and modify response properties in the mustache bat inferior colliculus. J. Neurophysiol. 68, 1760-1774.

Young, E.D., Robert, J-M., and Shofner, W.P. (1988) Regularity and Latency of Units in Ventral Cochlear Nucleus: Implications for unit classification and generation of response properties. J. Neurophysiol. 60, 1-29.

Comment by E.F. Evans

1) We have found what we think may be a non-specific (current effect ?) change in the many cell types in the cochlea nucleus towards the development of "chopper" response patterns. In your figure 4 you have controlled for this by application of strychnine, but it does inquire the use of current controls.

2) Have you seen changes in the receptive fields with application of strychnine?

3) In view of your finding (Evans and Nelson, 1973) that depressant anaesthetics (pentobarbitone, urethane e.g.) deleteriously affect inhibition in the cochlea nucleus, I was pleased to see plenty of evidence of inhibition in your data. Have you tried chloralose, which in the cochlea nucleus gave minimal alteration to inhibition compared with the unanaesthetized state?

Evans, E.F., and Nelson, P.G. (1973) The responses of single neurons in the cochlear nucleus of the cat as a function of their location and the anaesthetic state. Exp. Brain Res. 17, 402-427.

Reply

1) As you rightly point out, one must always be wary of non-specific responses when using iontophoresis, even when current balance is in operation. We do not believe we are seeing current effects for the following reasons: 1) the changes in discharge rate and regularity with strychnine were less marked than with bicuculline, even when the ejection currents used for strychinine were higher. 2) one would expect current effects to be instantaneous in their onset and reversed immediately the current was switched off. Our

bicuculline effects built up over several minutes (even with constant ejection current) and persisted for a few minutes after the current was switched off. 3) Where the holding time for the unit allows, we perform direct current and pH controls by passing current through another barrel containing 0.5 M NaCl, pH 3.5-4.0. Where we have applied this control, we have not seen any effects that are attributable to current.

2) We have only a small sample of 14 units in which we have been able to investigate the effects of both bicuculline and strychnine on frequency response areas. Six of these units showed small increases in area with strychnine. In only two of these units, however, were we able to match the firing rates of the cell with the two antagonists to enable us to compare their effects directly. For one unit, both strychnine and bicuculline produced a small increase (<25%) in area, while in the other the increase with bicuculline was twice that with strychnine.

3) Acting on a previous comment from you, we have now collected a sample of about 80 response areas under chloralose anaesthesia to compare with a similar number under urethane. We have not seen any response area types with chloralose that do not occur with urethane. More units show spontaneous activity with chloralose, but we cannot rule out the possibility that this is related to differences in the depth of anaesthesia under the two regimes rather than a specific effect of the drug.

Comment by R. Klinke

Is the pharmacology of inhibition in the monaural case the same as in the case of binaural stimulation?

Reply

We have not systematically studied responses to IIDs and ITDs in our experiments, but we have recorded a small sample of frequency response areas with binaural stimuli of equal level. Measurements of bandwidth changes with bicuculline, as reported in the written text, showed little difference between contra-aural and binaural stimulation. More recently we have calculated the change in the area of the excitatory region of the response area, as I described in my talk. These data show the same trend as the bandwidth measurements. Most of the group I units showed smaller changes in area than the group II units, and the shape of the excitatory response area of the group I units remained the same. But whereas with contra-aural stimulation none of the group I units showed a greater than 40% change in area, five units (17%) of the binuaral sample expanded by more than 50%. This suggests that binurally mediated GABA inhibibiton is frequency dependent in some units. I would emphasise that these are preliminary findings, based on a small sample of units, for which we made no attempt to optimise the IID or ITD for each unit. Other workers (eg. Faingold et al., 1991; Park and Pollak, 1993) have shown that binaural inhibition mediated by the stimulation of the ipsilateral ear is partially blocked by bicuculline, showing that inhibitory synapses intrinsic to the inferior colliculus are partly responsible for IID interactions.

Faingold, C.L., Boersma Anderson, C.A. and Caspary, D.M. (1991) Involvement of GABA in acoustically-evoked inhibition in inferior colliculus neurons. Hearing Res. 52, 201-216.

Park, T.J. and Pollak, G.D. (1993) GABA shapes sensitivity to interaural intensity disparities in the moustache bats inferior colliculus - implications for encoding sound location. J. Neurosci. 13, 2050-2067.

Physiological studies of the precedence effect in the inferior colliculus of the cat

T.C.T. Yin[1,2] and R.Y. Litovsky[1]

[1]*University of Wisconsin, Department of Neurophysiology, Madison, WI 53706, U.S.A.*
[2]*Vision, Touch and Hearing Research Centre, Univ. of Queensland, St. Lucia, Queensland, Australia.*

1 Introduction

From common experience we know that our ability to localize the direction of sound sources is preserved even in a reverberant environment, where the presence of echoes might be expected to create confusion about the sound source direction (Hartmann, 1983). In accordance with this ability to ignore echoes, psychophysical experiments have demonstrated that when two similar sounds are delivered from spatially separate locations with a time delay short enough that only a single sound is perceived, the localization of that sound is dominated by the location of the leading sound. This illusion is usually referred to as the *precedence effect* (PE), or law of the first wavefront, and the discovery of this effect is usually credited to either Wallach et al. (1949) or Haas (1951). While the psychophysical effect has been studied for almost 50 years, much less attention has been paid to the phenomenon by physiologists. We have therefore initiated a study of the PE and looked for physiological correlates of the psychophysical effects.

The PE can be easily demonstrated using stimuli delivered either in free field or dichotically with earphones (Blauert, 1983). In free field it is usually tested by placing a subject midway between two speakers that are stimulated with identical or similar sounds which are separated by a variable time delay (Fig. 1A). For click stimuli the perceived location of the source of sound as a function of the interclick delay (ICD) is shown in Fig. 1B. At long ICDs for values greater than the *echo threshold*, both clicks are heard and are localized to their respective locations in space. The value of echo threshold varies with the experimental conditions and with the stimulus: it is short for clicks (2-8 msec) and longer for speech (30-40 msec). For short ICDs, ($|ICD| < 1$ msec), a period of *summing localization* occurs in which only a single click is heard that is localized to a phantom source and both clicks contribute to the perceived location of the sound. If the stimuli are delivered simultaneously (ICD=0), the phantom source lies on the midline (Fig. 1A). Between the end of the summing localization period and the echo threshold is the time period during which the PE, or *echo suppression*, takes place. During the PE only a single sound localized to the position of the leading speaker is heard. Note that during the PE a leading sound source suppresses a lagging one, a forward masking effect, whereas during summing localization the lagging sound influences the perceived localization, a backward effect. Furthermore, PE and summing localization are active over different temporal windows: summing localization occurs for stimuli with ICDs of less than 1 msec while the PE develops for ICDs in the range of 2-40 msec. During the PE the lagging sound is not truly suppressed, since its absence is readily perceived by a change in the timbre and loudness of the sound when it is turned off, but rather its localization information is suppressed (Blauert, 1983).

Dichotic experiments have usually simulated the free field situation by delivering a pair of clicks to each ear with a variable ICD (Fig. 1C)(Zurek, 1980; Yost and Soderquist, 1984). To simulate the spatial location of each sound, a variable ITD is introduced to the leading and lagging pair of clicks. We have used both free field and dichotic conditions to look for correlates of the PE and summing localization in responses of cells in the central nucleus of the inferior colliculus (ICC) of the anesthetized cat. We chose the ICC as a possible source of such correlations because earlier studies using single clicks to each ear have shown that cells in the ICC exhibit both long-lasting forward and short-lasting backward masking effects (Carney and Yin, 1989). Two fundamental assumptions are that the cat experiences the PE and and that the discharge of ICC cells is related to the perceived location of the sound.

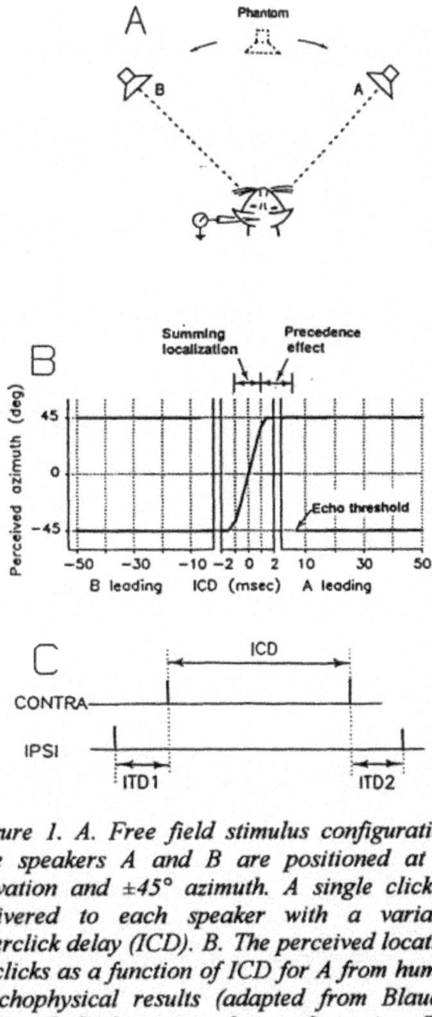

Figure 1. A. Free field stimulus configuration. The speakers A and B are positioned at 0° elevation and ±45° azimuth. A single click is delivered to each speaker with a variable interclick delay (ICD). B. The perceived location of clicks as a function of ICD for A from human psychophysical results (adapted from Blauert, 1983). C. Dichotic stimulus configuration. Two pairs of clicks, separated by an ICD, are delivered with an ITD1 in the leading and ITD2 in the lagging pair. By convention 0° azimuth is straight ahead, + angles are in the contralateral sound field, +ICDs correspond to delays of speaker B, and +ITDs represent delays of the ipsilateral ear. (From Yin, 1994).

2 Methods

The methods for most of these experiments are described in a recent paper (Yin, 1994). Briefly, single cells were recorded with metal microelectrodes from the ICC of the barbiturate anesthetized cat using either dichotic stimulation with a closed sound system or in free field in a sound proof room made anechoic with insulating foam. In our most recent work we have used an array of loudspeakers spaced at 15° intervals and placed in a hemicircle of 95 cm radius along the interaural and mid-sagittal plane. The levels of the clicks were usually about 5-15 dB above threshold.

3 Results

The data were obtained in two sets of experiments. One set came from free field recordings made at the University of Queensland while the first author was on sabbatical leave. The other came from dichotic and free field recordings made in Wisconsin. In all we studied 108 cells under dichotic and 145 cells in free field conditions. Initially we restricted our study to cells with low characteristic frequency (CF < 4 kHz) but in later experiments cells of all CFs were studied.

3.1 Responses to free field stimuli

Figure 2 shows responses of one cell in the ICC from free field recordings with speakers arranged as in Fig. 1A. Each set of 5 dot rasters shows responses in which the lagging click A was delayed with respect to the leading click B from 9.3 to 49.3 msec. The level of click B varied from 45 to 65 dB while A was held at 55 dB. At 55 dB in both ears (middle), this cell responded to clicks delivered from either speaker. Like most cells, for large values of ICD it responded to both clicks in the same way as it responded to each click by itself. As the |ICD| was shortened from 49 to 9 msec, there was gradual suppression of the lagging click with no change in the response to the leading click. The suppression depended upon the relative levels of the two clicks: it was stronger when the level of the leading click was increased (Fig. 2, 60, 65 dB) or when the level of the lagging click was decreased (not shown). In addition, there was suppression even if the initial click was

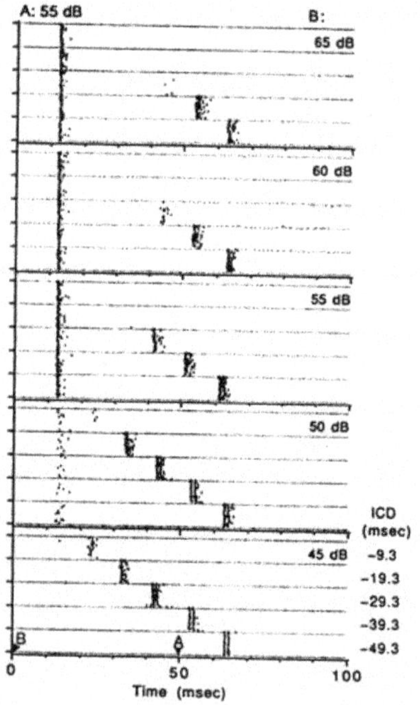

Figure 2. Echo suppression in the ICC to click pairs delivered in free field. In all cases click A was delayed by the value of ICD.

too weak to elicit a response (Fig. 2, 45 dB), which demonstrates that it is not fatigue or adaptation to the leading click that accounts for the suppression of the lagging click. Under both dichotic and free field stimulation almost all ICC cells exhibited such suppressive effects, though the degree of suppression varied considerably from cell to cell with 50% suppression in the 2-100 msec range.

In addition to the echo suppressive effect (Fig. 2), some ICC cells also exhibit a form of summing localization (Fig. 3). We first obtained the spatial sensitivity of the cell to click stimuli in the frontal field along the horizontal meridian (Fig. 3A). This cell responded to clicks delivered from each of the 13 frontal positions though, like most cells in the ICC, its best response came from the contralateral half of space (+ azimuths) with a peak at 0°. When speaker B led by 100 msec (ICD = -100 msec), the cell responded to both clicks with an early, weak response to speaker B followed 100 msec later by a

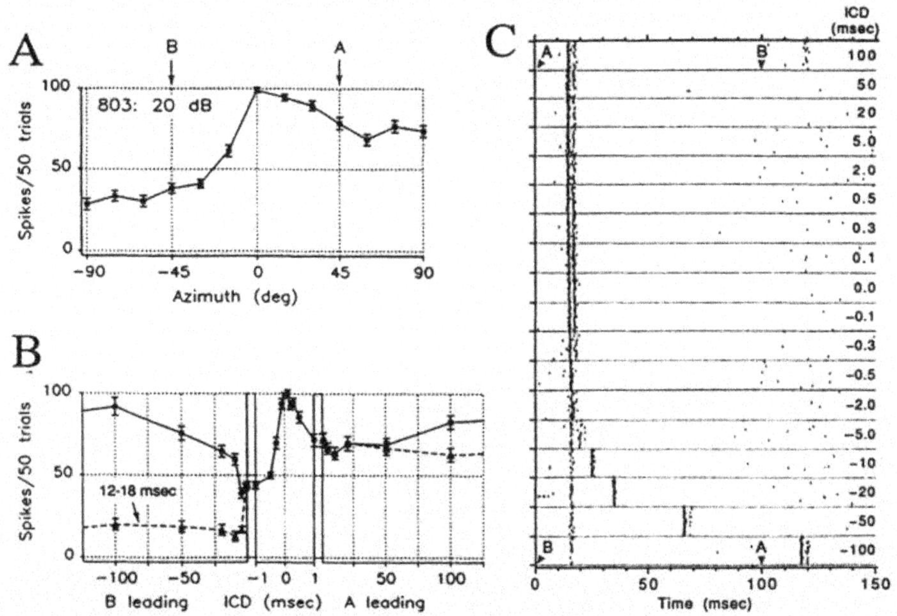

Figure 3. Responses of an ICC cell to single clicks as a function of azimuth (A), and double clicks as a function of ICD (B,C) in the free field. A. Arrows A and B indicate the speaker positions. Error bars in A and B represent ±1 S.E.M. over 50 repetitions. B. The total number of spikes, summed over the leading and lagging time windows is plotted as a function of ICD (full line) and the response to the leading click in the time window 12-18 msec after onset is plotted separately (dotted line). C. The same responses as in B are plotted as dot rasters. The small arrows A and B indicate the time that speakers A and B were activated for the two longest ICDs. CF = 0.8 kHz. (From Yin, 1994).

stronger response to A (Fig. 3C), as expected from the receptive field of the cell (Fig. 3A). As the ICD was shortened, the later response to A gradually became suppressed, while there was no change in the early response to B. Suppression of the response to speaker A was complete for ICDs shorter than 5 msec and its time course (full line) along with the onset response to speaker B (dotted line) are plotted in Fig. 3B. As the ICD is changed from -1 to +1 msec, the response increases reaching a maximum near ICD = 0 msec, which is more apparent in the spike counts (Fig. 3B) than in the dot rasters (Fig. 3C). At these short ICDs, the perceived location of the source moves from B to A, or from -45° to +45°, as the ICDs gradually increase from -1 to +1 msec. If the discharge of the cells is related to the *perceived* location of the sound source, we expect the azimuth axis of the receptive field profile from -45° to +45° to be mapped onto the time axis of the ICD function from -1 to +1 msec. In Fig. 3 this prediction is upheld.

3.2 Response to dichotic stimuli

Similar results were also obtained when we simulated the PE stimuli by delivering a pair of clicks to each ear under dichotic conditions (Fig. 1C). Responses from one cell are

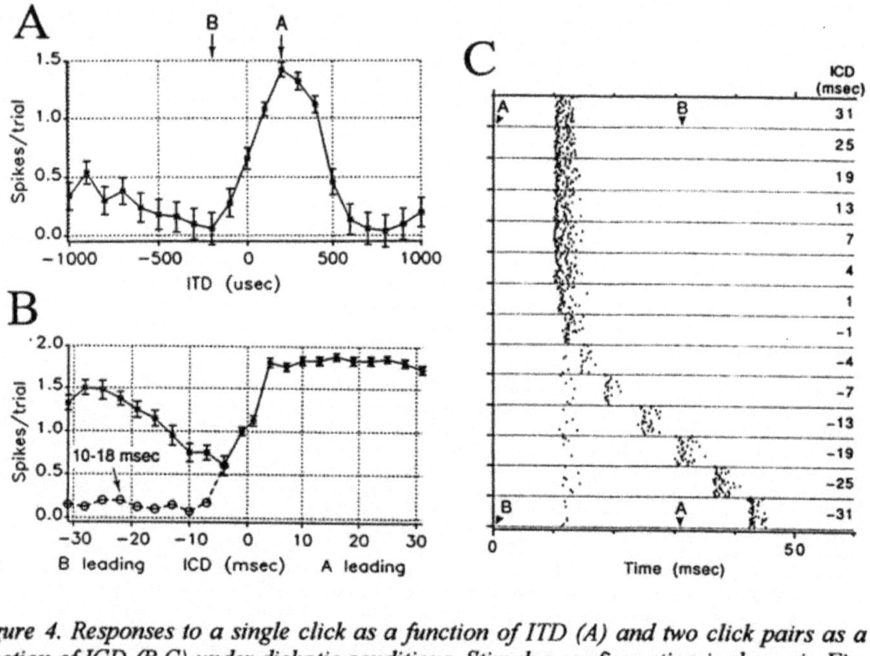

Figure 4. Responses to a single click as a function of ITD (A) and two click pairs as a function of ICD (B,C) under dichotic conditions. Stimulus configuration is shown in Fig. 1C with ITD1 = ITD$_B$ and ITD2 = ITD$_A$, respectively, as indicated by the arrows in A. Otherwise same format as Fig. 3. (From Yin, 1994).

shown in Fig. 4. In this case changes in azimuth were simulated by varying the interaural time difference (ITD). Fig. 4A shows that the cell was sensitive to variations in ITD of a single click pair (one click to each ear) with a maximal discharge for positive ITDs, corresponding to delays of the ipsilateral ear. Figs. 4B and 4C show the responses to two click pairs, with ITD_B = -200 msec and ITD_A = +200 msec, which were the maximal and minimal ITDs. The dot rasters of Fig. 4C show responses that are similar to those seen with free field stimuli. As expected from the cell's sensitivity to ITDs, when ITD_B led (- ICDs), there was a weak response to the leading click and a strong response to the lagging one which was gradually suppressed as the ICDs were shortened. At +ICDs when ITD_A was the leading click pair, there was only a strong onset response with no response to the lagging click even at the longest ICD (31 msec). At the shortest ICDs used (±1 msec) the response to the leading click pair is influenced by the lagging pair: at +1 msec, the response is weaker than that obtained at all other positive ICDs, and at -1 msec, the response was stronger than that expected from the summation of the weak onset response and the suppressed lagging response, indicating that the close proximity of the lagging click pair influences the response to the leading one. We interpret these responses at ±1 msec to be a reflection of summing localization: the response to the leading click pair at short ICDs was weakened when the lagging click was at an unfavorable ITD, which was the case at ICD = +1 msec) and strengthened when the lagging click was at a favorable ITD (ICD = -1 msec).

Several important features of ICC cells are evident in the responses of the two cells in Figs. 2-4. First, during the summing localization period, as ICDs were varied from -1 to +1 msec, the response in Fig. 3 was similar to that obtained when a single click stimulus was varied from -45° to +45°. Even the asymmetric shape of the receptive field in Fig. 3A is reflected in the summing localization response (Fig. 3B). Thus, the cell's response was that expected if the cat experienced summing localization and localized the sound source to a phantom speaker between the two fixed speakers. Second, there was a prominent suppression of the response to the lagging click for both cells when the ICDs were in the range of the psychophysically measured PE ($|ICD| < 10$ msec), though there was a difference between the time course and strength of the suppression in these two cells. In our sample of ICC cells almost all cells exhibited such suppression with considerable variability in its strength and time course. Third, the suppression was stronger when the leading click evoked a strong response.

3.3 Effect of position of the leading click

To explore this last point more thoroughly, we varied the position of the leading click while keeping the lagging click constant. Fig. 5 shows the response of one cell to such an experiment. Responses to single clicks (Fig. 5A, full line), the leading click (Fig. 5A, dotted, dashed lines) and the lagging click (Fig. 5B) as a function of the position of the leading click are shown at several different ICDs. The dot rasters (Fig. 5C) show responses to ICDs of 20 (top) and 10 (bottom) msec. In all cases the lagging speaker was placed at +30°, which is indicated by the arrow in 5A near the point of maximal discharge for single clicks. For ICD of 20 msec, there was little suppression of the lagging click

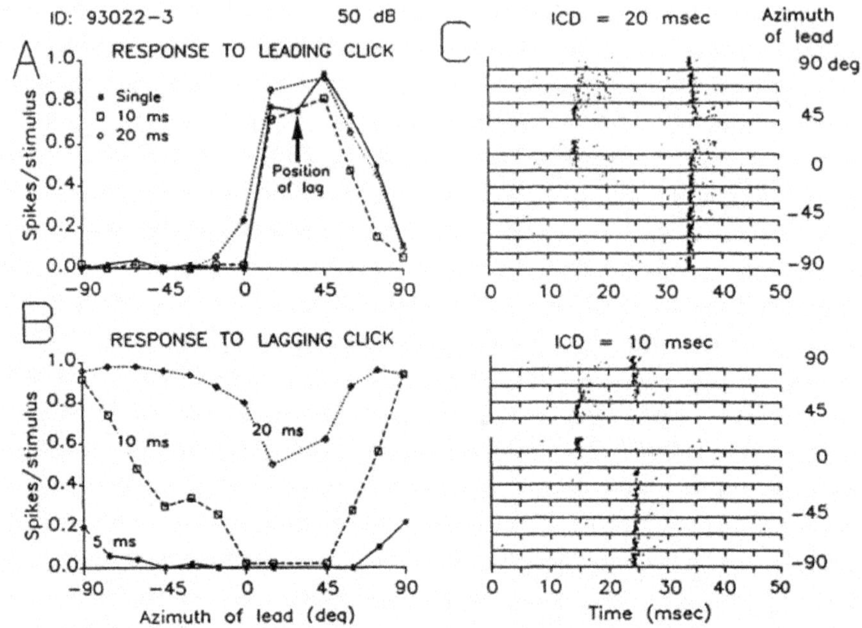

Figure 5. Effect of the position of the leading click on echo suppression. The location of the leading click was varied while holding the lagging click constant. A. Response to the leading click as a function of azimuth for single clicks and double clicks at two different ICDs. B. Response to the lagging click as a function of the position of the leading click at 3 different ICDs. C. Dot rasters of the same responses at two ICDs.

except when the leading click was near +30°. The zone of effective suppression is wider for ICD = 10 msec, with maximal suppression for positions near the leading speaker and with additional suppression at locations that elicit no response to the leading click (0°), and suppression is virtually complete for ICD = 5 msec at all locations. The overlapping curves in Fig. 5A indicate that the response to the leading click is not affected greatly by the presence of the lagging click for these ICDs. Most of the cells studied in this manner were similar to the one shown here in that the maximal suppression was obtained when the leading click was placed at a point of maximal response with a few exceptions in which maximal suppression occurred when the response to the leading click was low.

3.4 Echo suppression on the midsagittal plane

Most psychophysical studies of the PE have used stimuli displaced in the azimuth in which there are interaural differences in time and level, as illustrated above. However, Rakerd and Hartmann (1993) recently reported that such interaural differences are not necessary to produce the PE. To explore this question physiologically, we have used an array of speakers along the midsagittal plane from +90° (above the animal) to -30°. The intersection of the horizontal and vertical array of speakers was the speaker positioned straight ahead of the cat at 0° azimuth and 0° elevation. To compare the relative efficacy of suppression for speakers along azimuth and elevation, we used the common point at (0°,0°) as the lagging speaker. Figure 6 shows dot rasters of the responses as a function of ICD for a leading speaker at +90° azimuth (right) and +75° elevation (left). The positions of the leading speakers were chosen by the similarity in the response of the cell to single clicks at those two locations. It is evident from the dot rasters that nearly identical amounts of suppression are evoked when the leading and lagging speaker are displaced along the horizontal azimuth or vertical elevation. In general most cells tested in this paradigm behaved in a similar manner. Thus, interaural differences are not necessary to produce the echo suppression physiologically or psychophysically.

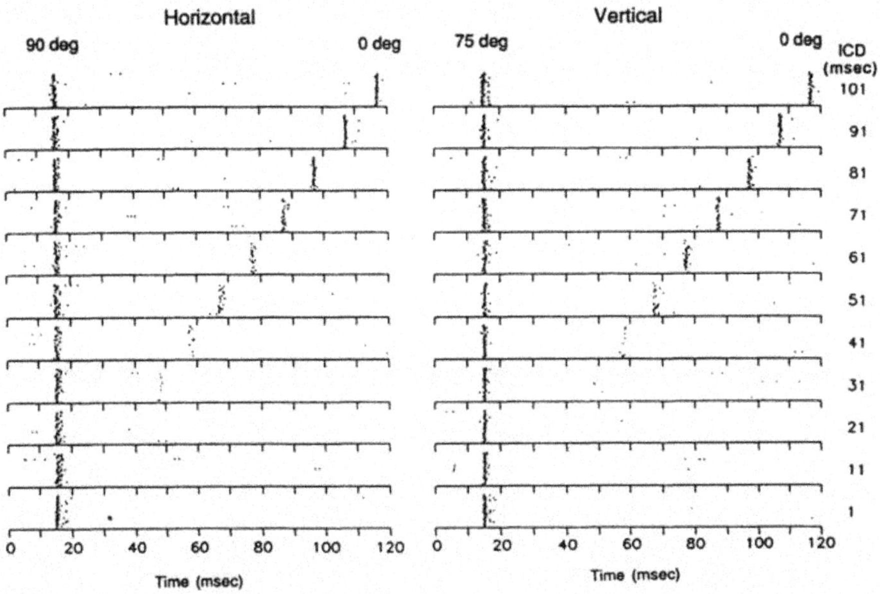

Figure 6. Comparison of the echo suppression evoked in one cell by a leading click on the horizontal and vertical plane. The lagging click was at the speaker directly ahead of the cat. The leading speakers were at +90° azimuth (left) and +75° elevation (right).

4 Discussion

These results represent the first descriptions of physiological responses to PE stimuli and suggest that many physiological correlates of the precedence effect and summing localization are present in the responses of cells in the ICC of the anesthetized cat. Almost all cells tested in the ICC exhibited some form of the echo suppression, though there was considerable variability from cell to cell in the strength and time course. Some cells also responded in a way consonant with summing localization. An important implication of these results is that the discharge of at least some cells in the ICC appears to be related to the perceived location of the sound source and that the cat experiences the PE and summing localization in a manner similar to human subjects (Cranford, 1982).

The suppression of the lagging sound by the presence of a leading one demonstrated in these experiments mirrors the psychophysical effect of the PE in a number of ways. The time course of the suppression is in the range expected from the PE, considering the variability in the population of cells. While a number of cells showed suppression over ICDs very much larger (> 40 msec) than that seen psychophysically, there were nonetheless many cells where complete suppression was not seen until ICDs < 5 msec, which is more similar to psychophysically measured echo thresholds with clicks. Since the psychophysical echo threshold is usually defined as the threshold at which the lagging sound is heard as a distinct source, this would be expected to reflect the shortest echo thresholds seen physiologically, just as the behavioral audiogram is predicted well by the lowest threshold auditory nerve fibers, even in the face of many fibers with much higher thresholds (Elliot et al., 1960; Liberman, 1978). Variations in the relative levels of the leading and lagging clicks also changed the cell's suppressive effect (Fig. 2) in the same manner as that seen psychophysically (Blodgett et al., 1956; Thurlow and Parks, 1961; Babkoff and Sutton, 1966).

From our results we cannot determine the origin of the suppression. In other experiments we have tested for echo suppression in auditory nerve fibers and cochlear nucleus cells. For both of these cell groups the strength of the suppression is markedly weaker than what we see in the ICC, suggesting that the suppression occurs at or above the level of the superior olive. Since suppression was seen even when the leading click did not evoke a response, the suppression cannot be due to an inhibitory recurrent collaterals circuit in the ICC itself.

Our findings of echo suppression for stimuli delivered in the midsagittal plane is consonant with some recent psychophysical tests of the PE in that plane. Rakerd and Hartmann (1993) reported that the echo threshold measured in the midsagittal plane was similar to that seen along the azimuthal plane. These results show that it is not necessary to have interaural differences to produce the PE.

5 Acknowledgements

This work was supported by grants DC00116 and DC00078 from NIH-NIDCD and TW01653 from the NIH Fogarty International Center. Thanks to the staff of the Dept. of Neurophysiology at the University of Wisconsin and of the Vision, Touch and Hearing Research Centre of the University of Queensland.

6 References

Babkoff, H. and Sutton, S. (1966) End point of lateralization for dichotic clicks. J. Acoust. Soc. Am. 39, 87-102.

Blauert, J. (1983) Spatial Hearing. The Psychophysics of Human Sound Localization. The MIT Press, Cambridge, MA.

Blodgett, H.C., Wilbanks, W.A. and Jeffress, L.A. (1956) Effect of large interaural time differences upon the judgement of sidedness. J. Acoust. Soc. Am. 28, 639-643.

Carney, L.H. and Yin, T.C.T. (1989) Responses of low-frequency cells in the inferior colliculus to interaural time differences of clicks: excitatory and inhibitory components. J. Neurophysiol. 62, 144-161.

Cranford, J. L. (1982) Localization of paired sound sources in cats: Effects of variable arrival times. J. Acoust. Soc. Am., 72, 1309-1311.

Elliott, D.N., Stein, L. and Harrison, M.J. (1960) Discrimination of absolute-intensity thresholds and frequency-difference thresholds in cats. J. Acoust. Soc. Am. 32, 380-384.

Gardner, M.B. (1968) Historical background of the Haas and/or precedence effect. J. Acoust. Soc. Am. 43: 1243-1248.

Haas, H. (1951) The influence of a single echo on the audibility of speech. Acoustica 1, 49-58.

Hartmann, W.M. (1983) Localization of sound in rooms. J. Acoust. Soc. Am. 74, 1380-1391.

Henry, J. (1851) Scientific writings of Joseph Henry (Smithsonian Institution, Washington D.C.), Part II, 1847-1878, pp. 295-296.

Liberman, M.C. (1978) Auditory-nerve response from cats raised in a low- noise chamber. J. Acoust. Soc. Am. 63, 442-455.

Rakerd, B. and Hartmann, W.M. (1993) Precedence effect with and without interaural differences - sound localization in three planes. J. Acoust. Soc. Am. 92: 2296 (abstract).

Thurlow, W.R. and Parks, T.E. (1961) Precedence-suppression effects for two click sources. Percep. and Motor Skills 13, 7-12.

Wallach, H., Newman, E.B. and Rosenzweig, M.R. (1949) The precedence effect in sound localization. Amer. J. Psychol. 57, 315-336.

Yin, T.C.T. (1994) Physiological correlates of the precedence effect and summing localization in the inferior colliculus of the cat. J. Neurosci. (in press).

Yost, W.A. and Soderquist, D.R. (1984) The precedence effect: revisited. J. Acoust. Soc. Am. 76, 1377-1383.

Zurek, P.M. (1980) The precedence effect and its possible role in the avoidance of interaural ambiguities. J. Acoust. Soc. Am. 67, 952- 964.

Comment by B. Scharf

How sharply tuned are the units you have been describing?

Reply

All of these recordings were made from the central nucleus of the inferior colliculus. Cells in the ICC are generally narrowly tuned with Q10dB values that are in the range of that seen in the auditory nerve. Thus these cells are not especially narrow or wide in their frequency tuning.

Performance of two models without explicit neuronal delay for binaural localization in the medial superior olive

B.H. Bonham and E.R. Lewis

Department of EECS, University of California
Berkeley, California/94720, USA

1 Introduction

The models of Shamma et al. (1989) and Jeffress (1948) present alternative schemes by which the CNS might use interaural time difference (ITD) to create a map of sound source azimuth. In both models, each element of the map (e.g., each binaural neuron) presents a response amplitude that depends on the azimuth, amplitude and frequency of the stimulus. Furthermore, in both models the computation of the response amplitude of a given map element is based on time delays imposed by the auditory system. It is the principal source of these delays that marks the difference between the models. In the Jeffress model, the sources of the delays are central rather than peripheral to the spiral ganglia (e.g., arising through axonal propagation times). The computation for each map element in this model is carried out through convergence of one monaural channel from each ear, each channel having the same characteristic frequency (CF) but a different time delay. In the Shamma (stereausis) model, the sources of the delays are peripheral to the spiral ganglia; the delays arise in the mechanical operations of the two cochleae. The computation for each map element in this model is carried out through convergence of monaural channels with different CFs.

The Stereausis model has been criticized occasionally for appearing to require convergence of monaural CFs that are too widely separated to be consistent with observed physiology of binaural neurons-- e.g., principal cells of the medial superior olivary nucleus (MSO). Part of the project reported in this paper was dedicated to testing this criticism with the idealized cochlear response functions published by Carney and Yin (1988). These functions are approximations to cochlear impulse responses that were estimated through reverse-correlation (REVCOR) analysis of spike trains from cat auditory nerve fibers responding to acoustic stimuli in the form of broad-band noise.

The remainder of the project reported here was dedicated to analysis of an alternative model for creation of a map of sound-source azimuth based on ITD. As in the maps created by the Jeffress and Shamma models, each element of the map arising from our model presents a response amplitude that depends on the azimuth, amplitude and frequency of the stimulus; and the computation of the response amplitude of a given map element is accomplished through convergence of monaural channels from both ears. As is true of the Jeffress model, the monaural tuning curves of each map element (each binaural neuron) in our model can exhibit identical CFs for the two ears. In our model, however, each of those tuning curves is derived by convergence of a population of neighboring cochlear channels, rather than a single cochlear channel. For each element, the distribution of channels is different for the two ears. This difference endows the element with a specific ITD sensitivity. The distributions also vary from element to element, and this variation provides a full range of ITD sensitivity over the map. The distributions of converging cochlear channels were derived directly and robustly from simulations of the development of afferent connections to the binaural neurons of the map. The simulations were based on Hebbian rules and on the idealized cochlear response functions published by Carney and Yin. It was, in fact, these simulations that led us to the alternative model.

2 The Stereausis Model with Carney-and-Yin Functions

2.1 Methods

The equations for the Carney-Yin model of a single cochlear channel are

$$h_k(t) = 0 \qquad t < t_k$$

$$h_k(t) = (t - t_k)^5 \, e^{-\frac{(t-t_k)}{T_k}} \sin[2\pi f_k (t - t_k)] \qquad t \geq t_k$$

$$t_k = 8.13 \, e^{-\frac{x}{6.44}}$$

$$T_k = 1.3 \, e^{-\frac{x}{2.0}} + 0.4 \, e^{-\frac{x}{15.0}} \tag{1}$$

where $h_k(t)$ is the impulse response of the channel; f_k is the CF of the channel; and x is the location of the cochlear origin of the channel, given in millimeters from the apex of the cochlea. Liberman (1982) gives the following relationship between f_k and distance (d) from the basal end of the cat cochlea:

$$f_k = 0.456\left(10^{0.021(100-d)} - 0.80\right) \tag{2}$$

where d is given as percent of total cochlear length. In our model of the cat cochlea, we assumed a total length of 25 mm:

$$x = 25\left(\frac{100 - d}{100}\right) \tag{3}$$

In our calculations, the impulse responses were normalized to yield constant total energy.

The normalizing factor, A_k, was

$$\tag{4}$$

To test the criticism of the stereausis model, we selected three ipsilateral CFs (500 Hz, 1.0 kHz and 2.0 kHz), five ITDs (0, 100 ms, 200 ms, 300 ms and 350 ms), and four binaural response functions R(·) of the general form

$$R[A_i h_i(t) * I_i(t),\ A_c h_c(t) * I_c(t)]$$

$$I_c(t) = I_i(t - t_d) \tag{5}$$

where the subscript i denotes the ipsilateral channel, c denotes the contralateral channel, I(t) is the input stimulus, t_d is the ITD, and * denotes the convolution operation. We used the following four response functions: (1) cross-correlation of the monaural responses, (2) cross-correlation of the rectified monaural responses, (3) maximum of the sum of the monaural responses, (4) time-difference between the peaks of the two monaural responses. Impulses, broad-band noise, and sinusoids served as stimulus waveforms (sinusoidal responses were presumed to be in steady state).

For impulses and broad-band noise stimuli, the goal of our computations was to identify points along the locus of maximum response (for a given ITD) of binaural elements when those elements are distributed over a plane in which the ordinate of each element is its contralateral CF and the abscissa is its ipsilateral CF. To do so, for each ipsilateral CF and each ITD we computed the contralateral CFs that would maximize response functions 1 to 3 and the contralateral CF that would minimize response function 4. These were taken to be four alternative criteria of maximum response. The realizability of each of them in neural circuitry has been argued in the neural modeling literature and will not be discussed here. For each alternative criterion, the computation was carried out for three ipsilateral CFs and thus yielded three pairs of coordinates (ipsilateral CF, contralateral CF), which we took to lie on the maximum-response locus based on that criterion.

For sinusoidal stimuli, the goal of our computations was to identify the stimulus frequency and ITD for which the abscissa of the maximum response was one of the preselected ipsilateral CFs (500 Hz, 1.0 kHz or 2.0 kHz). The contralateral CF that corresponded to that maximum was noted.

2.2 Results

The four alternative criteria led to very similar results, as did the click and broad-band noise stimuli. Thus results also were similar for the three ipsilateral CFs. Therefore, in this paper, we restrict our presentation to results based on criterion 1 (maximum correlation of the monaural responses) applied to click and tonal stimuli, and to 500 Hz ipsilateral CF. Figure 1a displays the computed points on a plane of constant ipsilateral CF, with ITD as the abscissa. This plot emphasizes the mapping of ITD onto contralateral CF (when the ipsilateral CF is fixed).

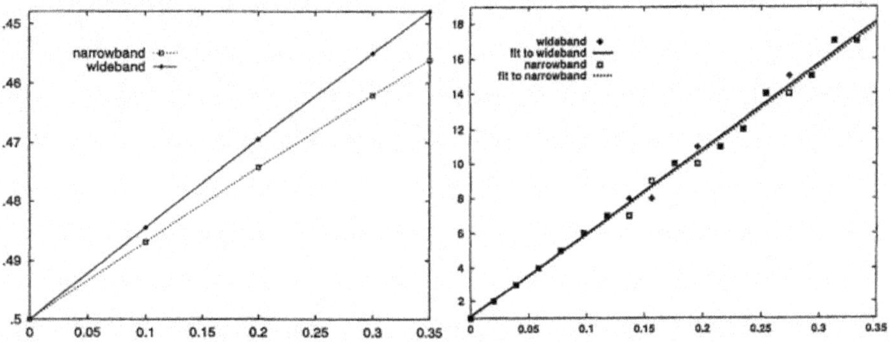

(a) (b)

Figure 1. Binaural elements responding maximally to tonal (narrow-band) and click (wide-band) stimuli. Horizontal axis is ITD (ms). (a) Stereausis model. Elements are identified by contralateral CF (vertical axis in kHz). Ipsilateral CF = 0.5 kHz. (b) Convergence model. Elements are identified by array index (vertical axis). Ipsilateral and contralateral CF = 0.5 kHz.

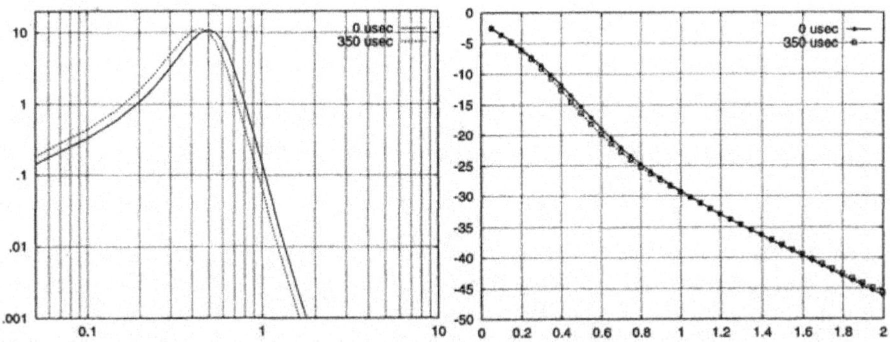

(a) (b)

Figure 2. Stereausis model. Contralateral monaural amplitude (a) and phase (b) response curves for binaural elements that respond maximally to clicks with ITDs of 0 and 350 us. Ipsilateral CF = 0.5 kHz. Horizontal axis is kHz; vertical axis is amplitude in (a) and radians in (b).

Note that, in Figure 1a, the full range of expected ITDs for the cat (0 to 350 ms) is covered by a contralateral CF range of approximately 0.2 octaves of ipsilateral CF. This is within the range of differences observed by Yin and Chan (1990) between ipsilateral and contralateral monaural CFs in binaural cells of the cat MSO. Thus the CF differences required by the Shamma model are consistent with the physiological data. A test of the Shamma model would have been provided by observation of dependence of ITD sensitivity on CF difference. Amplitude and phase responses for the contralateral monaural channels with best responses at ITDs of 0 and 350 ms are shown in Figure 2.

Notice that Figure 1a implies a disparity between the ITD map for click stimuli and that for tonal stimuli. The broad-band noise stimuli yielded the same ITD maps as the click stimuli, and thus the same disparity with respect to the tonal-stimuli maps.

3 A Convergence Model

3.1 Methods

In the developmental model employed here, the right and left monaural receptive fields of each binaural neuron were allowed to organize independently. As in our version of the Shamma model, the cochlea was represented here as an array of linear filters described by the Carney-Yin functions and weighted to have equal energies in response to clicks. Each binaural cell initially received connections (with random synaptic weights) from the outputs of a population of neighboring cochlear filters. Then the cochlear model was excited either by wide-band noise or by random tone pips, and the synaptic weights to the binaural cell were adjusted according to a Hebbian algorithm: the weight for a given filter channel being increased when the response of the binaural cell and the response of the filter were positively correlated, and being decreased otherwise. Both the initial distribution of connections and the final distributions of weights were constrained with respect to cochlear locale by truncated Gaussian density functions with the same mean and standard deviation, the latter ranging from less than 1% to as much as 12% of the cochlear length (see Figures 3a and 3b). The convergence (sum) of cochlear filter outputs in the final (developed) distribution yielded a particular linear monaural filter function for the binaural cell. In spite of the fact that the monaural mappings always comprised convergence of neighboring cochlear channels onto single binaural neurons, the monaural tuning curves of those neurons were not conspicuously less sharp than single-channel cochlear tuning curves (compare Figures 2a and 4a) except for a few of the tuning curves developed from the widest initial distributions.

Repetition of this process with different initial distributions of connections led to different final distributions of weights and different monaural filter functions. The CF of the final filter matched fairly well the CF of the cochlear filter at the center of the Gaussian constraint function. The principal differences among the filters were their phase properties; and each pair of different filter functions for a given CF (when combined and subjected to one of the four criteria of maximum response listed in Section 2.1) yielded a different sensitivity to ITD. This was the way in which we formed the models of binaural neurons in this study - by choosing one monaural filter function, and pairing it with other monaural filter functions with identical CFs (i.e., forcing the monaural CFs to be the same).

Next we ordered the paired filter functions (developed by our algorithm) according to ITD sensitivity (based on criterion 1 of section 2.1, with click stimuli)-- along an axis with a resolution of 20 ms. For the lowest CF, the total ITD range covered by the pairs was considerably greater than the physiological range (0-350 ms) for the cat. Also, a few (20-ms) gaps occurred in the ITD coverage. These tended to be filled as the number of development simulations was increased, but we did not run enough simulations to fill them all. Subsequently, these elements were tested for ITD sensitivity based on each of the criteria of Section 2.1, and for wide-band noise and tonal stimuli.

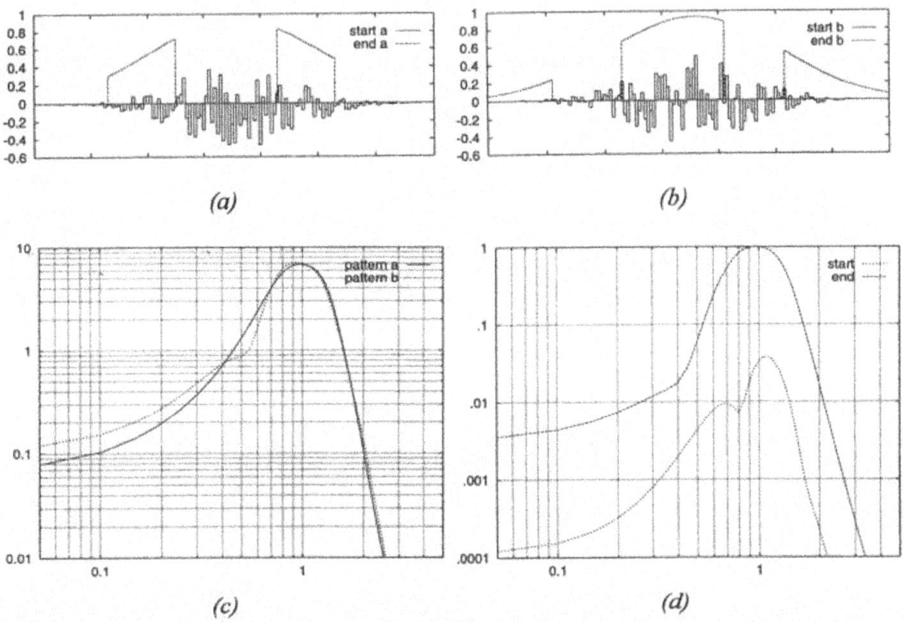

Figure 3. Development of tuning curves in the convergence model. (a) and (b) Initial (solid) and final (dashed) connection weights for two connection patterns that result in monaural responses with similar CF. Horizontal axis is cochlear position, and spans a range of 14% of the total cochlear length; vertical axis is connection weight (density of synapses). (c) Amplitude response curves for final distribution of connections weights in (a) and (b). (d) Amplitude response curves for initial (dotted) and final (dashed) connection weight patterns from another simulation run.

3.2 Results

As was true for the Shamma model, the four alternative criteria led to very similar results, as did the click stimuli and broad-band noise stimuli. Here we present results for criterion 1 - maximum correlation of the monaural responses, and for click and tonal stimuli. Figure 1b displays the computed points on planes of constant CF (both ipsilateral and contralateral), with ITD as the abscissa. Notice that Fig. 1b implies disparity between the ITD map for click stimuli and that for tonal stimuli, but that the disparity is less than that implied by Figure 1a for the Shamma model. Although this difference may favor our model with respect to fidelity of ITD mapping, it does not favor it with respect to its fidelity as a descriptor of the behavior of real binaural neurons. Indeed, it will remain neutral in that regard until there is physiological data concerning disparity in real binaural cells.

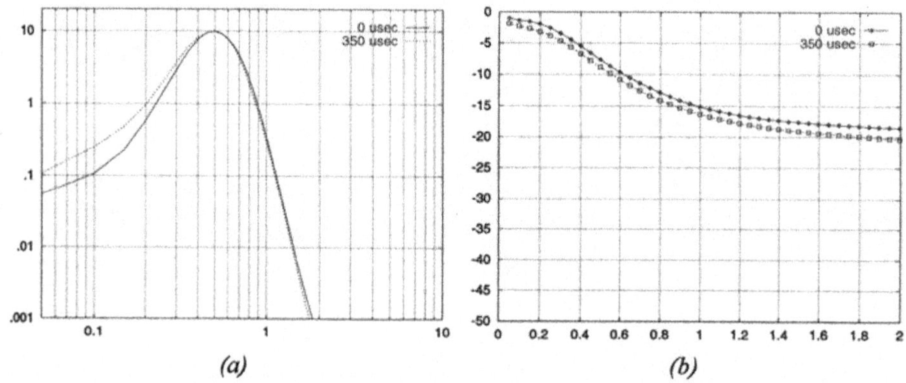

Figure 4. Convergence model. Contralateral monaural amplitude (a) and phase (b) response curves for binaural elements that respond maximally to clicks with ITDs of 0 and 350 us. Ipsilateral and contralateral CF = 0.5 kHz. Horizontal axis is kHz; vertical axis is amplitude in (a) and radians in (b).

4 Discussion

The cochlear delay model as we have implemented it does not incorporate any neuronal delays, but we do not mean to imply by this that neuronal delays are not present. Assuming that both axonal delay and cochlear delay were present, the extent to which each of these was used in the biological system could perhaps be determined by comparing CF-differences of binaural neurons to their best-ITD's. In a regression plot of these two characteristics, no trend (zero slope) would indicate that the system was not using any cochlear delay and was relying entirely on axonal delay. A non-zero slope in one direction would indicate that some cochlear delay was being used. (And a non-zero slope in the opposite direction would indicate that neuronal delay was being used to compensate for excessive cochlear delay, or vice versa!) If there is some convergence of auditory channels with different CF's onto a binaural cell (as in the convergence model), comparison of CF-difference and best-ITD no longer provides a measure of the extent to which neuronal and cochlear delays are used by the system. We have demonstrated that it is possible for a neuron to have non-zero best-ITD while having identical monaural CF's - without the use of specific neuronal delays. While the implementation of the convergence model presented here does not incorporate neuronal delays, the Hebbian algorithm we used would develop binaural cells that had a convergence of auditory channels with different CF's even if neuronal delays were present.

Perhaps the most exciting result of this work, though, is the demonstration that it is possible for a neuron to be actively "tuned" to a specific ITD without requiring modification of myelination, axon length, or properties of synaptic transmission. Instead, this tuning can be accomplished by an activity-dependent process similar to the well-established mechanism of long-term potentiation (LTP). Here we have presented this process as an alternative to the neuronal delay and cochlear delay models for ITD-based localization, but it is equally valuable as a mechanism by which initial inaccuracies in projection of bushy cells to binaural neurons might be counteracted.

5 Acknowledgements

The research reported here was supported by the Office of Naval Research, Grant N00014-91-J-1333 and by the National Institutes of Health, Grant DC00112.

6 References

Carney L.H. and Yin T.C.T. (1988) Temporal coding of resonances by low-frequency auditory nerve fibers: Single-fiber responses and a population model. J Neurophys. 60(5), 1653-77.

Jeffress L.A. (1948) A place theory of sound localization. J. Comp. Phys. Psych. 41, 1.

Liberman M.C. (1990) Effects of chronic cochlear de-efferentation on auditory-nerve response. Hearing Res. 49, 209-24.

Shamma S.A., Shen N. and Gopalaswamy P. (1989) Stereausis: Binaural processing without neural delays. JASA 86(3), 989-1006

Yin T.C.T. and Chan J.C.K., (1990) Interaural time sensitivity in medial superior olive of cat. J. Neurophys. 64(2), 465-88

Comment by P.W.J. van Hengel and H. Duifhuis

If we understand correctly, the Carney-Yin model you use for the impulse response of a single cochlear channel incorporates a delay time ranging from about 0.02 to 0.13 ms. We believe it is essentially wrong to assume a delay in this impulse response. Due to the incompressibility of the cochlear fluid, a stimulus presented at the stapes will immediately be "felt" by all sections of the cochlea, and the response will start without delay. The apparent delay should thus be interpreted as a more gradual onset which can be described by increasing the power 5 in the first term (after proper scaling of the argument).

Reply

Rather than describing the physical processes involved in the transduction of sound to nerve signals, the model of Carney and Yin is an input/output model designed to describe, in a simple manner, their observations of REVCOR-derived impulse responses. We chose the model because of this, and because of its ease of implementation.

Comment by Scharf

Of relevance to the question of just how different monaural CFs that converge on binaural units can be, I remind you of experiments showing that listeners can discriminate interaural onset time differences even when the frequencies to the two ears differ as much as a critical band (Scharf et al., 1976; Buus et al., 1984).

Scharf, B., Florentine, M., & Meiselman, C. H. (1976) Critical bandwidth in lateralization. Sensory Processes 1, 109-126

Buus, S., Scharf, B., & Florentine, M. (1984) Lateralization and frequency selectivity in normal and impaired hearing. J. Acoust. Soc. Amer. 76, 77-86

Comment by T. Yin

There are several features of the cochlear delay model that still appear to contradict existing physiological and anatomical data. First, Fig. 1A shows that the ITD at which the maximum response is obtained for wideband stimuli can differ from that for a pure tone by a considerable amount at large ITDs and furthermore it appears to deviate in a systematic direction, with maxima for tones peaking at higher IDTs. Our limited data from the MSO and our more considerable data from the inferior colliculus (Yin, Chan and Irvine, 1986) do not show large differences in the peaks of ITD curves for tones and noise, nor any systematic difference. Second, anatomical data on the projections of spherical bushy cells to the MSO of the cat show clear evidence for delay lines on the contralateral, but not the ipsilateral, side (Smith, Joris and Yin, 1993). All of the other relevant anatomical data, which come from studies in the chicken (Young and Rubel, 1983) and in the owl (Carr and Konishi, 1990), also show clear evidence for delay lines. Thus it does not seem parsimonious to propose that the auditory system uses cochlear delays when neural conduction delays are present.

With regard to the convergence model, there is also no evidence from the anatomical data of projections to the MSO that show the discontinuities seen in Fig. 3.

Carr, C.E., and Konishi, M. (1990). A circuit for detection of interaural time differences in the brainstem of the barn owl, J. Neurosci. 10, 3227-3246

Smith, P.H., Joris, P.X., and Yin, T.C.T. (1993). Projections of physiologically characterized spherical bushy cell axons from the cochlear nucleus of cat: evidence for delay lines to the medial superior olive, J. Comp. Neurol. 331, 245-260

Yin, T.C.T., Chan, J.C.K., and Irvine, D.R.F. (1987). Effects of interaural time delays of noise stimuli on low-frequency cells in the cat's inferior colliculus. I. Responses to wide-band noise, J. Neurophysiol. 58, 562-583

Young, S.R., and Rubel, E.W. (1983). Frequency-specific projections of individual neurons in chick brainstem auditory nuclei, J. Neurosci. 3, 1373-1378

Reply

With regard to the cochlear delay model:

The discrepancy in best-ITD's for tones and wideband noise that we have presented here is for the limiting case, in which no neuronal delays are present. For the opposite limiting case, in which only neuronal delays are used, no discrepancy in best-ITD would be observed. If both neuronal delays and cochlear delays were used, then the discrepancy in best-ITD's of a neuron for tones and for wideband noise would be less than those we have presented here, but still not zero. For formation of a map of ITD in the MSO, the neuronal delay model requires that there be a monotonic increase of the difference in the conduction times from the two ears. In its simplest form, this requires that delays to neurons from one ear (e.g., contralateral) be progressively longer, while delays to neurons from the other ear be monotonic (e.g., progressively shorter, Jeffress, 1948, or all exactly the same, Yin & Chan, 1990, Overholt, Rubel, & Hyson, 1992). Progressively longer axons from the contralateral ear appear to exist in barn owl, cat, and chick. A monotonic pattern of axon length from the ipsilateral ear appears to exist in the barn owl (Carr & Konishi, 1990). As far as we can see, published anatomical data show no evidence of monotonic pattern of axon length from the ipsilateral ear in the cat (Smith, Joris, & Yin, 1993) or in the chick (Overholt, Rubel & Hyson, 1992).

With regard to the convergence model:

The pattern of connections shown in Figure 3 describes the source of cochlear input to one side of an MSO neuron. This comprises both convergence/divergence onto bushy cells in the AVCN from the eighth nerve and convergence/divergence onto MSO cells from the bushy cells. I think that to truly identify the existence or absence of pattern discontinuities in the biological system like those exhibited by the model, it would be necessary to inject an MSO neuron with a trans-synaptic retrograde tracer and identify the exact positions in the cochlea that contribute input to the MSO neuron. Unfortunately, even this experiment may not totally illuminate the question of convergence for two reasons. First, some of our simulations (those with a narrow initial region of cochlear input to the developing MSO neuron) resulted in very closely spaced discontinuities and very narrow gaps, sometimes less than one percent of the cochlear length (less than 1/10 octave). Second, the exact pattern of synaptic densities that produces a tuning curve with a particular delay (or phase at CF) is not unique. The discontinuities evident in Figure 3 are a characteristic of our specific implementation of the Hebbian development algorithm; a different implementation would produce different patterns that would not necessarily exhibit discontinuities.

Overholt, E.M., Rubel, E.W., Hyson, R.L. (1992) A circuit for coding interaural time differences in the chick brainstem. J. Neurosci. 12, 1698-1708

Carr, C.E., and Konishi, M. (1990). A circuit for detection of interaural time differences in the brainstem of the barn owl, J. Neurosci. 10, 3227-3246

Smith, P.H., Joris, P.X., and Yin, T.C.T. (1993). Projections of physiologically characterized spherical bushy cell axons from the cochlear nucleus of cat: evidence for delay lines to the medial superior olive, J. Comp. Neurol. 331, 245-260

What do dichotic pitch phenomena tell us about binaural hearing ?

F. A. Bilsen

Perceptual Acoustics Lab., Applied Physics Department, Delft University of Technology P.O. Box 5046, 2600 GA Delft, The Netherlands

1 Introduction

Dichotic pitch phenomena have influenced our thinking about binaural interaction significantly. For as far as dichotic pitch values were concerned, Bilsen (1972) and Bilsen and Goldstein (1974) showed that the similarity of dichotic and monotic repetition pitch with the low-pitch of normal periodic signals (Houtsma and Goldstein, 1972) requires the existence of centrally generated spectral patterns with resolved (lower) harmonics. From such spectral patterns pitch is extracted by pattern recognition (Bilsen, 1977).

Later experiments on the lateralization of dichotic-pitch images for Huggins pitch (HP), Fourcin pitch (FP) and MPS-pitch (Raatgever and Bilsen, 1977; Raatgever, 1980) revealed that these pitch images behave like pure "time images" as postulated by Hafter and Jeffress (1968) for lateralized signals. This led us to conclude that, for wide band signals, the time image is the result of spectral-pattern recognition in which frequency information is pooled across frequency for particular interaural delays. Based on the Jeffress (1948) scheme, a Central Spectrum (CS) theory of binaural processing was developed (Bilsen, 1977; Raatgever and Bilsen, 1986) that stresses both interaural cross correlation and central spectrum recognition. Recently, the related concept of "straightness" was introduced by Stern and Trahiotis (1991).

Historically, it is remarkable that dichotic repetition pitch (DRP) triggered our thinking about central spectra (Bilsen, 1972; Bilsen and Goldstein, 1974), whereas it (still) is the dichotic pitch phenomenon that is not easily explained by the CS-theory in its present form. Recently, we discovered that DRP, contrary to the other dichotic pitch phenomena mentioned above, can be lateralized by means of an interaural level difference (ILD), though with a remarkable left-right asymmetry. This will be elaborated in the following sections. First, however, we will present new results of pitch matchings to reconfirm the older results, to determine the existence region, and to exclude the possibility of trivial cross-talk in the generation of DRP.

2 Properties of dichotic repetition pitch

2.1 Confirmation and extension of earlier results

Dichotic repetition pitch (DRP) can be heard if white noise is presented through headphones to the left and right ear of an observer with an interaural time delay (ITD) in the range of about 3 ms to 20 ms. The original results of DRP-matching experiments (Bilsen, 1972; Bilsen and Goldstein, 1974) have been confirmed in the past by Warren et al. (1981) and more recently by Hartmann (1993). All authors agree that DRP is difficult to hear. Warren et al. (1981) state: "This dichotic pitch is very difficult to hear, unlike monaural or diotic echo (repetition) pitch with the same delay periods, which is heard readily even by unpracticed listeners."

Other investigators, e.g. Fourcin (1970), have denied the existence of DRP. The present author always has had the impression that DRP is indeed a faint phenomenon, but that it is the problem of "finding" the pitch image in the head (separate from the diffuse noise image) and its low salience rather than the accuracy of pitch matchings. In order to reconcile these conflicting reports we started experiments to measure the existence region more precisely than we did before, to determine the accuracy of pitch matchings, and to look for conditions in which DRP was more difficult (or more easily?!) to perceive.

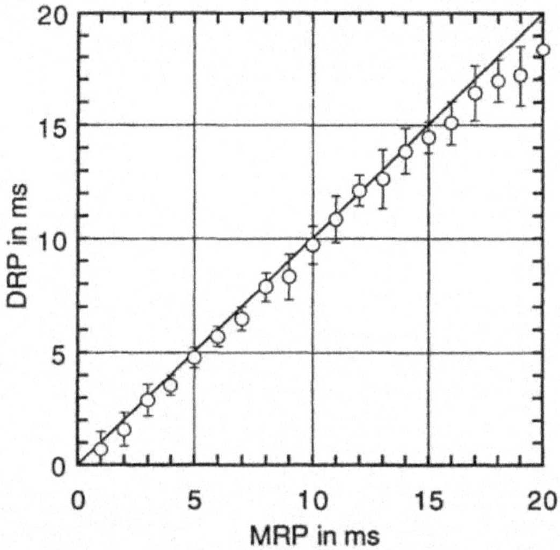

Figure 1. ITD (DRP) in ms matched against T (MRP) in ms for equal pitch.

Experiments were performed in which 3 subjects took part (For experimental details see section 4.1). They were instructed to match the pitch of a diotically presented MRP-stimulus (fixed time delay T) to a DRP by adjusting the ITD of the DRP-stimulus. They had 6 knobs to control three different in- and decrements in ITD, viz. ±1, ±0.1, and ±0.02 ms; they could switch between DRP and MRP at will. Each subject made 5 adjustments for each T (=1, 2, to 20 ms). The averaged results for all subjects are presented in Fig. 1. Similar matchings were performed with T adjustable and ITD fixed. These were judged less comfortable by the subjects, but appeared to give similar results. The solid line has been drawn through the origin under 45 degrees of arc. Though there seems to be a small deviation towards lower ITD values, the relation DRP=MRP appears to be confirmed.

The relative standard deviation, s(ΔITD)/ITD, from 15 matchings for each measured point is displayed in Fig. 2. The results clearly show that DRP can be matched with reasonable precision. The higher boundary of the existence region of DRP seems well determined by the steep decrease in matching accuracy for ITD=2 ms. The lower boundary is more diffuse. In fact DRP gradually changes into a periodicity sensation, called Infrapitch by Warren et al. (1981).

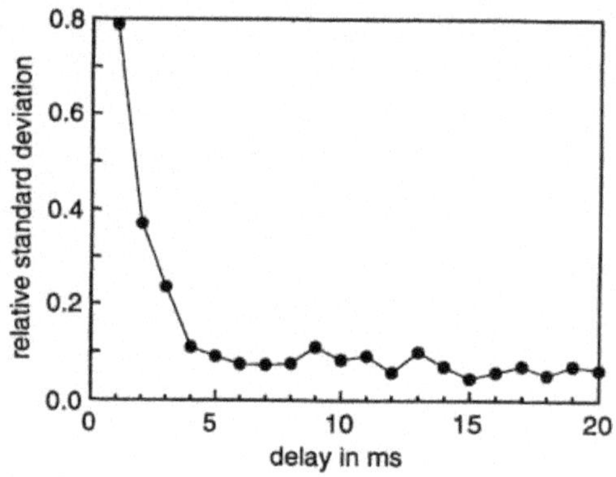

Figure 2. The relative standard deviation derived from the results of figure 1.

2.2 Arguments against cross-talk

It has been argued that DRP might be caused by a trivial form of interaural cross talk, e.g. bone conduction or air conduction, because: a) it sounds very similar to its monotic counter part (monotic repetition pitch); it has the same low pitch and the same timbre, b) it is probably the faintest dichotic pitch known, c) it behaves different from other dichotic pitch phenomena. One could imagine that the (un)delayed noise is fed to the contralateral ear by bone conduction or by cross-talk through a leaking headphone, thus producing a faint MRP in the left and/or right ear.

The following arguments and results of pilot experiments, however, exclude the possibility of an artefact by trivial cross-talk:

1) The DRP can be perceived and matched rather accurately at low over-all sensation levels. Even at a sensation level as low as 5 dB our subjects were able to match DRP to MRP. Such a result would be explainable by cross-talk only if cross-talk would be unrealistically strong. In audiology it is common practice to reckon with a rather low interaural cross-talk (40 to 50 dB),

2) If the signal to the left or right ear is attenuated with respect to the contralateral ear,

cross-talk, if effective, might result in different MRP's at the left and right ear. Attenuation of the undelayed signal might give rise to an MRP in the corresponding ear because the (delayed) signal from the contralateral ear will interfere optimally with the attenuated (undelayed) signal. In that case, however, one would expect a pitch lateralized to the undelayed ear and corresponding to ITD+ΔITD with ΔITD being the extra-interaural delay due to cross-talk. With the attenuation in the opposite channel, the pitch would correspond to ITD-ΔITD and it would be lateralized to the opposite ear. Such behaviour, however, has not been observed.

3) Possible cross-talk in the apparatus can be checked by measuring autocorrelation functions or (comb) spectra for the left and right ear signal. In our case the signals appeared to be perfectly white.

3 DRP and the central spectrum theory

The central spectrum (CS) theory was developed as a simplified analytical model for the processing of interaural delay or phase differences for low-frequency (<1500 Hz) signals. Following the Jeffress (1948) scheme of binaural interaction, filtered cochlear signals from one ear are added along internal (neural) tapped-delay lines to the undelayed signals from corresponding cochlear outputs of the contralateral ear. After squaring, a continuum arises of power (mimicking neural activity) versus frequency and internal delay, the so-called central activity pattern (CAP).

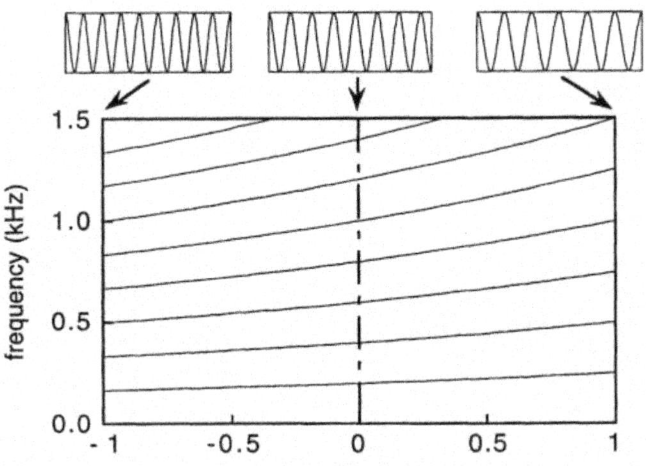

Figure 3. The CAP of DRP for ITD=T= 5ms. Only lines of maximum activity (P=2) have been plotted. At the top of the figure, central spectra are given for three different cross sections.

For a dichotic signal with an interaural phase function $\Phi(f)$, the CAP is shown (Raatgever and Bilsen, 1986) to be equal to

$$P(f,\tau_i) = 1 + \cos\{\Phi(f) - 2\pi f\tau_i\} \quad (1)$$

where f is frequency and τ_i is the internal delay along the (cross-correlation) time axis. For a DRP-signal with ITD = T the CAP takes the form:

$$P(f,\tau_i) = 1 + \cos\{2\pi f(T - \tau_i\} \quad (2)$$

As an example of the CAP illustrative for DRP, curves of maximum activity (P=2) have been plotted in Fig. 3 for T=5 ms.

In the CS-theory, the central spectrum corresponding to the perceived pitch is given by the cross-section of the CAP at the internal delay τ_i =0 (dash-dotted line) which corresponds to the perceived position of the DRP-image. From Eq.(2) and Fig. 3 it might be clear that he DRP-value is correctly predicted. However, one should wonder why all the other candidate harmonic spectra at the other internal delays cannot be heard. Is the DRP the result of another mechanism, or is DRP the result of averaging central spectra across internal delay?

4 Lateralization of DRP

4.1 Experimental set-up

DRP-stimuli derived from lowpass-filtered gaussian noise with a high-cutoff frequency of 2300 Hz, were generated in a digital signal processor (Loughborough DSP 96002; sample frequency 25 kHz; (program) code generated by a Comdisco SPW system). Thus a dichotic stimulus (see simplified block diagram in Fig. 4) with an ITD and

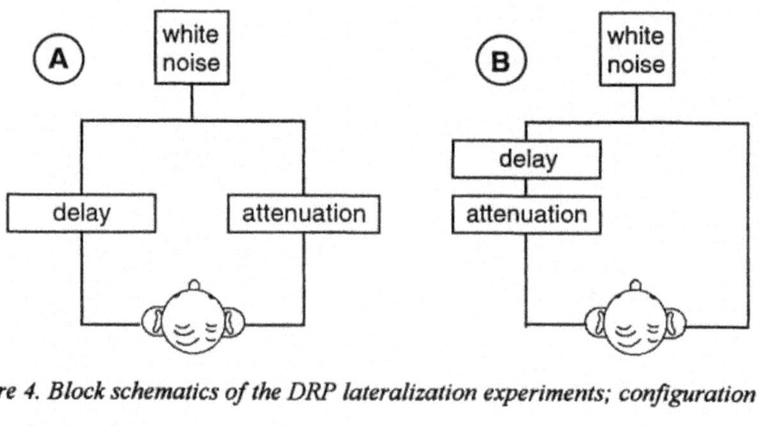

Figure 4. Block schematics of the DRP lateralization experiments; configuration A and B.

an ILD in either the same (configuration B) or the opposite-ear signal channel (configuration A) was obtained.

In order to have a comfortable perception of DRP the ITD was programmed such that an 8 note equally-tempered musical scale was played ranging from C (130.8 Hz; ITD=7.65 ms) to c (261.6 Hz; ITD=3.82 ms) with a stimulus duration of 1 second for each note; the noise itself was not switched on and off but was present continuously. The musical scale was played repeatedly, each time with a particular ILD in a range of 0 to 20 dB. For each ILD, the subject, seated in a sound proof booth and listening with headphones (Beyer DT 770) at a sensation level of about 40 dB, had to indicate the in-head position of the DRP-melody image on a linear scale ranging from -5 (left ear position) to +5 (right ear position) with 0 center position (compare Blauert, 1983, for standard lateralization procedures).

4.2 Results

Two experienced subjects participated in this experiment, in a total of four separate sessions for each subject: two sessions with configuration A of which one with left and right headphones interchanged to average out a possible bias in perceived lateralization, and the same for configuration B. Their averaged results are presented in Fig. 5; thus each measured point is the average of four observations.

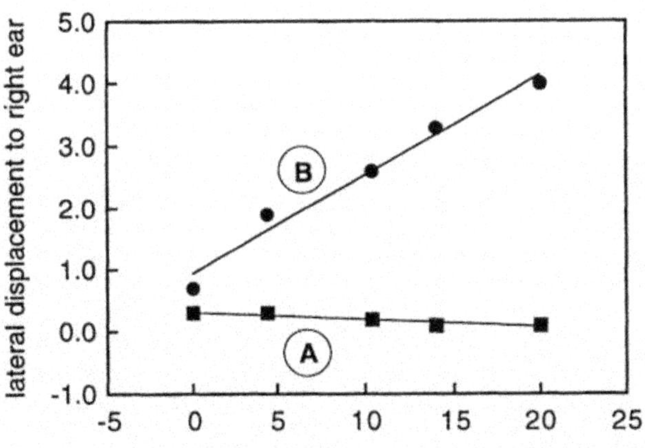

Figure 5. DRP-lateralization results for configurations A and B.

It was reported by the subjects that the DRP-image did not move within a scale, thus it was confirmed that the value of T seems to have no influence on the position of DRP. They also reported that the DRP was experienced more salient for ILD 10 dB than for 0 dB.

4.3 Discussion

The results of Fig. 5 are very remarkable because of their asymmetry. Configuration A hardly shows any shift in DRP-position with changing ILD, whereas configuration B shows a substantial shift with changing ILD. In the latter case, the relation between perceived position and ILD is about comparable to the function one observes for the lateralization of diotic noise with changing ILD (Blauert, 1983). A simple explanation for this asymmetry could not be found.

An explanation by the advocate of the devil stressing cross-talk clearly fails. If simple cross talk (by air or bone conduction) were to play a significant role, one would expect the strongest DRP in the ear provided with the attenuated signal, because the intensity of delayed and undelayed signal are more equal than in the unattenuated ear, thus providing the best-modulated comb spectrum and consequently the strongest MRP in the attenuated ear. In case B one thus would expect lateralization towards the attenuated ear. However, one observes the opposite.

5 General discussion

Dichotic repetition pitch (DRP) is a faint binaural pitch phenomenon, evoked by the interaural delay of a single (white) noise signal. It appears not to be an artefact due to trivial interaural cross-talk. It has been shown in the past that its pitch behaviour provides evidence for a central-spectrum processing of pitch, rather than cross-correlation processing for which (according to Fourcin) two uncorrelated noise sources would be required. Nevertheless, as discussed in section 3, DRP-extraction is still not fully understood. The present experiments were intended to get further understanding of the binaural processes involved.

The present results on the accuracy of DRP matchings show that its existence region is sharply limited to ITD's larger than 2 ms, whereas the lower border is more diffuse and extends into the region of rattle- or infra-pitch. This is not unexpected since the lateralization of binaural signals in general is limited to ITD's smaller than 1 ms. Note that the CS-concept correspondingly has no need for (neural) internal delays longer than say 1 ms.

In former papers, it has been shown that the dichotic-pitch images of HP, FP, and MPS can be lateralized by an (extra) ITD. The lateralization shows great similarity with the behaviour of the time image. ILD's, on the contrary, are ineffective in lateralizing these dichotic pitches; they only affect their salience. In the present paper, it is shown that, of course, an extra ITD does not influence the lateralization of DRP (How would the binaural system, for a change in ITD, be able to discriminate between a change in pitch and a change in lateralization?). However, for DRP, ILD's are effective in lateralizing the pitch image, be it in an asymmetric way and with an unexpected increase in salience for ILD's in the order of 10 dB.

The final tempting conclusion, thus, should be that there are two separate mechanisms: a mechanism to evaluate ITD's and a mechanism to evaluate ILD's. DRP could very well be the product of the ILD-mechanism exclusively, contrary to HP, FP and

MPS that are clear exponents of the ITD-mechanism.

6 Acknowledgements

The experiments described in section 2 were performed by Han Dols in fulfilment of his master's thesis. Thanks go to the subjects JR, HD and FB for their persistence.

7 References

Bilsen, F.A. and Goldstein, J.L. (1974) Pitch of dichotically delayed noise and its possible spectral basis. J.Acoust. Soc. Am. 55, 292-296.

Bilsen, F.A. (1972) Pitch of dichotically delayed noise. In: E. de Boer, B.L. Cardozo and R. Plomp (Eds.), Hearing Theory 1972, I.P.O., Eindhoven, the Netherlands, pp. 5-8.

Bilsen, F.A. (1976) Pronounced binaural pitch phenomenon. J. acoust. Soc. Am. 59, 467-468.

Bilsen, F.A. (1977) Pitch of noise signals: Evidence for a "central spectrum". J. Acoust. Soc. Am. 61, 150-161.

Blauert, J. (1983) Spatial Hearing. MIT Press, Cambridge, U.S.A..

Cramer, E.M. and Huggins, W.H. (1958) Creation of pitch through binaural interaction. J. Acoust. Soc. Am. 30, 413-417.

Fourcin, A.J. (1970) Central pitch and auditory lateralization. In: R. Plomp and G.F. Smoorenburg (Eds.), Frequency Analysis and Periodicity Detection in Hearing, Sijthoff, the Netherlands, pp. 319-328.

Hafter, E.R. and Jeffress, L.A. (1968) Two image lateralization of tones and clicks. J. Acoust. Soc. Am. 44, 563-569.

Hartmann, W.M. (1993) Personal communication.

Houtsma, A.J.M. and Goldstein, J.L. (1972) The central origin of the pitch of complex tones: Evidence from musical interval recognition. J. Acoust. Soc. Am. 51, 520-529.

Jeffress, L.A. (1948) A place theory of sound localization. J. Comp. Physiol. 41, 35-39.

Klein, M.A. and Hartmann, W.M. (1981) Binaural edge pitch. J. Acoust. Soc. Am. 70, 51-61.

Raatgever, J. and Bilsen, F.A. (1977) Lateralization and dichotic pitch as a result of spectral pattern recognition. In: E.F. Evans and J.P. Wilson (Eds.), Psychophysics and Physiology of Hearing, Academic, London, pp. 443-453.

Raatgever, J. (1980) Binaural time processing and time-intensity trading. In: G. van den Brink and F.A. Bilsen (Eds.), Psychophysics, Physiology and Behavioural Studies in Hearing, D.U.Press, Delft, the Netherlands, pp. 425-428.

Raatgever, J. and Bilsen, F.A. (1986) A central spectrum theory of binaural processing. Evidence from dichotic pitch. J. Acoust. Soc. Am. 80, 429-441.

Stern, R.M. and Trahiotis, C. (1991) The role of consistency of interaural timing over frequency in binaural lateralization. In: Y. Cazals, K. Horner and L. Demany (Eds.), Auditory Physiology and Perception, Pergamon, Oxford, pp.547-554.

Warren, R.M., Bashford, J.A. and Wrightson, J.M. (1981) Detection of long interaural delays for broadband noise. J. Acoust. Soc. Am. 69, 1510-1514.

Comment by J. Culling

A distinction must be made between across-frequency grouping and across-frequency integration. The former groups frequency channels sharing common features which are likely to be associated with a common sound-source. The latter gathers channels together indiscriminately. Stern & Trahiotis (1991) demonstrated across-frequency integration of interaural timing information in lateralization, but Culling and Summerfield (1994) found no evidence of across-frequency *grouping* by common interaural delay in a speech identification task. Conventional models of binarual masking release simply detect frequency channels which display interaural decorrelation and can explain Huggins-pitch, MPS-pitch and binaural edge pitch without using across-frequency grouping. Why, therefore, is it necessary to invoke across-frequency grouping (as described in the spoken presentation) in order to explain these phenomena?

Culling, J.F. and Summerfield, Q. (1994) Proceedings of 127th Meeting of the Acoustical Society of America.

Reply

I agree that conventional models like the EC-model can explain Huggins pitch, or generally: the generation of "central spectrum peaks". But, in order to correctly predict both the low-pitch and its (lateralized) image of e.g. MPS, we postulated a mechanism that "takes together" (groups, not integrates) the CS-peaks at the proper common internal delay. We did not study or encounter dichotic low-pitch phenomena inconsistent with that view so far.

A new approach to study binaural interaction at high frequencies

A. Kohlrausch, S. v. d. Par, A. J. M. Houtsma

Institute for Perception Research (IPO)
P.O. Box 513, 5600 MB Eindhoven, The Netherlands

1 Introduction

The fact that the auditory system receives input from two receivers which have some spatial separation forms the main basis for our ability to localize sound sources. Depending on the direction of the source, the input signals at the two eardrums show interaural differences in time and amplitude as well as in spectral detail. Besides helping in localization, these two receivers help in the perceptual separation of auditory events if they originate from differently located sources.They also allow detection of signals at a lower signal-to-noise ratio than when someone is listening with only one ear (e.g., Bronkhorst and Plomp, 1988).

In the laboratory this latter ability is studied in masking experiments leading to a Binaural Masking Level Difference (BMLD). In a typical BMLD condition, the subject listens through headphones to a noise masker which is identical in the right and the left ear (No). The test signal to be detected is a sinusoid that has an interaural phase difference of 180 degrees (Sπ). In such a condition, the masked threshold (i.e., the level of the test signal at its threshold) can be more than 15 dB below the value in a reference condition without an interaural phase difference (So).

It has already been observed at a very early stage that the BMLD seems to be a low-frequency phenomenon (Hirsh, 1948). More specifically, if the masker is a broadband noise, the BMLD decreases for higher signal frequencies and amounts to no more than 3 dB above 2 kHz (Colburn and Durlach, 1978). This observation was explained with the decrease of phase locking in auditory nerve fibers above about 1 kHz. As pointed out, for instance by Durlach (1964), this loss of fine-structure information destroys the cues based on interaural time differences. What remain are rapidly fluctuating interaural intensity differences, which result in the 3-dB improvement at high frequencies.

This view was changed by a series of experiments which demonstrated that interaural time differences could be used quite well at high frequencies for lateralization as well as for detection (e.g., Henning, 1974; McFadden and Pasanen, 1978). The important new aspect was that the authors of these experiments used high-frequency stimuli with a narrow bandwidth, either amplitude-modulated sinusoids or narrowband noise with a typical bandwidth of 50 Hz. The envelopes of these stimuli fluctuated at a low rate, since the rate of envelope fluctuation is limited to approximately half the bandwidth of the signals. Thus, interaural time differences can be utilized at high frequencies if they are conveyed through differences in the envelopes.

The combined effects of signal frequency and masker bandwidth on the BMLD can be summarized as follows: In a broadband noise masker, the BMLD has a maximum of about 15 dB around 300 Hz. Towards higher frequencies, it decreases rapidly and is only about 3 dB above 2 kHz. In a narrowband masker, the low-frequency BMLD is even larger and can amount to 24 dB (Metz et al., 1968). Towards higher frequencies, the value decreases somewhat, but for a noise 50 Hz wide centered at 4 kHz, it still amounts to 10-15 dB (McFadden and Pasanen, 1978; Zurek and Durlach, 1987; Bernstein and Trahiotis, 1992a). Besides the loss of fine structure, the increase of the critical bandwidth with frequency has been discussed as a possible source for the decrease of the BMLD at high frequencies. As mentioned above, the maximum rate of envelope fluctuation in a bandpass signal is proportional to the bandwidth of the signal. Therefore, the maximum rate of envelope fluctuation within one auditory filter is higher at a high center frequency compared with a low-frequency filter. This also results in an increasing rate of fluctuation of interaural time and intensity differences in the envelope of high-frequency auditory channels of broadband signals. It has been concluded from several binaural experiments that the hearing system is not able to evaluate such fast fluctuations efficiently (Grantham and Wightman, 1979; Zurek and Durlach, 1987; Bernstein and Trahiotis, 1992a).

A new approach to investigate BMLDs at high frequencies was introduced by Bernstein and Trahiotis (1992a). They related the BMLD to changes in interaural cross-correlation rather than worrying about whether in the BMLD task the listener's decision is based on the statistics of interaural amplitude or time differences. Since their signals were centered at 4 kHz, they could not use the classical full-waveform correlation measure (e.g., Durlach et al., 1986), because the fine structure is not coded in the neural activity. Instead, they calculated the interaural correlation as correlation of the *envelopes*. As a general law valid for many conditions relevant in this context, they found that the correlation of the envelopes is approximately the square of the full-waveform correlation. With this measure, the high-frequency $NoS\pi$ thresholds could be predicted by the listener's sensitivity to changes in interaural correlation of the resulting envelopes.

The rationale for the present study is closely related to this way of reasoning. We derive the stimulus envelope for a high-frequency masking condition (thereafter called transposed stimulus) from the half-wave rectified version of a low-frequency reference condition. After the first steps of peripheral transduction (corresponding to the output of the inner hair cell) the interaural correlation of the envelope (for the high-frequency transposed stimulus) will have the same value as the full-waveform correlation of the (rectified) low-frequency reference. If the sensitivity to interaural differences is the same at low and high frequencies (as assumed for the sensitivity to interaural time differences by Colburn and Esquissaud, 1976) and our modelling of the peripheral transduction is sufficiently exact, the BMLD for the transposed signal condition should be of an amount similar to that for a standard low-frequency condition.

2 Method

2.1 Threshold procedure

Masked thresholds were determined using a 3-Interval Forced-Choice procedure with adaptive level adjustment. The three masker intervals of 400 ms duration were separated by pauses of 200 ms. In one interval, a 300-ms signal was added temporally centered in the masker interval. The subject had to indicate which of the three intervals contained the signal. The signal level was adjusted following a two-down one-up rule (Levitt, 1971). The step size for level changes was 8 dB in the beginning of each run. It was reduced after each second reversal of the signal level by a factor two, until a step size of 1 dB was reached. A run was extended over 14 reversals. The first six reversals were discarded and the median value of the last eight reversals was used as the threshold value. Four threshold values were obtained for each parameter value and subject. In total five subjects participated in these experiment. They were all members of the hearing and speech group at IPO.

2.2 Stimuli

All stimuli were generated digitally and converted to analog signals with a two-channel, 16 bit D/A converter at a sampling rate of 32 kHz. The bandpass noise maskers were generated in the frequency domain. The amplitudes of the spectral components in the passband were set to a constant value and the phases were uniformly distributed between 0 and 2π. After an inverse Fourier transform, a noise buffer of 2 s duration was obtained. From this buffer, different 400-ms sections were chosen for every interval by randomly selecting one sample as starting value. For each run, a new noise buffer was calculated by randomly choosing a new set of phase values for the complex spectrum. The signals were sinusoids with a frequency equal to the center frequency of the corresponding noise passband. Signal and masker were gated with 20-ms raised-cosine ramps. Six center frequencies between 125 Hz and 4 kHz (octave steps) were included in the measurements. The bandwidth of the masker had one of the following values: 5, 10, 25, 50, 100, 250, 500, 1000, 2000, 4000, or 8000 Hz with the additional restriction that the maximum bandwidth was equal to twice the center frequency. The noise was always presented without any interaural phase difference (No). The signal was either presented interaurally in phase (So) or out of phase ($S\pi$). The Binaural Masking Level Difference (BMLD) was calculated as threshold difference between the NoSo and $NoS\pi$ conditions. The masker had a constant overall sound pressure level of 70 dB at all bandwidths. Masked thresholds are expressed as signal-to-overall-noise ratio (S/N). The procedure for generating the transposed stimuli of Experiment 2 will be described below.

3 Experiment 1

In the first experiment, the combined influence of both the center frequency and the masker bandwidth was investigated. The results are presented in Fig. 1, which shows the influence of the center frequency on the BMLD for two different bandwidths. The narrowband masker was 10 Hz wide, a bandwidth clearly below the critical bandwidth at all signal frequencies. The wideband masker had a bandwidth equal to twice the signal frequency which is clearly wider than the critical bandwidth. The plotted values are the averages of three subjects.

The dependence of BMLD on frequency is very similar for the two bandwidths. The difference between the two curves lies between an average of 9 dB for the three lowest frequencies and an average of 11 dB for the three highest frequencies. This result limits the possible contribution of the increasing auditory-filter bandwidth to the high-frequency decrease of the BMLD in broadband noise to only a few dB.

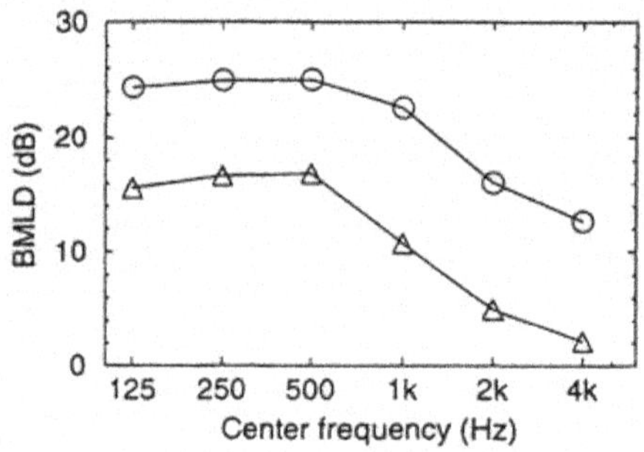

Figure 1. BMLDs in the condition NoSπ at several center frequencies for narrowband noise (10 Hz, O) and broadband noise (Δ). Average of 3 subjects.

4 Experiment 2

4.1 Signal processing

In order to motivate the specific signal configuration used in our second experiment, we first discuss what kind of binaural cues are available in masking conditions at low and at high frequencies. The upper two panels of Fig. 2 depict two such conditions for a center frequency of 125 Hz (top panel) and 4 kHz (middle panel). The first interval (0 to 100 ms) in both panels shows the waveform of a noise with a bandwidth of 25 Hz at the respective center frequencies. In the second interval (100 to 200 ms), a sinusoidal signal with a frequency equal to the center frequency of the noise is added to the noise waveform shown in the first interval. Its level is 10 dB below the rms value of the noise, a S/N value that is well *above* the masked threshold in the condition NoSπ. This signal is added in phase (solid curve) or out of phase (dashed curve) in the top panel. For reasons of visual clarity, the addition is shown in the middle panel for only *one* signal phase. The signals shown in the interval 100 to 200 ms thus represent the acoustic waveforms presented to the right and left ear in a signal interval in the condition NoSπ.

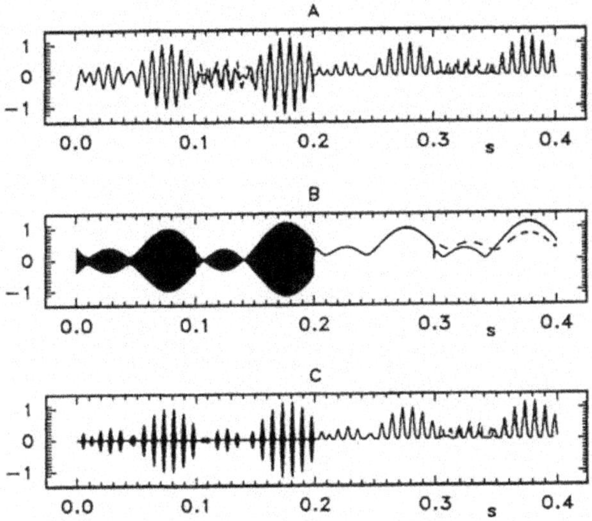

Figure 2. Waveforms for three stimulus conditions before (0 to 200 ms intervals) and after the first stages of peripheral transduction (200 to 400 ms intervals). Panel A: a 125-Hz condition; panel B: a 4-kHz condition; panel C: a 125-Hz transposed condition with 4 kHz center frequency. The intervals ranging from 0 to 100 ms show a 25-Hz-wide masker alone. In the interval from 100 to 200 ms, a sinusoidal signal is added in 0 phase (solid line in panel A), and, for panel A, also in π phase (dashed line). See text for further details.

In the inner ear, these signals are modified by the basilar-membrane and hair-cell properties, which we model by a half-wave rectifier and a low-pass filter with a cut-off frequency of 500 Hz. The bandpass filtering is omitted in this figure, since the acoustic stimuli have a subcritical bandwidth. The result of such a transformation for the waveforms in intervals 1 and 2 is shown in intervals 3 (0.2 to 0.3 s) and 4 (0.3 to 0.4 s). The finestructure of the masker is clearly preserved in panel A. Interval 4 shows that the interaural differences in the acoustic signals are also available after the hair-cell transformation; the continuous and dashed curves differ in interaural intensity and interaural timing in the finestructure. These interaural differences will become smaller with decreasing signal level.

At 4 kHz (panel B), the information about the finestructure is lost after hair-cell tranduction (see interval 3). Interval 4 shows that only interaural differences in the slowly varying *envelope* remain available as possible cues for binaural processing. By comparing intervals 4 from panel A and B, it is obvious that at a high frequency, less interaural information is available for any central processing stage following the peripheral transduction. Since our first experiment revealed a continuous decrease in BMLD above 500 Hz for all bandwidths, it is very likely that this decrease is at least in part due to the loss of finestructure information.

If we want to present the same interaural differences as in panel A in a high-frequency channel, we have to construct our signals in a very specific way, as illustrated in panel C. We generate a *transposed* signal-masker condition by using the two signals from interval 4 in panel A to modulate a 4-kHz carrier signal. This transposed signal is presented in panel C in an analog way as in panel B (i.e., only one of the two possible signal phases is shown in interval 2). In the transposed signal there is a 4-kHz as well as a 125-Hz finestructure. Due to the loss of high-frequency finestructure information in the hair cells, only the last one is coded in the neural system. This is indicated in interval 4 of panel C. We can see that the same interaural differences as in the low-frequency condition (panel A) result from the peripheral transduction. By measuring BMLDs for these transposed stimuli and comparing the results with the outcome of the first experiment, one can test how much the extra finestructure information in the transposed stimuli improves binaural interaction at high frequencies.

The signal processing for our transposed stimuli bears some similarity with the stimuli used by Bernstein and Trahiotis (1992b), but has at least one major advantage. If *we* reduce the signal level relative to the noise masker, the difference between masker-alone and masker-plus-signal interval becomes inaudible. Therefore, the present signal configuration allows us to measure diotic and dichotic thresholds which in addition can be expressed with the same measure (signal-to-overall-noise ratio) as in the original low-frequency condition.

Our original motivation for creating these stimuli was derived from the work of Colburn and Esquissaud (1976). They had investigated a model for the processing of interaural time differences that was based on the assumption that the *central* processing of interaural differences was basically the same at all frequencies. In such a case, the BMLDs of transposed stimuli should be as large as in the low-frequency condition. There is, however, also a different interpretation of the thresholds for transposed stimuli, if one relates dichotic thresholds to sensitivity for changes in interaural crosscorrelation. For subcritical masker bandwidths, the S/N ratio in an NoSπ condition can be easily related to the interaural crosscorrelation (cf., Durlach et al., 1986). In a simulation (using ten independent noise samples of 200 ms duration and an Sπ signal of the same duration) we found a relation between S/N and an average $\Delta\rho$ (equal to $1 - \rho$), which is shown by the crosses in Fig. 3. The circles show the average value of $\Delta\rho$ derived from the interaural correlation of the *envelope* for the same stimuli. In this simulation, the correlation of the envelopes is always higher ($\Delta\rho$ being smaller) than the full-waveform correlation, and the difference in ρ corresponds over a wide range of S/N values to a change in S/N of about 3 dB. Readers familiar with the paper by Bernstein and Trahiotis (1992a) will remember that they found as a practical rule that the correlation of the envelope corresponded to approximately the square of the full-waveform correlation, thus it was always smaller. The reason for this opposite result is that we calculated the normalized crosscorrelation value, while Bernstein and Trahiotis calculated the Pearson Product Correlation.

Applying the result of Fig. 3 to high-frequency BMLD experiments with standard and with transposed stimuli, one can expect a gain of about 3 dB in S/N ratio for the transposed stimuli relative to the standard high-frequency BMLD. This decrease in dichotic thresholds (or, correspondingly, the increase in BMLD) should occur independently of the exact amount of the high-frequency BMLD found for an individual subject.

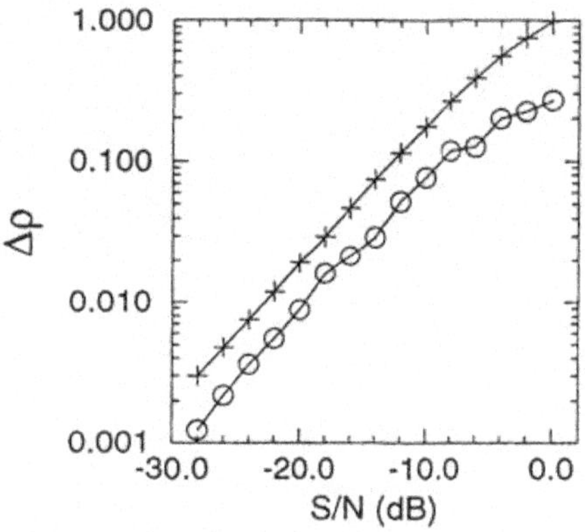

Fig. 3: Change in the normalized interaural crosscorrelation ($\Delta\rho = 1 - \rho$) in the condition NoSπ as a function of the signal-to-overall-noise ratio. Crosses indicate correlation values for the full waveform, circles indicate correlation values for the (Hilbert) envelope. Average of ten independent estimates for 200-ms stimuli.

4.2 Results

We first want to compare the threshold values in the transposed and standard conditions for a diotic condition. Fig. 4 shows masked threshold values as a function of masker bandwidth for three conditions: 250-Hz low-frequency (O), 4-kHz high-frequency (◊) and a transposed high-frequency condition derived from the 250-Hz condition (□). Thresholds are the averages of five subjects. For bandwidths between 5 and 50 Hz, all thresholds are nearly identical, and decrease by about 4 dB for a tenfold increase in noise bandwidth. This result is in good agreement with many other experiments back to Bos and de Boer (1966) and is generally related to the decreased variance of the energy estimate for noise samples with a larger bandwidth. Between 50 and 500 Hz bandwidth, 4-kHz and transposed data continue to decrease at this rate because the noise bandwidth is still below the critical bandwidth at 4 kHz. The 250-Hz low-frequency data decrease at a rate of about 10 dB per tenfold increase in bandwidth, which is equivalent to a constant signal-to-noise ratio in a band of 50-Hz width around the signal frequency. This result shows that our way of transposing the low-frequency information onto a high-frequency carrier allows the detection of the signal at exactly the same signal-to-noise ratio as in a standard procedure, provided the noise bandwidth remains below the critical bandwith at the corresponding carrier (or center) frequency.

In Fig. 5 we plot the BMLD values for the same three spectral conditions. Again, the results are the averages of five subjects. BMLDs are largest for the 250-Hz condition and tend to be smallest for the 4-kHz condition, especially for bandwidths less than 50 Hz. Although the 4-kHz stimuli and the transposed stimuli are both centered at 4 kHz, the BMLDs for transposed stimuli are clearly larger than those for the 4-kHz stimuli at the smaller bandwidths. Thus, the extra fine-structure information in the transposed stimuli is beneficial for binaural detection. For larger bandwidths there does not seem to be such a benefit.

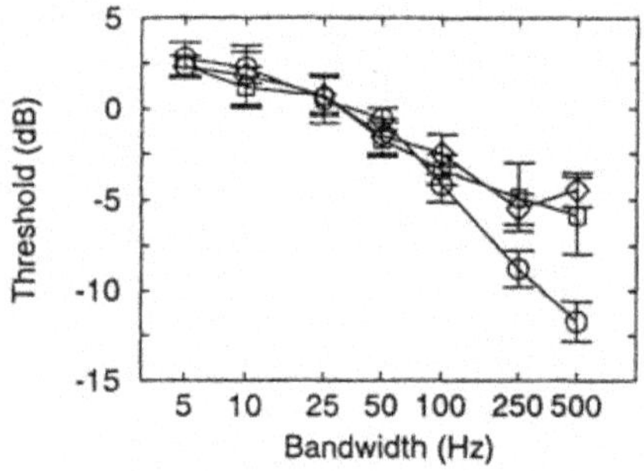

Figure 4. Masked thresholds for NoSo as a function of masker bandwidth for three spectral conditions: standard low-frequency (centered at 250 Hz, O) and high-frequency condition (centered at 4 kHz, ◊) and transposed condition derived from 250 Hz and centered at 4 kHz (□). Average results of five subjects.

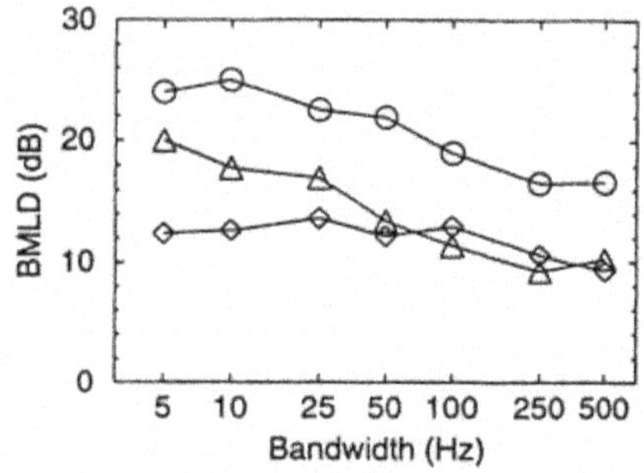

Figure 5. BMLDs for NoSπ as a function of masker bandwidth for three spectral conditions: standard low-frequency (centered at 250 Hz, O) and high-frequency condition (centered at 4 kHz, ◊) and transposed condition derived from 250 Hz and centered at 4 kHz (Δ). Average results of five subjects.

On average, BMLDs for transposed stimuli are smaller than for the 250-Hz stimuli. This observation does not hold to the same degree for each individual subject. The two most extreme examples are shown in Figs. 6 and 7. For the smaller bandwidths, the BMLDs for transposed and low-frequency conditions for subject SP differ by approximately 4 dB whereas subject AK shows a difference of about 10 dB. For subject AK, however, the 4-kHz BMLDs are much lower than for subject SP. This difference suggests that binaural processing at 4 kHz is in general less effective for subject AK, but that there still is a benefit for binaural interaction provided by the extra finestructure information.

Experiment 2 was repeated with the center frequency of the low-frequency stimuli shifted from 250 to 125 Hz, which was also used to derive the transposed stimuli. Since the bandwidth of the transposed stimuli is about twice the center frequency (plus the noise bandwidth) of the original stimuli, this change in frequency leads to a smaller bandwidth of the transposed stimuli. Therefore, the spectrally more narrow transposed stimuli derived from 125 Hz should be less affected by the auditory filter at the 4-kHz carrier frequency. The results of two subjects are shown in Figs. 8 and 9. The transposed and the low-frequency BMLDs match to within a few dBs for both subjects. For subject SP there is an advantage for the transposed condition with respect to the 4 kHz condition at all bandwidths, while for subject MH this is only the case at small bandwidths.

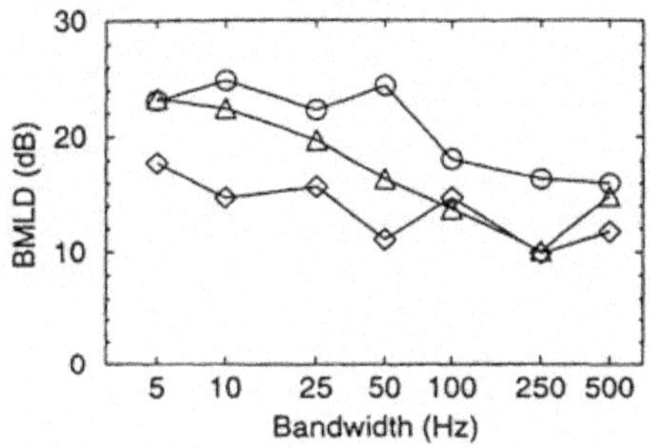

Figure 6. BMLDs for several bandwidths for 250 Hz (O), 250 Hz transposed (Δ) and 4 kHz (◊). Subject SP.

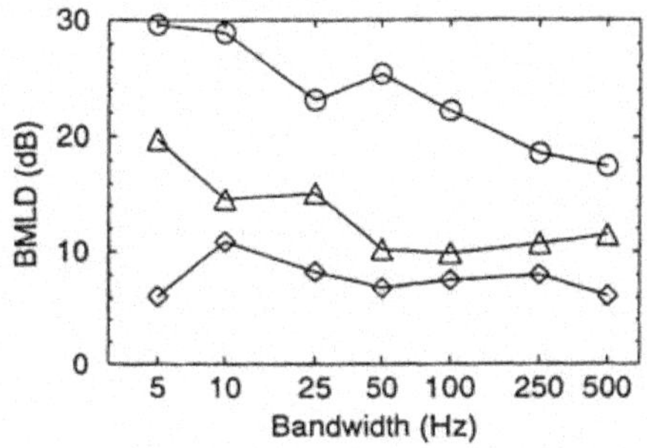

Figure 7. BMLDs for several bandwidths for 250 Hz (O), 250 Hz transposed (Δ) and 4 kHz (◊). Subject AK.

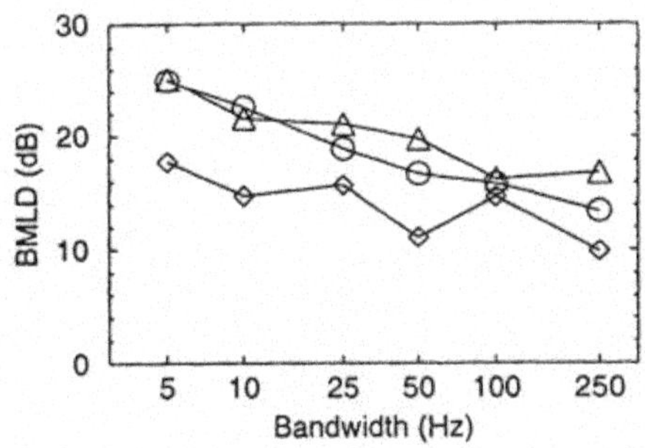

Figure 8. BMLDs for several bandwidths for 125 Hz (O), 125 Hz transposed (Δ) and 4 kHz (◊). Subject SP.

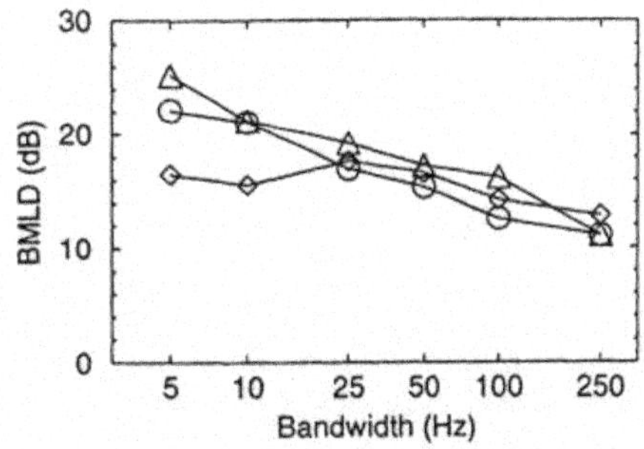

Figure 9. BMLDs for several bandwidths for 125 Hz (O), 125 Hz transposed (Δ) and 4 kHz (◊). Subject MH.

5 Discussion

As shown in Fig. 1, the change in the BMLD with increasing center frequency is nearly the same for a narrowband and a broadband masker. This is remarkable since one would expect that the increasing auditory-filter bandwidth (and the corresponding higher rate of fluctuation of binaural cues) would reduce the high-frequency BMLD more for a broadband noise than for a narrowband noise. In addition, together with the analysis shown in Fig. 3, it becomes obvious that the loss of fine structure alone cannot explain the high-frequency decrease in BMLD. If we assume that the interaural crosscorrelation as calculated in Fig. 3 is a reasonable predictor for $NoS\pi$ thresholds, then we must conclude that, in contrast to the assumption of Colburn and Esquissaud for interaural time differences, the sensitivity to correlation changes decreases with frequency. Such a decrease has been reported by Koehnke et al. (1986), who observed an average increase in $\Delta\rho$, using a reference correlation of one, by a factor of four going from 500 to 4000 Hz center frequency.

The data in Figs. 5 to 9 show that the addition of 'fine-structure' information in the envelope increases high-frequency BMLDs at small bandwidths. When the fine-structure information imposed on the envelope was at a 250-Hz rate (Figs. 5 to 7), the benefit was absent for larger bandwidths of the noise masker (> 50 Hz). This lack of benefit occurred even though the rates of envelope fluctuation caused by the larger masker bandwidths remained at or below 250 Hz.

6 References

Bernstein, L.R., and Trahiotis, C. (1992a) Discrimination of interaural envelope correlation and its relation to binaural unmasking at high frequencies. J. Acoust. Soc. Am. 91, 306-316

Bernstein, L.R., and Trahiotis, C. (1992b) Detection of antiphasic sinusoids added to the envelopes of high-frequency bands of noise. Hear. Res. 62,157-165

Bos, C.E., and de Boer, E. (1966) Masking and discrimination. J. Acoust. Soc. Am. 39, 708-715

Bronkhorst, A.W., and Plomp, R. (1988). The effect of head-induced interaural time and level differences on speech intelligibility in noise. J. Acoust. Soc. Am. 83, 1508-1516

Colburn, H.S., and Durlach, N.I. (1978) Models of binaural interaction. Handbook of Perception, Vol. IV, Hearing. edited by E.C. Carterette and M.P. Friedman (Academic, New York), pp. 467-518

Colburn, H.S., and Esquissaud P. (1976) An auditory-nerve model for interaural time discrimination of high-frequency complex stimuli. J. Acoust. Soc. Am. 59, S23

Durlach, N.I. (1964) Note on binaural masking-level differences at high frequencies. J. Acoust. Soc. Am. 36, 576-581

Durlach, N.I., Gabriel, K.J., Colburn, H.S., and Trahiotis, C. (1986) Interaural correlation discrimination: II.Relation to binaural unmasking. J. Acoust. Soc. Am. 79, 1548-1557

Grantham, D.W., and Wightman, L. (1979) Detectability of a pulsed tone in the presence of a masker with time-varying interaural correlation. J. Acoust. Soc. Am. 65, 1509-1517

Henning, G.B. (1974) Detectability of interaural delay in high-frequency complex waveforms. J. Acoust. Soc. Am. 55, 84-90

Hirsh, I.J. (1948) The role of interaural phase on interaural summation and inhibition. J. Acoust. Soc. Am. 20, 761-766

Koehnke, J., Colburn, H.S., and Durlach, N.I. (1986) Performance in several binaural-interaction experiments. J. Acoust. Soc. Am. 79, 1558-1562

Levitt, H. (1971) Transformed up-down methods in psychoacoustics. J. Acoust. Soc. Am. 49, 467-477

McFadden, D., and Pasanen, E.G. (1978) Binaural detection at high frequencies with time-delayed waveforms. J. Acoust. Soc. Am. 63, 1120-1131

Metz, P.J., Bismarck, G. von, and Durlach, N.I. (1968) Further results on binaural unmasking and the EC model. J. Acoust. Soc. Am. 43, 1085-1091

Zurek, P., and Durlach, N.I. (1987) Masker-bandwidth dependence in homophasic and antiphasic tone detection. J. Acoust. Soc. Am. 81, 459-464

Binaural spectral interference in detection and discrimination paradigms

Leslie R. Bernstein and Constantine Trahiotis

Center for Neurological Sciences, Surgical Research Center, Department of Surgery (Otolaryngology), University of Connecticut Health Center, Farmington, CT 06030

1 Introduction

Several recent experiments have demonstrated that sensitivity to interaural disparities presented within restricted spectral regions can be degraded by the presence of energy in other, even quite remote, spectral regions. Such degradations in performance have been called "interference," a term that serves to differentiate these phenomena from masking.

Binaural interference was first demonstrated by McFadden and Pasanen (1976). They found that a diotic, narrow band of noise centered at 500 Hz (the interferer) degraded their listeners' abilities to discriminate interaural temporal disparities (ITDs) presented within a second narrow band of noise centered at 4 kHz (the target). Importantly, the converse was not true. That is, the ability to discriminate ITDs within a narrow band of noise centered at 500 Hz was *unaffected* by the presence of a diotic, narrow band of noise centered at 4 kHz. Thus, binaural interference appeared to be characterized by a spectral *asymmetry*.

More recently, Zurek (1985) reported what he termed "spectral dominance" in sensitivity to ITDs which occurred only within narrow spectral portions of a broadband noise. Zurek utilized noises that were diotic save for the spectral regions containing the delay. These regions, what Zurek termed "target bands," had a bandwidth of 40% of their center frequency. Data were collected for target bands whose center frequencies ranged from 250 Hz to 4 kHz. Thus, the target bands were always flanked, spectrally, by diotic noise. Although some interference was observed for targets centered at 1 kHz and below, sensitivity to ITD was drastically reduced for targets centered at 2 kHz to 4 kHz.

The purpose of this report is to present the results of recent experiments conducted in our laboratory that demonstrate binaural interference in several experimental contexts.

2 Interference in the discrimination of ITDs

Our first experiments (Trahiotis and Bernstein, 1990) extended Zurek's observations. Like Zurek, we studied the detectability of ITDs presented within a restricted "target" region of a broadband noise whose spectral extent was always 40% of its center frequency. The broadband interfering noise that flanked the target region was either gated coincidentally with the target region (as was the case in McFadden and Pasanen's and Zurek's studies) or was presented continuously. In the latter case, the target region was gated "into" the continuous flanking noise. A second departure was to present interfering information that was either interaurally uncorrelated or diotic.

Figure 1 contains the data averaged across six listeners. The most salient aspect of the data is the extremely large threshold obtained for targets centered at 4 kHz in the presence of gated, diotic, flanking noise (open square).

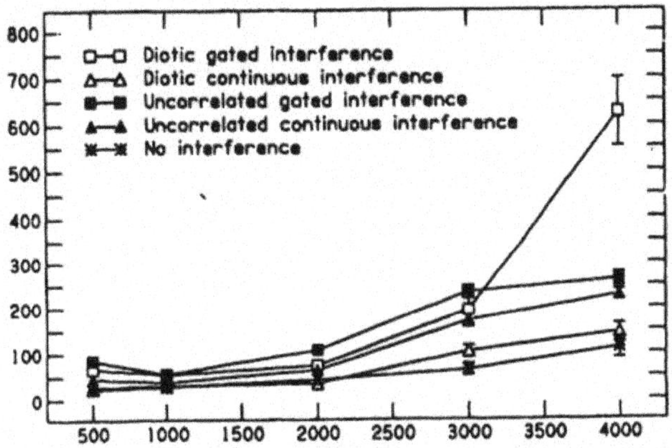

Figure 1. Threshold ITD as a function of the center frequency of the target band. Closed symbols denote uncorrelated interferers; open symbols denote diotic interferers. Squares denote gated interference; triangles denote continuous interference. Asterisks denote targets presented with no interference. Each point represents the average across six listeners; error bars represent ± 1 s.e.m. (from Trahiotis and Bernstein, 1990, with permission)

This outcome essentially replicates Zurek's result. Importantly, when the interferer was presented continuously and/or when the interferer was interaurally uncorrelated, thresholds were greatly reduced or were essentially identical to those obtained when the targets were presented in isolation. The vanishingly small amount of interference produced by the continuous, diotic flanking noise, appears to preclude any explanation of interference based on a *simple* notion of spectral dominance. In that view, the binaural images produced by low-frequency stimuli predominate over those produced by high-frequency stimuli. In addition, the differing amounts of interference produced by diotic and interaurally uncorrelated interferers appear to preclude explanations of interference based solely on strictly monaural interactions or mechanisms. Both outcomes also argue strongly that interference is not due to masking.

We have recently extended the measurements of binaural interference in several ways. First, we measured interference when the listeners were uncertain as to which of four target regions (centered on 300 Hz, 1200 Hz, 2400 Hz, or 4800 Hz) within the broadband noise could contain an ITD (Buell and Trahiotis, 1994). A single-interval paradigm was employed. The target region was gated coincidentally with the diotic, flanking interfering noise. Under conditions of spectral uncertainty, performance was degraded for *all* target regions, and some listeners were unable to detect even a 1-ms ITD presented within the two highest frequency regions.

Second, we again measured degradations in sensitivity to ITDs produced by diotic and uncorrelated interferers that were either gated coincidentally with the target or were continuous (Bernstein and Trahiotis, 1994). The target was a 100-Hz-wide band of noise centered at 4 kHz. The interferer was a 100-Hz-wide narrow band of noise centered at 500 Hz. Figure 2 shows the amount of interference produced in each condition.

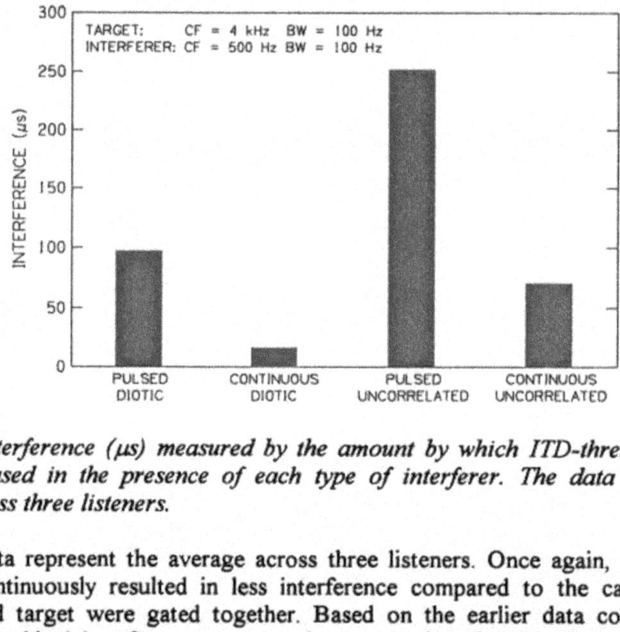

Figure 2. Interference (μs) measured by the amount by which ITD-thresholds for the target increased in the presence of each type of interferer. The data represent the average across three listeners.

The data represent the average across three listeners. Once again, presenting the interferer continuously resulted in less interference compared to the cases when the interferer and target were gated together. Based on the earlier data collected with a broadband (flanking) interferer, we were quite surprised to find that the greatest amount of interference was produced when the interferer was gated coincidentally with the target, *but was interaurally uncorrelated.* At this time we are investigating other stimulus conditions that may provide some explanation for the divergent outcomes.

Third, we measured listeners' abilities to detect ITDs within a 100% sinusoidally amplitude-modulated (SAM) tone consisting of a 4 kHz carrier modulated at 250 Hz (Heller and Trahiotis, 1994a). Under conditions of interference, a second SAM tone, also 100%-modulated at 250 Hz and centered at either 500 Hz, 1 kHz, or 2 kHz was also present. Greater amounts of interference were produced by the SAM tones centered at 500 Hz or 1 kHz than by the spectrally more proximate SAM tone centered at 2 kHz.

Thresholds measured with the interferers either in-phase or out-of-phase with the target were essentially equivalent. These two outcomes, taken together, argue strongly that interference is not due to a monaural disruption of the traveling-wave envelope of the higher frequency target by the lower frequency interferer as discussed by McFadden and Pasanen (1976). Heller and Trahiotis also found that the amount of interference was reduced when the interfering information was presented continuously rather than coincidentally with the target.

3 Interference and the masking level-difference

We wondered whether degradations in performance similar to those described above would be observable in a binaural masking level-difference (MLD) paradigm. For interaural signal/masker configurations (e.g., N_0S_π) that produce an MLD, detection of the signal is, presumably, based upon time-varying interaural disparities produced when the signal is added to the masking noise. In one set of experiments, we measured interference for a low-frequency target (Bernstein, 1991; Bernstein and Trahiotis, 1993). In that case, binaural timing information is presumably conveyed by the fine-structure of the stimuli. Recently, we measured interference with a high-frequency target where binaural timing information is presumably conveyed by the envelope of the stimuli (Bernstein and Trahiotis, 1994).

For the low-frequency experiments, we explored whether the detectability of an 800-Hz tone (the target) masked either by wide-band or by a 100-Hz-wide band of noise in the N_0S_π configuration would be affected by the presence of a 400-Hz tone (the interferer). Because the N_0S_π threshold is much lower under narrow-band masking, this narrow-band condition allowed us a larger range over which to assess the effects of the interferer.

Figure 3 illustrates some of our results and displays the thresholds (E/No in dB) averaged across four listeners (Bernstein and Trahiotis, 1993). The left-most pair of histograms within each grouping represents the conditions in which the 800-Hz target was presented, homophasically (N_0S_0) or antiphasically (N_0S_π), with no interfering stimulus. The right-most pair represents two conditions in which the pulsed tonal interferer was present either interaurally in-phase ($N_0S_\pi I_0$) or interaurally out-of-phase ($N_0S_\pi I_\pi$). Note the larger MLD obtained for N_0S_π with the narrow-band as compared to the wide-band noise. Also note that more interference occurs with the narrow-band masker (about 9 dB) than for the wide-band masker (about 5 dB). Two aspects of the data argue very strongly that the interference observed is a *binaural* phenomenon. First, even thresholds obtained in the presence of the interferer are *lower* than the thresholds obtained in the N_0S_0 baseline condition. That is, an MLD persists under interference. Secondly, although not shown in the figure, data collected in $N_0S_0I_0$ and $N_0S_0I_\pi$ conditions, where detection is based on monaural cues, revealed no interference effects. Two other aspects of the large set of data we collected deserve mention. First, when the roles of the target and

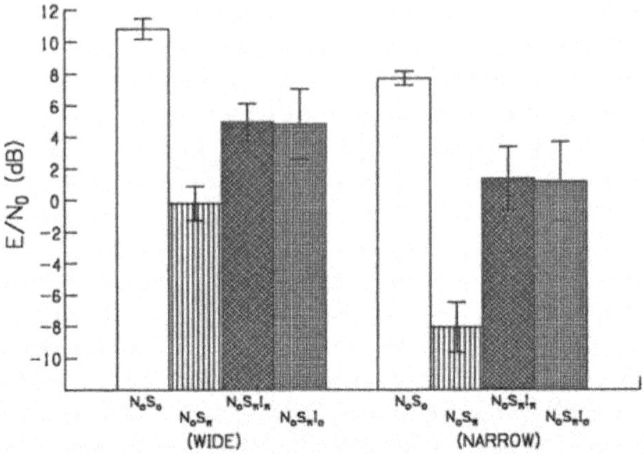

Figure 3. E/N$_0$(dB) at threshold required for detection of an 800-Hz tonal target masked by wide-band and narrow-band noise. Open and striped bars represent thresholds for the N_0S_0 and N_0S_π conditions, respectively. Diamond- and square-hatched bars represent thresholds obtained when the I_π and I_0 interferers, respectively, were pulsed with the 800-Hz S_π target. The data represent the mean across four listeners. Error bars represent ± 1 s.e.m. (adapted from Bernstein and Trahiotis, 1993, with permission)

interfering tones were reversed (400-Hz target, 800-Hz interferer) much less interference was observed. This finding is consistent with the spectral asymmetry of interference discussed earlier. Second, also in accord with ITD-discrimination data discussed earlier, presenting the 400-Hz tonal interferer continuously substantially reduced the amount of interference. However, we were impressed to find that providing a "forward fringe" (by turning on the interferer prior to the onset of the 800-Hz target) did not lead to a reduction in the potency of the interferer. In fact, thresholds were essentially unchanged as the duration of the forward fringe was varied from 10 to 320 ms! This finding is consistent with the data reported by Stellmack and Dye (1989) and by Woods and Colburn (1992) who measured the detectability of static ITDs for pure-tone targets in the presence of "fringed" interferers. We believe these outcomes rule out explanations of binaural interference based on perceptual "fusion," or lack of segregation of the target and interferer. In this regard, it is important to note that Woods and Colburn stated that all their listeners "reported hearing more than one sound object in response to the stimulus (pg. 2900)" even though substantial interference was observed. Perhaps as discussed by Yost (1991), the fusion/segregation of auditory sources depends upon predominately *monaural* processes.

For the high-frequency experiments, we obtained data when the target was a 4 kHz tone masked by a 100-Hz-wide band of noise in the N_0S_π configuration. The interferer was a 100-Hz-wide band of noise centered at 500 Hz that was either diotic or was

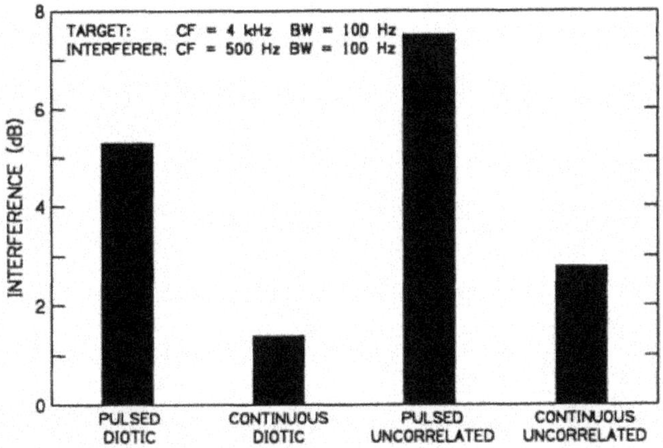

Figure 4. Interference (dB) measured by the amount by which detection-thresholds for the target in the N_0S_π increased in the presence of each type of interferer. The data represent the average across four listeners.

interaurally uncorrelated and was either gated coincidentally with the target or was presented continuously. These conditions parallel those used by McFadden and Pasanen (1976), Trahiotis and Bernstein (1990), and those used to generate the data in Figure 2. Figure 4 shows that the amount of interference, averaged across four listeners, was, as has been true in several other contexts, reduced when the interferer was presented continuously. In accord with the ITD-discrimination data shown in Figure 2, the greatest amount of interference was obtained when the interferer was interaurally uncorrelated as was pulsed on and off with the target. Thus, it appears that the relative amount of interference obtained with pulsed-diotic versus pulsed-interaurally uncorrelated interferers can vary. It depends upon whether the interferer is spectrally remote from the target or whether it is broadband and contains energy in spectral regions adjacent to the target region. However, more data are necessary to pinpoint which spectral relations between targets and interferers are really responsible for these differences.

4 Related findings

Data collected recently in our laboratory, as well as those recently collected by Heller and Richards (1991), indicate that binaural interference can also occur when listeners are required to discriminate interaural intensitive differences (IIDs). Unlike the large spectral asymmetries observed with ITDs and with MLDs, interference measured with IIDs appears to be quite symmetric. Data obtained from some listeners even indicate a spectral asymmetry *opposite* to that observed with ITDs and MLDs. That is, remote, high-frequency energy can cause threshold-IIDs for low-frequency targets to increase by equivalent, or even greater, amounts than the increases in threshold observed for high-frequency targets and low-frequency interferers.

The interference effects found with measurements of ITDs, IIDs and MLDs lead naturally to the question of whether spectrally-remote information could affect the lateral position of the intracranial image produced by the target. We have recently completed such measurements and found that low-frequency, spectrally-remote diotic information can produce large displacements of the intracranial position of a high-frequency target (Heller and Trahiotis, 1994b). For example, for one of the listeners, an ITD of 800 μs in an SAM tone centered at 4 kHz (the target) produced an intracranial image located far toward one ear. When an SAM tone centered at 500 Hz was gated coincidentally with the 4-kHz target, the listener's judgments indicated that the image was now very close to the mid-line! This general result appears to hold for other listeners as well.

The reader should not be left with the impression that combining binaural information across spectral regions always leads to decrements in performance. Listeners, who are unable to ignore non-informative, diotic, information in one spectral region while attempting to detect an ITD in a higher spectral region, are able to combine, *optimally*, ITDs that are simultaneously present in both regions (Buell and Trahiotis, 1993).

5 Acknowledgments

This work was supported by grants from NIH (DC-00527, DC-00234) and a grant from AFOSR (89-0030).

6 References

Bernstein, L. R. (1991). Spectral interference in a binaural detection task, J. Acoust. Soc Am., 89, 1306-1313.

Bernstein, L. R. and Trahiotis, C. (1993). Spectral interference in a binaural detection task: Effects of masker bandwidth and temporal fringe, J. Acoust. Soc Am., 94, 735-742.

Bernstein, L. R. and Trahiotis, C. (1994). Interference effects in binaural discrimination and masking-level difference paradigms, in preparation.

Buell, T. N. and Trahiotis, C. (1993). Interaural temporal discrimination using two sinusoidally amplitude-modulated, high-frequency tones: Conditions of summation and interference, J. Acoust. Soc Am., 93, 480-487.

Buell, T. N. and Trahiotis, C. (1994). Detection of interaural delay in bands of noise: Effects of spectral interference combined with spectral uncertainty, J. Acoust. Soc Am., in press.

Heller, L. M. and Richards, V. M. (1991). Differential lateralization interference for interaural time and interaural level differences, J. Acoust. Soc Am., 89, 1995.

Heller, L. M. and Trahiotis, C. (1994a). Interference in detection of interaural delay in a SAM tone produced by a second, spectrally remote SAM tone, presentation at the seventeenth meeting of the Association for Research in Otolaryngology (abstract #283).

Heller, L. M. and Trahiotis, C. (1994b). The effects on the lateralization of a SAM tone produced by a second, spectrally remote SAM tone, in preparation.

McFadden, D. and Pasanen, E. G. (1976). Lateralization at high frequencies based on interaural time differences, J. Acoust. Soc. Am. 59, 634-639.

Stellmack, M. A. and Dye, R. H. (1989). The effect of onset asynchronies between components on the ability to detect a delayed component embedded in a diotic complex, J. Acoust. Soc Am. 86, S11.

Trahiotis, C. and Bernstein, L. R. (1990). Detectability of interaural delays over select spectral regions: Effects of flanking noise, J. Acoust. Soc Am. 87, 810-813.

Woods, W. S. and Colburn, H. S. (1992). Test of a model of auditory object formation using intensity and ITD discrimination, J. Acoust. Soc Am., 91, 2894-2902.

Yost, W. A. (1991). Auditory image perception and analysis: The basis for hearing, Hear. Res. 56, 8-18.

Zurek, P. M. (1985). Spectral dominance in sensitivity to interaural delay for broadband stimuli, J. Acoust. Soc. Am. 78 Suppl. 1, S18.

Excitation patterns

Adaptation and attention in psychoacoustics

Bertram Scharf

Auditory Perception Laboratory Northeastern University, Boston, MA 02115-5096, USA and
Laboratoire de Mécanique et d'Acoustique, 13402 Marseille Cedex 20, France

1 Introduction

The research on adaptation and attention that I shall review has become over the years more and more closely informed by neurophysiological considerations. Accordingly, it is easy to adhere to the original inspiration of these meetings which was, at least in part, to bring together concepts from psychoacoustics and from auditory physiology. I shall not attempt to review the whole literature on auditory adaptation, let alone on attention. I shall concentrate on loudness adaptation and on selective attention in the frequency domain, relating loudness adaptation to the spread of excitation in the auditory system and selective attention to the role of the olivocochlear bundle.

Although liaisons exist between adaptation and attention, they have not been in the forefront of this research. Nonetheless, some of the work on attention was motivated by questions posed relative to common observations of effects that could be taken to be the result of adaptation, as well as from our laboratory findings on loudness adaptation. For example, one of our principal discoveries concerning adaptation was that pure tones below approximately 10 kHz show loudness adaptation at low sensation levels (SL) but not above 30 dB or so. Some colleagues suggested that perhaps weak sounds easily passed out of the field of attention and so seemed to become softer. This is not the case. First of all, no amount of conscious effort restores the loudness of an adapted low-level tone once it has declined. Second, white noise at 10 dB SL adapts very little, much less than a pure tone even though its loudness level is initially lower than that of the tone (Scharf, 1978), which ought to make it more vulnerable to decreased attention.

Nonetheless, constant sounds often do go unnoticed after a short period of exposure, and that could be taken as evidence for strong adaptation. Apparent inaudibility under such conditions would not qualify as an example of *sensory* adaptation because the listener can readily bring the unnoticed sounds to full consciousness and to their original loudness. Sensory adaptation refers to the decline over time in the perceived magnitude of an unchanging stimulus, a decline that can be reversed by changing the stimulus condition but not by changing how one listens.

Most of the rest of this paper treats adaptation and attention separately.

2 Loudness Adaptation

2.1 Background

Casual observation suggests that steady sounds do not decline in loudness as long as we listen (i.e. attend) to them. Yet, many laboratory studies (e.g. Békésy, 1929; Hood, 1950; Palva and Kärjä, 1969) suggested the opposite. In his influential paper, Hood (1950) reported that loudness level declined as much as 50 phons within 2 to 3 min. These measurements were made by dichotic loudness matching--a continuous sound in one ear was matched in loudness to a brief or intermittent sound in the other. Thus, under some conditions Hood found that after a few minutes of exposure to a continuous tone in one ear, an intermittent tone in the other ear had to be set 50 dB lower to match the continuous tone in loudness. Several authors (cf. Ward, 1973) pointed out the likely role of interaural interactions in such procedures so that any measured decline in loudness was not necessarily the result simply of prolonged exposure to a continuous sound.

Further research made it clear that loudness adaptation comes in several guises. *Simple loudness adaptation*, the decline in loudness that results from sustained exposure to a sound, was shown to be restricted to pure tones at low levels (Scharf, 1983), except for tones at very high frequencies which adapt also at high stimulus levels (Miskiewicz et al., 1993). *Ipsilaterally induced adaptation* is the adaptation induced by a temporary increment in the level of a sound or by the introduction of another more intense, intermittent sound to the same ear or ears (Canévet et al., 1983). *Contralaterally induced adaptation* is the adaptation measured in the presence of an intermittent contralateral sound (Botte et al., 1982).

2.2 Simple Loudness Adaptation

Pure tones seem to be the only sounds that decline in loudness to a significant degree as a direct and unique result of continuous exposure. And they show such declines only at low levels, within about 30 dB of threshold, unless they are at frequencies higher than about 10 kHz, where they also show adaptation above 30 dB SL. Noises, even narrow-band noise, adapt much less than tones. Thus, given that pure tones are restricted to the laboratory, simple loudness adaptation must be a rare natural phenomenon. In this respect loudness is unlike most other sensory modalities, such as brightness, odor, taste, and touch, which do adapt over time. The question arises as to why loudness is different. A functional reason would be that exposure to loud sounds for long periods leads to reduced sensitivity. Organisms that adapted to loud sounds would be less likely to leave noisy environments (because loudness is the main component of sound annoyance) and so would be more likely to develop impaired hearing, temporarily if not permanently. Uncovering the conditions under which loudness does adapt should help clarify how loudness usually avoids adaptation.

Not all pure tones are equally prone to loudness adaptation. Figure 1 shows how the amount of loudness adaptation after 2 or 3 min of exposure to a pure tone depends on the tone's frequency, at 10 dB SL (filled symbols) and at 30 or 40 dB SL (unfilled symbols).

[These data were obtained by the method of successive magnitude estimation which requires the listener to assign numbers to express the loudness of a sustained sound at regular intervals (e.g. every 20 s).] At 10 dB SL, the degree of adaptation increases nearly monotonically with frequency, with a steep rise beyond about 10 kHz. At 30 and 40 dB, adaptation is virtually absent at all frequencies below approximately 10 kHz, beyond which it again increases very rapidly. (The inverted unfilled triangles at 0% represent data for only seven listeners who, on the average, showed a small *increase* in loudness with exposure time; however, the precise value is not available and so zero is used.) Scharf (1983, Fig. 7) showed at frequencies from 0.25 to 4 kHz that loudness adaptation (measured as the percentage decline in loudness) decreases nearly linearly as sensation level increases up to 30 dB. In contrast, at 16 kHz, as Fig. 1 shows, adaptation is essentially the same at 10 and 40 dB SL. The few data on adaptation at levels lower than 10 dB show that at 5 dB SL, tones between 0.25 and 4 kHz decline in loudness by close to 80% after 2 min (Scharf, 1983). Overall, loudness adaptation for pure tones depends strongly on level at lower frequencies, but hardly at all at 16 kHz where adaptation is nearly as strong at 40 dB SL as at 10 dB SL (Miskiewicz et al., 1993; Scharf, 1992).

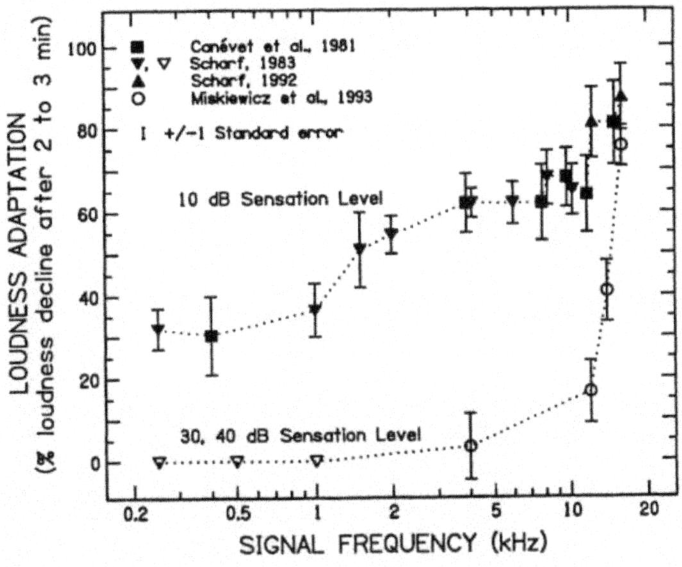

Figure 1. The dependence of loudness adaptation, measured as the percentage decline in loudness after an exposure of 2 to 3 min, on signal frequency. Data at 30 and 40 dB SL are combined for comparison to data at 10 dB SL.

The measurements in Fig. 1 were carried out to durations of only 2 or 3 min because earlier data had suggested that adaptation reaches an asymptote within 3 min. However, recent measurements suggest that adaptation may continue over longer exposure periods even if most of it does occur during the first few minutes. Not only is the duration of the exposure important in adaptation, but also the temporal signature of the stimulus. Adaptation can be eliminated or reduced by introducing beating between two tones or amplitude modulating a single tone (Scharf, 1983). Two beating tones around 4 kHz at 10 dB SL showed almost no adaptation. As the two tones were set further apart in frequency, adaptation increased until for two tones more than a critical band apart, adaptation was as great as for a single tone at 10 dB. Also a narrow-band noise at 10 dB SL shows much less adaptation than a pure tone. It is likely that the amplitude fluctuations inherent in noise keep most noises, both narrow band and broadband, from adapting. However, no measures are available for noise below 10 dB SL, so it may well be that noise adapts when weak enough. Moreover, preliminary measurements suggest that neither amplitude modulation nor beating at a rate of 5 Hz causes much of a decline in the adaptation of a weak 16-kHz tone.

Individuals vary greatly in the amount of adaptation they report. Some of the variability can be ascribed to differences in criterion and in the listener's interpretation of just what loudness represents. However, the lack of any interaction between adaptation in one ear and that in the other suggests that simple adaptation could take place largely in the cochlea. For example, strong adaptation in one ear over a 90-s exposure has no effect on the loudness of a tone presented immediately afterward to the other ear (Scharf, 1983). In the same vein, the lack of adaptation in one ear stimulated by a 4-kHz tone at 40 dB SL does not prevent strong adaptation in the other ear stimulated simultaneously at 10 dB SL. Nonetheless, central and even cognitive influences cannot be entirely excluded. For example, musicians adapt less than non-musicians (Baruch and Botte, 1989) which probably suggests central rather than sensory factors.

The key to the occurrence of adaptation appears to be a stimulus that gives rise to steady stimulation over a restricted region of the auditory nervous system. We refer to this notion as the *restricted-excitation-pattern hypothesis*. This hypothesis followed from the finding that signals, such as strong tones and broadband noise (even at low levels) that evoke broad excitation patterns, adapt little, whereas weak tones adapt markedly. It was also noted that a high-pass noise causes a simultaneous 4-kHz tone near 60 dB SPL to adapt; this could be due to the restriction of excitation by the presence of the noise, which also raises the threshold for the tone. Most compelling are the recent findings of Miskiewicz et al. (1993) showing that loudness adaptation increases with frequency so that at 16 kHz, adaptation is very strong even in the quiet at 56 dB SL. At very high frequencies, excitation is restricted by the upper limit of hearing. Indeed, Fig. 2 shows how adaptation at 14 kHz depends on threshold at 16 kHz. Listeners who were less sensitive at 16 kHz adapted more at 14 kHz than listeners who were more sensitive; the implication is that the less sensitive listeners had more restricted excitation patterns at 14 kHz.

The restricted-excitation-pattern hypothesis is reminiscent of the multiband version of Zwicker's (1956) excitation-pattern model for intensity discrimination as developed by Florentine and Buus (1981). The model handles nicely phenomena like the divergence between intensity discrimination at 1 kHz and at 14 kHz and its increase with sound pressure level (Florentine, 1983). According to the model, discrimination improves markedly with level at 1 kHz and hardly at all at 14 kHz because the listener bases his/her decision upon input from all the critical bands covered by the excitation pattern which broadens with increasing level very much at a low frequency but very little at a high frequency. Florentine (1983) also showed that intensity discrimination became poorer when the excitation pattern was restricted by a high-pass noise (cf. Hellman, 1978, re loudness growth and Scharf, 1983, re loudness adaptation) or by higher thresholds at very high frequencies (cf. Fig. 2 and Miskiewicz et al., 1993).

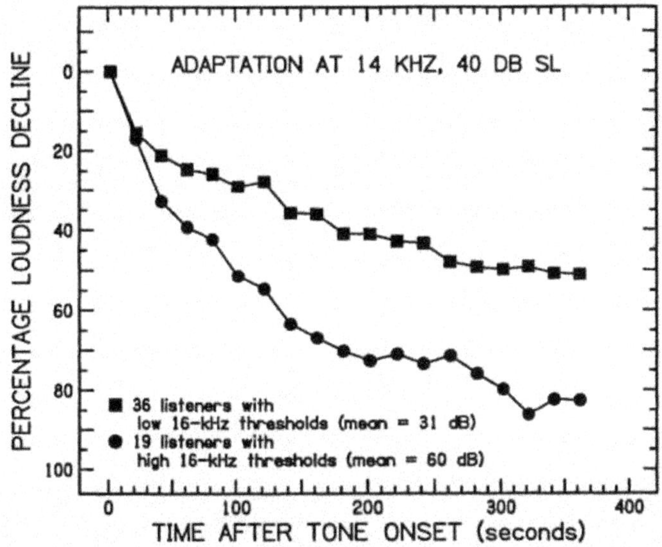

Figure 2. The percentage decline in the loudness of a 14-kHz tone at 40 dB SL as a function of tone duration. One curve is for a group of listeners with thresholds at 16 kHz that are lower than 50 dB SPL and the other is for a group with thresholds that are higher than 50 dB.

As noted above, adaptation is reduced when the stimulus is modulated. In other sensory modalities, fluctuation is essential in avoiding adaptation. In vision, adaptation is greatly increased by fixating a light stimulus on the retina, thereby circumventing nystagmus and saccades which effectively modulate the stimulus (Riggs et al., 1953). In taste, adaptation is reduced by making a steadily flowing taste stimulus intermittent (Meiselman and Halpern, 1973). So it is not surprising that in hearing, adaptation is weak for temporally varying stimuli such as beating tones and most noises. Perhaps sounds that evoke broad excitation patterns do not adapt because the effective neural activation across critical bands is asynchronous and, in effect, fluctuating.

2.3 Ipsilaterally Induced Adaptation

Another kind of adaptation occurs when a sound is incremented intermittently or another sound, the inducer, is presented intermittently to the same ear. The loudness of the sound during its weaker periods declines by an amount that depends on a number of stimulus factors. The increment must be 5 dB or more, and the greater the increment, the greater is the loudness adaptation (Canévet et al., 1983). Although 5-s increments every 30 s reduce loudness more than do 1-s increments, further increases in the duration or repetition rate of the increments have little effect on the amount of adaptation (Scharf et al., 1983a). The induced adaptation does not depend on tone frequency (Charron and Botte, 1988). It is stronger for a tone than for a noise (Scharf and Canévet, 1989). However, for both tones and noise the adaptation becomes greater as the base level decreases, at least below 40 dB SPL (Scharf and Canévet, 1989).

The adaptation induced by an intermittent tone at a different frequency than the continuous tone follows more or less the same rules as that induced by a simple increment in level. However, at moderate stimulus levels the amount of adaptation declines markedly as the frequency difference between the inducer and the continuous tone increases, revealing strong frequency selectivity with a bandwidth close to the critical band (Charron and Botte, 1988; Baruch and Botte, 1989).

Ipsilaterally induced adaptation (IIA) is probably closer to auditory fatigue than to adaptation. It is correlated with temporary threshold shift; listeners who are more susceptible to IIA also have larger threshold shifts after exposure to a high-level tone (Botte et al., 1988). Moreover, at moderate inducer levels, IIA is greatest when the continuous tone is at the same frequency as the intermittent inducer tone, but as the inducer level increases from 75 to 95 dB, adaptation is greatest when the continuous tone is at a higher frequency than the inducer (Charron and Botte, 1988). This shift is like the well-known half-octave shift seen in auditory fatigue at higher levels. Unlike fatigue, however, IIA does not increase with inducer level--below 50 dB it goes the other way, increasing as threshold is neared--nor with inducer duration beyond 5 s or so. This type of loudness decline may well involve both adaptation and fatigue (cf. Botte and Mönikheim, in press).

2.4 Contralaterally Induced Adaptation

Contralaterally induced adaptation (CIA) takes place when a continuous sound in one ear is accompanied by an intermittent sound in the other. The stimulus variables that control this type of adaptation are reasonably well understood, but the underlying mechanism remains unclear. Such adaptation increases somewhat with the frequency of the continuous tone, but not as much as simple adaptation does (Botte et al., 1982); the increase occurs at combinations of frequencies and levels where simple adaptation does not take place. Although CIA occurs at high as well as at moderate levels, it is stronger for a 50-dB tone than for an 80-dB tone (Scharf, 1983). Most of the induced decline in loudness takes place within the first 2 to 3 min of exposure to the inducer.

Rather surprisingly, within wide limits the characteristics of the inducer have little effect on the amount of induced adaptation. Adaptation is induced even when the inducer differs widely in frequency from the continuous tone (Botte et al., 1982, 1986). When the frequencies of the continuous and inducer tones are the same, the amount of induced adaptation varies little with the rate of intermittency (Botte et al., 1982; Canévet et al., 1985; Scharf et al., 1983). The level of the inducer can also vary over a wide range, from 20 dB weaker than the continuous tone to 20 or 30 dB stronger with little change in the amount of adaptation (Botte et al., 1982).

Recovery from CIA is difficult to achieve (Scharf et al., 1983b). Turning off the intermittent inducer tone altogether and the continuous tone for 5 s results in only a partial recovery of loudness, which then precedes to decline again despite the absence of the intermittent tone. Even after 30 s of silence, the continuous tone, when reintroduced, shows strong adaptation in the absence of contralateral stimulation. Such marked resistance to complete recovery has not been noted in simple adaptation.

For several reasons, it would seem that the restricted-excitation-pattern hypothesis does not apply to CIA. (1) The amount of adaptation does not relate to stimulus factors that would be associated with a reduced spread of excitation. (2) The adaptation does not appear to be peripheral. (3) Recovery from CIA is very different from that in simple adaptation. The more central neural locus of CIA is suggested by its very nature, which involves interaction between the two ears, and by its close relationship to auditory lateralization (Botte et al., 1986). Moreover, Botte et al. (1982) showed that while the loudness of a continuous tone declined in the presence of a contralateral inducer, the masking by that tone of a pulsed higher-frequency tone remained constant, which would mean--to the extent that masking is peripheral--that the excitation evoked in the cochlea was not affected and the loudness decline must have taken place more centrally.

3 Attention

The modern era of research on attention was ushered in with the publication of Broadbent's book, *Perception and Communication*, in 1958. Broadbent drew most of his empirical inspiration from research on hearing, largely concerned with the simultaneous processing of multiple messages. Nonetheless, vision soon took center stage in research on attention. Aside from the large literature on the effects of attention on evoked auditory potentials, research on auditory attention has been limited. Issues of central importance in vision, such as late vs. early selection in the filtering of sensory input and automatic vs. controlled processing (cf. Allport, 1993), have hardly been addressed in hearing, least of all in psychoacoustics. Filtering has, of course, been a primary issue in psychoacoustics, but it has been almost exclusively a question of peripheral filtering and frequency selectivity. Accordingly, most of the studies of attention in psychoacoustics have been in the frequency domain and have concentrated on the detection of signals in noise.

Two experimental approaches are distinguished, one that measures detection when signal frequency is unpredictable, the other when attention is focused on a designated frequency region. I begin with a brief discussion of frequency uncertainty. That discussion is followed by a review of those studies that sought to determine how focusing attention on a given frequency region (or regions) affected detection outside that region (or those regions). Finally, research with human patients is reported that seems to implicate the olivocochlear bundle in attentional filtering.

3.1 Frequency Uncertainty

In experiments on frequency uncertainty, listeners are presented tonal signals in noise at unpredictable frequencies chosen from a wide range of values. Green (1961), in what has become the classic reference, noted the wide inter-subject variability in results of earlier studies. He reduced variability by letting his three well-trained observers listen to the extremes and the center of the frequency range from which the signals were chosen. The major outcome was that widening the frequency range from 1 Hz (same frequency on every trial) to 1 kHz increased threshold only about 1 dB; widening the range to 3.5 kHz increased threshold another 2 dB. Thus, the largest measured effect of frequency uncertainty on threshold was 3 dB, much less than expected if the observer had been listening in a single, narrow frequency region under all conditions, as per the single-band model, or had been listening in many different regions, as per the multi-band model. The single-band model predicts an increase in threshold of the order of 10 dB because under maximum uncertainty the observer would have been listening in the wrong band most of the time. The multi-band model predicts a similar increase because the signal falls in only one band while noise comes from all the monitored bands thereby decreasing the effective signal-to-noise ratio. Green argued that both models failed because they assumed no uncertainty in the fixed-frequency condition. He proposed that even when the frequency is always the same "the observer has a considerable amount of initial uncertainty."

More recently, Buus et al. (1986) have proposed a modified multi-band model that comes closer to predicting the data. Nonetheless, it seems that observers can adopt different listening strategies when faced with frequency uncertainty, as suggested by Swets (1963, 1984).

Gundy (1961) showed that the strategy can be modified by providing the listener with prior information about the stimuli. He measured detection of a 1-kHz tone in broadband noise. To one group of naive listeners, he presented the signal at a clearly audible level several times before each block of trials. To another group, he made it obvious that the same signal would be presented throughout the experiment but did not let them hear it beforehand at the higher level. The uninformed listeners were initially unable to detect the tone at all, d' was near 0 (50% correct) at the end of the first 50 trials. Informed listeners had a d' close to 1.5 (85% correct). [That difference may be equivalent to at least 5 or 6 dB (Dai et al., 1991).] Whereas Green's listeners knew that many different frequencies were to be presented and so probably adopted a multi-band listening strategy, Gundy's uncued listeners, knowing that the signal would always be the same, may have adopted a single-band strategy, listening for a single frequency in various parts of the spectrum. Focusing attention in the wrong place (wrong frequency region) is more detrimental to detection, it would seem, then spreading attention over a wide range--at least initially. After 200 trials, d' increased to around 0.7 for the uncued listeners. For a different group also tested without cues but with the signal 2 dB stronger, the d' increased from an initial value near 0.7 to 2.0 after 250 trials. Cued listeners, who started with a d' above 2.0, showed hardly any improvement over 200 trials.

These results seem quite reasonable, i.e. that a weak sound at an unknown frequency is more difficult to hear just as a dim point of light at an unknown location is more difficult to spot. And Gundy's data show how readily listeners adopt what seems like a single-band strategy when explicitly informed about the frequency to listen for. One should like to measure the width and shape of the listening or attentional band by determining the detectability of signals outside as well as within the targeted band. The probe-signal procedures yield such measures.

3.2 Probe-Signal Procedures

The essence of the probe-signal procedure is to focus the listener's attention on one or more specific frequency regions while measuring detection there and also at one or more other, unspecified regions. This approach has the great advantage of yielding a measure of the detectability of unattended signals. The results have shown how finely tuned, yet flexible the auditory system is.

An early example of a kind of probe-signal procedure was in a report by Tanner and Norman (1954). On a four-interval forced-choice test, their listeners scored 65% correct for the detection of a 1-kHz tone burst in white noise. After an unannounced change in signal frequency to 1.3 kHz, the listeners scored 25%, at chance. Telling the four listeners about the frequency change soon brought performance back to 65%.

It may have been this report that led Greenberg and Larkin (1968) to develop an explicit procedure for measuring frequency selectivity by assessing performance at unexpected frequencies. They led their listeners to focus attention on 1 kHz, usually by presenting that frequency at a higher level before each block of trials. In the ensuing trials, they presented the signal at the expected, target frequency of 1 kHz on 77% of the trials and at a different, probe frequency on 23% of the trials. Presented against a continuous wide-band noise, both the target signal, at 1 kHz, and the probe signal, at the other frequency, were presented at signal-to-noise ratios that would normally yield approximately 80% correct detection (2IFC). Listeners scored near 80% correct when the signal was at the target frequency or close to it. Percentage correct declined rapidly as the signal frequency moved further away from the target until at a frequency approximately half a critical band away, performance was near chance. Yama and Robinson (1982) reported similar results for a target signal at 500 Hz.

Unlike these earlier studies, which tested highly experienced listeners over many sessions, Scharf et al. (1987) tested untrained listeners in a single session. Listeners were led to focus on 1 kHz by a cue presented at that frequency at the beginning of every trial. The cue was 8 dB above the SPL required for 75% correct detection (2IFC); the signal was 4 dB above that level. Listeners scored near 90% at 1 kHz and close to 50% at distant probe frequencies. The data fit nicely the ROEX filter derived from notch-noise experiments (Patterson and Moore, 1986). Control measurements showed that listeners scored 90% correct on those same probe frequencies when they were subsequently presented as the only signals.

Listeners can be led to focus on more than a single frequency region. Macmillan and

Schwartz (1976) gave higher-level samples of two frequencies several critical bands apart and told their listeners that signals would occur at either one of those frequencies. Detection was highest for signals at either target frequency and declined as the signal frequency moved away from the targets, reaching near-chance levels at distant frequencies including those falling between the targets. Schlauch and Hafter (1991) used a four-tone cue to promote four-band listening. Detection was highest at frequencies corresponding to the components of the cue and fell at other frequencies. In both studies, performance at the targeted frequencies declined somewhat as their number increased from one to two to four.

Listeners sometimes adopt a two-frequency listening strategy even when they are not supposed to and are not so instructed. Usually it is not clear why that occurs. Sometimes it is because the probe level was too high. To reduce the likelihood of that happening and to speed up data collection, Dai et al. (1991) developed a multi-probe procedure in which the target is presented on 75% of 64 trials and eight other probe frequencies on the other 25% (16 trials). Thus, in a block of trials each probe frequency is presented twice. This procedure was used with four experienced listeners at five target frequencies from 250 to 4000 Hz. The data showed sharp filtering; bandwidths were somewhat narrower than the critical band. Like the single-probe procedure, the multi-probe version does not require trained listeners. Figure 3 shows more recent, unpublished

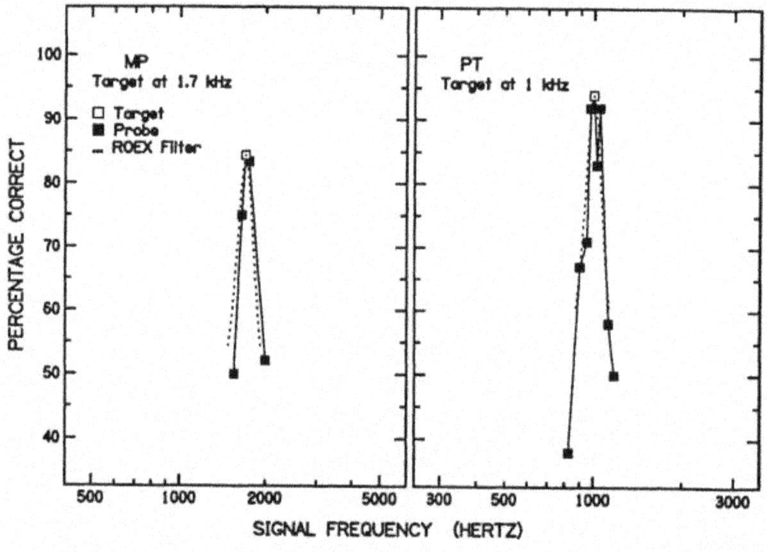

Figure 3. Percentage correct in a 2IFC multi-probe task plotted as a function of signal frequency. Listener MP was presented four probe frequencies around a target at 1.7 kHz; listener PT was presented eight probes around a target at 1 kHz. The ROEX filter was derived from notched-noise experiments.

data for two relatively inexperienced listeners. In these tests, probes were presented on 50% of the trials, every trial beginning with a cue at the target frequency. Listener MP was given four probe frequencies, each one presented eight times at random in a block of 64 trials, yielding a total of 48 trials per probe in six blocks. Listener PT was given eight probe frequencies over six blocks for a total of 24 trials per probe. These observers, like most others in multi-probe tests, listen through a single filter, very much like the auditory filter (represented by the ROEX filter in Fig. 3) measured in notched-noise experiments.

Two questions often arise about undetected probe frequencies. (1) Are the probes undetected because they are not heard or because they are not recognized as signals? (2) At what level can they be detected; that is, how much are the probes "attenuated"?

3.2.1 Are probes heard but not heeded?

Scharf et al. (1987) used the term "heard-but-not-heeded hypothesis" to identify the hypothesis that listeners hear probes but misidentify them as part of the noise, and ignore them. They presented experimental evidence refuting this hypothesis and supporting a single-band model, according to which observers usually listen through a single auditory filter in the probe-signal procedure. I review briefly that evidence and present some new data.

If listeners misidentify signals because they expect only the target frequency, then telling listeners about the presence of probes should improve the detection of probes. However, when we told one of our groups of untrained listeners that signals other than the target would be presented, the detection of distant probes stayed down near chance (Scharf et al., 1987). Knowledge about probes does not matter much to trained listeners either. Dai et al. (1991) continued to obtain approximately the same results from a listener, who had completed many hundreds of trials with eight probes, after telling her about the presence of probes. Moreover, in that study the results for the experimenter who served as one of the four observers were like those of the other observers.

Another prediction of the heard-but-not-heeded hypothesis would be that removing the cue from every trial would make it less likely that the listener ignore probe frequencies. However, results show that once a listener has become set to listen in a particular frequency region, removing the cue does not improve the detection of distant probes (Greenberg and Larkin, 1968; Scharf et al., 1987).

The heard-but-not-heeded hypothesis should also mean that listeners who were not heeding a probe signal that occurred on only a minority of trials should be more likely to respond to the probe if it occurred more often. Such is not the case. The same probe can be presented on as many trials as the target without affecting performance. Figure 4 gives the mean percentage correct for four listeners as a function of signal frequency. Filled symbols are for probes, and unfilled symbols are for the target at 1.7 kHz and for the probe frequencies presented as expected signals in control conditions. Filled squares are for blocks of trials in which the target was presented 75% of the time, which is the approximate percentage used in most of the published experiments using the probe-signal method; filled circles are for blocks in which targets were presented 50% of the time. In each block of 100 trials, a single probe frequency was presented on 25 or 50 trials. The

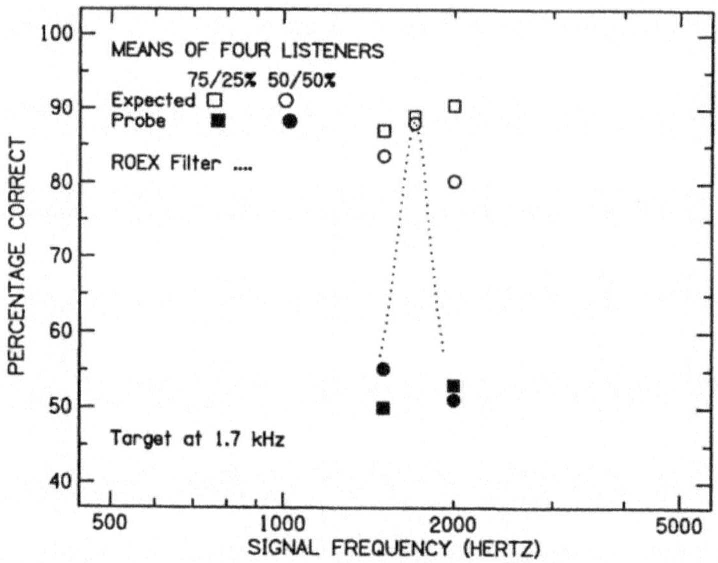

Figure 4. Percentage correct as a function of signal frequency in a single-probe task. In half the probe conditions, the probe was presented on 25% of the trials (squares), and in the other half on 50% of the trials (circles).

cue was always at the target frequency of 1.7 kHz, except in control conditions. No clear difference emerges from these data between the 50% and 75% conditions. Probes were detected about as poorly in both conditions by the four listeners. (However, two other listeners did score better on some probes in the 50% condition than in the 75% condition.)

Another test of the heard-but-not-heeded hypothesis is to vary the quality of the signal without changing its frequency locus. The filter model implies that the quality of the signal matters little and that the frequency locus is the primary, perhaps the sole determinant of how detection will vary with signal level. Frequency locus would matter for the heard-but-not-heeded hypothesis in so far as it means that the probe sounds more or less like the target, but other stimulus attributes like bandwidth and temporal pattern would also matter. To test these differing predictions, Ebata and Scharf (1992) presented a 1-kHz tone as cue and target and a narrow band of noise centered on 1 kHz as the probe. In a separate experiment, the converse held, that is, the noise was the cue and target, and the tone was the probe. Under both arrangements, 14 listeners in one experiment and 15 in the other detected the probes just as well as the targets despite the large perceptual difference between a tone and a band of noise. Huanping Dai and I also varied quality by using different temporal patterns. In one experiment, the target was a 1-kHz tone burst repeated three times every 130 ms for 30 ms. The probe was repeated eight times every 42 ms for 12 ms. In one block, the probe burst had the same frequency,

1 kHz, as the target, and in another block it had a different frequency, 1.7 kHz. The 1-kHz probe bursts were detected just as well as the target, despite the difference in temporal pattern, whereas the 1.7-kHz probe bursts were not detected (56% correct). In another experiment, the target and probe had the same temporal pattern but different frequencies. Despite having the same pattern as the target, the probes were poorly detected (60% correct). If observers responded only to signals that were like the cue and target, they ought not to have heeded a band of noise when the target was a tone; unlike temporal patterns should also have gone unheeded. Still another way to vary the nature of a sound is to change its direction in space. Scharf et al. (1989) reported that 1-kHz probe signals from a loudspeaker 45° to the right were detected as well as 1-kHz targets from a loudspeaker 45° to the left. So far, it seems that the only stimulus attribute to influence detection scores for constant-level probes is tonal frequency.

Schlauch and Hafter (1991) provide some of the clearest evidence against the heard-but-not-heeded hypothesis. In one experiment their cues, presented on every trial, were made up of four simultaneous tones, each separated from its neighbors by a frequency ratio of at least 1.4. (The component frequencies were chosen randomly from trial to trial from a range of nearly 3 kHz.) The individual tonal components seldom stood out perceptually from the overall complex. Nonetheless, listeners detected probes at or near the component frequenies but not distant probes including those falling between the component frequencies. The observers appeared to listen through four bands simultaneously. It is difficult to believe that they ignored probes--especially in-between ones--because they were unlike any one of the cue components, which were not heard separately to begin with. These results seem especially difficult to square with the heard-but-not-heeded hypothesis.

3.2.2 How much are probes attenuated?

The probe-signal method is usually applied with probes set to a constant level. Percentage correct is measured as a function of signal frequency. When the percentage correct is at chance, the question arises as to how much the probe level must be increased to permit detection. That value would give an approximation of the amount of effective attenuation the probes undergo. To obtain that estimate, Dai et al. (1991) measured psychometric functions by presenting probes at various sound pressure levels. Classical psychometric functions were also obtained for the signals presented alone at the probe frequencies. The psychometric functions for the signal presented alone and for it presented as a probe could then be compared. Their difference in level at some criterion value of percentage correct provides an estimation of the effective attenuation of the probe. However, measuring psychometric functions for probe signals raises the possibility that the listener changes to a two-band strategy after having been exposed to more intense probes which are readily audible. To mitigate that problem, Dai et al. (1991) presented probes at 24 different frequencies as well as at 6 different levels in each block of trials. After taking into account the likely effect of higher-level probes, Dai et al. (1991) estimated 7 to 8 dB as the likely amount of effective attenuation of distant probes. In other words, to be detected as well when presented as a distant probe as when presented as a fully attended signal, a probe must be increased 7 or 8 dB.

An estimate of 7 to 8 dB is congruent with the outcome of a study by Ebata et al. (1968) who measured psychometric functions for tones presented in the quiet. Thresholds were 6 to 8 dB higher when the tones were unexpected than when expected. An 8-dB value is also buttressed by anecdotal evidence. In our single-probe experiments, occasionally listeners did not hear a new cue, usually in a control condition with a signal frequency, which had previously been a probe, presented as both cue and target. The unexpected cue went undetected although it was set 8 dB above 75% detection level. Finally, in a study of auditory evoked potentials, Squires et al. (1973) reported that a tone in noise had to be increased 8 dB to evoke potentials at the same amplitude in an active-reading (visual) condition as in an active-listening condition. Paying full attention to the signal was equivalent to increasing its level by 8 dB.

3.3.3 On making probes detectable

Probes can be made more detectable in several ways other than by increasing their level. Gating the masker so that it comes on 300 ms before the signal (or potential signal) in each observation interval resulted in the detection of distant probes at an average of 65 to 75% correct whereas the same probes in a continuous noise were detected with scores between 50 and 65% (Dai and Buus, 1991). Reducing the duration of the signals from 295 ms to 5 ms had a similar effect (Wright and Dai, 1994). These stimulus changes appear to have caused observers to focus on more than one attentional band. Just why gating the masker or shortening the signal disrupts selective listening is unclear. Another, more radical procedure that results in the detection of probe signals is the sectioning of the olivocochlear bundle, which is discussed after the next section.

3.3.4 Controlled vs. automatic listening; early vs. late selection

Swets (1963) suggested that listeners can control their listening strategy and thereby modify auditory filtering, e.g. by widening the critical band. Many of the data reviewed above seem to indicate that stimulus conditions control whether a single band is primarily monitored or a number of bands. Gated maskers and brief signals are particularly good examples. Furthermore, the four-tone cues of Schlauch and Hafter (1991) led to the monitoring of four narrow and separated bands in spite of the lack of salience for any of the components that would permit the listener to focus easily on them. The fact that explicit knowledge about the probes does not influence performance could be taken as further evidence for automatic processing. Evidence in the other direction comes from a paper by Hafter and Schlauch (1992). They instructed listeners to detect tonal signals at the musical fifth above a cue tone presented at the beginning of every trial. The frequency of the cue was changed from trial to trial. Listeners with musical training gave results that looked much like the attentional filtering seen with the usual cues that require listening at the cue frequency, itself. Hafter and Schlauch also gave visual cues to musicians with absolute pitch to indicate in which frequency region to listen. Cues given as notes in musical notation worked nearly as well as auditory cues. These results would suggest that the listener can explicitly determine which frequency region to focus upon.

Whether controlled or automatic or sometimes one, sometimes the other, attentional filtering could occur early or late in the auditory system, that is, closer or farther from the cochlea. Even if completely controlled, the strong efferent input to the cochlea provides the neural hardware for top-down processing. The evidence suggests automatic processing with some central control. Cognitive input could possibly prepare the cochlea for responding in different ways depending upon the acoustic input. The next section addresses these questions experimentally.

3.3.5 Selective attention without efferent input

If efferent input to the cochlea plays a role in the selective listening seen in probe-signal tasks, then listeners whose olivocochlear bundle (OCB) has been sectioned should give different results in those tasks. Such observers are available for study when the vestibular nerve, which contains the OCB, is sectioned by vestibular neurotomy to relieve severe vertigo, usually resulting from Ménière's disease. So far, probe-signal measurements are available from 13 such patients, ten of whom were operated on by Professor J. Magnan or Dr. A. Chays in Marseille, and three by Professor J. Nadol in Boston. Eleven of them have an audiometric hearing level at the tested frequency of less than 30 dB, and two have hearing levels greater than 30 dB.

Before presenting results, I address two sets of questions. The first concerns the evidence that the OCB has been sectioned in these patients. Is the whole OCB severed together with the vestibular nerve? Animal studies suggest the whole OCB travels within the inferior vestibular nerve, and human studies give no evidence for a different anatomical arrangement (Arnesen, 1985; Gacek, 1961). Is the whole vestibular nerve sectioned? Caloric tests of vestibular function, subjective reports, photomicrographs taken during the operation, and the surgeon's report all favor the notion that the whole vestibular nerve was sectioned in these patients (cf. Scharf et al., 1994).

Other questions concern the implication of studying an impaired auditory system. Is the function of the efferent input the same in an ear with Ménière's disease as in a normal ear? The best answer to this question is to study patients before the operation as well as after. Could any measured changes be the result of side effects of the operation that have nothing to do with the OCB? In most patients, hearing thresholds do not change after the operation, and in fact other auditory functions show little or no change. Could the hearing loss usually associated with Ménière's disease obscure effects of efferent input? Most of the patients studied had a mild hearing loss in the frequency region examined, and several had nearly normal thresholds over much of the audible frequency range.

The most difficult problem in this research is the variability in the effect of the vestibular neurotomy on selective attention. In some patients, a clear difference emerges either between test results before the neurotomy and those after or between their normal ear and their operated ear. In others, the differences are much smaller.

Selective attention was measured by single-probe and multi-probe procedures. Owing to the limited time usually available with each patient, probes were presented in almost all cases on 50% of the trials. Prior to the application of the probe-signal method, masked thresholds were usually measured by an 2IFC adaptive procedure using a five-down/one-up rule which asymptotes on approximately 87% correct. These measurements permitted an evaluation of the critical ratio and hence of frequency selectivity in broadband masking. Of 16 patients for whom such values are available (including three who could not be tested for selective attention), only one had abnormal critical ratios (cf. Scharf et al., 1993). Four patients whose critical ratios were measured before and after the operation showed no increase in the ratio. Accordingly, most probe-signal measurements could be made with signals and noise set to the same levels before and after the operation or in the normal and in the operated ears of the same patient.

Before-after comparisons of selective attention are available for three patients, all of whom had nearly normal thresholds in the tested frequency range around 1 kHz. Because the patients came to the laboratory for the tests the day before the operation for only a couple of hours, pre-operative results are limited, especially for two of them. Nonetheless, all three gave some evidence of better detection of probes after the operation than before. For one patient, SB, the data are impressive. Many other psychoacoustic tests were carried out on him and are the subject of an extensive paper (Scharf et al., 1994) which includes a portion on selective attention. Figure 5 is taken from that paper. These results are from the single-probe version of the probe-signal procedure. The before-after contrast

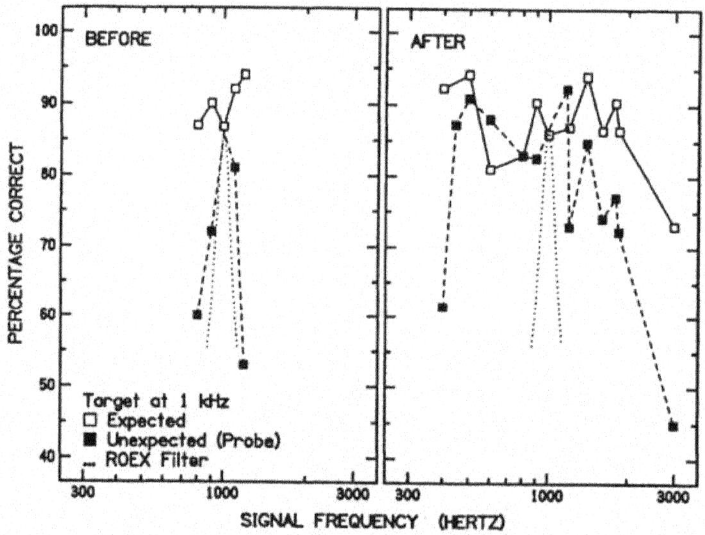

Figure 5. Performance on a single-probe task before and after sectioning of the olivocochlear bundle during a vestibular neurotomy. Data were collected one day before the operation and over a period of ten months afterwards. The patient had hearing levels within 20 dB of normal at the audiometric frequencies (from Scharf et al., 1994).

is striking. Before the neurotomy, his performance follows closely the ROEX filter; afterwards, it deviates widely. Probes that were detected near chance before were detected well above chance one week later and over the next ten months during which tests were continued. The patient also detected probes when the target frequency was 4 kHz. Figure 5 would seem to suggest that SB's attentional filter became much wider after the neurotomy. Before discussing why such a widening probably did not occur, I present data from two other patients.

Figure 6 shows the results for patient LG who has a 25-dB loss at the target frequency of 1 kHz, and for CA who has approximately a 40-dB loss at the target frequency of 500 Hz, at which she was tested. Percentage correct is shown by circles for the normal ear and by squares for the operated ear. Owing to the limited data for LG, we do not know just how far out he detects probes. Patient CA detects probes over a wide range of frequencies, both below and above the target. Three other patients, in addition to the three in Figs. 5 and 6, give evidence of detecting probes at frequencies both above and below the target. Other patients show less symmetry. Two patients detected lower-frequency probes but not higher-frequency ones; three others detected probes only toward higher frequencies. For the remaining two patients, data were too variable or sparse to permit any conclusions about symmetry.

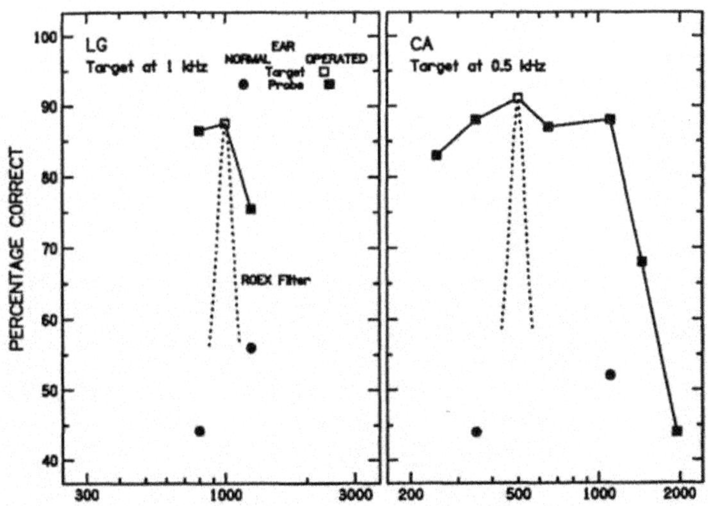

Figure 6. Performance on a single-probe task by two patients whose vestibular nerve and olivocochlear bundle had been sectioned. Circles are for the normal ear, and squares for the operated ear.

The data from the three patients whose data are shown in Figs. 5 and 6 provide particularly clear evidence for an effect of the vestibular neurotomy on the detection of probe signals in the single-probe task. Data from the other ten patients also show better detection of probes relative to pre-operative performance (two cases) or to the unoperated ear (eight cases).

Despite large variability in the behavior of patients, some conclusions about the role of the OCB in selective attention are possible. It is almost certain that sectioning the OCB does not widen the cochlear filter. First of all, the critical ratio was normal in 15 of 16 patients. Second, the auditory filter as measured in notched noise (Patterson and Moore, 1986) in six patients was the same in the operated ear as in the normal ear in four of them and was about twice as wide in two. (It is possible that the filter was wider in these two patients before the operation, but it had not been measured.) It is also clear that the attentional filter, to the extent that it is distinct from the auditory filter, is not wider after the neurotomy. The most telling evidence is that measurements by the multi-probe procedure (usually with eight probe frequencies, sometimes with four) have revealed selectivity--in the seven patients for whom such tests were made--that is much closer to normal than the single-probe measurements. For example, SB scored 90% correct when a 600-Hz tone was presented as the only probe frequency in the single-probe task (Fig. 5) and scored 57% correct when it was presented as the lowest of eight probe frequencies in a multi-probe task. If detection of the 600-Hz probe in the single-probe task reflected an abnormally wide filter at the target frequency of 1 kHz, then detection in the multi-probe task ought to have been equally good despite the presence of additional signals.

Why, in most patients, is probe detection in the single-probe task better than in the multi-probe task? One possibility is that without efferent input, probe frequencies are still effectively attenuated, but less so. Hence, when a single probe is presented, its effective level is high enough that the patient often hears it and so adopts a two-band strategy. When many probes are presented, their pitch varies too much to permit the listener to adopt readily a multi-band or even a two-band strategy. Even so, the hypothesized reduction in the effective attenuation of probes would explain why patients detect multiple probes somewhat better than normal. One piece of evidence in support of this explanation is that patient SB detected some distant probes better than normal in his *unoperated* ear. These measurements were made only after the neurotomy and after a number of tests on the operated ear. It is possible that SB came to use a two-band strategy as his normal listening mode in our tests.

The role of efferent input to the cochlea appears to be rather small. But it almost surely plays some role in selective attention, as suggested also by reports of small but significant effects of manipulations of attention on otoacoustic emissions (Giard et al., 1994; Puel et al., 1988). However, the change in selective attention following the elimination of efferent input depends much on the individual patient. Already in a normal population, we find that listeners differ in just how poorly they detect probes, especially in the single-probe version. Perhaps people differ in the amount of effective attenuation of probe signals, which in turn reflects differences in the potency of efferent input to the cochlea. Such variability was noted in the cat with respect to contralateral suppression, via the OCB, of auditory-nerve responses (Liberman, 1989).

With respect to auditory attention in general, these results suggest that much of it is automatic, at least in the frequency domain. However, cognitive control is possible as shown in visual cuing, cuing to the 5th, the ability of listeners to adopt a two-frequency strategy, and so forth. The similarity of the attentional and auditory filters suggest further that the filtering is largely if not entirely cochlear. The finding that efferent input modulates the filtering, however weakly, lends further support to that idea.

4 Acknowledgements

I thank M.-C. Botte, R. Hellman, G. Canévet, and A. Miskiewicz for many helpful comments on parts of an earlier version of this article. I thank E. Hafter for many stimulating discussions about selective attention. I am deeply grateful to J. Magnan and A. Chays at the Hôspital Nord in Marseille and to J. Nadol at the Massachusetts Eye and Ear Infirmary in Boston for having made possible the testing of their patients. The U. S. Public Health Service, through NIH grant 2 RO1NS07270, provided partial support for this research.

5 References

Allport, A. (1993) Attention and control: Have we been asking the wrong questions? A critical review of twenty-five years. In: D. E. Meyer and S. Kornblum (Eds.), Attention and Performance XIV, The MIT Press, Cambridge, MA, pp. 183-218.

Arnesen, A. (1985) Anastomosis in humans. Acta Otolaryngol., Supplement 423, 81-84.

Baruch, C. and Botte, M.-C. (1989) Individual differences in adaptation: The musicians' case. In: G. Canévet, B. Scharf, A.-M. Bonnel, and C.-A. Possamaï (Eds.), Proc. 5th Meeting Interntl. Soc. Psychophysics, CNRS, Marseille, pp. 102-107.

Békésy, G. von (1929) Zur Theorie des Hörens; Ueber die Bestimmung des einem reinen Tonempfinden entsprechenden Erregungsgebietes der Basilarmembran vermittelst Ermündungserscheinungen, Phys. Z. 30, 115-125.

Botte, M.-C., Baruch, C., and Scharf, B. (1986) Loudness reduction and adaptation induced by a contralateral tone. J. Acoust. Soc. Am., 80, 73-81.

Botte, M.-C., Canévet, G., and Scharf, B. (1982) Loudness adaptation induced by an intermittent tone. J. Acoust. Soc. Am., 72, 727-739.

Botte, M.-C., Charron, S., Mönikheim, S., and Scharf, B. (1988) Predicting susceptibility to auditory fatigue on the basis of loudness adaptation. In: B. Berglund, U. Berglund, J. Karlsson, and T. Lindvall (Eds.), Noise as a Public Helath Problem, Vol. 2. Swedish Council for Bldg. Res., Stockholm, 39-44.

Botte, M.-C. and Mönikheim, S. (in press) New data on the short-term effects of tone exposure. J. Acoust. Soc. Am.

Broadbent, D. E. (1958) Perception and Communication. Pergamon Press, London.

Buus, S., Schorer, E., Florentine, M., and Zwicker, E. (1986) Decision rules in detection of simple and complex tones. J. Acoust. Soc. Am. 80, 1646-1657.

Canévet, G., Scharf, B., and Botte, M.-C. (1983) Loudness adaptation, when induced, is real. Brit. J. Audiol. 17, 49-57.

Canévet, G., Scharf, B., and Botte, M.-C. (1985) Simple and induced loudness adaptation. Audiol. 24, 430-436.

Charron, S. and Botte, M.-C. (1988) Frequency selectivity in loudness adaptation and auditory fatigue. J.

Acoust. Soc. Am. 83, 178-187.

Dai, H. and Buus, S. (1991) Effect of gating the masker on frequency-selective listening. J. Acoust. Soc. Am. 89, 1816-1818.

Dai, H., Scharf, B., and Buus, S. (1991) Effective attenuation of signals in noise under focused attention. J. Acoust. Soc. Am. 89, 2837-2842.

Ebata, M. and Scharf, B. (1992) The effect of selective attention on auditory detection. J. Acoust. Soc. Jpn. (E) 13, 59-61.

Ebata, M., Sone, T., and Nimura, T. (1968) Improvement of hearing ability by directional information. J. Acoust. Soc. Am. 43, 289-297.

Florentine, M. (1983) Intensity discrimination as a function of level and frequency and its relation to high-frequency hearing. J. Acoust. Soc. Am. 74, 1375-1379.

Florentine, M. and Buus, S. (1981) An excitation-pattern model for intensity discrimination. J. Acoust. Soc. Am. 70, 1646-1654.

Gacek, R. R. (1961) The efferent cochlear bundle in man. Archiv. Otolaryngol. (Chicago) 74, 690-694.

Giard, M-H, Collet, L., Bouchet, P., and Pernier, J. (1994) Auditory selective attention in the human cochlea. Brain Res. 633, 353-356.

Green, D. M. (1961) Detection of auditory sinusoids of uncertain frequency. J. Acoust. Soc. Am. 33, 897-903.

Greenberg, G. and Larkin, W. (1968) Frequency-response characteristic of auditory observers detecting signals of a single frequency in noise: The probe-signal method. J. Acoust. Soc. Am. 44, 1513-1523.

Gundy, R. (1961) Auditory detection of an unspecified signal. J. Acoust. Soc. Am. 33, 1008-1012.

Hafter, E. R. and Schlauch, R. S. (1992) Cognitive factors and selection of auditory listening bands. In: A. L. Dancer, D. Henderson, R. J. Salvi, and R. P. Hamernik (Eds.), Noise-Induced Hearing Loss, Mosby Year Book, St. Louis, pp. 303-310.

Hellman, R. P. (1978) Dependence of loudness growth on skirts of excitation patterns. J. Acoust. Soc. Am. 63, 1114-1119.

Hood, J.D. (1950) Studies in auditory fatigue and adaptation. Acta Oto-Laryngol. S92.

Liberman, M. C. (1989) Rapid assesment of sound-evoked olivocochlear feedback: Suppression of compound action potentials by contralateral sound. Hear. Res. 38, 47-56.

Macmillan, N. A. and Schwartz, M. (1975) A probe-signal investigation of uncertain-frequency detection. J. Acoust. Soc. Am. 58, 1051-1058.

Meiselman, H. L. and Halpern, B. P. (1973) Enhancement of taste intensity through pulsatile stimulation. Physiol. Behav. 11, 713-716.

Miskiewicz, A., Scharf, B., Hellman, R., and Meiselman, C. (1993) Loudness adaptation at high frequencies. J. Acoust. Soc. Am. 94, 1281-1286.

Palva, T. and Kärjä, J. (1969) Suprathreshold auditory adaptation. J. Acoust. Soc. Am. 45, 1018-1021.

Patterson, R. D. and Moore, B. C. J. (1986) Auditory filters and excitation patterns as representations of frequency resolution. In Moore, B. C. J. (Ed.) Frequency Selectivity in Hearing, Academic Press, London, 123-177.

Puel, J. L., Bonfils, P., and Pujol, R. (1988) Selective attention modifies the active micromechanical properties of the cochlea. Brain Res. 447, 380-383.

Riggs, L. A., Ratliff, F., Cornsweet, J. C., and Cornsweet, T. N. (1953) The disappearance of steadily fixated visual test objects. J. Opt. Soc. Am. 43, 495-501.

Scharf, B. (1978) Loudness. In E. C. Carterette and M. P. Friedman (Eds.), Handbook of Perception. Vol. 4. Hearing. Academic Press, New York, pp. 187-242.

Scharf, B. (1983) Loudness adaptation. In J. V. Tobias, and E. D. Schuber (Eds.), Hearing Research and Theory. Academic Press, New York.

Scharf, B. (1991) Loudness adaptation measured by the method of successive magnitude estimation. In Ratio Scaling of Psychological Magnitudes. Edited by G. A. Gescheider and S. J. Bolanowski. Hillsdale, NJ: L. Erlbaum, pp. 199-214.

Scharf, B. (1992) Recent measurements of loudness adaptation and the definition of loudness. In Proceedings of the 14th International Congress on Acoustics, Volume 3. Edited by L. Peizi. Beijing, H1-5.

Scharf, B., Botte, M.-C., and Canévet, G. (1983a) Loudness adaptation induced interaurally and monaurally. In R. Klinke and R. Hartmann (Eds.), Hearing--Physiological Basis and Psychophysics. New York: Springer Verlag.

Scharf, B., Botte, M.-C., and Canévet, G. (1983b) Récupération après adaptation induite de sonie. L'Année Psychologique, 83, 9-24.

Scharf, B. and Canévet, G. (1989) Loudness adaptation, loudness functions, and decruitment: In G. Canévet, B. Scharf, A.-M. Bonnel, and C.-A. Possamaï (Eds.) Fechner Day 89, Proceedings of the 5th Meeting of the International Society for Psychophysics. CNRS, Marseille, pp 137-142.

Scharf, B., Magnan, J., Collet, L., Ulmer, E., and Chays, A. (1994) On the role of the olivocochlear bundle in hearing: A case study. Hear. Res., 75, 11-26.

Scharf, B., Nadol, J., Magnan, J., Chays, A., and Marchioni, A. (1993) Does efferent input improve the detection of tones in monaural noise? In: R. Verrillo (Ed.), Sensory Research: Multimodal Perspectives. L. Erlbaum, Hillsdale, NJ, pp. 299-306.

Scharf, B., Possamaï, C., and Bonnel, A. (1989) Deceptive psychophysics: The probe-signal method and focused attention. In S. Dornic and G. Ljunggren (Eds.) Psychophysics in Action. Springer Verlag, Berlin, pp. 67-80.

Scharf, B., Quigley, S., Aoki, C., Peachey, N., and Reeves, A. (1987) Focused auditory attention and frequency selectivity. Percept. Psychophys. 42, 215-223.

Schlauch, R. S. and Hafter, E. R. (1991) Listening bandwidths and frequency uncertainty in pure-tone signal detection. J. Acoust. Soc. Am. 90, 1332-1339.

Squires, K. C., Hillyard, S. A. and Lindsay, P. H. (1973) Vertex potentials evoked during auditory signal detection: Relation to decision criteria. Percept. Psychophys. 14, 265-272.

Swets, J. A. (1963) Central factors in auditory frequency selectivity. Psychol. Bull. 60, 429-440.

Swets, J. A. (1984) Mathematical models of attention. In R. Parasuraman and D. R. Davies (Eds.) Varieties of Attention. Academic Press, New York, pp. 183-242.

Tanner, W. and Norman, R. (1954) The human use of information: II. Signal detection for the case of an unknown signal parameter. Transactions of the Inst. of Radio Engin., Prof. Group on Infor. Theory PGIT-4, 222-227.

Ward, W.D. (1973) Adaptation and fatigue, in J. Jerger (ed.), Modern Developments in Audiology, 2nd Ed., Academic Press, New York.

Wright, B. A. and Dai, H. (1994) Detection of unexpected tones in noise. I: The effect of signal duration. J. Acoust. Soc. Am. 95, 931-938.

Yama, M. and Robinson, D. (1982) Comparison of frequency selectivity for the monaural and binaural hearing systems. J. Acoust. Soc. Am. 71, 694-700.

Zwicker, E. (1956) Die elementaren Grundlagen zur Bestimmung der Informationskapazität des Gehörs. Acustica 6, 365-381.

Comment by A.J.M. Houtsma

In Fig. 7 you show up to 90% loudness adaptation at high frequencies. This means that the tones loudness has declined to a level very close to the loudness that corresponds to detection thresholds (1/16 sone). This, in turn, seems to imply that the threshold must increase with loudness adaptation. Is there any direct evidence that this happens?

Reply

We have measured thresholds by Békésy tracking beginning after the end of tones at 10 dB SL. Thresholds appear to be elevated immediately afterwards, but we are not sure how much of this elevation reflects the change in stimulus and task. A better answer requires more data but conceptally you are entirely right.

Auditory frequency resolution in mammals: From neuronal representation to perception

G. Ehret

Abteilung Vergleichende Neurobiologie, Universität Ulm,
D - 89069 Ulm, Germany

1 Introduction

Most animal communication calls and human speech sounds are complex in the frequency domain, that is, they are composed of many simultaneously occurring frequency components. It has been shown in many studies of acoustic behavior of animals from insects to frogs, birds, and mammals that the spectral composition of a sound conveys information important for shaping the responses of a receiver. Likewise, the formant structure in human speech gives rise to vowel identification and discrimination. The use of frequency information in communication sounds is meaningful only on the basis of a sufficient frequency resolution in the auditory systems. In fact, frequency resolution is one of the fundamental built-in properties of the auditory systems from insects to humans (e.g. Zwicker and Feldtkeller, 1967; Scharf, 1970; Saunders et al., 1979; Ehret and Gerhardt, 1980; Dooling, 1980; Ehret et al. 1982; Ehret, 1983).

Measurements of frequency resolution require that at least two (often many) frequency components interact and influence some perceptual aspect of the sound (psychophysics) or some response feature of neurons in the auditory system (physiology). In both cases, the measured quantity, expressing the quality of frequency resolution, is called the "critical bandwidth" or "critical band". Originally (Fletcher, 1940), critical bands have been determined in experiments on the perception of tones in noise and, therefore, are psychophysical measures. Fletcher's concept, which is still valid today, says that frequency resolution in the auditory system is accomplished by a bank of bandpass filters with continuously variable center frequencies which are instantaneously brought into coincidence with spectral peaks of a heard sound signal. The peaks will be detected if their energy is greater than the sum of the noise energy within the critical bandwidth around the frequency of the peak. Thus, the larger the critical bands are, the lower is the probability that two spectral peaks in a sound can be resolved (e. g. detected separately) and the higher is the probability that spectral peaks are masked by noise also passing the critical band. It follows that critical bands comprise two processes: filtering in the frequency domain and summation of sound energy within the filter bandpass. In other words, critical bands are a measure in terms of spectral distance of the ability of the auditory system to resolve frequency components in complex sounds by spectral integration.

Critical bandwidths have been determined in many types of psychophysical tests (Zwicker and Feldtkeller, 1967; Scharf, 1970; Moore, 1982; Greenwood, 1991b) such as masking of a tone by narrowband noise centered around tone frequency (e. g. Fletcher, 1940; Greenwood, 1961b; Ehret, 1976), masking of a tone centered in a notch of a noise (e. g. Patterson, 1976; Weber, 1977), masked tonal thresholds in comb-filtered noise (Houtgast, 1977; Pick, 1980), loudness summation (Gässler, 1954; Zwicker et al., 1957; Scharf, 1959), phase perception of amplitude-modulated tones (Zwicker, 1952; Schorer, 1986), perception of tonal consonance (Plomp and Levelt, 1965; Greenwood, 1991a), fusion of lateralized sound images (Scharf et al., 1976). Most of the studies showed that critical bands appear to be linear filters (spectral integration independent of the type and intensity of sound passing through the filter). Their bandwidths depend on the method of measurement and on the species used. In experiments in which critical bands were determined by bandwidth variations of a filter-centered sound (e. g. narrowband masking, loudness summation, lateralization) they are of constant, intensity-independent bandwidths over a broad intensity range, often up to 70 - 80 dB above the detection threshold for the sound, whereas critical bands increase and/or their filter slopes decrease with increasing sound intensity in experiments in which sound energy outside a critical band could influence processing inside the filter (e. g. masking by comb- or notch-filtered noise).

2 Peripheral Origin of Frequency Resolution

In the original approach (Fletcher, 1940), critical band filtering was attributed to the frequency-place transformation and frequency tuning in the cochlea. It has been shown for various mammals and humans that psychophysically determined critical bandwidths are related to the cochlear tonotopy in a way that they cover equal distances on the basilar membrane (e.g. Greenwood, 1961a, 1990; Ehret, 1989). The fact that frequency resolution and critical band filtering has its origin in the spacial frequency resolution within the cochlea leads to a certain relationship between the widths of critical band filters and frequency (the center frequency of the filters). If critical band filtering is closely related to frequency filtering in the cochlea, one may expect properties of critical bands in the responses of auditory nerve fibers. On the other hand, critical bands are empirical perceptual phenomena measured in psychophysical tests as filters that divide a sound spectrum into units of perceived sound quality. Therefore, it is conceivable that characteristics of critical bands may emerge from processing in higher auditory centers of the brain. So we have to ask which of the features of critical bandwidths as determined psychophysically are found in the responses of auditory nerve fibers.

Only one set of data is available and shown in Fig. 1A. Critical bandwidths in cats were measured psychophysically by masking the perception of a tone with narrowband noise of variable bandwidths (Pickels, 1975; Nienhuys and Clark, 1979) and, with a very similar procedure, electrophysiologically in auditory nerve fibers (Pickles and Comis, 1976). A discharge-rate criterion was used to determine changes of the neuronal response to the tone when the bandwidth of the masking noise was varied. As Fig. 1A demonstrates, neural and psychophysical critical bands show a similar average frequency dependence. This can be expected considering that critical bands have their origin in the frequency resolution within the cochlea. The filter bandwidths of most auditory nerve fibers are, however, narrower by a factor of about 4 than those of the behavioral tests.

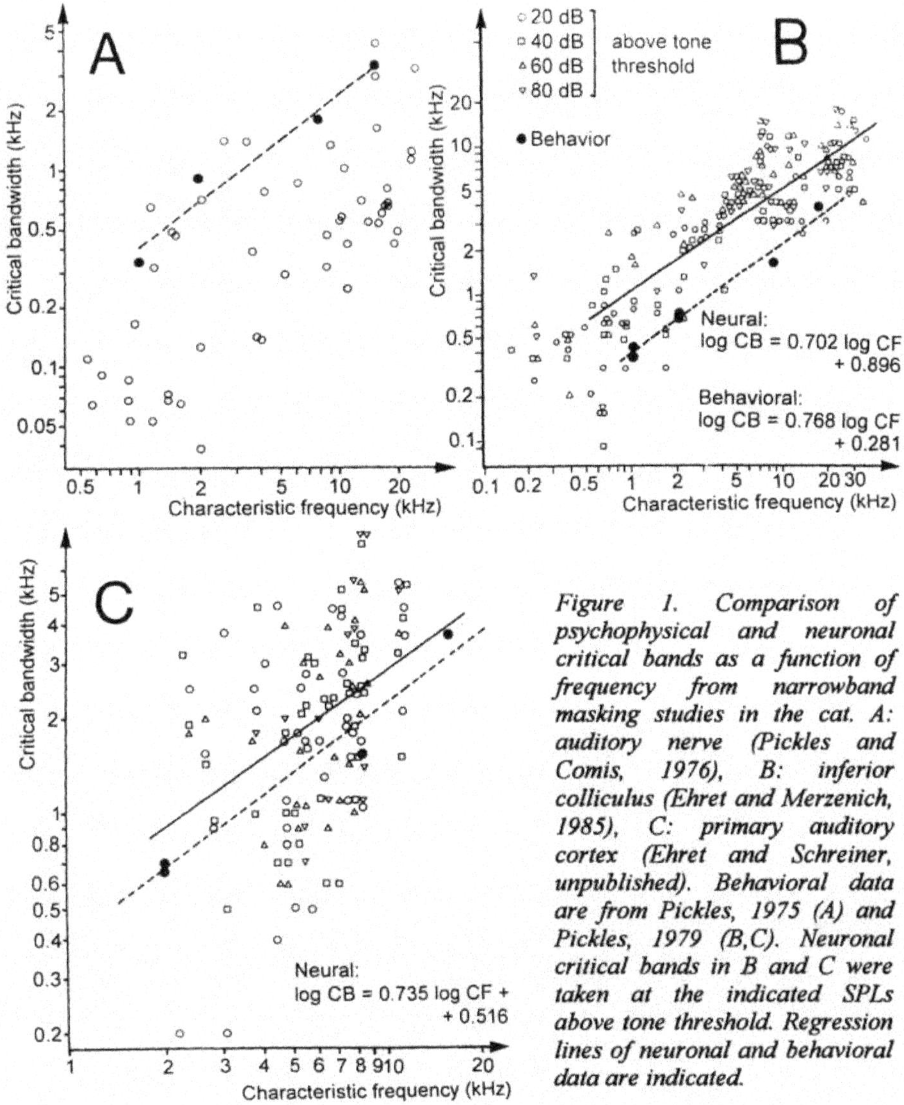

Figure 1. Comparison of psychophysical and neuronal critical bands as a function of frequency from narrowband masking studies in the cat. A: auditory nerve (Pickles and Comis, 1976), B: inferior colliculus (Ehret and Merzenich, 1985), C: primary auditory cortex (Ehret and Schreiner, unpublished). Behavioral data are from Pickles, 1975 (A) and Pickles, 1979 (B,C). Neuronal critical bands in B and C were taken at the indicated SPLs above tone threshold. Regression lines of neuronal and behavioral data are indicated.

This means that frequency resolution at the level of single auditory nerve fibers is both absolutely and on the average better than the animal can make use of in perception tests. It has not been tested with narrowband masking paradigms whether neuronal critical bandwidths remain constant with increasing sound intensity as psychophysical critical bands do. Indirect evidence for a widening of neuronal critical bandwidths and/or nonlinear spectral integration in the filters comes from measurements of tone response threshold in a background of broadband noise (Ehret and Moffat, 1984). The ratio of the tone intensity at the masked threshold and the spectral intensity of the masking noise (critical ratio) is considered to be proportional to the width of the filter that filters out the effective masking noise band from the broadband spectrum (Fletcher, 1940; Scharf, 1970). This critical ratio, determined in auditory nerve fibers of the mouse, increases by about 30 times (the filter bandwidths may become 30 times wider) if the tone level is increased from absolute response threshold to 40 dB above this threshold of the fibers.

In conclusion, the few available data of noise masking of tone responses of auditory nerve fibers indicate that critical band filters of appropriate, intensity-independent bandwidths are not present at the level of the auditory nerve although the filter characteristics of cochlear nerve fibers and psychophysically determined critical bands certainly have a common source in the cochlear filter, the origin of tonotopy.

3 Frequency Resolution in Centers of the Auditory Pathway

Physiological measurements of frequency resolution corresponding in methodology with psychophysical studies of critical bands have been made in the inferior colliculus of cats (Ehret and Merzenich, 1985, 1988) and humans (Zerlin, 1986) and primary auditory cortex of cats (Ehret and Schreiner, to be published).

3.1 Inferior colliculus

The following measures of filter equivalence have been taken from single neurons in the central nucleus of the inferior colliculus (ICC) by using discharge rate changes and overall temporal response patterns (Ehret and Merzenich, 1988): conventional single-tone frequency tuning curves together with inhibitory areas; effective bandwidths which are critical ratios at the absolute response threshold of the neurons; critical ratios centered at the characteristic frequency (CF) up to 80 dB above tone response threshold; critical bands from narrowband masking procedures centered at the CF of the neuron up to 80 dB above tone response threshold (these measurements are equivalent to those from behavioral tests in cats mentioned before); critical bands from two-tone response integration in which the frequency distance was determined over which stimulation by two phase-locked tones elicited a summed excitatory response in the neuron (these measurements are related to critical bands from loudness summation).

All these measures corresponding to filter bandwidths showed the same frequency dependence as the critical bands from the behavioral and auditory nerve fiber studies (Fig. 1A, B). The bandwidths of the neurons with the smallest critical bands coincide with the psychophysically measured critical bands while the average values differ by a factor of 2.8 (about 4.5 dB) (Fig. 1B). Since in the behavioral tests the noise was about 4.5 dB louder than in the neuronal ones, ICC neurons were overmasked by 4.5 dB in the behavioral study. Therefore, the cats used the neurons least sensitive to masking, those with the smallest filter bandwidths for perception of the tone. It seems that in psychophysical critical band measurements the frequency resolution in the midbrain is fully exploited, while the sharper frequency resolution in the auditory nerve cannot be used. This suggestion may apply only to low sound intensities at which the data from the auditory nerve were taken (Pickles and Comis, 1976), because at higher intensities frequency resolution in the auditory nerve deteriorates (e. g. Evans, 1977; Møller, 1981) while it does not change in the inferior colliculus (Ehret and Merzenich, 1985, 1988; comp. Fig. 1B). Why the average frequency resolution as determined by narrowband noise-masking tests at low sound intensities worsens going from the auditory nerve to the inferior colliculus, is not clear. One reason is that neurons in the ICC can have areas of response facilitation around the tuning curves, mainly close to their tips (Ehret and Merzenich, 1988; Ehret, 1988). Noise energy in the facilitation areas, without being excitatory by itself, enhances the responses to tones and noise within the excitatory tuning curve and thus contributes to the masking so that parts of the facilitatory area belong to the critical band filters (unit 26 in Fig. 2B). Since not all neurons studied had facilitation areas close to the tips of their excitatory tuning curves, further studies have to clarify the causes for the differences in critical bandwidths of neurons in the auditory nerve and ICC.

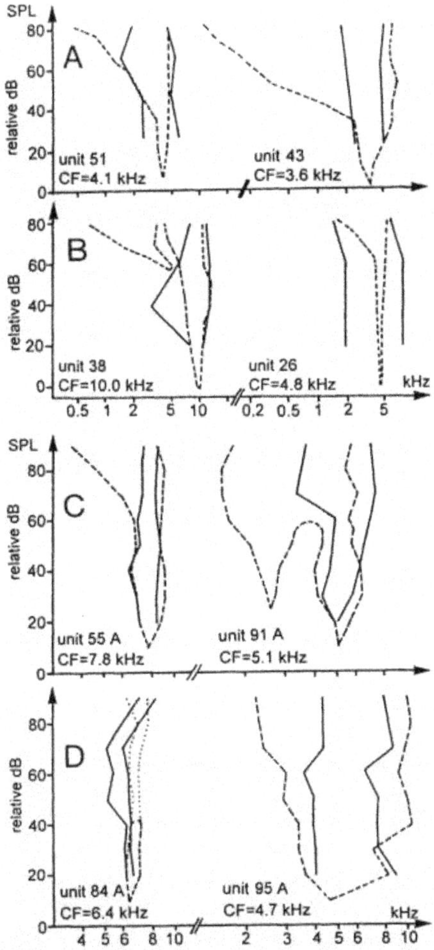

Figure 2. Single-tone excitatory tuning curves (dashed lines) and critical band filters (solid lines) determined by narrowband masking in 4 neurons of the inferior colliculus (A, B) and primary auditory cortex (C, D) of the cat. Unit 84A has a closed tuning curve without noise which changes to the dotted line when a noise is added. From Ehret and Merzenich (1988) and Ehret and Schreiner, unpublished.

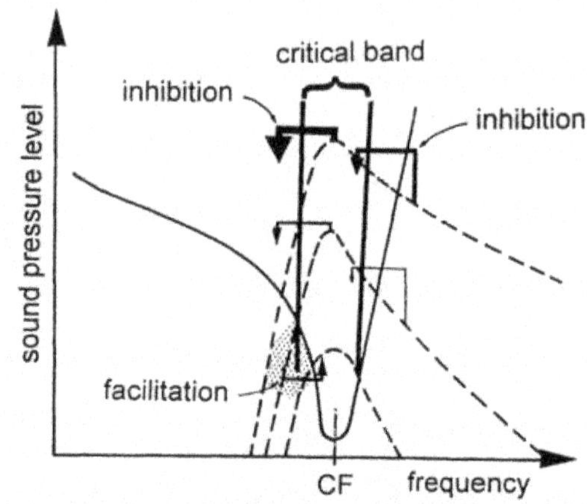

Figure 3. The diagram shows how lateral inhibition and facilitation can influence the critical band filter (determined in a narrowband masking paradigm) of a neuron in the inferior colliculus (IC). Thin line: single-tone excitatory tuning curve; thick line: borders of the critical band; dashed lines: input excitation patterns to the IC induced by tonal stimulation at CF at 3 different SPLs. Strength of inhibition is indicated by the thickness of the lines. The excitation patterns give rise to the shown inhibitory and facilitatory effects and thus shape the critical band (see text).

In most individual neurons of the ICC, critical bandwidths (narrowband masking) did not increase with increasing sound level (Fig. 2A, B) and also, on the average, critical bandwidths were intensity-independent. Lateral inhibition seems to be the major mechanism responsible for the intensity-independence of these critical bands (Ehret and Merzenich, 1988; Ehret, 1988). Most neurons in the ICC have inhibitory bands on both sides of the excitatory tuning curve. Inhibition by frequencies lower than the CF of the neuron is rather weak, by frequencies higher than CF stronger, whereby the strength of inhibition increases with increasing sound intensity. As shown in Fig. 3, such inhibitory effects can shape the critical band of a neuron to an intensity-independent filter at its output. Consider a neuron in the ICC is stimulated by a critical-band wide narrowband noise centered at its CF. This noise should just mask the response to a CF tone. The tone and noise response of the neuron exerts a strong inhibition (mainly at high intensities) beyond the lower border of the critical band, so that if the noise band is widened towards lower frequencies, by keeping the spectrum level of the noise constant, all excitation outside the critical band is cancelled out by inhibiton. With the increase of the noise band, no excitation is actually present to be summed up from outside the critical band so that the bandwidth remains constant. Thus, the lower boundary of the critical bandwidth does not change with intensity although it may be set within the excitatory tuning curve of the neuron. On the other hand, if the noise band is widened towards higher frequencies, the inhibitory influence from high frequency areas on the excitation within the critical band is increased. It has been shown that lateral inhibition exerts a stronger effect on the edges of the excitatory area (the high-frequency border of the filter) than on the tone in its center (Ryan and Miller, 1978; Le Beau et al., this volume) so that this increased inhibition (which gets stronger with increasing sound intensity) acts mainly on the noise within the critical band and reduces its masking influence on the tone. Thus, the tone response is released from being masked. On this basis, lateral inhibition from outside the processing within the critical band prevents the bandwidth from being widened along the upper border of the excitatory tuning curve. It is evident that the excitatory single-tone tuning curve of the neuron in the ICC does not represent the filter relevant for the analysis of a complex sound like tones in noise (Fig. 2A, B).

Taking this evidence on critical bands of single neurons in the inferior colliculus (narrowband masking) together, we find that critical bands have the right bandwidths and the intensity-independence found in behavioral tests. These features are established by facilitatory and inhibitory influences on the responses of these neurons. It follows, therefore, that critical bands with psychophysically determined features are not present in the auditory nerve but can be found in single neurons of the auditory midbrain. Support for this conclusion comes from a two-tone integration study on humans (Zerlin, 1986). Wave V but not waves I-IV of the auditory brainstem tone-evoked response shows a sudden increase if the frequency distance between two simultaneously presented tones becomes equal or smaller than the psychophysically determined critical bandwidth.

3.2 Auditory Cortex (AI)

If psychophysically relevant frequency resolution is established in the auditory pathway to or at the inferior colliculus, how is this information, including characteristics of critical bands, represented in higher auditory centers like the primary auditory cortex (AI)? Recent measurements on masking of tone responses by narrowband noise in single neurons of AI of the cat (Ehret and Schreiner, to be published; similar procedures as in Ehret and Merzenich, 1985, 1988) provide some first data.

Fig. 4 shows a lateral view on the cat neocortex with AI and other areas and, enlarged, 33 recording sites where critical bands from 48 neurons have been determined. The recording sites on this cortex covered isofrequency contours with characteristic frequencies between about 3 and 6 kHz. Average neural critical bandwidths, measured 20 and 50 dB above the tone response thresholds respectively, within 0.5 mm dorso-ventral sections of AI are also indicated (Fig. 4). It is evident that average bandwidths have different values depending on the location of the neurons on the dorso-ventral extension of AI. Average critical bandwidths coming close to the psychophysical value of 0.97 kHz at a center frequency of 4 kHz (interpolated from Pickles, 1975) are found in neurons of central and ventral sections of the isofrequency contours. In the center of an isofrequency contour, neurons are usually most sharply tuned in terms of $Q_{10\ dB}$-and $Q_{40\ dB}$-values (Schreiner and Mendelson, 1990; Q = CF divided by the bandwidth of the excitatory tuning curve at the respective tone level above absolute threshold). Thus, there is a correspondence between the average sharpness of tuning to a single tone and average bandwidth of frequency resolution in the dorso-ventral center of AI.

Critical bandwidths from neurons of the central AI of 4 cats are shown in Fig. 1C as a function of CF and sound level above tone response threshold. As in the auditory nerve and inferior colliculus, the frequency dependence of average neural critical bands is the same as in the behavioral measurements. Similar to the ICC, average critical bands in AI do not change with sound intensity (comp. Fig. 1C, 2C,D). The bandwidths of single

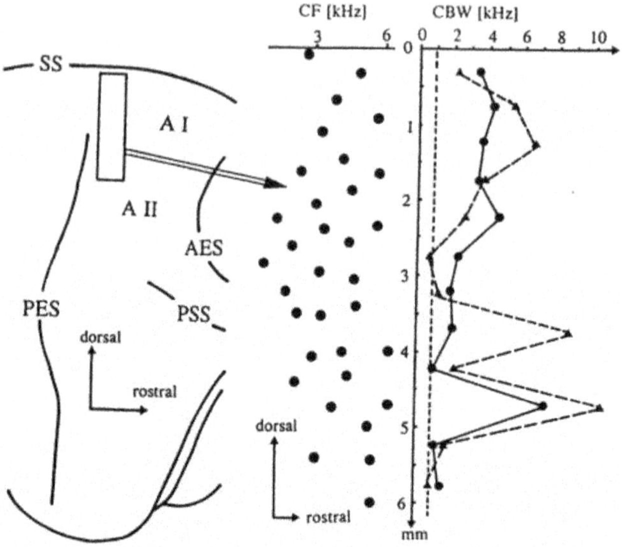

Figure 4. Lateral view on the auditory cortex of a cat. Recording area in the primary auditory cortex (AI) is enlarged and recording sites representing neurons with CFs of about 3 - 6 kHz are shown by dots. Critical bandwidths (CBW) averaged from neurons within 0.5 mm dorso-ventral sections are shown from measurements 20 dB (circles) and 50 dB (triangles) above tone response thresholds. Dotted vertical line: behavioral value at a CF of 4 kHz (from Pickles, 1975). AII: secondary auditory cortex, AES: anterior ectosylvian sulcus, PES: posterior ectosylvian sulcus, PSS: pseudosylvian sulcus, SS: suprasylvian sulcus.

neurons in AI show about the same variation as in the ICC but are, on the average, smaller. A comparison of average single-tone tuning curves with critical bands in the same neurons (Fig. 2C,D) shows discrepancies between both measures of frequency resolution similar to those found in the ICC.

Taking this preliminary evidence form critical band measurements in AI together, one may conclude that perceptually relevant information on critical band filtering is present at the level of the primary auditory cortex.

4 Conclusion

One may hypothesize that frequency resolution represented by critical band information is distributed from the inferior colliculus to higher auditory centers in which this information is combined with other products of auditory analysis to provide the basis for sound pattern discrimination and learning. One example for species-specific call recognition based primarily on frequency resolution and the outputs of critical bands is shown in Fig. 5 (see Ehret, 1989). Since most animal communication calls are complex in the frequency domain, many more examples will be discovered in which critical bands play a major role in call discrimination and recognition.

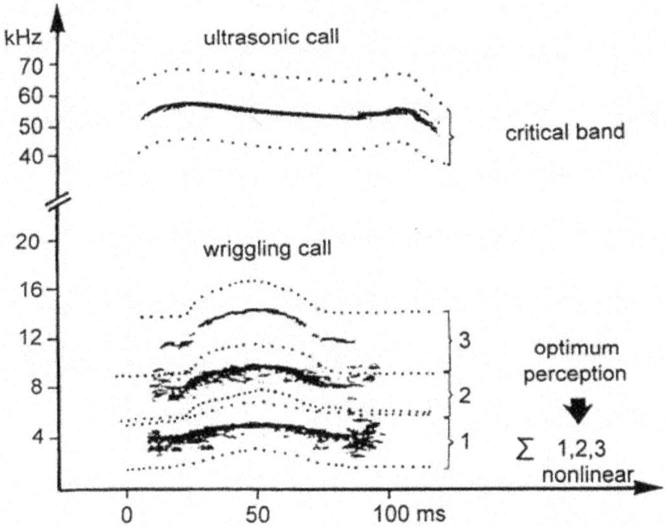

Figure 5. Sonagrams of ultrasonic and wriggling calls of mouse pups. Critical bandwidths of the mouse auditory system are indicated by dotted lines. The calls are recognized by adult mice on the basis of a spectral analysis using critical band information. Wriggling calls are perceived optimally if the weighted outputs of three critical bands are summed up. The output of the critical band around the lowest harmonic is most important (from Ehret, 1989).

5 Acknowledgement

The original studies on critical bands in the inferior colliculus and auditory cortex were done in collaboration with Drs. Merzenich and Schreiner at UCSF and supported by the Coleman Fund, the Deutsche Forschungsgemeinschaft and the Human Frontier Science Program.

6 References

Dooling, R. J. (1980) Behaviour and psychophysics of birds. In: A. N. Popper and R. R. Fay (Eds.), *Comparative Studies of Hearing in Vertebrates*, Springer-Verlag, New York, pp. 261 - 288.

Ehret, G. (1976) Critical bands and filter characteristics of the ear of the house mouse (Mus musculus). Biol. Cybern. 2, 35 - 42.

Ehret, G. (1983) Psychoacoustics. In: J. F. Willott (Ed.), *The Auditory Psychobiology of the Mouse*, Thomas, Springfield (Ill.), pp. 13 - 56.

Ehret, G. (1988) Frequency resolution, spectral filtering, and integration on the neuronal level. In: G. M. Edelman, W. E. Gall, W. M. Cowan (Eds.), *Auditory Function. Neurobiological Bases of Hearing*, Wiley, New York, pp. 363 - 384.

Ehret, G. (1989) Hearing in the mouse. In: R. J. Dooling, S. H. Hulse (Eds.), *The Comparative Psychology of Audition. Perceiving Complex Sounds*, Erlbaum, Hillsdale, pp. 3 - 32.

Ehret, G. and Gerhardt, H. C. (1980) Auditory masking and effects of noise on responses of the green treefrog (Hyla cinerea) to synthetic mating calls. J. Comp. Physiol. 141, 13 - 18.

Ehret, G. and Merzenich, M. M. (1985) Auditory midbrain responses parallel spectral integration phenomena. Science 227, 1245 - 1247.

Ehret, G. and Merzenich, M. M. (1988) Complex sound analysis (frequency resolution, filtering and spectral integration) by single units of the inferior colliculus of the cat. Brain Res. Revs. 13, 139 - 163.

Ehret, G. and Moffat, A. J. M. (1984) Noise masking of tone responses and critical ratios in single units of the mouse cochlear nerve and cochlear nucleus. Hear. Res. 14, 45 - 57.

Ehret, G., Moffat, A. J. M. and Tautz, J. (1982) Behavioral determination of frequency resolution in the ear of the cricket, Teleogryllus oceanicus. J. Comp. Physiol. 148, 237 - 244.

Evans, E. F. (1977) Frequency selectivity at high signal levels at single units in cochlear nerve and nucleus. In: E. F. Evans, J. P. Wilson (Eds.), *Psychophysics and Physiology of Hearing*, Academic Press, London, pp. 185 - 192.

Fletcher, H. (1940) Auditory patterns. Rev. Mod. Phys. 12, 47 - 65.

Gässler, H. (1954) Über die Hörschwelle für Schallereignisse mit verschieden breitem Frequenzspektrum. Acustica 4, 408 - 414.

Greenwood, D. D. (1961a) Critical bandwidth and the frequency coordinates of the basilar membrane. J. Acoust. Soc. Am. 33, 1344 - 1356.

Greenwood, D. D. (1961b) Auditory masking and the critical band. J. Acoust. Soc. Am. 33, 484 - 502.

Greenwood, D. D. (1990) A cochlear frequency-position function for several species - 29 years later. J. Acoust. Soc. Am. 87, 2592-2605.

Greenwood, D. D. (1991a) Critical bandwidth and consonance in relation to cochlear frequency-position coordinates. Hear. Res. 54, 164 - 208.

Greenwood, D. D. (1991b) Critcial bandwidth and consonance: Their operational definition in relation to cochlear nonlinearity and combination tones. Hear. Res. 54, 209 - 246.

Houtgast, T. (1977) Auditory-filter characteristics derived from direct-masking data and pulsation-threshold data with a rippled-noise masker. J. Acoust. Soc. Am. 62, 409 - 415.

Møller, A. R. (1981) Coding of complex sounds in the auditory nervous system. In: J. Syka, L. Aitkin (Eds.), *Neuronal Mechanisms of Hearing*, Plenum Press, New York, pp. 87 - 103.

Moore, B. C. J. (1982) *An Introduction to the Psychology of Hearing*. 2nd Ed., Academic Press, London.

Nienhuys, T. G. W. and Clark, G. M. (1979) Critical bands following the selective destruction of cochlear inner and outer hair cells. Acta Otolaryngol. 88, 350 - 358.

Patterson, R. D. (1976) Auditory filter shapes derived with noise stimuli. J. Acoust. Soc. Am. 59, 640 - 654.

Pick. G. F. (1980) Level dependence of psychophysical frequency resolution and auditory filter shape. J. Acoust. Soc. Am. 68, 1085 - 1095.

Pickles, J. O. (1975) Normal critical bands in the cat. Acta Otolaryngol. 80, 245 - 254.

Pickles, J. O. (1979) Psychophysical frequency resolution in the cat as determined by simultaneous masking and its relation to auditory-nerve resolution. J. Acoust. Soc. Am. 66, 1725 - 1732.

Pickles, J. O. and Comis, S. D. (1976) Auditory-nerve-fiber bandwidths and critical bandwidths in the cat. J. Acoust. Soc. Am. 60, 1151 - 1156.

Plomp, R. and Levelt, W. J. M. (1965) Tonal consonance and critical bandwidth. J. Acoust. Soc. Am. 37, 548 -560.

Ryan, A. and Miller, J. (1978) Single unit responses in the inferior colliculus of the awake and performing rhesus monkey. Exp. Brain. Res. 32, 389 - 407.

Saunders, J. C., Rintelmann, W. E. and Bock, G. R. (1979) Frequency selectivity in bird and man: A comparison among critical ratios, critical bands and psychophysical tuning curves. Hear. Res. 1, 303 -323.

Scharf, B. (1959) Critical bands and the loudness of complex sounds near threshold. J. Acoust. Soc. Am. 31, 365 - 370.

Scharf, B. (1970) Critical bands. In: J. V. Tobias (Ed.) *Foundations of Modern Auditory Theory*, Vol. 1, Academic Press, New York, pp. 159 - 202.

Scharf, B., Florentine M. and Meiselman, C. H. (1976) Critical bands in auditory lateralization. Sens. Processes 1, 109 - 126.

Schorer, E. (1986) Critical modulation frequency based on detection of AM versus FM tones. J. Acoust. Soc. Am. 79, 1054 - 1057.

Schreiner, C. E. and Mendelson, J. R. (1990) Functional topography of cat primary auditory cortex: Dis-- tribution of integrated excitation. J. Neurophysiol. 64, 1442 - 1459.

Weber, D. L. (1977) Growth of masking and the auditory filter. J. Acoust. Soc. Am. 62, 424 - 429.

Zerlin, S. (1986) Electrophysiological evidence of the critical band in humans. J. Acoust. Soc. Am. 79, 1612 - 1616.

Zwicker, E. (1952) Die Grenzen der Hörbarkeit der Amplitudenmodulation und der Frequenzmodulation eines Tones. Acustica 2, Acust. Beih. 3, 125 - 133.

Zwicker, E. and Feldtkeller, R. (1967) *Das Ohr als Nachrichtenempfänger*. Hirzel, Stuttgart.

Zwicker, E. Flottorp, G. and Stevens, S. S. (1957) Critical bandwidth in loudness summation. J. Acoust. Soc. Am. 29, 548 - 557.

Comment by E.V. Evans

Since Pat Wilson and I started making comparisons between psychophysical critical band and effective bandwidths of cochlear nerve fibres (e.g. Evans and Wilson, 1973), I have been increasingly unhappy about the comparison for two main reasons:

a) The traditional critical band is a difficult measure for animal behavioural experiments, and has been overtaken, especially in human psychophysics, by the Equivalent Rectangular Bandwidth (ERB) from masking experiments using spectrally architectured noise (e.g. band-stop noise: Patterson, 1976; Moore et al., 1983; filtered noise: Pick, Evans and Wilson, 1977).

b) The comparisons are made difficult by the large variance of the physiological bandwidths if animals are not selected for optimal physiological condition.

Figure 1 shows a comparison, in the same strain of guinea pigs, between behavioural ERBs using band-stop (notch) noise masking (+) and comb-filtered noise masking (bracketed points) and the physiological ERBs (circles) of single cochlear nerve fibres from guinea pigs selected for normal physiological condition according to mean arterial blood pressure and round window recorded click CAP threshold criteria (for details of behavioural and physiological data see Evans et al., 1992). The physiological data in figure 1 are the ERB`s measured from the mean of these fit Gaussian and rounded exponential filter shapes to the FTC`s, just as was done in the behavioural case, whereas the ERB`s of Evans et al. (1992) are from the raw FTC data.

The physiological data now have little variance, and the correspondence with the behavioural frequency selectivity is excellent. Thus we have concluded that auditory frequency selectivity at least measured in this manner, is already limited by the physiological bandwidths at the cochlear nerve level.

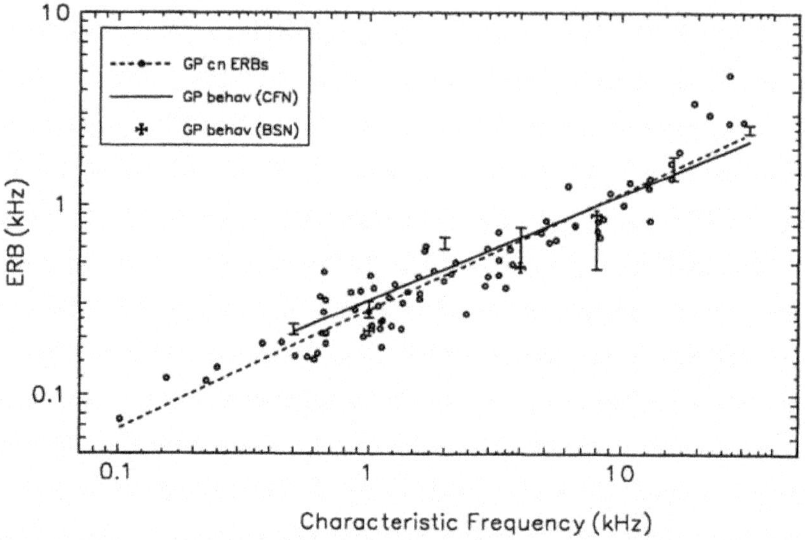

Figure 1. Comparison between physiological and psychophysical (behavioural) frequency selectivity in the guinea pig. Open circles: physiological measures of equivalent rectangular bandwidths (ERB) of 80 cochlear nerve fibres recorded in 9 guinea pigs under normal conditions of sytemic arterial blood pressure and cochlear action potential threshold, plotted against their characteristic frequencies; dashed line: regression through physiological data. Bracketted symbols: behavioural ERBs derived from comb-filtered noise masking respectively +/- 1 SE; cross symbols: behavioural ERBs derived from band-stop noise masking; solid line: regression through behavioural (CFN) data. In all data, ERBs are computed from the mean of the best fitted Gaussian and rounded exponential filters.

Evans, E.F., Wilson, J.P. (1973) Frequency selectivity of the cochlea. In: A.R. Moller (Ed)., *Basic Mechanisms in Hearing*, Academic Press, NY, pp. 519-551

Evans E.F., Pratt, S.R., Spenner, H., Cooper, N.P. (1992) Comparisons of physiological and behavioural properties: auditory frequency selectivity. In: Y. Cazals K. Horner, L Demany (Eds) *Advances in the Biosciences: Vol 83: Auditory Physiology and Perception*, Pergamon Press Oxford, pp. 159-169

Moore, B.C.J. & Glasberg, B.R. (1983). Suggested formulae for calculating auditory-filter bandwidths and excitation patterns. J. Acoust. Soc. Am. 74, 750-764.

Patterson, R. (1976). Auditory filter shapes derived with noise stimuli. J. Acoust. Soc. Am. 59, 640-654.

Pick G.F., Evans E.F., Wilson J.P. (1977) Frequency resolution of patients with hearing loss of cochlear origin. In: E.F. Evans and J.P.Wilson (Eds) *Psychophysics and Physiology of Hearing*, Academic Press London, pp. 273-281

Reply

The comment by Evans raises the extremely important issue of the comparability between physiological and psychophysical (behavioral) studies for our understanding of mechanisms of auditory processing. I think that only those measurements, for example on critical band-widths, are truly comparable and thus lead to significant statements, that are taken with the same kind of acoustical stimulation and, in addition, are based on the same kind of data evaluation. Both acoustical stimulation and data handling, however, differ between the behavioral and physiological studies on equivalent rectangular bandwidths (ERBs) of which the results are shown in Evans' Fig. 1 (from Evans et al. 1992). ERBs of cochlear nerve fibers were not measured in masking tests as in the behavioral paradigm but were calculated under certain filter-shape assumptions from excitatory frequency tuning curves. Such a calculation seems to be allowed only for low excitation levels, because the asymmetries and tails of tuning curves at higher levels (which both also depend on frequency) indicate that the ERB may not adequately represent the cochlear filter at these levels. In the behavioral tests the tone sensation was masked either by comb-filtered or band-stop noise of about 50 dB sensation level and threshold differences were used to fit theoretical filter shapes from which the ERB values were calculated. In view of the mentioned differences between physiological and psychophysical filter assessments, the good fit of both sets of data (Fig. 1 of Evans) seems to be rather accidental than reflecting properties of the same filters. An additional complication of Evans' behavioral paradigm is due to the fact that noise energy from outside the filter (notch) was influencing the processing and threshold estimation of the tone within the filter. Suppression areas at the sides of excitatory tuning curves of auditory nerve fibers (e.g. Sachs and Kiang, 1968), tone-response enhancement by noise as found in auditory nerve fibers (e.g. Ehret and Moffat, 1984), and areas of lateral inhibition and facilitation of neurons in higher auditory centers (e.g. Ehret and Merzenich, 1988) all influence the signal-to-noise ratio within the auditory filters and, therefore, the estimation of filter bandwidths via masked thresholds in notched-noise and comb-filtered noise masking paradigms. Since inhibitory effects, on the average, dominate especially at higher sound levels, filter bandwidths measured with these masking paradigms may be smaller than those determined by narrowband masking procedures (e.g. Ehret, 1976) in which sound (noise + tone) excitation is concentrated within the filter bandwidth to be determined.

Ehret, G. (1976) Critical bands and filter characteristics of the house mouse (Mus musculus). Biol. Cybernetics 24, 35 - 42.

Ehret, G. and Merzenich, M. M. (1988) Complex sound analysis (frequency resolution, filtering and spectral integration) by single units of the inferior colliculus of the cat. Brain Res. Revs. 13, 139 - 163.

Ehret, G. and Moffat, A. J. M. (1984) Noise masking of tone responses and critical ratios in single units of the mouse cochlear nerve and cochlear nucleus. Hear. Res. 14, 45 - 57.

Evans, E. F. Pratt, S. R., Spenner, H. and Cooper, N. P. (1992) Comparisons of physiological and behavioural properties: auditory frequency selectivity. In: Advances in the Biosciences, Vol. 83, Pergamon Press, London, pp. 159 - 164.

Sachs, M. B. and Kiang, N. Y.-S. (1968) Two-tone inhibition in auditory nerve fibers. J. Acoust. Soc. Am. 43, 1120 - 1128.□

Comment by A. Rees

In a study of rate-level functions to tones in noise in the inferior colliculus of the guinea pig, Alan Palmer and I (Rees and Palmer, 1988) showed that the maximum driven firing rate of many neurones to a tone in low levels of noise was greater than in the tone alone condition. This might support your finding of facilitatory areas for neurones in the IC. In what percentage of neurons do you find such facilitation?

Rees, A. and Palmer, A.R. (1988) Rate-intensity function and their modification by broadband noise for neurons in the guinea-pig inferior colliculus. J Acoust. Soc. Am. 83, 1488-1498.

Reply

In a study on the inferior colliculus (IC) of the mouse (Ehret and Moffat, 1985) we found 13 - 21 % (depending on the area in the IC), in a study on the IC of the cat (Ehret and Merzenich, 1988) 43 % neurons that showed tone-response enhancement at some level of background noise. Of the IC neurons in the cat, however, only 12 % had facilitation areas at the sides of their excitatory single-tone tuning curve. This means that enhancement of tone reponses by noise in the IC is not necessarily linked to facilitation areas but may be due to other mechanisms already present at the level of the auditory nerve and cochlear nucleus where tone-reponse enhancement is found in 17 % (cochlear nerve) and about 30 % (cochlear nucleus) of the neurons (Ehret and Moffat, 1984).

Ehret, G. and Merzenich, M. M. (1988) Complex sound analysis (frequency resolution, filtering and spectral integration) by single units of the inferior colliculus of the cat. Brain Res. Revs. 13, 139 - 163.

Ehret, G. and Moffat, A. J. M. (1984) Noise masking of tone responses and critical ratios in single units of the mouse cochlear nerve and cochlear nucleus. Hear. Res. 14, 45 - 57.

Ehret, G. and Moffat, A. J. M. (1985) Inferior colliculus of the house mouse II. Single-unit responses to tones, noise and tone-noise combinations as a function of sound intensity. J. Comp. Physiol. 156, 619 - 635.

Sensitivity to excitation-level differences within a fixed number of channels as a function of level and frequency

Søren Buus[1] and Mary Florentine[2]

[1]*Communication and Digital Signal Processing Center, Dept. of Electrical and Computer Engineering (409 DA), Northeastern University, 360 Huntington Avenue, Boston, MA 02115-5096, U.S.A.*

[2]*Communication Research Laboratory, Department of Speech-Language Pathology and Audiology (133 FR), Northeastern University, 360 Huntington Avenue, Boston, MA 02115-5096, U.S.A.*

1 Introduction

This paper examines how differential sensitivity to excitation levels of two successive stimuli varies with excitation level and frequency. Many models of auditory discrimination assume that detection of modulation and/or discrimination of small differences between successive stimuli may be based on a change in àctivity within one or more frequency-selective auditory channels (e.g., Zwicker 1956, 1970; Maiwald, 1967; Florentine and Buus, 1981; Moore and Glasberg, 1986; Siebert, 1968; Delgutte, 1987; Viemeister, 1988). It has often been assumed that the sensitivity to such a change is independent of the excitation level in the channel and its center frequency. For example, Zwicker (1956, 1970) assumed that the just-noticeable amount of amplitude or frequency modulation was the amount of modulation necessary to produce a 1-dB variation in excitation level in any critical band. Likewise, the multi-band excitation-pattern model for level discrimination (Florentine and Buus, 1981), which is based on Zwicker's excitation-pattern model, assumes that the sensitivity, d', within a critical band is proportional to the excitation-level difference, ΔL_E, in the band. Similar assumptions are evident in physiologically-based models. For example, Delgutte (1987) and Viemeister (1988) investigated whether a group of auditory-nerve fibers tuned to approximately the same frequency could be expected to yield Weber's law, as assumed in the excitation-pattern models.

The assumption of Weber's law within a single frequency-selective channel was based on data showing that difference limens, ΔL_{DL}s (=20 log[1+$\Delta p_{DL}/p$], where p is sound pressure), are roughly independent of level for stimuli that excite a constant number of channels. For example, broadband noise excites all available channels once its level is well above threshold and ΔL_{DL}s for broadband noise are approximately independent of level above 20 dB SL or so (e.g., Viemeister, 1974; Moore and Raab, 1975; Houtsma *et al.*, 1980). Further support for the assumption of Weber's law comes from data obtained for stimuli presented with maskers chosen to confine the discriminable information to channels tuned to a limited range of frequencies. For example, Viemeister (1972) found that ΔL_{DL}s for a 0.95-kHz tone presented with an intense bandpass noise centered at 1.9 kHz did not change appreciably between 30 and 85 dB SPL. Likewise, Moore and Raab (1974) found that ΔL_{DL}s for a 1-kHz tone presented in a notched noise with a two-octave wide notch centered on the signal were nearly identical for tone levels near 40 and 75 dB SL. Finally, ΔL_{DL}s for broadband noise presented with notched-noise maskers closely followed Weber's law over a 60- to 80-dB range of levels (Viemeister, 1974, 1983; Moore and Raab, 1975).

One problem in the interpretation of these studies is that the data for bandlimited stimuli may reflect properties of simultaneous across-frequency comparisons as employed in profile analysis [see Green (1988) for review]. The maskers used to limit the spread of excitation could have provided a reference for simultaneous comparisons of excitation levels in different critical bands and allow the presence of the level increment to be detected as an increase in the signal-to-masker ratio. If so, Weber's law may be a property of profile analysis and does not necessarily reflect the auditory system's ability to detect a small difference in level between two successive stimuli.

Another problem is that intensity coding may depend on frequency. In most previous studies, the findings of Weber's law were obtained for stimuli that limited the discriminable information to the mid-frequency range. It is also unclear if the constant ΔL_{DL}s obtained for broadband noise indicate that all channels follow Weber's law. They could result because variations in sensitivity within separate channels tend to average out over the many channels excited by the broadband noise.

In fact, several experiments on level discrimination with high-frequency tones and noises indicate that Weber's law may not hold within a single critical band. Carlyon and Moore (1984) reported that ΔL_{DL}s for brief 6.5-kHz tones were much larger at moderate levels than at low or high levels, especially when the tone was presented in notched noise. Likewise, ΔL_{DL}s for 100–500-ms tones between 6 and 10 kHz often vary non-monotonically with level and are largest at moderate levels (e.g., Penner *et al.*, 1974; Long and Cullen, 1985; Florentine, 1986; Florentine *et al.*, 1987). Florentine *et al.* (1987) concluded that the non-monotonic behavior of the ΔL_{DL}s at moderately high frequencies could only be predicted if the sensitivity within a single channel varied with level. Finally, Buus (1990) found that ΔL_{DL}s for noise bands centered at 3 kHz were larger at 60 dB SPL than at 30 or 90 dB SPL for noise bandwidths between 1 and 24 Barks (critical bands). This indicates that Weber's law is unlikely to hold, at least at high frequencies.

The present experiment examines whether the sensitivity to a difference in excitation level within a single auditory channel varies with both level and frequency. Comprehensive measurements of the channel sensitivity for a wide range of levels and frequencies were obtained for six listeners and compared across individuals.

2 Method

2.1 Stimuli

The sensitivity was derived from measurements of ΔL_{DL}s as a function of level and frequency of signals presented in notched noise. Because bandlimited stimuli at high levels cause excitation over a wide range of frequencies, notched-noise maskers were used to limit the spread of excitation. To avoid excessive intrusion of the masking noise into the signal band, the notch was three critical bands wide. In contrast to previous experiments, the masker level was varied randomly between presentations. This reduced the likelihood that the level increment was detected by simultaneous across-frequency comparisons (i.e., profile analysis; see Green, 1988) and increased the chance that the discrimination thresholds reflect successive comparisons (Buus and Florentine, 1994).

The signal was composed of three equally intense tones separated by one critical band. This ensured that the signal bands were excited directly by acoustic energy. The frequency of the middle component was 0.25, 1, 4, 8, or 14 kHz and the overall pedestal level varied from about 10 dB SL to 90 dB SPL in 10-dB steps. The notched noise consisted of two bands of uniformly masking noise, which were three critical bands wide. (Only the lower masker band was presented with the 14-kHz signal and the lower masker band was a one critical band wide lowpass noise for the 0.25-kHz signal.) The upper cutoff frequency of the lower band was one-half critical band below the lowest of the three components and the lower cutoff frequency of the upper band was one-half critical band above the frequency of the highest component. The cutoffs were very steep and the attenuation in the notch exceeded 50 dB for frequencies more than 70 Hz away from the cutoff frequencies, which were specified as the 6-dB down points. On each presentation, the level of the masker, measured within one critical band, was chosen randomly from a uniform distribution between -5 and -15 dB *re* the pedestal level. This combination of signal and masker was chosen to reduce the chance that the ΔL_{DL}s would be affected by masking in channels tuned to the signal frequency, while eliminating spread of excitation. The 10-dB range of random masker levels ensures that ΔL_{DL}s less than 3.6 dB cannot be obtained by profile analysis (see Green, 1988).

The signal duration was 500 ms. Signals were separated by a 300-ms interstimulus interval. The masker came on 200 ms before the signal and went off 50 ms after it, such that the total masker duration was 750 ms. All times were measured between the half-amplitude points of the 20-ms raised-cosine rise and fall of the stimuli.

2.2 Apparatus

A PDP 11/73 computer controlled the stimuli, sampled the listeners' responses, and executed the adaptive procedure. The three-tone signal was produced by a 16-bit D/A converter (Boys Town Institute), whose output was low-pass filtered (Frequency Devices 848E, 190 dB/octave), and divided into a pedestal channel and an increment channel. Each channel was gated by an electronic relay followed by an electronic switch (Wilsonics BSIT) and attenuated (Wilsonics PATT) before they were added in phase in the headphone amplifier, which fed one earpiece of the Sony MDR-V6 headphone. The notched-noise masker was produced by a noise generator (Brüel and Kjaer 1405) followed by a uniformly-masking-noise filter, a lowpass filter (Frequency Devices 848E), and a digital Finite Impulse Response filter (Fern Developments EF8, 512 taps). The masker was gated (Wilsonics BSIT), attenuated (Wilsonics PATT), amplified, and added to the signal.

2.3 Procedure

The ΔL_{DL}s were measured in a 2I,2AFC paradigm using a three-down/one-up adaptive procedure, which converges on the ΔL necessary to produce 79.4% correct responses (Levitt, 1971). Assuming unbiased responses, this corresponds to a d' of about 1.16. The level of the increment (i.e., $20\log[\Delta p/p]$) decreased following three consecutive correct responses and increased following one incorrect response. The step size was 5 dB initially and was reduced to 2 dB after the second reversal. Reversals occurred whenever the level difference in successive trials changed from increasing to decreasing or vice versa. As in several of our previous experiments (e.g., Florentine, 1986; Florentine *et al.*, 1987), a single measurement of ΔL_{DL} consisted of three brief, consecutive tracks. Each track terminated after five reversals and the ΔL_{DL} was calculated from the average increment level at the last two reversals for each of the three tracks. Three such ΔL_{DL}s were obtained for each listener and condition and the average ΔL_{DL} was calculated as the geometric mean across repetitions. Conditions were presented in mixed order.

2.4 Listeners

Six listeners participated in the experiment. Five were university students (18 to 25 years old) with no history of hearing difficulties. The sixth listener, DI, is a member of the laboratory staff and is about 15 years older. All listeners had audiometric thresholds less than 15 dB HL between 0.25 and 8 kHz and, except PP, had normal thresholds at 14 kHz as defined by our laboratory standard. Except DI, all listeners were paid to participate in the experiments. Before the onset of data collection, the listeners practiced the task until no systematic improvement in performance was apparent. Each listener received at least 8 hours of training. DI had extensive previous experience in psychoacoustic experiments, including other experiments on level discrimination.

3 Results

The ΔL_{DL}s obtained for each of the six listeners are shown in Fig. 1. The average ΔL_{DL}s are plotted as a function of the overall level of the three-tone signal with center frequency as the parameter. For clarity, error bars are omitted for individual data points. As illustrated in the middle left panel, the average standard error of the means for individual listeners and conditions is about 13% of the means. Considerable variation

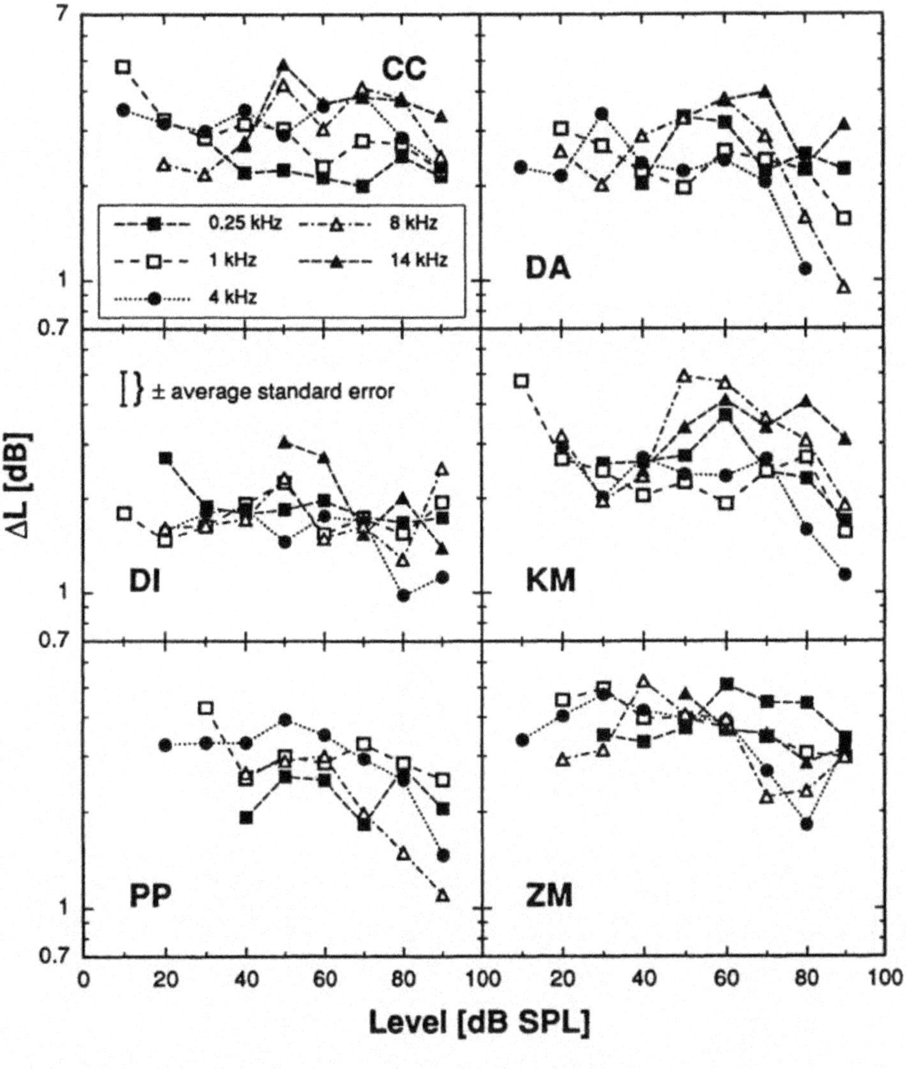

Figure 1. *ΔL_{DL}s for three-tone signals masked by notched noise plotted as a function of pedestal level. Each panel shows the geometric means of ΔL_{DL}s obtained at 0.25, 1, 4, 8, and 14 kHz for one listener. Symbols are shown in the inset at the top left panel. The range encompassed by two average standard errors of the mean for a single listener and condition is illustrated by the error bar in the middle left panel.*

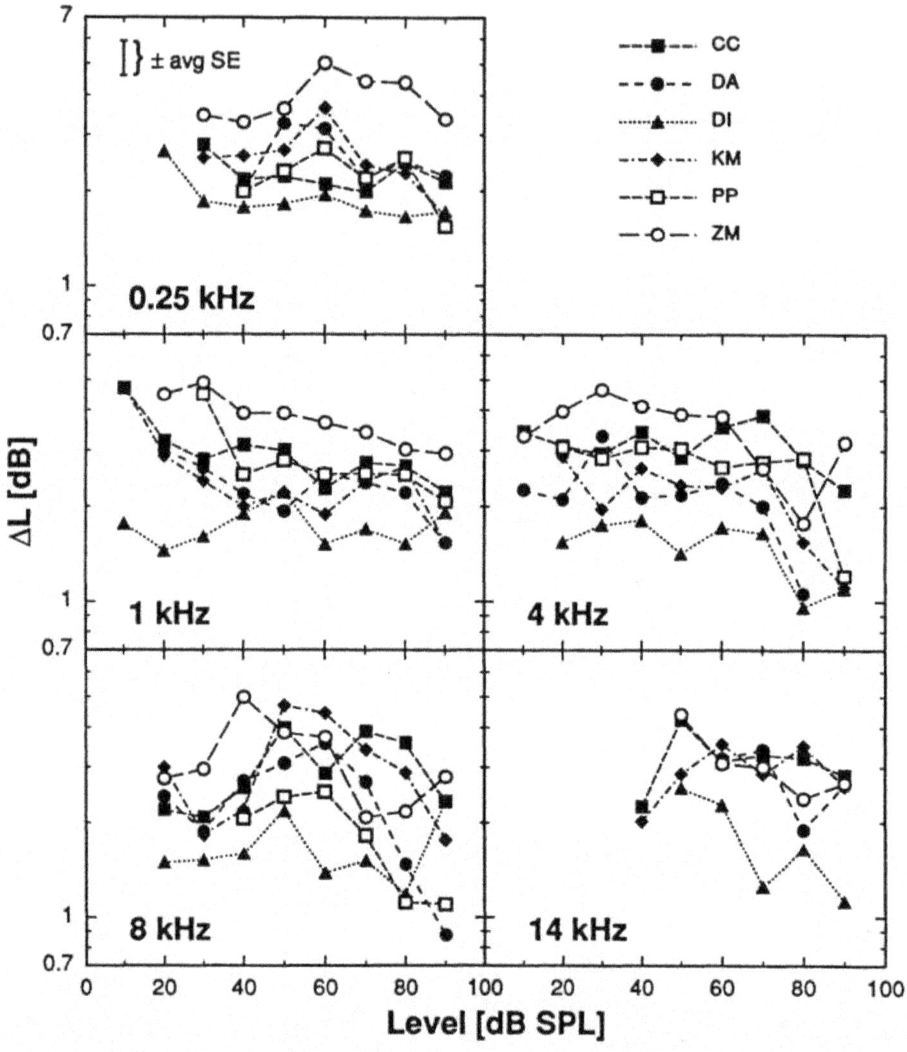

Figure 2. ΔL_{DL}s for individual listeners plotted as a function of pedestal level. Each panel shows data obtained at one center frequency. Symbols indicate different listeners as shown at the top right. The range encompassed by two average standard errors for a single listener and condition is shown in the top left panel.

among the listeners is apparent. For example, DI generally has the smallest ΔL_{DL}s and ZM tends to have the largest. The shapes of the functions also vary. For example, CC and DI tend to have relatively flat functions below 8 kHz, whereas PP and KM tend to have functions that decrease at high levels.

Figure 2 shows the same data as Fig. 1, but it is plotted with listener as the parameter. Data for each signal frequency are shown in separate panels. Comparison of Figs. 1 and 2 indicates that differences across listeners for a single center frequency are considerably larger than differences across frequency for a single listener. Nevertheless, it is clear that the ΔL_{DL}s at 0.25 and, especially, 1 kHz tend to vary relatively little with level. In other words, Weber's law may be considered a reasonable first approximation to the data at low frequencies. As the frequency increases, however, the ΔL_{DL}s appear to deviate from Weber's law. At 4 kHz, the ΔL_{DL}s for most listeners decrease considerably as the pedestal level increases above about 70 dB SPL. At 8 kHz, all listeners show clearly non-monotonic functions and the ΔL_{DL}s generally are two to three times larger at moderate levels than at low or high levels. The level at which the ΔL_{DL}s reach maximum varies considerably across listeners. For example, maximal ΔL_{DL}s are obtained at 40 dB SPL for ZM and at 70 dB SPL for CC. At 14 kHz, the ΔL_{DL}s for four of the five listeners for whom data could be obtained vary relatively little with level, except at low sensation levels; the ΔL_{DL}s for DI tend to decrease with increasing level.

Altogether, Figs. 1 and 2 show that the ΔL_{DL}s obtained in the absence of spread of excitation vary considerably with level and frequency as well as across listeners. It is noteworthy that expressing the pedestal level in terms of sensation level does not make the data more orderly, neither within listeners nor within center frequencies. Thus, the data are presented as functions of SPL, which is the way in which they were obtained.

The large individual differences make averaging across listeners tenuous. The idiosyncratic shapes obtained for individual listeners tend to disappear and the resulting averages are likely to show considerably less variation across levels and frequencies than those for any individual. However, most studies on level discrimination present group means, despite that considerable individual differences often are present (see Florentine *et al.*, 1987). Therefore, the group means of the present data, although imperfect, are likely to provide the most reasonable basis for discussing the extent to which they allow the multi-band excitation-pattern model to predict previous data. Accordingly, Fig. 3 shows the geometric means across the listeners. As expected, the average functions vary considerably less with level and frequency than those for individual listeners and are unlikely to be truly representative of a single listener. Nevertheless, some interesting patterns emerge. At 0.25 and 1 kHz, the ΔL_{DL}s closely follow Weber's law, hovering around 2.5 dB. At 4 kHz, the ΔL_{DL}s hover around 2.7 dB up to 70 dB SPL, but decrease sharply to about 1.7 dB at higher levels. At 8 and 14 kHz, the functions are clearly non-monotonic, reaching maxima of about 3.3 dB around 50 dB SPL and decreasing at higher levels. The ratio of the maximum to the minimum of the group mean ΔL_{DL}s at 8 kHz is 1.9, similar to that found for the listeners with the flattest functions. At 14 kHz, the ΔL_{DL}s decrease slightly less than a factor 1.5 as the level increases from 50 to 90 dB SPL, in large part due to DI's sharply decreasing ΔL_{DL}s.

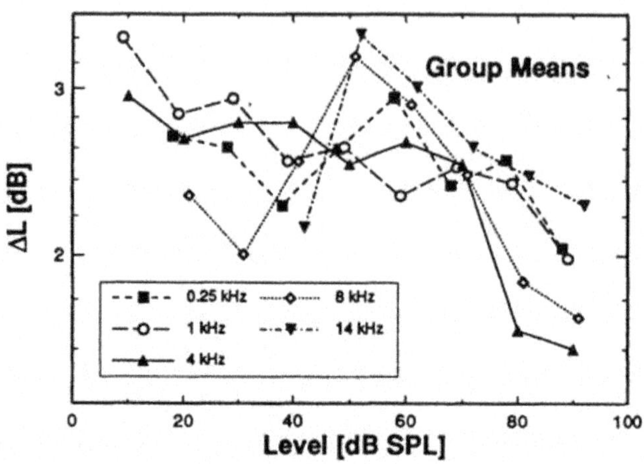

Figure 3. Geometric means of $\Delta L_{DL}s$ for the group of six listeners. The $\Delta L_{DL}s$ are plotted as a function of pedestal level in dB SPL. For clarity, the data have been shifted slightly to the left for 0.25 and 1 kHz and to the right for 8 and 14 kHz.

4 Discussion

Several questions warrant discussion. First, how do the present data compare to previous data on level discrimination for tones in conditions with limited spread of excitation? Second, to what extent could the previous and present data be influenced by profile analysis? Third, what is the sensitivity to an excitation-level increment within a single frequency-selective auditory channel and how does it vary with excitation-level and characteristic frequency of the channel? Fourth, how do predictions obtained with these sensitivity functions agree with previous data on level discrimination? These questions are considered below.

4.1 Comparison with previous studies

Two studies measured $\Delta L_{DL}s$ for tones near 1 kHz in the presence of maskers, which limited spread of excitation. Viemeister (1972) showed that an intense noise one octave above a 0.95-kHz signal nearly eliminated the "near-miss" to Weber's law. The average $\Delta L_{DL}s$ for two listeners decreased from 1.2 to 0.95 dB as the signal level increased from 30 to 85 dB SPL. Likewise Moore and Raab (1974) found $\Delta L_{DL}s$ of 1.7 dB around 40 dB SL and 1.5 dB at 72 dB SPL. The slight decrease of about 10% over a 30–40-dB range of pedestal levels is well within the range obtained for individuals in the present study. Altogether, it seems that the available data agree that sensitivity in channels tuned near 1 kHz is largely independent of level or may improve slightly as level increases.

4.2 Influence of profile analysis

In the present experiment, the level of the notched-noise maskers varied randomly to reduce the chance that the ΔL_{DL}s would be affected by profile analysis. The 10-dB range used for the randomization would produce ΔL_{DL}s of about 3.6 dB for an ideal observer using profile analysis. For five of our six listeners, the ΔL_{DL}s obtained at and below 4 kHz are smaller. Thus, it seems unlikely that profile analysis affected the results appreciably. At 8 and 14 kHz, several ΔL_{DL}s are around or above 3.6 dB and we cannot exclude that profile analysis may have affected the results. However, profile analysis deteriorates markedly at high frequencies (Green *et al.*, 1987), and our ΔL_{DL}s are smaller than those they reported for profile analysis with a 9-kHz signal. Thus, it seems unlikely that profile analysis affected our data materially, even at the highest frequencies. Given that profile analysis did not have any palpable effect on our data and that our data at 1 kHz are in excellent qualitative agreement with those obtained in previous studies (Viemeister, 1972; Moore and Raab, 1974), it also seems unlikely that those data are affected by profile analysis to any great extent.

4.3 Sensitivity to an excitation-level increment: Effect of excitation level and frequency

Whereas it seems clear that the sensitivity of a single channel tuned near 1 kHz closely follows Weber's law, the present data show that Weber's law does not hold at all frequencies. This is particularly true in individual listeners who tend to show considerable differences in the ΔL_{DL}s obtained at various frequencies and levels. Even the average data show sizable variation across levels, especially at the higher frequencies. This is evident in Fig. 4, which shows how the sensitivity to a 1-dB increment in excitation level within a single critical band varies with excitation level in the band. The excitation levels are obtained by adjusting the SPL at each frequency such that the average thresholds for our listeners coincide with the excitation level thresholds in Zwicker's (1956) model. The sensitivity is derived from the ΔL_{DL}s in Fig. 3 under the assumption that the three critical bands excited by our three-tone signals contributed equally to the overall sensitivity and making use of the finding that the sensitivity to a level difference is proportional to the level difference (Buus and Florentine, 1991). Accordingly, a 1-dB level increment yields

$$d' = \frac{1.16}{\sqrt{3}\,\Delta L_{E,DL}} \tag{1}$$

where $\Delta L_{E,DL}$ is the excitation-level increment corresponding to a d' of 1.16. At high levels, $\Delta L_{E,DL}$ is equal to ΔL_{DL}. At low levels, however, the continuously-present noise floor, which accounts for absolute thresholds in the model, "dilutes" the excitation-level increment for two reasons. First, the combined excitation intensity of the threshold noise and the pedestal is higher than the excitation intensity of the pedestal alone; thus, the relative level of excitation for the increment ("signal") is less than that of the acoustic stimulus. Second, the increment is uncorrelated with the threshold noise, which reduces the level increase produced for a given signal-to-masker ratio (where the "masker" is the combined excitation caused by the pedestal and the threshold noise).

The functions in Fig. 4 show that the sensitivity is fairly independent of frequency and level at moderate excitation levels. At high levels, the sensitivity increases somewhat at all frequencies. In addition, the sensitivity at 14 and 8 kHz reaches a minimum for excitation levels of 20 and 40 dB and increases considerably with decreasing level at low levels. In part, the increased sensitivity reflects the relatively small ΔL_{DL}s obtained at the lowest levels tested at 8 and 14 kHz. However, it also depends on the assumed effect of the threshold noise, which is critically dependent on the transfer function used to obtain excitation levels from acoustic levels. Changing the transfer function a few dB changes the low-level sensitivity by 20–30% for the ΔL_{DL}s obtained. Thus, these low-level sensitivities should be interpreted with caution.

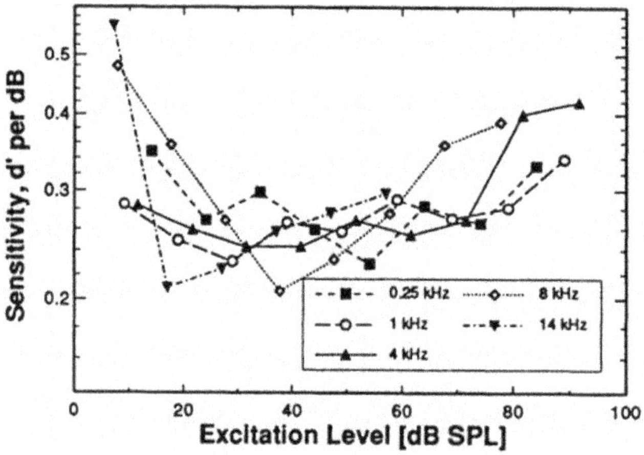

Figure 4. Sensitivity to a 1-dB increment in excitation level within a single auditory channel as a function of excitation level in the channel.

4.4 Model predictions with new sensitivity functions

The sensitivity functions obtained in the present study allow the multi-band excitation-pattern model for intensity discrimination (Florentine and Buus, 1981) to predict many features of the data. The typical sensitivity of about 0.25 per dB yields predicted ΔL_{DL}s whose magnitude is in excellent agreement with those obtained for different listeners by Florentine *et al.* (1987). The new sensitivity functions also help predict features of data for level discrimination for pure tones, that could not be predicted with the assumption of Weber's law within a single channel. In particular, the precipitous improvement at higher levels obtained for tones between 6 and 12 kHz becomes understandable in view of the sensitivity functions obtained in the present study. For example, the marked increase in sensitivity at high levels at 4 and 8 kHz allows the model to predict the relatively small ΔL_{DL}s obtained at high levels for these frequencies, despite the limited spread of excitation. In effect, the increasing sensitivity within a single high-frequency channel largely compensates for the lack of numerous channels tuned to frequencies above these high stimulus frequencies. Likewise, the low sensitivity obtained at low-to-moderate levels at 8 and 14 kHz help increase the predicted ΔL_{DL}s at moderate levels. However, the minimum in the sensitivity functions is not low enough to allow the predicted ΔL_{DL}s at 8 kHz to show a distinct maximum at moderate levels—unlike the data. In fact, the predicted ΔL_{DL} at 50 dB SPL is nearly half that obtained by Florentine *et al.* (1987). This discrepancy indicates that the true sensitivity functions may have considerably lower minima than those shown in Fig. 4.

One possible explanation of the discrepancy is that the notched-noise masker is likely to modify the intensity coding in channels tuned to the signal. For example, Evans (1974) has shown that the rate/intensity function of a single auditory-nerve fiber responding to a tone at the characteristic frequency can be shifted considerably by the presence of flanking noise bands. Thus, the notched-noise masker may have improved the sensitivity by shifting the response function of fibers that would be saturated if the signal was presented in isolation. Another explanation is that a very low sensitivity in one channel is "masked" by higher sensitivities in adjacent channels. For example, if one channel has a sensitivity of 0 (i.e., an infinite difference limen) but two adjacent channels have normal sensitivity, the measured ΔL_{DL} for the three channels would increase only 25%. Thus, it is likely that the "averaging" over three channels used in the present study caused our estimated sensitivity to vary less with level and frequency than the true sensitivity functions. Accordingly, our data must be interpreted with caution. Despite these problems, the estimated functions in Fig. 4 point out many important features that are likely to hold for the true functions and they provide direct evidence that the sensitivity in a single auditory channel should not be assumed to be independent of level and frequency.

5 Acknowledgments

Debra Ingenito helped with data collection. Research was supported by NIDCD Grant R01DC00187.

6 References

Buus, S. (1990) Level discrimination of frozen and random noise. J. Acoust. Soc. Am. 87, 2643-2654.

Buus, S. and Florentine, M. (1991) Psychometric functions for level discrimination. J. Acoust. Soc. Am. 90, 1371-1380.

Buus, S. and Florentine, M (1994) Effect of masker bandwidth and rove range on level discrimination of signals in notched noise. J. Acoust. Soc. Am. 94.

Carlyon, R.P. and Moore, B.C.J. (1984) Intensity discrimination: A severe departure from Weber's law. J. Acoust. Soc. Am. 76, 1369-1376.

Delgutte, B. (1987) Peripheral auditory processing of speech information: Implications from a physiological study of intensity discrimination. In M.E.H. Schouten (Ed.), The Psychophysics of Speech Perception. Nijhoff, Dordrecht, the Netherlands, pp. 333-353.

Evans, E. F. (1974) Auditory frequency selectivity and the cochlear nerve. In: E. Zwicker and E. Terhardt (Eds.): Facts and Models in Hearing, Springer, Heidelberg, pp 118-129.

Florentine, M. (1986) Level discrimination of tones as a function of duration. J. Acoust. Soc. Am. 79, 792-798.

Florentine, M. and Buus, S. (1981) An excitation-pattern model for intensity discrimination. J. Acoust. Soc. Am. 70, 1646-1654.

Florentine, M., Buus, S., and Mason, C.R. (1987) Level discrimination as a function of level from 0.25 to 16 kHz. J. Acoust. Soc. Am. 81, 1528-1541.

Green, D.M., Osnan, Z.A., and Forrest, T.G. (1987) Frequency effects in profile analysis and detecting complex spectral changes. J. Acoust. Soc. Am. 81, 692-699.

Green, D.M. (1988) Auditory profile analysis, Oxford University Press, Oxford, England.

Houtsma, A.J.M., Durlach, N.I., and Braida, L.D. (1980) Intensity perception. XI. Experimental results on the relation of intensity resolution to loudness matching. J. Acoust. Soc. Am. 68, 807-813.

Levitt, H. (1971) Transformed up-down methods in psychoacoustics. J. Acoust. Soc. Am. 49, 467-477.

Long, G.R. and Cullen, J.K., Jr. (1985) Intensity difference limens at high frequencies. J. Acoust. Soc. Am. 78, 507-513.

Maiwald, D. (1967) Ein Funktionsschema des Gehörs zur Beschreibung der Erkennbarkeit kleiner Frequenz-und Amplitudenänderungen. Acustica 18, 81-92.

Moore, B.C.J. and Glasberg, B.R. (1986) The role of frequency selectivity in the perception of loudness, pitch and time. In: B.C.J. Moore (Ed.) Frequency Selectivity in Hearing. Academic, New York.

Moore, B.C.J. and Raab, D.H. (1974) Pure-tone intensity discrimination: Some experiments relating to the "near-miss" to Weber's law. J. Acoust. Soc. Am. 55, 1049-1054.

Moore, B.C.J. and Raab, D.H. (1975) Intensity discrimination for noise bursts in the presence of a continuous bandstop background: Effects of level, width of the bandstop, and duration. J. Acoust. Soc. Am. 57, 400-405.

Penner, M.J., Leshowitz, B., Cudahy, E., and Ricard, R. (1974) Intensity discrimination for pulsed sinusoids of various frequencies. Percept. Psychophys. 15, 568-570.

Siebert, W.M. (1968) Stimulus transformations in the peripheral auditory system. In: P.A. Kolers and M. Eden (Eds.), Recognizing Patterns. MIT Press, Cambridge, MA, pp. 104-133.

Viemeister, N.F. (1972) Intensity discrimination of pulsed sinusoids: The effects of filtered noise. J. Acoust. Soc. Am. 51, 1265-1269.

Viemeister, N.F. (1974) Intensity discrimination of noise in the presence of band-reject noise. J. Acoust. Soc. Am. 56, 1594-1600.

Viemeister, N.F. (1983) Auditory intensity discrimination at high frequencies in the presence of noise. Science 221, 1206-1208.

Viemeister, N.F. (1988) Psychophysical aspects of auditory intensity coding. In: G.M. Edelman, W.E. Gall, and W.M. Cowan (Eds.), The Auditory System: Development, Physiology, and Psychophysics. Wiley, New York.

Zwicker, E. (1956) Die Elementaren Grundlagen zur Bestimmung der Informationskapazität des Gehörs. Acustica 5, 365-381.

Zwicker, E. (1970) Masking and psychological excitation as consequences of the ear's frequency analysis. In R. Plomp and G.F. Smoorenburg (Eds.), Frequency Analysis and Periodicity Detection in Hearing. A.W. Sijthoff, Leiden, pp. 376-396.

Comment by H. Dai

Your model predictions are generated based on the assumption that internal noise is independent across frequency channels. In a profile-analysis study (Dai and Green, 1992), we needed to assume high correlation among the frequency channels in order to account for our data. Would you elaborate how would the model generate predictions assuming a high correlation among the channels.

Dai, H. and Green, D.M. (1992). Auditory intensity perception: Simultaneous versus successive across channel comparison. J.Acoust.Soc.Am. 91, 2845-2854.

Reply

To a first approximation, the predicitons would become similar to those of Zwicker's (1956; 1970) original single-band model, which does not account for the superior discrimination obtained for wideband stimuli at moderate levels (see, Florentine and Buus, 1981; Buus, 1990). It is not clear that the correlation found for profile discrimination applies to simple level discrimination. It seems possible that the across-channel correlation results from the roving-level procedure used for profile discrimination.

Comment by N.F. Viemeister

The use of band-reject noise to restrict information to a limited number of channels is appealing but requires caution in interpretation of the data. The general problem is that band-reject noise may do more than simply mask information within its passband. It may, and very likely does, affect the response of channels tuned to frequencies within the notch. This has been a concern about the many studies of intensity discrimination that have used band-reject maskers (see Viemeister, 1988; Plack and Viemeister, 1993). It is a particular concern in the present study which uses band-reject noise to evaluate limited-channel intensity discrimination and then uses these data in a model that permits generalisation to a wide variety of stimuli situations. The question, of course, is whether the behaviour seen in band reject noise is a valid indication of that of a limited number of truly isolated channels, channels isolated without the use of band-reject noise.

The immediate concern is the possible role of suppression (e.g. see Evans and Zhao, this volume). If the response to the test-stimulus (the three component complex) is significantly suppressed by the band-reject noise, than the data may not be valid description of that of isolated channels. As an extreme example, the band-reject noise may suppress the response to the test stimulus to an approximately constant value. This, like an automatic gain control, may in itself produce the Webers-Law behaviour shown (approximately) by the data.

Although suppression is likely to be involved in this and other experiments using band-reject noise, there are some indications that it is not a major problem. Unpublished data from my laboratory indicates that roving the relative level of the band-reject noise over a 20 dB range does not appreciably affect intensity discrimination of a pure tone. If the band-reject noise significantly suppressed the response to the tone, then roving the noise level should rove the effective level of the tone and thus should produce elevated Δ Ls. In the present study and in a study presented by the authors at an ASA meeting (June 1994), the relative level of the band-reject noise was roved to eliminate profile analysis. The data also indicate no appreciable effect of roving. As argued above, this also suggests no appreciable effect of suppression.

While the results described above suggest no major effect on suppression, this possibility requires more thorough examination. More generally, the possible effects of band-reject noise on putatively isolated channels needs further consideration. Until these effects are understood, considerable caution should be applied in interpreting data such as those presented here as indicative of the behaviour of isolated channels.

Plack, C.J. and Viemeister, N.F. (1993) Suppression and the dynamic range of hearing. J. Acoust. Soc. Am. 93, 976-982.

Viemeister, N.F. (1988) Psychophysical aspects of auditory intensity coding. In: Edelman, G.M., Gall, W.E. and Cowan, W.M. (Eds.) Auditory Function: Neurobiological Bases of Hearing. Wiley, New York, pp. 213-241.

Reply

We agree that one should be careful in interpreting results for stimuli presented in notched noise. As discussed in our paper, one cannot assume that the operation of channels tuned to the signal frequency is unaffected by the presence of the masker. The finding that the sensitivity functions that we obtained produced quite reasonable, although not perfect, predictions of ΔL_{DL}s for tones presented in isolation indicates that the effects of the notched noise on the signal channel, in our experiment, probably are small in most cases. Indeed, the relatively good discrimation obtained in most of our conditions indicates, as you note, that suppression is unlikely to have affected our results appreciably.

Detection of combinations of frequency modulation: An application of the IWAIF model

Lawrence L. Feth, Ashok K. Krishnamurthy* and Tao Zhang

*Speech and Hearing Science and *Electrical Engineering, The Ohio State University Columbus, Ohio 43210 USA*

1 Introduction

Our work has been guided by the underlying assumption that human auditory communication is a modulation - demodulation process. That is, we assume that sources produce a complex stream of sound pressure waves with information encoded as variations (i.e., modulation) of signal amplitude and frequency. Speech, music and most environmentally important sounds can be described in this way. Recently, Maragos, et al., (1992) have shown that an energy-tracking operator can be applied to speech signals to produce an algorithm that tracks speech formant amplitude and frequency. The result of the energy-tracking operation is an amplitude-by-frequency product that is quite similar to the EWAIF-IWAIF calculations used in our previous work (Anantharaman, et al., 1993). Earlier work by Teager and Teager (1990) showed that the production of speech could be modeled as the modulation of amplitude and frequency of each formant. Fineberg, et al., (1992) have also begun to apply the modulation model to speech recognition problems.

The human listener's task is then modeled as one of demodulating the sound stream. Much of the past work in psychoacoustics might be characterized as "spectrum picture processing." That is, complex sounds are Fourier-analyzed into an amplitude-by-frequency picture. The experimenter then models auditory perception as a process of analyzing this "spectrum picture". The work on "profile analysis" (see Green, 1988) could be described in this manner. The spectrum picture processing approach leads to studies of broad bandwidth, complex sounds in masking or discrimination experiments. Our "mo-dem" approach leads us to investigate time-varying, complex sounds. We suggest that understanding the auditory processing of such signals with dynamic spectra is essential to better understanding human auditory perception.

1.1 Previous work with STEP-GLIDE signals

The Envelope-Weighted Average of Instantaneous Frequency (EWAIF) model was originally developed to predict the spectral pitch of narrow bandwidth signals for normal hearing human listeners (Feth, 1974; Feth, et al., 1982). We moved to the study of frequency transitions (Feth, et al., 1989) because formant transitions are essential in the description of consonants in speech (e.g., Liberman, et al., 1956). Our experimental work was first designed to determine the appropriate width of the ear's temporal window for the processing of such signals. Several determinations of the limits of auditory temporal acuity are given in the literature (e.g., Green, 1991, 1973 a & b, 1985). Moore and his colleagues have reported the equivalent rectangular duration (ERD) for a temporal window that is the time-domain analog of the roex filter shape of the peripheral filter bank (Moore, et al., 1988; Plack and Moore, 1990, 1991). Little of this previous work has used dynamic signals, that is, signals with frequency transitions. To determine a measure of temporal acuity for such signals, we devised a discrimination task in which listeners were asked to distinguish between a tone frequency modulated over a linear trajectory (a GLIDE) and one covering the same frequency change via a multiple-step trajectory (the STEP). Details are given in Madden and Feth (1992), but the essential result was that the just-discriminable step was approximately 7 to 10 ms for frequencies of 2 kHz and below. Above 2 kHz, the just-discriminable step becomes longer.

Application of the original EWAIF model to dynamic signals proved to be difficult because of the complexity of the EWAIF calculation. The result was the IWAIF model (Anantharaman, et al., 1993). Here, intensity is used to weight the frequency values. The advantage is that the IWAIF can be calculated in the frequency domain using an FFT, whereas the EWAIF was calculated in the time domain. In addition to the great improvement in computational efficiency, the IWAIF form of the model has led to an interpretation of the model output that appears to have wide applicability in our further understanding of auditory signal processing. The result of the IWAIF calculation is the "center of gravity" of the signal spectrum. Such a simple concept has great intuitive appeal for predicting the locus of spectral pitch for many sounds. It is also the basis for the "perceptual formant" suggested by Chistovitch (1979) as the determinant of vowel quality.

A short-term model (ST-IWAIF) can be applied to signals with frequency transitions (Krishnamurthy and Feth, 1993). For example, the STEP and GLIDE signals have nearly the same long-term spectrum, and consequently, the same long-term IWAIF values. Nonetheless, they are easily discriminable, indicating that human listeners are able to utilize cues that are more short-term in nature. To explain such data, it is necessary to introduce the ST-IWAIF model. The model is based on the assumption that the listener can track the changing IWAIF of a dynamic signal and use it as a potential cue for discriminating between two signals. The ST-IWAIF of a signal at time t_0 is determined by the spectral properties of the signal in a small time window of duration T_w around t_0. Let $s_1(t)$ and $s_2(t)$ be the two signals, both of duration T that are to be discriminated. The listener is assumed to track the ST-IWAIF values $I_1(t)$ and $I_2(t)$, $0 \le t \le T$, of $s_1(t)$ and $s_2(t)$, respectively. Further, we assume that there is internal noise in the auditory system that limits our ability to track frequency. This internal noise is modeled as an additive noise $w(t)$ that corrupts the true ST-IWAIF values. We assume that $w(t)$ is white, zero-mean, Gaussian noise with a power spectral density of $N_0/2$. Since the IWAIF is essentially a signal frequency parameter, we suggest that pure tone frequency-difference limen data be used for that purpose. Thus, if the frequency DL for a tone of duration T at the IWAIF frequency is Δ, we suggest that

$$\frac{N_0}{2} = \Delta^2 . \tag{1}$$

Given the above assumptions, the d' for this model is given by

$$d' = \sqrt{\frac{1}{\Delta^2}\int_0^T (I_2(t) - I_1(t))^2 dt}. \quad (2)$$

The ST-IWAIF model was applied to the results of the original STEP-GLIDE discrimination task with good results. Figure 1 shows the duration of an individual step for STEP signals that were discriminable from GLIDE signals on 75% of the trials. Open symbols represent results averaged for four listeners over signal duration ranging from 25 to 100 ms. Performance is collapsed over signal duration and overall frequency excursion, to be characterized by the rate of transition. Transition rates were 2-, 4- and 8-Hz/ms. Filled symbols represent the performance predicted by the ST-IWAIF model. Model parameters were adjusted so that predictions and data were matched at 1 kHz for the 8 Hz/ms conditions. Those same parameters were then used to predict performance for all

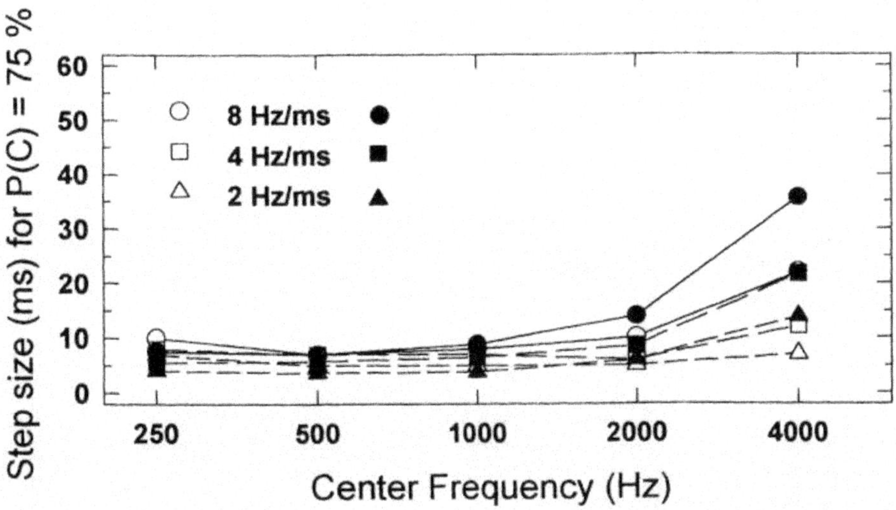

Figure 1. Just-discriminable step size in ms. Open symbols are averaged for four listeners with normal hearing. Circles are for a sweep rate of 8 Hz/ms, squares are 4 Hz/ms and triangles are 2 Hz/ms. Filled symbols are the predicted values obtained from the ST-IWAIF model.

other conditions. In general, the model predicts average listener performance very well. At 250 Hz it predicts better performance (i.e., shorter step size). At 4 kHz, the model predicts poorer performance (larger step size) than our listeners obtained.

1.2 Madden's model for FM glide discrimination

Recently, Madden (1994) extended the investigation of temporal processing of FM glides. Using an adaptive 2AFC task, he determined the smallest frequency increase between successive steps at which the STEP signal could just be distinguished from the GLIDE. Madden modeled his results using an intensity-based model: A bank of bandpass filters each followed by a non-linearity, temporal window and level detector. Similar models have been used by several investigators of auditory temporal acuity (e.g., Viemeister, 1979; Forrest and Green, 1987; Shailer and Moore, 1987; Green and Forrest, 1988). Madden's modeling indicated that the equivalent rectangular duration (ERD) of the temporal window was about 5 ms for signals ranging from 250 Hz to 6 kHz. However, he was forced to allow detector efficiency to vary substantially over the frequency range to obtain a fit to his data. This is in marked contrast to the detector efficiency reported for temporal acuity of signals without FM.

1.3 IWAIF model predictions of Madden's results

The ST-IWAIF model was applied to Madden's results. The model predictions are shown in Figure 2 along with the averaged data from Madden's paper. The ST-IWAIF model predicts slightly better performance than Madden's listeners obtained. Given that the listeners may not be 100% efficient, the prediction of slightly better performance is not unexpected. Behavior of the model predictions is in line with expectations, except for signals with a large number of steps. For the difficult discrimination of nine, ten or eleven steps versus the seventeen steps in the standard signal, Madden's adaptive procedure apparently drove the listeners to extremely large frequency increments between steps. We assume that they were using a different cue to reach criterion when the increment per step was over 100 Hz.

2 Detection of sinusoidal plus ramp FM

There are some concerns about the influence of subtle spectral differences between the glide and the step signals with the use of the STEP-GLIDE discrimination task. To minimize the possible contamination of "splatter" at each step, Madden used a 17-STEP signal as the standard rather than a true linear glide. Further, the transitions were "rounded" to reduce the spread of energy when the signal frequency was abruptly changed to a new value.

Consider the STEP signal used in the previous work. It can be described as a triangular wave modulator added to a linear ramp before the combined waveform is used to modulate the frequency of a carrier tone. It can be difficult to specify the modulation index of such a combined modulation waveform. If, instead, a sinusoid is added to a linear ramp to produce the combined modulator, the resulting modulator is easy to specify. This new target signal replaces the STEP signal used previously. If the slope of the ramp is

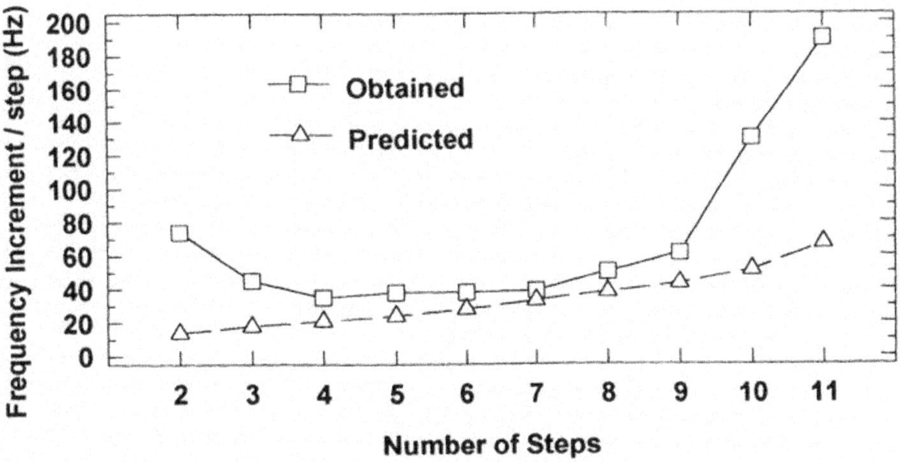

Figure 2. Comparison of Madden's results at 1 kHz with ST-IWAIF model predictions.

zero (i.e., no change in base frequency), the listener's task is simply detection of sinusoidal FM. When the sinusoidal FM is added to a linear ramp, the listener's task is similar to that in the discrimination of STEP versus GLIDE signals (Zhang et al., 1994).

2.1 Method

Listeners with normal hearing were asked to determine which of two tones was sinusoidally frequency modulated. In one set of experimental conditions, the standard signal was a steady tone, and the target signal was generated by frequency modulating the standard with a sinusoid at 4, 8, 16, 32, 64, 128 or 256 Hz. In other conditions, the standard signal was frequency modulated by a linear ramp. The target was then generated by adding the sinusoidal FM to the linear FM. To avoid the possibility of anchoring effects, the frequency of each signal was chosen from a uniform random distribution. This is commonly called a roving-frequency condition.

2.2 Signal generation

All signals were generated using the TDT System II. Three listeners were tested at one time. Separate channels from the four-channel D-to-A converter delivered signals to one side of a Sennheiser HD 414 headset. Individual detection thresholds for the standard signals were determined using an adaptive 2AFC procedure; the FM detection task was conducted at 50 dB SL. Signal duration was 250 ms with rise-fall times of 5 ms.

2.3 Procedures

Data were collected in blocks of 50 trials using an adaptive 2Q, 2AFC procedure. A 3-up, 1-down rule was used (Levitt, 1971) to estimate the 79.4 % point on the listeners' psychometric functions. Data were collected from at least six blocks of trials before averaging the results. When the results appeared to be too variable, an additional three blocks were run and the "best" six were averaged.

3 Results

3.1 Sinusoidal FM detection: with or without glide

Figure 3 shows the results for detection of sinusoidal FM at f_c = 1 kHz averaged for three listeners. The abscissa displays modulation frequency, ranging from 4 to 256 Hz. The ordinate is β, the index of modulation required to obtain 79.4% correct detection. Results for detection of sinusoidal FM added to a linear ramp FM are also shown. Here the ramp rises 800 Hz over 250 ms. In general, listeners have more difficulty detecting the sinusoidal FM in the presence of the ramp than they do when the standard is an unmodulated tone. The data displayed in Figure 3 were averaged over the four roving-frequency ranges tested. Remarkably, there is no effect of roving on the listeners' ability to detect the sinusoidal FM, either for the steady base-line, or for the ramped one.

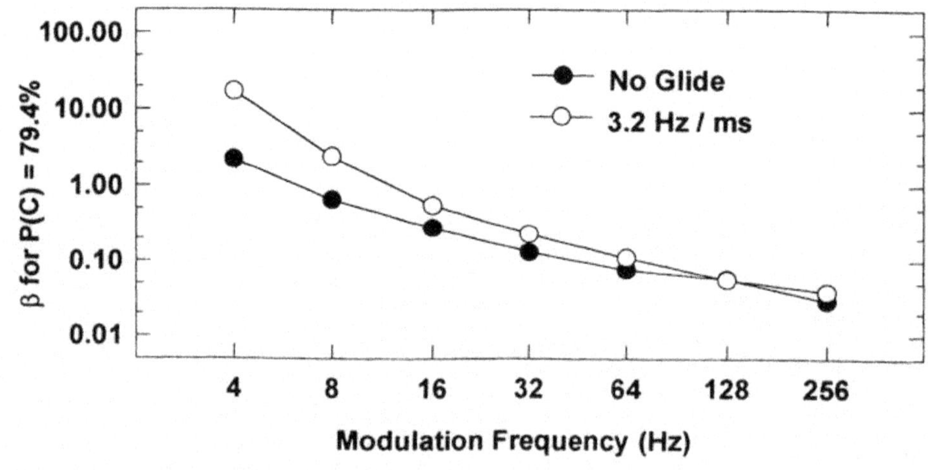

Figure 3. Detection of sinusoidal FM modulation averaged for three listeners. Circles are for simple FM detection; filled squares are for detection of the sine FM added to a linear glide. Starting frequency rove range: none, 200, 400 and 800 Hz.

3.2 Sine wave analog to STEP-GLIDE discrimination

Three listeners with normal hearing were tested in an FM detection task constrained to be analogous to the earlier STEP-GLIDE discrimination task. The STEP signal was replaced by a sinusoidal FM plus GLIDE modulator. Signal duration was set to 100 ms and the transition rate was 4 Hz/ms. The sinusoidal FM was added to the linear ramp with starting phase at 180^0 to better approximate the STEP signal. Detection thresholds for the sine FM were obtained at octave frequencies from 250 Hz through 4 kHz, plus 6 kHz. An adaptive, 3-up, 1-down rule (Levitt, 1971) was used to adjust the period of the sinusoidal FM to approximate the discrete steps used earlier. Thus, for a 100 ms signal, a modulation rate of 10 Hz completes one cycle in 100 ms. To approximate 2 steps, the rate was changed to 20 Hz. For each new modulation rate, the amplitude of the sinusoid was adjusted so that it would have the same power as the triangular modulator that produced the original step function. This is only one of several constraints that might be placed on the sinusoid to "match" it to the triangular waveform.

Discrimination results for three listeners are shown in Figure 4 along with the performance predicted for each one using the ST-IWAIF model. As with the earlier STEP-GLIDE results, the just-detectable period is approximately uniform from 250 Hz to 2 kHz. Performance is poorer at 4 kHz but at 6 kHz it appears to have leveled off.

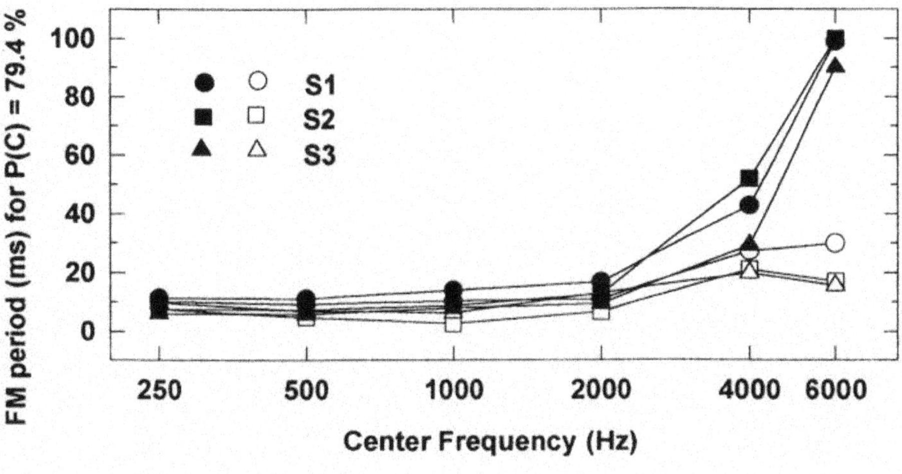

Figure 4. Individual results for the listeners detecting a sinusoidal FM added to a linear glide. Filled symbols are ST-IWAIF predictions for listener performance.

4 Discussion

Our original set of STEP-GLIDE signals led us to conclude that the width of the temporal processing window was approximately constant across signal frequencies below 2 kHz. We attributed listeners' poorer performance in STEP-GLIDE discrimination at higher frequencies to the ear's inability to follow the frequency transition, perhaps due to the loss of phase-locking in the primary neural units. Madden's extension of that work (1994) introduced an adaptive testing procedure and modeled the results using the "traditional" intensity based model used in previous temporal acuity measurements such as gap detection or temporal modulation transfer functions. Madden's adaptive procedure kept the signal duration and number of steps fixed over a block of experimental trials and varied the frequency excursion of the signal pairs. The adaptive procedure determined the frequency interval (FI) for which listeners could distinguish the STEP from the GLIDE. Recent work by Hsu (1993) has shown that the just-discriminable change in frequency-transition slope obeys Weber's law. That is, $\Delta F/F$ in Madden's procedure changes with each change required by the adaptive rule.

The intensity model used by Madden matched listener performance fairly well for the mid-range of signal frequencies tested. The model had to be allowed poorer detector efficiency to reproduce the upturn in just-discriminable frequency increment at the smallest and largest number of steps. The large increase in frequency increment required to achieve discrimination performance at 79.4% for the large number of steps is difficult to explain within the limits of the assumed task presented to the listeners. In essence, they are asked to distinguish a transition containing 9, 10 or 11 discrete steps over 50 ms from a standard containing 17 steps over that same duration. The very large frequency increment required to "satisfy" the adaptive procedure suggests that perhaps at this end of the discrimination task, listeners were using a different cue to make the distinction. Certainly, the increments were large enough to suggest that simple frequency discrimination of the initial frequency jump might be the cue.

At the other end of Madden's FI vs. step-number curve, there is a drop in FI with increasing numbers of steps. For 2, 3 and 4 steps the overall frequency excursion is approximately 150 Hz. In the earlier work, we found that the duration of a single step remained constant for criterion performance over a wide range of signal duration and frequency excursions. The falling FI vs. step-number curve may not reflect that same behavior.

We have shown above that a ST-IWAIF model can account for Madden's results about as well as the intensity-based model he proposed. There remain some reservations about signal artifacts (energy splatter at the transitions) and problems with the adaptive procedure as implemented by Madden. Thus, we have proposed that sinusoidal FM added to a linear ramp be used to further test the IWAIF model.

Our initial results indicate that the ST-IWAIF model can account for listener performance in the detection of sinusoidal FM. When the ramp has zero slope, our task is the familiar FMDL task. For that task, we have indicated that introducing a roving-frequency paradigm has little or no effect on listener performance. Our results appear to be reasonable when compared with previous determinations of the FMDL (Moore and

Glasberg, 1989) given differences in psychophysical procedures and signal parameters.

When the sinusoidal FM is added to a ramp modulation, listener performance in the detection of FM is somewhat poorer at the lowest FM rates. In the "traditional" FMDL task, the baseline for comparison is fixed in frequency over the duration of the signal. For our ramp-plus-sine FM task, the baseline is moving.

Finally, when we use the sinusoidal FM plus GLIDE signal to replicate the earlier STEP-GLIDE discrimination results, listener performance is consistent with our earlier findings. We suggest that the listener's inability to "follow" the changing baseline at higher frequencies (perhaps due to the loss of phase locking in the auditory nerve) probably accounts for the poorer performance in both STEP-GLIDE discrimination and in FM detection. The ST-IWAIF model predicts progressively poorer performance above 2 kHz than our listeners achieve. This may indicate that such discriminations are not based on the listeners' ability to follow rapid frequency transitions, as the model assumes. However, since the model uses the listener's DLF to estimate variance in the tracking task, model performance is degraded as the DLF increases at higher signal frequencies.

5 Acknowledgement

This work was supported by a grant from the AFOSR.

6 References

Anantharaman, J. N., Krishnamurthy, A. K. and Feth, L. L. (1993) Intensity weighted average of instantaneous frequency as a model for frequency discrimination. J. Acoust. Soc. Amer. 94, 723-729.

Chistovitch, L. A. and Lubinskaya, V. V. (1979) The 'center of gravity' effect in vowel spectra and critical distance between formants: Psychoacoustical study of perception of vowel-like stimuli. Hearing Research 1, 185-195.

Cullen, J. K., Houtsma, A. J. M. and Collier, R. (1992) Discrimination of brief tone-glides with high rates of frequency change. Fifteenth Midwinter Research Meeting of the ARO, 67.

Feth, L. L. (1974) Frequency discrimination of complex periodic tones. Perception and Psychophysics 15, 375-378.

Feth, L. L., Neill, M. E. and Krishnamurthy, A. K. (1989) Auditory temporal acuity for dynamic signals. J. Acoust. Soc. Amer. 86, S122-123.

Feth, L. L., O'Malley, H. and Ramsey, Jr. J. (1982) Pitch of unresolved, two component complex tones. J. Acoust. Soc. Amer. 72, 1403-1412.

Fineberg, A. B., Mammone, R. J. and Flannagan, J. L. (1992) Application of the modulation model to speech recognition. In Proceedings of the ICASSP, I-541-I544.

Forrest, T. G. and Green, D. M. (1987) Detection of partially filled gaps in noise and the temporal modulation transfer function. J. Acoust. Soc. Amer. 82, 1933-1943.

Green, D. M. (1971) Temporal auditory acuity. Psychological Review 78, 540-551.

Green, D. M. (1973a) Minimum integration time. In: Basic Mechanisms in Hearing, H. Duifuis, J. W. Horst and H. P. Wit (eds.), Academic Press, NY, 829-846.

Green, D. M. (1973b) Temporal acuity as a function of frequency. J. Acoust. Soc. Amer. 54, 373-379.

Green, D. M. (1985) Temporal factors in psychoacoustics. In: Time Resolution in Auditory Systems, A. Michelsen (ed.), Springer Verlag, NY, 122-140.

Green, D. M. (1985) Profile Analysis: Auditory Intensity Discrimination. Oxford Science Publications, NY.

Green, D. M. and Forrest, T. G. (1988) Detection of amplitude modulation and gaps in noise. In: Basic Mechanisms in Hearing, H. Duifuis, J. W. Horst and H. P. Wit (eds.), Academic Press, NY, 323-331.

Hsu, C.-Y. (1993) Auditory discrimination of frequency transitions by human listeners and a computational model. Unpublished Ph. D. Dissertation, Ohio State University.

Krishnamurthy, A. K. and Feth, L. L. (1993) Short-term IWAIF model for frequency discrimination. J. Acoust. Soc. Amer. 93, 2387.

Levitt, H. (1971) Transformed up-down methods in psychoacoustics. J. Acoust. Soc. Amer. 49, 476-477.

Liberman, A. M., Delattre, P. C., Gerstman, L. J. and Cooper, F. S. (1956) Tempo of frequency change as a cue for distinguishing classes of speech sounds. J. Exptl. Psych. 52, 127-137.

Madden, J. P. (1994) The role of frequency resolution and temporal resolution in the detection of frequency modulation. J. Acoust. Soc. Amer. 95, 454-462.

Madden, J. P. and Feth, L. L. (1992) Temporal resolution in normal-hearing and hearing-impaired listeners using frequency-modulated stimuli. J. Speech Hear. Res. 35, 436-442.

Maragos, P. Kaiser, J. F. and Quatieri, T. F. (1992) On separating amplitude from frequency modulations using energy operators. In Proceedings of the ICASSP, II-1 - II-4.

Moore, B. C. J., Glasberg, B. R., Plack, C. J. and Biswas, A. K. (1988) The shape of the ear's temporal window. J. Acoust. Soc. Amer. 83, 1102-1116.

Moore, B. C. J. and Glasberg, B. R. (1989) Mechanisms underlying the frequency discrimination of pulsed tones and the detection of frequency modulation. J. Acoust. Soc. Amer. 86, 1722-1732.

Plack, C. J. and Moore, B. C. J. (1990) Temporal window shape as a function of frequency and level. J. Acoust. Soc. Amer. 87, 2178-2187.

Plack, C. J. and Moore, B. C. J. (1991) Decrement detection in normal and impaired ears. J. Acoust. Soc. Amer. 90, 3069-3076.

Teager, H. M. and Teager, S. M. (1990) Evidence for non-linear sound production mechanisms in the larynx. In: NATO Advanced Study Institute on Speech Production and Speech Modeling, Kluwer Press, 241-261.

Viemeister, N. F. (1979) Temporal modulation transfer functions based upon modulation thresholds. J. Acoust. Soc. Amer. 66, 1354-1380.

Zhang, T., Feth, L. L. and Krishnamurthy, A. K. (1994) Detection of frequency modulation in steady and gliding tones. J. Acoust. Soc. Amer. 95, 2965.

Auditory filtering and the critical bandwidth at low frequencies

Brian C.J. Moore and Aleksander Sek

Department of Experimental Psychology, University of Cambridge, Downing Street, Cambridge CB2 3EB, England

1 Introduction

The critical bandwidth (CB) is a measure of the frequency resolution of the auditory system that can be derived using many different tasks. It can be defined empirically as "that bandwidth at which subjective responses change rather abruptly" (Scharf, 1970). It is generally assumed that the CB reflects the characteristics of the filtering that takes place in the auditory periphery, and that the CB is related to the bandwidth of the auditory filter. Indeed, it is common for researchers to talk of "critical band filters".

Measures of the critical bandwidth obtained from a variety of experiments generally agree reasonably well for centre frequencies above about 1 kHz. However, at lower centre frequencies there are considerable discrepancies among the different measures. The "traditional" function relating the CB to centre frequency (Zwicker, 1961; Scharf, 1970; Zwicker and Terhardt, 1980) flattens off for centre frequencies below 500 Hz at a value of about 100 Hz. However, when this function was first suggested, the data at low frequencies were rather sparse, and the estimates were based principally on only two types of measurements: the critical ratio and the critical modulation frequency (more details of these will be given later). In contrast, more recent measurements, based mainly on notched-noise or rippled-noise masking, indicate that the CB continues to decrease below 500 Hz (Moore and Glasberg, 1983, 1987; Glasberg and Moore, 1990; Moore et al., 1990). This paper examines some of the reasons for the discrepancies between different methods, and argues that the weight of evidence from a variety of experiments supports the idea that the CB does continue to decrease down to very low centre frequencies.

There have been two basic approaches to estimating the values of CBs from experimental data. The first is "empirical"; there is no explicit model of the underlying process. The researcher merely tries to estimate a "breakpoint" in the data relating performance to bandwidth - a point at which subjective responses change "abruptly". Typically, the data are fitted with two straight lines, one for narrow bandwidths and the other for wider bandwidths, and the intersection point of the two lines defines the CB (Fletcher, 1940; Zwicker et al., 1957). While this approach might be described as "neutral", in not being tied to a specific model, it is fraught with difficulty. Firstly, most of the tasks that have been used to estimate the CB do not reveal any abrupt changes as a function of bandwidth. Rather, performance tends to change smoothly and progressively as bandwidth is altered (Moore and Glasberg, 1986; Patterson and Moore, 1986). Secondly, the estimated CB can be strongly influenced by the axes on which the data are plotted (e.g. a linear or logarithmic axis for bandwidth), but the choice of axes is largely arbitrary in the absence of a theoretical model. Finally, the estimated value of the CB can be strongly influenced by small errors in the data (Moore and Glasberg, 1986).

An alternative approach is to try to fit the data with a specific theoretical model. For example, a certain general form can be assumed for the shape of the auditory filter, and the data can then be used to estimate the bandwidth of the filter (Patterson and Moore, 1986). Typically, the filter is assumed to have the form of a rounded exponential (Patterson et al., 1982; see Eq. 1 below) and the filter bandwidth is specified as its equivalent rectangular bandwidth (ERB).

This paper takes the second of the two approaches outlined above. It assumes that variations in performance with bandwidth depend primarily, but not exclusively, on the properties of the auditory filter. Data from a variety experiments are shown to be consistent with an auditory filter whose bandwidth decreases with decreasing frequency down to very low frequencies. The paper concentrates on data obtained at low centre frequencies.

2 Measures of the Critical Bandwidth Based on Masking

Almost all estimates of the auditory filter shape and bandwidth derived from masking experiments are based on the assumptions of the power spectrum model of masking (Fletcher, 1940; Patterson and Moore, 1986), and particularly the assumption that threshold at a given signal frequency corresponds to a fixed signal-to-masker ratio at the output of an auditory filter centred close to the signal frequency. There are clearly some situations where this assumption is not valid and these situations should be avoided if valid estimates of the auditory filter shape are to be obtained. Generally, this means avoiding maskers with very narrow bandwidths or strong temporal fluctuations; for reviews see Moore and Glasberg (1987) and Moore (1994). In this paper, we assume that the auditory filter has one of the general forms suggested by Patterson et al. (1982):

$$W(g) = (1-r)(1+pg)\exp(-pg) + r \tag{1}$$

where g is the deviation from the centre frequency of the filter divided by the centre frequency, $W(g)$ is the intensity-weighting function describing the shape of the filter, p is a parameter that determines the sharpness of the passband of the filter, and r is a parameter that flattens the filter skirts at frequencies remote from the centre frequency, by imposing a dynamic range limitation. In many cases, the term r is very small and can be ignored. Although our analyses are based on this filter shape, the basic conclusions would be the same if other filter shapes were assumed, such as a Gaussian. The assumed filter shape affects the exact bandwidth value obtained (Glasberg et al., 1984), but does not affect estimates of how the filter bandwidth varies with frequency.

2.1 Notched-noise Masking

The notched-noise method was developed by Patterson (1976) and has been reviewed in several publications (Patterson and Moore, 1986; Moore and Glasberg, 1987; Glasberg and Moore, 1990). The threshold for detecting a sinusoidal signal is measured as a function of the width of a spectral notch in the noise masker. The notch can be positioned both symmetrically and asymmetrically about the signal frequency. The method has the advantage of avoiding obvious strong violations of the assumptions of the power-spectrum model. Measurements at low centre frequencies have been obtained by several authors (Fidell et al., 1983; Shailer and Moore, 1983; Moore et al., 1990; Peters and Moore, 1992; Rosen and Stock, 1992). Glasberg and Moore (1990) have described methods of analyzing the data that take into account transmission of sound through the outer and middle ear. All of these papers are in agreement, showing that even a relatively small notch in the noise can produce a significant decrease in signal threshold. For example, a 40-Hz wide notch centred at 100 Hz typically produces a decrease in threshold, relative to that obtained with no notch, of 8-14 dB. This is inconsistent with the "traditional" CB value of 100 Hz, since a 40-Hz notch would produce only a 2-dB decrease in power at the output of a 100-Hz wide filter. Application of the auditory-filter model to these data indicates that the ERB of the auditory filter decreases with decreasing frequency below 500 Hz, reaching a value of 25-45 Hz (mean about 36 Hz) at a centre frequency of 100 Hz. Glasberg and Moore (1990) proposed the following equation to describe the variation of the ERB with centre frequency (F, in kHz):

$$\mathrm{ERB} = 24.7(4.37F + 1) \tag{2}$$

2.2 Rippled-noise Masking

This method may suffer from the problem of "off-frequency listening" (the use of auditory filters centred away from the signal frequency; see Patterson and Moore, 1986), but otherwise it avoids obvious strong violations of the assumptions of the power-spectrum model. The masker has a spectrum with a sinusoidal ripple on a linear frequency scale. The threshold of the signal is measured as a function of ripple density, with the spectrum constructed so that either a peak or a dip in the spectrum falls at the signal frequency. Houtgast (1977) estimated auditory filter shapes with this method over a wide range of centre frequencies. The results were in very good agreement with those obtained using the notched-noise method, showing a continuing decrease in auditory filter bandwidth below 500 Hz (Moore and Glasberg, 1983).

2.3 Two-tone Masking

In this method, the task is to detect a narrowband signal centred between two sinusoidal tones, as a function of the frequency separation of the two tones. This method can be affected by the detection of combination products produced by the interaction of the signal and the lower masker tone. It can also be influenced by beats, whose detectability varies with the frequency separation of the masker and signal; this violates one of the assumptions of the power spectrum model. The problem of beats can be reduced, but not eliminated, by using narrowband noise as the signal. Hence, auditory-filter bandwidths obtained using this method are probably not as accurate as those obtained using the notched-noise method.

Fastl and Schorer (1986) presented results of two-tone masking for low centre frequencies. If the results are fitted with the auditory filter model (see the comment by Moore following the paper of Fastl and Schorer), the bandwidths estimated using this method show a clear decrease with decreasing centre frequency down to 125 Hz. At 125 Hz, the estimated ERB is 41 Hz for a sinusoidal signal and 58 Hz for a 30-Hz wide noise signal. These values are slightly larger than the values estimated using notched-noise or rippled-noise maskers, but still considerably smaller than the traditional value of the CB. The wider value obtained for the noise signal may be explained by the fact that the signal bandwidth was comparable to the ERB at 125 Hz.

2.4 The Critical Ratio

This is an indirect method for estimating the auditory filter bandwidth, based on the assumption that, at threshold, the ratio of signal power to masker power at the output of the auditory filter, K, is constant, and independent of frequency. The threshold of a sinusoidal signal is measured in broadband white noise. If the power of the signal at threshold is P_t, and the noise power density is N_0, then this assumption is described by the equation

$$P_t/(N_0.ERB) = K, \tag{3}$$

which can be rearranged to give

$$ERB = P_t/(N_0.K). \tag{4}$$

If K were independent of frequency, then the ERB would be proportional to the ratio P_t/N_0, which is often known as the critical ratio. This ratio actually increases at very low centre frequencies (Hawkins and Stevens, 1950), and this had a strong influence on early estimates of the CB. However, recent data suggest that K is not independent of frequency, but increases markedly at low centre frequencies. The notched-noise method allows separate estimates of the auditory filter shape and of the quantity K, which is often referred to as "detection efficiency". The data of Moore et al. (1990) and of Rosen and Stock (1992) indicate that the value of K increases by a factor of 3-5 (5-7 dB) as the centre frequency decreases from 800 to 100 Hz. The critical ratio is about a factor of 1.25 (1 dB) larger at 100 than at 800 Hz (Hawkins and Stevens, 1950). Using Eq. 4, this implies that the ERB is about a factor of 3 smaller at 100 than at 800 Hz, in reasonable agreement with Eq. 2, but very different from the traditional CB values.

2.5 Summary of Results from Masking Experiments

When interpreted in terms of the auditory filter model, the results of all the experiments reviewed above are consistent in showing that the ERB continues to decrease with decreasing centre frequency below 500 Hz. For centre frequencies of 100 - 125 Hz, the ERB estimates mostly fall in the range 24 - 45 Hz.

3 The Critical Modulation Frequency (CMF)

This method had a strong influence on early estimates of the CB (Zwicker, 1952), and it has been argued to be one of the best methods for estimating the CB at low frequencies (Fastl and Schorer, 1986; Schorer, 1986; Zwicker and Fastl, 1990), so it is considered in some detail here. An amplitude modulated (AM) sinewave with modulation index m, and a frequency modulated (FM) sinewave with modulation index β, may each be considered as composed of three sinusoidal components, corresponding to the carrier frequency, f_c, and two sidebands (an FM wave actually contains many components but for small modulation indices only the first two sidebands are important). When the modulation indices are numerically equal ($m = \beta$), and when the carrier frequencies and modulation frequencies are the same, the components of an AM wave and an FM wave are identical in frequency and amplitude, the only difference between them being in the relative phase of the components. If, then, the two types of wave are perceived differently, the difference is likely to arise from a sensitivity to the relative phase of the components.

Zwicker (1952), Schorer (1986) and Sek (1994) measured the just-detectable amounts of amplitude or frequency modulation, for various rates of modulation. They found that for high rates of modulation, where the frequency components were widely spaced, the detectability of FM and AM was equal when the components in each type of wave were of equal amplitude ($m = \beta$). However, for low rates of modulation, when all three components fell within a narrow frequency range, AM could be detected when the relative levels of the sidebands were lower than for a wave with a just-detectable amount of FM ($m < \beta$). This is illustrated in the upper panel of Fig. 1 (data from Sek, 1994).

If the threshold for detecting modulation is expressed in terms of the modulation index, m or β, the ratio β/m decreases as the modulation frequency increases, and approaches an asymptotic value of unity. This is illustrated in the lower panel of Fig. 1. The modulation frequency at which the ratio first becomes unity is the CMF. Zwicker (1952) and Schorer (1986) suggested that the CMF is reached when the spectral sidebands in the stimulus first become detectable. Once the modulation is detected in this way, the relative phases of the components do not play a role. Zwicker (1952) and Schorer (1986) suggested further that the CMF corresponded to half the value of the CB; essentially, the CMF was assumed to be reached when the overall stimulus bandwidth reached the CB. If this is correct, then the CMF may be regarded as providing an estimate of the CB at the carrier frequency.

Sek and Moore (1994) have presented evidence that the interpretation of the CMF proposed by Zwicker (1952) and by Schorer (1986) is not correct. For medium to high carrier frequencies, the CMF appears to correspond to the point where the lower sideband in the spectrum first becomes detectable (Hartmann and Hnath, 1982). However, Sek and Moore (1994) showed that, for very low carrier frequencies, the upper sideband becomes detectable before the lower sideband.

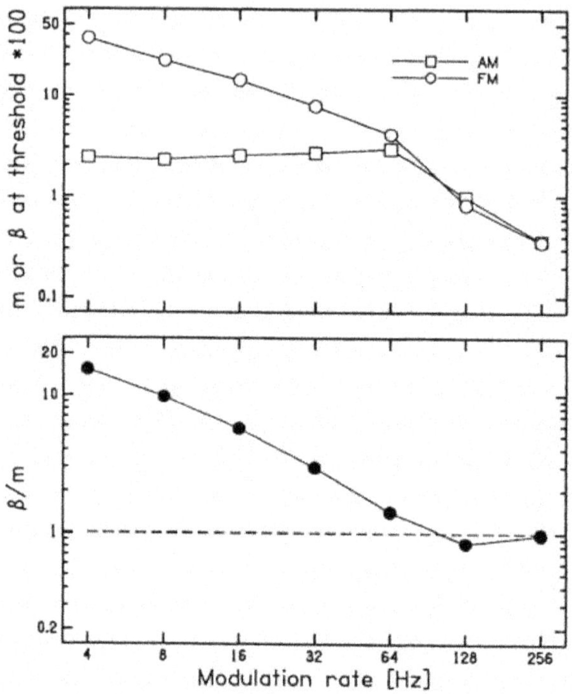

Figure 1. The upper panel shows the thresholds for detecting sinusoidal AM or FM, expressed as the respective modulation indices, m or β, plotted as a function of modulation rate. The carrier frequency was 1000 Hz. The lower panel shows the ratio m/β. Data from Sek (1994).

To determine which sideband was used for detection, Sek and Moore compared the results from two experiments. In the first experiment, thresholds were measured for the detection of AM and FM, using several different (low) carrier frequencies and a range of modulation rates around the CMF. The thresholds were expressed in terms of the levels of the sidebands at threshold. In the second experiment, thresholds were measured for detecting a single sinusoid, corresponding to either the upper or lower sideband of the modulated signals used in experiment 1, in the presence of a sinusoidal masker corresponding to the carrier frequency. If a component corresponding to a given sideband, say the upper one, has a lower threshold than a component corresponding to the other sideband, then the given sideband should be more detectable in a situation where both sidebands are present (as in the modulation-detection task). Furthermore, if modulation detection thresholds are determined by the threshold for the most-detectable sideband, then the thresholds determined for that sideband in experiment 2 should correspond with those determined in experiment 1.

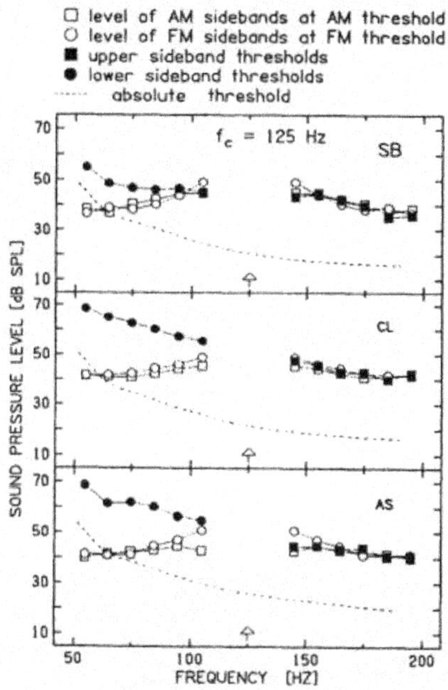

Figure 2. Results for a carrier frequency of 125 Hz. Modulation detection thresholds are expressed in terms of the levels of the sidebands at threshold (open squares - AM thresholds; open circles FM thresholds). Filled symbols show thresholds for detecting a single sinusoidal signal below (circles) or above (squares) the masker frequency. Dashed curves show absolute thresholds. Each panel shows results for one subject.

An example of the results for f_c = 125 Hz, is shown in Fig. 2. Each panel shows results for one subject, and the value of f_c is indicated by an arrow. Dashed lines show absolute thresholds. The open symbols show the results of experiment 1; the level of each sideband at the modulation detection threshold is plotted as a function of frequency. Since the upper and lower sidebands were always equal in level, each measured theshold is presented twice, giving a pattern of thresholds symmetrical about f_c. For the higher modulation frequencies used, the AM and FM thresholds coincide, whereas for the lower values used (sidebands closest to f_c), the FM thresholds are higher than the AM thresholds. This reflects the fact that the modulation frequencies were chosen to span the CMF. These results are consistent with earlier results showing that the CMF for low carrier frequencies is typically about 40 Hz (Zwicker, 1952; Schorer, 1986; Sek, 1994).

The filled symbols show the results of experiment 2, where thresholds were measured for single sinusoids corresponding to the upper and lower sidebands in experiment 1. The thresholds obtained for signals with frequencies below f_c (filled circles) were generally higher than those for signals with frequencies above f_c. This suggests that, when both sidebands were present simultaneously (as in experiment 1), detection was based on the upper sideband rather than the lower sideband.

Comparing the results of experiments 1 and 2, it is clear that the thresholds for the lower sideband alone (filled circles) are markedly higher than the levels of the lower sideband at the modulation detection threshold (open symbols). This indicates that, at the modulation detection threshold, the lower sideband would have been undetectable. Indeed, for the highest modulation frequency used, the lower sideband (at 55 Hz) would have been below absolute threshold. In contrast, for modulation rates above the CMF, the levels of the upper sideband at the modulation detection threshold are almost identical with the detection thresholds of the upper sideband when presented alone (filled squares). Taken together, these results indicate that modulation detection thresholds for modulation rates above the CMF were determined by the threshold for detection of the upper sideband.

The results of Sek and Moore (1994) suggest that carrier frequencies from 200 to 250 Hz lie in a transition region. For carriers below that region, modulation detection thresholds for rates above the CMF are determined by the threshold for detecting the upper sideband. For carriers above that region, detection is probably based mainly on the threshold for detecting the lower sideband (Hartmann and Hnath, 1982; Ozimek and Sek, 1987; Moore and Sek, 1992). Within that region, both sidebands may contribute to detection of the modulation. The fact that the most detectable sideband switches from the lower one to the upper one as the carrier frequency decreases means that the CMF is confounded as a measure of frequency selectivity, since the auditory filter centred on the upper sideband has a greater bandwidth than the auditory filter centred on the lower sideband.

Sek and Moore (1994) discussed several factors that might cause the lower sideband to become less detectable for low carrier frequencies. These included; the effect of the transfer function of the middle ear (Zwislocki, 1975; Rosowski, 1991); the possibility that the cochlea is characterized by a relatively high level of internal noise at low frequencies (Nedzelnitsky, 1980); and the possibility that the signal-to-masker ratio required for threshold increases at low frequencies. It seems likely that the main cue used for signal detection when a single sideband was present was the beating produced by the interaction of the signal and masker. Riesz (1928) and Harris (1963) showed that the beat "depth" required for threshold increased markedly at low frequencies. In addition, the detectability of beats decreases with increasing beat rate (above 3-4 Hz) and with decreasing sensation level (Riesz, 1928; Harris, 1963).

These factors provide further justification for our claim that the CMF is confounded as a measure of frequency selectivity; none of these factors is directly connected with frequency selectivity, yet all may influence the value of the CMF for low carrier frequencies. Sek and Moore showed that, taking these factors into account, the values of the CMF for low carrier frequencies can be reconciled, at least to a first approximation, with the estimates of auditory filter bandwidth and shape summarised by Glasberg and Moore (1990).

4 The Audibility of Partials in Complex Sounds

Under some conditions, listeners are able to "hear out" individual partials in complex tones, i.e, they can hear pitches corresponding to frequencies of individual components. Plomp (1964) and Plomp and Mimpen (1968) suggested that in order for a partial to be heard out in this way, it has to be separated from neighbouring partials by at least one CB. If this is the case, then the CB can be estimated as the smallest frequency separation from it's neighbours at which a partial can be heard out. As is the case for other methods of estimating the CB, the data do not show a distinct breakpoint; rather the ability to hear out a given partial increases progressively as its frequency separation from neighbouring partials increases. Hence, the value of the CB estimated by this method is somewhat arbitrary, depending on the criterion level of performance chosen. Nevertheless, the method may give an appropriate indication of the way that the CB varies with frequency.

The data of Plomp and Mimpen indicate that, for harmonic complex tones, about the first five to eight harmonics can be heard out, almost independently of fundamental frequency. Taking the separation between the seventh and eighth harmonics as a limiting value, this suggests a CB of about 13% of the centre frequency, which is comparable with estimates of the ERB of the auditory filter at medium to high centre frequencies, but suggests smaller values at lower centre frequencies. Moore and Ohgushi (1993) constructed inharmonic complex tones with partials equally spaced on the ERB scale proposed by Glasberg and Moore (1990). If this scale correctly describes the variation of the ERB with centre frequency, and if the ability to hear out a partial depends only on its separation in ERBs from neighbouring partials, then all of the partials in the complex tones should have been heard out equally well. In fact, the lowest and highest partials within the complexes were heard out better than partials within the complexes. In addition, for partials within the complexes, partials below 1000 Hz tended to be heard out better than partials above 1000 Hz.

Taken at face value, these results suggest that the CB at low frequencies is *smaller* than the ERB values proposed by Glasberg and Moore (1990). However, Moore and Ohgushi (1993) suggested that this task is affected by factors other than peripheral filtering. One factor is musical experience (Soderquist, 1970; Fine and Moore, 1993). The other is phase locking to the frequencies of individual partials, which may play a role in determining the pitches of components at low frequencies but not at high frequencies. Overall, though, results on the audibility of partials in complex tones clearly indicate that the CB continues to decrease with decreasing centre frequency below 500 Hz.

5 Summary and Conclusions

The "traditional" CB function flattens off below 500 Hz at a constant value of about 100 Hz. However, the values below 500 Hz were based largely on two types of measures, the critical ratio and the critical modulation frequency, which are confounded as estimates of frequency selectivity. Estimates of the auditory filter bandwidth based on notched-noise, rippled-noise and two-tone masking consistently show that the ERB of the auditory filter continues to decrease below 500 Hz. Data on the audibility of partials in complex tones also show a continuing decrease in the CB for centre frequncies below 500 Hz. The function describing the variation of the ERB with centre frequency proposed by Glasberg and Moore (1990; Eq. 2 of this paper) is consistent with the data discussed here, and is also consistent with early data on tonal consonance and dissonance (Meyer, 1898; Plomp and Levelt, 1965), and with the CB function proposed by Greenwood (1961), based on the assumption that each CB corresponds to a constant distance on the basilar membrane.

6 Acknowledgements

This work was supported by the Medical Research Council (UK) and by Fellowships awarded to A. Sek by the Royal Society and the Wellcome Trust.

7 References

Fastl, H. and Schorer, E. (1986) Critical bandwidth at low frequencies reconsidered. In: B. C. J. Moore and R. D. Patterson (Eds.) Auditory Frequency Selectivity, Plenum, New York, pp. 311-318.

Fidell, S., Horonjeff, R., Teffeteller, S. and Green, D. M. (1983) Effective masking bandwidths at low frequencies. J. Acoust. Soc. Am. 73, 628-638.

Fine, P. A. and Moore, B. C. J. (1993) Frequency analysis and musical ability. Music Percept. 11, 39-53.

Fletcher, H. (1940) Auditory patterns. Rev. Mod. Phys. 12, 47-65.

Glasberg, B. R. and Moore, B. C. J. (1990) Derivation of auditory filter shapes from notched-noise data. Hear. Res. 47, 103-138.

Glasberg, B. R., Moore, B. C. J. and Nimmo-Smith, I. (1984) Comparison of auditory filter shapes derived with three different maskers. J. Acoust. Soc. Am. 75, 536-544.

Greenwood, D. D. (1961) Critical bandwidth and the frequency coordinates of the basilar membrane. J. Acoust. Soc. Am. 33, 1344-1356.

Harris, J. D. (1963) Loudness discrimination. J. Speech. Hear. Dis. Monographs, Supplement 11, 1-63.

Hartmann, W. M. and Hnath, G. M. (1982) Detection of mixed modulation. Acustica 50, 297-312.

Hawkins, J. E., Jr. and Stevens, S. S. (1950) The masking of pure tones and of speech by white noise. J. Acoust. Soc. Am. 22, 6-13.

Houtgast, T. (1977) Auditory-filter characteristics derived from direct-masking data and pulsation-threshold data with a rippled-noise masker. J. Acoust. Soc. Am. 62, 409-415.

Meyer, M. (1898) Zur Theorie der Differenztöne und der Gehörsempfindungen überhaubt. Beitr. Akust. Musikwiss 2, 25-65.

Moore, B. C. J. (1994) Frequency analysis and masking. In: B. C. J. Moore (Ed.) Handbook of Perception and Cognition, Volume 6. Hearing, Academic Press, Orlando, Florida (in press).

Moore, B. C. J. and Glasberg, B. R. (1983) Suggested formulae for calculating auditory-filter bandwidths and excitation patterns. J. Acoust. Soc. Am. 74, 750-753.

Moore, B. C. J. and Glasberg, B. R. (1986) The role of frequency selectivity in the perception of loudness, pitch and time. In: B. C. J. Moore (Ed.) Frequency Selectivity in Hearing, Academic, London, pp. 251-308.

Moore, B. C. J. and Glasberg, B. R. (1987) Formulae describing frequency selectivity as a function of frequency and level and their use in calculating excitation patterns. Hear. Res. 28, 209-225.

Moore, B. C. J. and Ohgushi, K. (1993) Audibility of partials in inharmonic complex tones. J. Acoust. Soc. Am. 93, 452-461.

Moore, B. C. J., Peters, R. W. and Glasberg, B. R. (1990) Auditory filter shapes at low center frequencies. J. Acoust. Soc. Am. 88, 132-140.

Moore, B. C. J. and Sek, A. (1992) Detection of combined frequency and amplitude modulation. J. Acoust. Soc. Am. 92, 3119-3131.

Nedzelnitsky, V. (1980) Sound pressures in the basal turn of the cat cochlea. J. Acoust. Soc. Am. 68, 1676-1689.

Ozimek, E. and Sek, A. (1987) Perception of amplitude and frequency modulated signals (mixed modulation). J. Acoust. Soc. Am. 82, 1598-1603.

Patterson, R. D. (1976) Auditory filter shapes derived with noise stimuli. J. Acoust. Soc. Am. 59, 640-654.

Patterson, R. D. and Moore, B. C. J. (1986) Auditory filters and excitation patterns as representations of frequency resolution. In: B. C. J. Moore (Ed.) Frequency Selectivity in Hearing, Academic, London, pp. 123-177.

Patterson, R. D., Nimmo-Smith, I., Weber, D. L. and Milroy, R. (1982) The deterioration of hearing with age: frequency selectivity, the critical ratio, the audiogram, and speech threshold. J. Acoust. Soc. Am. 72, 1788-1803.

Peters, R. W. and Moore, B. C. J. (1992) Auditory filter shapes at low center frequencies in young and elderly hearing-impaired subjects. J. Acoust. Soc. Am. 91, 256-266.

Plomp, R. (1964) The ear as a frequency analyzer. J. Acoust. Soc. Am. 36, 1628-1636.

Plomp, R. and Levelt, W. J. M. (1965) Tonal consonance and critical bandwidth. J. Acoust. Soc. Am. 38, 548-560.

Plomp, R. and Mimpen, A. M. (1968) The ear as a frequency analyzer II. J. Acoust. Soc. Am. 43, 764-767.

Riesz, R. R. (1928) Differential intensity sensitivity of the ear for pure tones. Phys. Rev. 31, 867-875.

Rosen, S. and Stock, D. (1992) Auditory filter bandwidths as a function of level at low frequencies (125 Hz-1 kHz). J. Acoust. Soc. Am. 92, 773-781.

Rosowski, J. J. (1991) The effects of external- and middle-ear filtering on auditory threshold and noise-induced hearing loss. J. Acoust. Soc. Am. 90, 124-135.

Scharf, B. (1970) Critical bands. In: J. V. Tobias (Ed.) Foundations of Modern Auditory Theory, Academic Press, New York, pp. 157-202.

Schorer, E. (1986) Critical modulation frequency based on detection of AM versus FM tones. J. Acoust. Soc. Am. 79, 1054-1057.

Sek, A. (1994) Modulation detection thresholds and critical modulation frequency based on random amplitude and frequency changes. J. Acoust. Soc. Jpn. (E) 15, 67-75.

Sek, A. and Moore, B. C. J. (1994) The critical modulation frequency and its relationship to auditory filtering at low frequencies. J. Acoust. Soc. Am. 95, 2606-2615.

Shailer, M. J. and Moore, B. C. J. (1983) Gap detection as a function of frequency, bandwidth and level. J. Acoust. Soc. Am. 74, 467-473.

Soderquist, D. R. (1970) Frequency analysis and the critical band. Psychon. Sci. 21, 117-119.

Zwicker, E. (1952) Die Grenzen der Hörbarkeit der Amplitudenmodulation und der Frequenzmodulation eines Tones. Acustica 2, 125-133.

Zwicker, E. (1961) Subdivision of the audible frequency range into critical bands (Frequenzgruppen). J. Acoust. Soc. Am. 33, 248.

Zwicker, E. and Fastl, H. (1990) Psychoacoustics - Facts and Models, Springer-Verlag, Berlin.

Zwicker, E., Flottorp, G. and Stevens, S. S. (1957) Critical bandwidth in loudness summation. J. Acoust. Soc. Am. 29, 548-557.

Zwicker, E. and Terhardt, E. (1980) Analytical expressions for critical band rate and critical bandwidth as a function of frequency. J. Acoust. Soc. Am. 68, 1523-1525.

Zwislocki, J. J. (1975) The role of the external and middle ear in sound transmission. In: D. B. Tower and E.L. Eagles (Eds.) The Nervous System, Vol. 3. Human Communication and its Disorders, Raven Press, New York, pp. 45-55

Comment by E.F. Evans

Consistent with your psychophysical conclusions, the ERBs of cochlear nerve fibres are still reducing with reducing frequency below 500 Hz (see Evans et al. 1992 and Fig. 1 of my comment to Ehret, this volume).

Comment by H. Dai

The idea that the critical band continues to decrease down to a low centre frequency is also supported by the result on attention filter measured using the probe-signal method of Greenberg and Larkin (1968). Dai, Scharf and Buus (1991, Fig. 3) showed that the attention filter changes width with centre frequency in a similar manner as the notched-noise filter. There are two potential advantages associated with the probe-signal method for measuring the shape of the auditory filter. First, the filter's weighting function is obtained without changing the masker, which may be considered as a "nondestructive" method. Second, as Hafter (personal communication) pointed out, filter shape measured with the probe-signal method is most reliable around the centre frequency of the filter, which provides a relatively reliable estimate of the 3-dB down bandwidth. For these reasons, the probe-signal method should be considered at least as reasonable as the other discussed methods for measuring the critical-band.

Dai, H., Scharf, B. and Buus, S. (1991) Effective attenuation of signals in noise under focused attention.. J. Acoust. Soc. Am. 89, 2837-2842.

Greenberg, G. and Larkin, W. (1968) Frequency-response characteristic of auditory observers detecting signals of a single frequency in noise: The probe-signal method. J. Acoust. Soc. Am. 44, 1513-1523.

Reply

I am not convinced that the probe-signal method provides a reliable means for estimating the shape or bandwidth of the auditory filter. However, the results probably do depend partly on the auditory-filter bandwidth, so the continuing decrease in bandwidth at low centre frequencies found using the probe-signal method can be taken as support for the arguments presented in our paper.

Comment by D. Green

I certainly agree with your bandwidth estimates at low frequencies, because our masking experiments produced low estimates (Fidell et al. 1983). I would like to submit an approximation to Eq. 2 for those who like simple expressions. The formula

$$ERB_{approx.} = (1/10)\ F + 25\ \text{Hz}$$

where F is in Hertz. This agrees with Eq. 2 within 10% over the range of F from 100 to 10 000.

For those who wish better accuracy the expression

$$ERB_{approx.} = (11/100)\ F + 25\ \text{Hz}$$

approximates Eq. 2 within 2% for the same range.

Reply

Your approximations may be useful to those who want a simple expression to memorise. However, I will happily provide you with a handy card with Eq. 2 written on it. This, plus a hand calculator, will give the "correct" answer and will keep Don Greenwood happy.

Comment by A. Kohlrausch

While referring to the publications of Moore et al. (1990) and Rosen and Stock (1992) you state that the parameter K which is equivalent to the ratio between signal and masker power at the output of the auditory filter, increases significantly (5 to 7 dB) as the centre frequency decreases from 800 Hz to 100 Hz. Because "K provides a measure of the efficiency of the detection process following the auditory filter" (Moore et al., 1990), this finding implies that the S/N values for signals in any kind of masker (provided the masker's bandwidth is subcritical) should increase by 5 to 7 dB as the signal frequency is lowered from 800 to 100 Hz. This is in contradiction with data from our laboratory which are shown in the figure. These data were obtained with the procedure described in Kohlrausch et al. (this volume) and show N_0S_0 masked thresholds in narrowband-noise maskers, expressed as signal-to-overall-noise ratio, as a function of the centre frequency of the noise. The four curves indicate data for 4 different noise bandwidths between 5 and

50 Hz. There is no threshold increase between 1000 and 125 Hz for the 5 and 10 Hz data and an increase of only 1.5 dB for 25 and 50 Hz masker bandwidths. The increase in threshold with decreasing masker bandwidth is in line with the predictions of an energy-detector model.

Your statement that the increase in K just reflects the fact that you have a narrower noise bandwidth (and thus following an energy detector argument, a higher S/N value) at the output of a low-frequency auditory filter, is unsatisfactory for the following reasons:

1.) This argument applies only to broadband conditions where the masker bandwidth is at least as wide as the auditory filter at the corresponding signal frequency. This is certainly an important qualification compared to the rather general statements of the increasing detector efficiency in Moore et al. (1990), a statement repeated by Rosen and Stock (1992).

2.) If the increase in K at low frequencies is indeed a consequence of the reduced "effective" masker bandwidth an the output of a low frequency filter as compared to a high frequency filter, then the factor K is obviously more dependent on the statistics of the masker than on the efficiency of auditory processing. In short, if you would use a deterministic masker (tone, complex tone, frozen noise), the argument of the role of envelope fluctuations would not be applicable and, for these conditions, based on your arguments in the discussion, one has to expect a *constant* S/N value at all frequencies. This, again, is in contradiction with the generality of the statements about the detector efficiency. One might also wonder, to what extent your argument is applicable to other than Gaussian noise maskers with that of a Gaussian noise.

3.) A more general point: the philosophy behind the derivation of RoEx filter shapes from notched noise data is that masking is only dependent on the S/N ratio after a filtering process. This is a pure spectral view of masking by noise bands that explicitly rejects only influences of temporal fluctuations in the envelopes of a noise masker, despite experimental evidence that envelope fluctuations *do* play a role in "spectral masking" conditions (Buus, 1985; Mott and Feth, 1986; v.d. Heijden and Kohlrausch, 1994).What you do by allowing a frequency dependent value for the detector efficiency, is to re-introduce the consequences of *temporal* fluctuations of the masker into a pure *spectral* model of masking.

Attributing the role of temporal fluctuations exclusively to the centre frequency of the auditory filter (via the value of K), instead of to the actual statistics of the masker at the output of the auditory filter, is in my view a wrong solution.

Buus, S. (1985) Release from masking caused by envelope fluctuations. J. Acoust. Soc. Am 78, 1958-1965.

Heijden, M. v.d. and Kohlrausch, A. (1994) Using an excitation-pattern model to predict auditory masking. Hear. Res. 80,38-52.

Mott, J.B. and Feth, L.L. (1986) Effects of the temporal properties of a masker upon simultaneous-masking patterns. In: B.C.J. Moore and R.D. Patterson (Eds.) Auditory frequency selectivity. Plenum Press, New York, 381-386.

Reply

We do not wish to claim that the value of K reflects only central decision processes. Indeed, to the contrary, we have suggested that fluctuations in the masker do play an important role. Thus, K should not be taken as a constant that would be the same for "any kind of masker", as you suggest. The important point for the arguments presented in our paper is whether the value of K is similar for a broadband masker (when measuring the critical ratio) and for a notched-noise masker. We believe that it is reasonable to assume this to be approximately true.

The increase of K with decreasing frequency when broadband or notched-noise maskers are used is probably related to the rapidity of fluctuations at the output of the auditory filter. These fluctuations are slower, and have a more deleterious effect on performance, at low frequencies because of the narrower bandwidth of the auditory filter. When the masker has a very narrow bandwidth, less than the ERB of the auditory filter, performance will be determined mainly by the stimulus statistics, and the effect of auditory filtering will be small. Hence if a masker has a subcritical bandwidth at all centre frequencies tested, performance will be independent of centre frequency, consistent with your results.

I think that the differences between us arise primarily from the way that the term "detection efficiency" is used. If several subjects are tested with identical stimuli, for example in a notched-noise experiment, it its often found that the value of K varies across subjects. In this case, it seems appropriate to describe the variation in terms of detection efficiency. It is in this context that the term was first used. However, the term may be less appropriate when K changes because of a change in the properties of the masker or signal.

I want to emphasize once again that I have never claimed that temporal fluctuations in the masker are unimportant. Indeed, I have several publications that specifically address the role of fluctuations. The important point when choosing stimuli for estimating the auditory filter shape is that the temporal fluctuations should play a small role, or that their effects should not alter markedly when the spectral characteristics of the masker are changed.

Comment by B. Scharf

What do measurements of loudness summation across frequency show as the critical bandwidth at low frequencies, below 500 Hz?

Reply

We are aware of only a very few measures of the critical bandwidth for loudness at frequencies below 500 Hz. These measures, like similar measures at higher center frequencies, usually do not show a distinct "breakpoint" as a function of bandwidth, making it hard to determine a value for the critical bandwidth. The interpretation of the results is also complicated by the fact that absolute sensitivity changes markedly with frequency for frequencies below 500 Hz.

Loudness estimation and compensation for impaired listeners employing a categorical scale

Birger Kollmeier, Volker Hohmann

AG Medizinische Physik, FB Physik, Universität Oldenburg, 26111 Oldenburg, Germany

1 Introduction

The traditional measurement method for loudness perception requires the subject to judge the loudness of a given stimulus in relation to the perceived loudness of a reference stimulus. It is based on the work by Stevens (1956) and Zwicker (1960) and has found a wide application (e.g., the sone scale, loudness measurements based on ISO 532 B, estimation of loudness growth functions for normal and impaired listeners). However, the ratio scale established with such a psychophysical experiment seems not to be well suited to the listener's capabilities in loudness judgements. Heller (1991) even demonstrated that a random number generator with only very few additional assumptions can exactly generate most of the power-law relationships demonstrated by Stevens (1956).

Instead, native listeners are capable of rating the perceived loudness in coarse categories, such as the loudness categories used in music from pianissimo to fortissimo. Heller therefore derived a categorical loudness estimation procedure, the "Würzburger Hörfeldskalierung", which was first used in clinical measurements by Hellbrück and Moser (1985) and later modified for practical clinical applications in a german joint research project (Kollmeier et al., 1993, Hohmann, 1993). A similar categorical loudness scaling procedure was developed by Pascoe (1988) and Allen (1990). In this method, a narrow-band stimulus is presented to the subject at a presentation level randomly selected in a predefined range. The subject's task is to judge the perceived loudness in categories ranging from "very soft", "soft", "neither loud nor soft", "loud", to "very loud". In the original Heller approach the stimulus is presented a second time and the coarse categories are subdivided into ten divisions each. The method was therefore named "Kategorial-Unterteilungs (KU)-Lautheit" (i.e., categorical subdivided loudness) in order not to be confused with the "loudness" measured with a ratio scale.

The problem with this categorical loudness scale, however, is the lack of a theoretical model to predict the perceived categorical loudness for a given acoustical input signal. In addition, the relation between the categorical loudness scale and the sone scale (with the related theoretical background) is yet unclear. In this paper, therefore a model for categorical loudness perception is developed which is a modification of the model developed by Zwicker (1960). In addition, first results of the application of this model to loudness restoration in impaired listeners are given.

2 Method

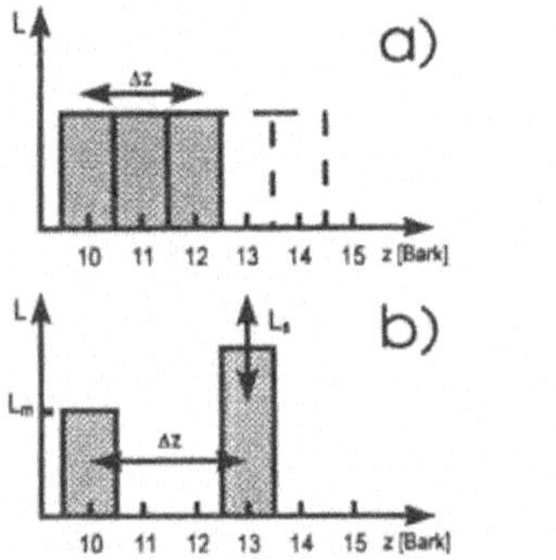

Figure 1: Sketch of the stimuli employed.

In order to study these effects in detail and to derive a loudness model for categorical loudness perception, two different experimental configurations were used: In the first configuration, the categorical loudness of six narrow-band noise samples with a bandwidth of one critical band each was measured for each band individually and for combinations of the bands. The stimuli had a duration of two seconds and a center frequency between 1375 and 2925 Hz, corresponding to the critical band rates z = 10 Bark and z = 15 Bark, respectively. Five combination signals were generated from these six bands by adding up the critical-band noise samples for z = 10-11, 10-12, ... until 10-15 (c.f., Fig. 1a). The signals were presented at 7 levels between 0 dB and 100 dB HL.

The influence of mutual masking of critical bands for loudness estimation was measured with a signal configuration given in Fig. 1b. One of the critical-band noise samples was used as a "masker" with a constant level and an additional critical-band noise sample was used as "probe" signal, exhibiting a predetermined frequency distance to the masker and a randomly selected presentation level which varied in a broad range. The masker was either the signal with the lowest center frequency 1375 Hz (corresponding to z=10) or the narrow-band noise with the highest center frequency of 2925 Hz (i.e., z=15) presented at 40, 60 or 80 dB HL. Each of the remaining four respective critical-band noise signals was used as probe signal. The duration of all stimuli was 2 seconds. They were presented twice to the subjects who had to judge the overall loudness.

Six normal listeners participated voluntarily in this study. They had clinical normal hearing and were trained with different psychophysical experiments.

A personal computer HP Vectra 386 was used to control the experiment. Stimuli were generated off-line using an FFT-approach to filter 3 s of a Gaussian noise at a sampling rate of 44.1 kHz. For each center frequency, a different 2-second section (including 50-ms raised-cosine ramps) of the appropriately filtered noise was converted to analog with a 16-bit D/A converter on an Ariel DSP 32C coprocessor board. The signals were low-pass filtered and adjusted to the appropriate presentation level with a computer-controlled audiometer developed within a German joint research project. The signals were presented monaurally to the subject's ear using DT 48 headphones. The appropriate hearing level correction factor for the headphone employed was used for all center frequencies of the noise bands. The subject was situated in a sound-insulated listening chamber. An Epson hand-held computer EHT-10 with LCD-touch screen was used as a flexible instruction and response box for the subject. On the LCD screen, a bottom-up-triangle was displayed to the subjects as a graphical representation of the perceived loudness. The five main categories were equally-spaced written along the triangle together with the two limiting categories (from bottom to top: inaudible, very soft, soft, intermediate, loud, very loud, too loud). Between each pair of the five main categories, an intermediate category could be selected. Thus, a total number of eleven categories were selectable for the subject. After the presentation of each stimulus of 2 seconds duration, the subjects had an arbitrary amount of time to select the appropriate response category and were allowed to change their judgements within 1 second after their first selection.

3 Results

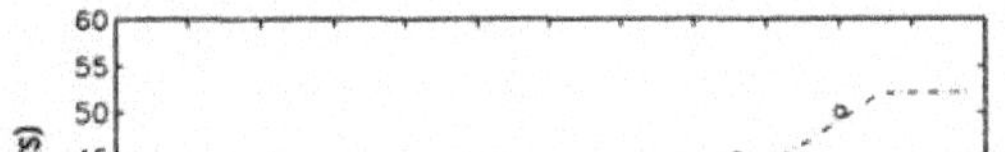

Figure 2. Observed categorical loudness (circles) vs. stimulus level. A straight line is fitted to the data characterized by m, L_{25} and the pedestal.

Fig. 2 gives a typical result of a loudness scaling experiment for one subject employing a critical-band noise at z=10 Bark. The categorical loudness values reported by the subject are transformed to a scale between 0 and 50 linearly. This scale was developed by Heller (1985) who uses ten subdivisions of each of the five main categories. For the individual results of each scaling experiment, a straight line was fitted to the data which is indicated by the dashed-dotted line in Fig. 2. The slope m of the dashed-dotted line and the level L_{25} (i.e., the level corresponding to a categorical loudness of 25 units) are fitted to the data. For small levels of the probe noise, the value of a "pedestal" loudness is fitted to the data, especially in the "masked" conditions. Our approach to fit a straight line as a "target" function for the result of a all loudness scaling experiments in this study was motivated by the simplicity of the fitting procedure as well as the empirical results from a large number of normal and impaired subjects whose data were collected and evaluated in a German joint research project (Kollmeier et al., 1993).

Table 1. Mean (and Std.-Dev.) of the fitted parameters for 6 subjects. The upper part gives the results for single critical-band noise samples. The lower part gives the results for increasing the bandwith (c.f. Fig. 1 a).

Center Frequ. (Hz)	Bandwidth (Bark)	Slope m (units/dB)	Level L_{25} (dB HL)
1375	1	.52 (.10)	61.6 (7.8)
1600	1	.56 (.10)	63.6 (7.1)
1860	1	.55 (.13)	65.4 (7.2)
2160	1	.54 (.19)	68.5 (10.9)
2500	1	.53 (.15)	70.8 (9.1)
2925	1	.53 (.14)	68.4 (5.7)
1480	2	.51 (.06)	57.3 (6.2)
1635	3	.52 (.10)	59.1 (6.4)
1795	4	.52 (.09)	59.1 (5.9)
1985	5	.50 (.09)	58.5 (4.2)
2210	6	.51 (.14)	60.6 (7.0)

Table 1 gives average values and standard deviations of the fitted parameters m and L_{25} averaged across the individually fitted results for six normal subjects. The upper part of Table 1 gives the values obtained for single critical-band noise samples, whereas the lower part of the table gives the value for the combined bands (i.e., configuration sketched in Fig. 1a). Only small variations of L_{25} and m are observed across the frequencies tested. However, the combined noise bands (lower part of Tab1) yield somewhat smaller values of m and considerably lower L_{25}-values than for individual critical-band noise bands at the comparable center frequency. This difference ranges between 4.3 dB and 7.9 dB with increasing bandwidth of the combined signals. It is in qualitative agreement with the data on loudness summation published in the literature (cf. Zwicker & Fastl, 1990, p. 189). Since the combined signals exhibit a slightly shallower slope, the difference in loudness judgement between broad-band and narrow-band signals is more pronounced for small loudness values. A quantitative analysis of the data given here is performed with a modified loudness model after Zwicker (cf., section 4.)

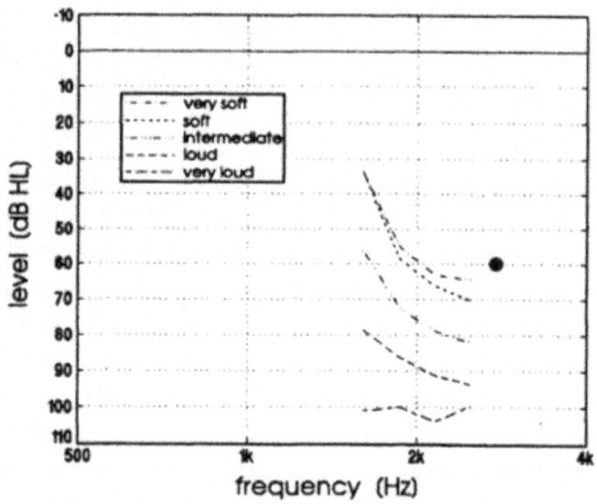

Figure 3. Isoloudness curves for the masked condition (c.f., Fig. 1b) for one subject employing a 2925-Hz masker at 60 dB HL (large dot).

Fig. 3 gives the scaled loudness of a "Probe" critical-band noise for one subject employing a 60-dB masker at 2925 Hz (i.e., z=15 Bark). The level and frequency of the masker is represented by a black dot. The scaling results for different frequencies of the probe signal are represented by isoloudness curves (i.e., curves connecting the stimulus level belonging to the same categorical loudness impression). Obviously, the effect of the masker on the scaled loudness decreases with increasing frequency separation between masker and probe noise band. The slope of the isoloudness curves for small loudness values thus averages to about 8 dB/Bark, whereas a shallower slope of 4 dB/Bark was obtained for the case of a low-frequency masker (z= 10 Bark) and a high-frequency probe noise band. These slopes are considerably shallower than the slopes of about 25 dB/Bark usually connected with downward spread of masking and 10 dB/Bark for upward spread of masking. Note, however, that the slopes decrease with increasing distance from the masked threshold and even vanish at the highest probe levels employed.

Another important effect relates to the "pedestal" categorical loudness values in the "masked" conditions for small "probe" levels: The observed loudness deviates substantially from the "expected" values from the conditions without masking. Table 2 gives for each masker condition employed the expected and observed average categorical loudness value in units. The highest deviations occur for a high masker level and the high-frequency masker. An explanation for this effect is the tendency of the subjects to match the predefined categorical scale with the dynamic range of the stimuli actually presented within a measurement block. Thus, the average categorical loudness of a constant stimulus is underestimated in this configuration and the range of the additional noise is overestimated. This effect clearly demonstrates the limits of the loudness scaling method in estimating the "absolute" subjective loudness.

Table 2. Expected and observed pedestal loudness for the six "masked" conditions.

Masker		Loudness pedestal (units)	
Frequency (Hz)	Level (dB HL)	expected	observed
1375	40	14.6	13.1
1375	60	25.0	20.6
1375	80	35.5	32.5
2925	40	11.4	11.0
2925	60	22.0	16.4
2925	80	32.7	27.3

4 Development of a categorical loudness model

A well-established model to predict the loudness of stimuli configurations similar to those employed in this study is the model by Zwicker (1960) which is the basis for the ISO 532 B. This model is based on a ratio scale, i.e., the loudness of two different signals is assessd by the subject by associating it with a ratio of numerals.The loudness of a 1-kHz sinusoid at 40 dB SPL is defined to be 1 sone. To calculate the loudness of an arbitrary stationary acoustical signal, the following steps are performed:

- A spectral analysis is performed where the respective energy in each critical band is calculated after a correction of the outer ear and middle ear transfer function.
- The spectral energy distribution is converted into an excitation pattern by taking into account the average absolute threshold of normal listeners and by accounting for upward and downward spread of masking by including ramps with a slope of about 25 dB/Bark towards lower frequencies and -10 dB/Bark towards high frequencies.
- The loudness in sone is calculated with a power law with an exponent of 0.3. This exponent is slightly increased for low input levels. Based on these empirical data the excitation level in each critical band is converted into specific loudness.
- The total loudness is calculated as the sum of the specific loudness integrated across all critical bands.
- A time-dependent version of the model was developed by Zwicker (1977). The temporal smoothing of the time-dependent total loudness is performed in a way which approximates the integration properties and the forward masking properties of the ear.

The loudness model as described above was implemented off-line. It was applied to each of the stimuli configurations and presentation levels employed in this study. Fig. 4 gives the resulting scatter plot of the computed loudness in sone plotted on the x-axis versus the empirical categorical loudness value (in categorical units) given on the y-axis. For each experimental condition, the parameter L_{25} and m fitted to each listener's data were averaged across subjects. The loudness growth functions employing these averaged parameters for each stimulus configruation were sampled at equal level steps. The results for the critical-band noise samples are given as trapezoids and the results with increasing bandwidth (c. f., Fig. 1a) are given as crosses. The computed loudness is given as 20 log(sone). For small stimulus levels, the empirical loudness is restricted to a small range between 0 and 5 units and hence varies less than the predicted loudness. Hence, the corresponding measurement points at low stimulus levels are generally not very well represented by the straight lines fitted to the data. Despite this discrepancy, the relation between the categorical loudness and the logarithm of the computed loudness is very well represented by one straight line. In particular, all different measurement configurations and bandwidths produce approximately the same relation between the computed and the observed loudness. The deviations between the curves with different center frequencies of the single noise bands are only about three categorical loudness units which corresponds to a level variation of about 6 dB.

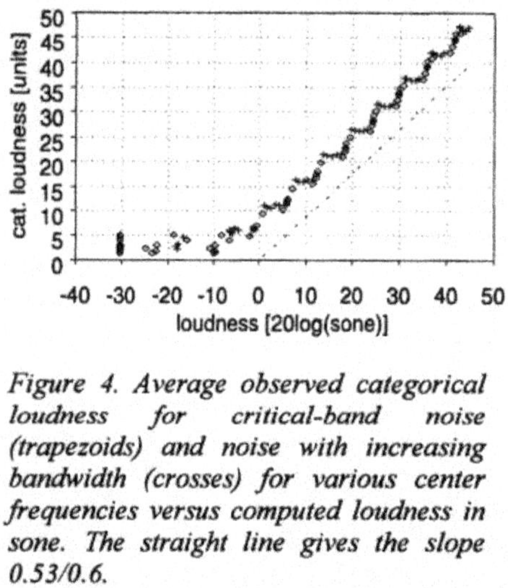

Figure 4. Average observed categorical loudness for critical-band noise (trapezoids) and noise with increasing bandwidth (crosses) for various center frequencies versus computed loudness in sone. The straight line gives the slope 0.53/0.6.

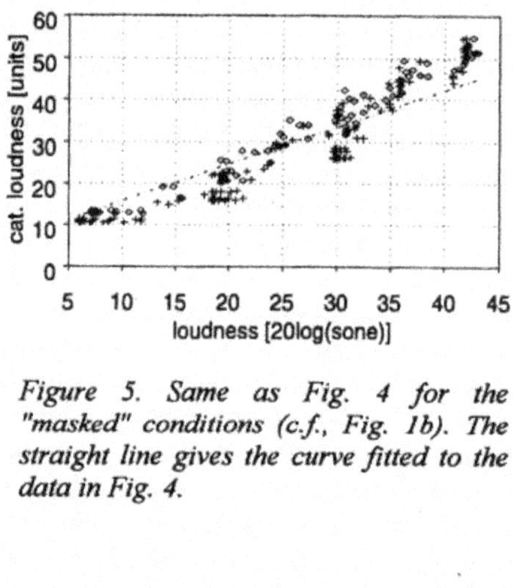

Figure 5. Same as Fig. 4 for the "masked" conditions (c.f., Fig. 1b). The straight line gives the curve fitted to the data in Fig. 4.

The exact linear relation between the observed and predicted loudness is due to the power law of the computed loudness in sone and the assumed linear increase of categorical loudness with stimulus level. If we assume an exponent of 0.3 for the power law and an average slope of the best fitted straight line in Fig. 4 with 0.53, then the following relation between the computed loudness N, the categorical loudness KU, and the sound intensity I (with I_0 being the absolute hearing threshold) applies:

$$N \sim (I/I_0)^{0.3}, \quad KU \sim 0.53 \times 10 \log (I/I_0) \tag{1}$$

By eliminating the intensity I/I_0 from both equations, the following relation between N and KU is obtained:

$$KU = 0.53/0.6 \times 20 \log(N) + \text{const.} \tag{2}$$

This linear relation is plotted as dashed line in Fig. 4 for const=0, wheras const=7 provides the best fit to the data.

The equivalence of observation and prediction across different narrowband stimuli (trapezoids in Fig 4) does not neccessarily coincide with the results from the bandwidth-increasing experiment. The crosses in Fig. 4 give the comparison between the observed categorical loudness values and the computed loudness values predicted by the Zwicker model. Obviously, the data exhibit the same slope as for the critical-band noise samples. However, they are shifted towards somewhat higher categorical loudness values by about two categorical units which corresponds to about 4 dB. This effect is small in relation to the comparatively large effect stimulus bandwidth on the fitted parameters m and L_{25} (c.f., Tab. 1). Thus, the model appears to describe the effect of bandwidth correctly within the limits of measurement accuracy.

Fig. 5 gives the results for the "masked" condition both for the low-frequency masker at 1375 Hz (trapezoids) and the high-frequency masker at 2925 Hz (crosses).The average relation between categorical loudness and loudness in sone derived above (c.f., Eq. 2) is given as a dashed-dotted line. Obviously, the data in Fig. 5 deviate more from this "predicted" relation in sone than for the data in Fig. 4. In addition, the average slope of the data in Fig. 5 is steeper than the slope derived from Fig. 4. Both effects can be explained by the subject's bias in estimating the constant categorical loudness of the "masker" while being instructed to judge the total loudness of the combination of probe and masker. If the probe is inaudible in the presence of the masker, the loudness of the masker is consistently underestimated in comparison with the masker-alone scaling experiment. This effect can explain the deviation from the expected straight line in Fig. 5 at small loudness values. For higher loudness values, however, the loudness model appears to overestimate the mutual masking effect of probe and masker, since the observed categorical loudness values are considerably higher than expected from Fig. 4. However, a precise estimate of the amount of mutual masking involved in loudness judgements can not be given on the basis of our data.

Similar deviations between predicted and observed loudness values can also be observed when employing the high-frequency-masker (i.e., crosses in Fig. 5). The largest deviations from the expected straight line are observed for the highest masker level of 80dB (right-hand side of Fig. 5), where large variability occur across different frequency separations between masker and signal. However, this effect might at least partially be caused by the subjects' variability and bias in assessing the total loudness of the complete stimulus rather than certain components of the stimulus.

5 Discussion

For the stationary signals employed in our study, the empirical categorical loudness and the loudness model after Zwicker both yield a measure of the perceived loudness which appears to be consistent across a considerable variety of signal configurations. Thus, a simple transformation between both measures of perceived loudness was derived. The observed deviations from this relation can be explained as follows: For very small sensation levels, the loudness scaling procedure restricts the subject's choice. Hence, the results do not represent the actual loudness impression and, in addition, do not coincide with the Zwicker model. Additional deviations for both small and large sensation levels may be due to one of the following two effects:

1) In the "masked" condition, the subject did not give a consistent scaling impression for the "masker" which was always presented at the same sensation level. Obviously, they had difficulties to judge the overall loudness of the complete stimulus and underestimated the loudness of the masker if the masked signal was very soft. This effect relates to the "context effect" known from loudness scaling experiments (Kollmeier et al., 1993), i.e., the subject's tendency to match the range of the available loudness scale into the dynamic range of the stimuli presented. This effect yields steeper loudness growth functions if the range of stimulus levels is reduced.

2) The limited coincidence between the empirical categorical loudness and the calculated loudness after Zwicker may also be due to an inadequate model. In particular, the model derives its description of the additivity of loudness in different frequency bands on the spread of masking across frequency bands. However, masking relates to the loss of audibility of one spectral component in the presence of another component, whereas loudness summation typically takes place if both components are both audible. Thus, the interaction between adjacent spectral bands during the loudness summation process might deviate from the Zwicker model.

Overall, however, the deviations between the loudness model and the observed loudness are comparatively small. Thus, the categorical loudness can be predicted from the loudness model using Eq.2 with an average error of about 2.5 scaling units which corresponds to 5 dB. This deviation is small in comparison with the intraindividual reproducibility of loudness scaling experiments.The good correspondence between both measures of the perceived loudness does not infer that both loudness scales are identical. While the loudness in sone after Zwicker is measured on a ratio scale with an infinite possible values, the categorical scale only encompasses a very limited set of values. This leads to the above-mentioned effect that the categorical loudness does not yield a high variability at low stimulus levels. A satisfactory correspondence between both scales can be achieved by a linear interpolation between the obtained categorical loudness values.

For practical purposes in clinical audiology as well as for using the loudness model in a digital hearing aid (see below), an extention of the experiments described here to sensorineurally hearing-impaired listeners is desirable. First results indicate that a satisfactory agreement between loudness scaling data and a loudness model can be found if the audiogram, the increased critical band filters and the increased slope of loudness growth in the individual impaired listener is accounted for (Launer et al., 1994). As already pointed out in the introduction, the loudness scaling method appears to be a simple, robust and reliable method especially adapted for native subjects without extensive training. Thus it is suited well for the purposes of clinical audiology and hearing aid fitting. This is particularly true if this method is supplemented by a theoretical model to predict its outcome for a given stimulus.

6 Application to a digital hearing aid

The principal problem for fitting hearing aids to impaired listeners is to match the loudness sensation of the individual impaired listener for a given input acoustical signal with the loudness sensation of a normal listener. Although this goal has been tried to achieve with different methods to prescribe the frequency gain in hearing aids (see working group on communication aids, 1991, for a review), until now no satisfactory rule has been established for the input-level and frequency-dependent gain of an "ideal" hearing aid. The modified loudness model derived so far seems to be a good basis for such a goal. Therefore, it was incorporated in a digital, binaural hearing aid that tries to compensate for the "recruitment" phenomenon, i.e., the distorted loudness perception for sensorineurally hearing-impaired patients. Since the details of this approach are described elsewhere (Hohmann, 1993), only a short overview of this approach and the first results are reported here.

A loudness scaling procedure employing narrow-band noise stimuli is typically performed at different center frequency with each individual impaired subject in order to assess the "effective" frequency-dependent hearing loss and the recruitment phenomenon. Thus, for each narrow-band noise, the appropriate gain factor for restoring the impaired listener's loudness impression can be derived from comparing the scaling curves of the impaired listener with the average curve of normal listeners. This principle is used in multiband dynamic compression algorithm where the gain in each frequency band is derived independently from the adjacent bands. For broad band input signals (such as speech), however, this procedure yields a wrong total gain for the impaired listener, since it does not account for the mutual masking and loudness summation of adjacent frequency bands. Thus, multiband dynamic compression algorithms usually do not provide the correct gain for speech over a wide range of input levels and frequency spectra even if their narrow-band gain is adjusted correctly.

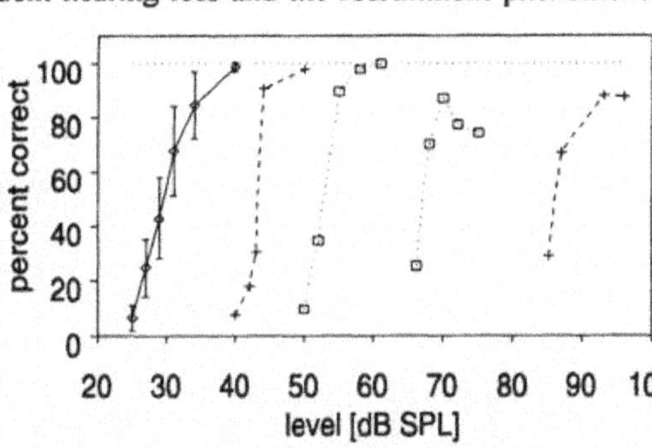

Figure 6. Percent sentence intelligibility vs. speech level for normal listeners (diamonds) and two sensorineurally impaired listeners without hearing aid (curves to the right) and with a simulated loudness compensating aid (curves in the middle).

To compensate for this effect and to improve the performance of multiband dynamic compression algorithms, a loudness-model-based multiband dynamic compression algorithm was developed and implemented in real time which performs the following operations: First, the critical-band spectrum is analysed at each time frame to yield the input level within each frequency band. Then, the amount of mutual interaction between adjacent bands is determined using a loudness model. Further, the "reduced" input level is calculated for each frequency band that correspond to that fraction of the partial loudness in the respective band which is due to the stimulus energy within this band. If a band is totally masked by adjacent bands, the reduced level is set to zero, whereas no change in the input level is performed if the band under consideration is not even partially masked by adjacent bands. Subsequently, these "reduced" input levels are used as input to the critical-band-specific gain tables which are derived for each individual impaired listener by the loudness scaling data at different frequencies. This procedure guarantees that a correct gain is obtained both for narrow-band signals and for broad-band signals. In addition, the procedure yields no spectral smearing of the input signal's spectral shape. A digital hearing aid operating on a binaural input and providing a binaural output in real time was simulated with a system using three DSP 32C signal processors in a personal computer (cf., Kollmeier et al., 1993).

Fig. 6 shows speech intelligibility results in quiet using a german sentence test for two sensorineurally impaired listeners. The leftmost curve denotes the intelligibility performance as a function of speech level for six normal listeners, whereas the two curves to the right denote the performance-intensity curves for two impaired listeners without amplification and without any hearing aid. The curves in the middle denote the aided condition for the same impaired listeners. Obviously, the overall gain of the speech was not quite correct. This effect is due to the comparatively poor accuracy of the loudness scaling method for small loudness values. Unfortunately, this aspect of the scaling data is important for selecting the correct gain for speech understanding in quiet. However, the most striking effect of the algorithm is its ability to increase the maximum performance of the two impaired listeners from 90 % (without aid) back to 100 %. Obviously, the algorithm is capable of compensating the "distortion component" of the hearing loss which is due to the distorted internal signal representation even if the signal is amplified enough to be audible. Thus, the algorithm seems to restore the impaired listener's speech perception in quiet in a rather impressive way. This supports the general approach of applying psychoacoustic knowledge to speech processing techniques.

7 Acknowledgement

Work supported by BMFT - PT FDG. Thanks to the members of the Medical Physics group for their contributions to this paper and to A. Sievers and K. Bramstedt for typing and styling the manuscript.

8 References

Allen, J.B., Hall, J.L., and Jeng, P.S. (1990) Loudness growth in 1/2-octave bands (LGOB) - A procedure for the assessment of loudness. J. Acoust. Soc. Am. 88, 745-753.

Hellbrück, J. and Moser, L.M. (1985) Hörgeräte-Audiometrie: Ein computerunterstütztes psychologisches Verfahren zur Hörgeräteanpassung. Psychol. Beiträge 27, 494-508.

Heller, O. (1991). Oriented category scaling of loudness and speech audiometric validation. In: Schick, A. et al. (eds.), Contributions to Psychological Acoustics, BIS Oldenburg, Germany.

Hohmann, V. (1993). Dynamikkompression für Hörgeräte - Psychoakustische Grundlagen und Algorithmen. VDI Reihe 17 Nr. 93. Düsseldorf:VDI-Verlag 1993.

Kollmeier, B. et al. (1993) Erprobung und Validisierung von sprachaudiometrischen und anderen Testverfahren für die klinische Audiometrie. BMFT-Zwischenbericht, Universität Göttingen.

Launer, S., Hohmann, V., Kollmeier, B. (1994) Experimente und Modellvorstellungen zur Lautstärkeskalierung bei Schwerhörenden. In: Fortschritte der Akustik, DAGA '94, Bad Honeff.

Pascoe, D.P. (1988) Clinical measurements of the auditory dynamic range and their relation to formulas for hearing aid gain. In: Jensen, J.H. (ed.). Hearing Aid fitting, 13th Danavox Symposium.

Stevens, S.S. (1956) The Direct Estimation of Sensory Magnitudes - Loudness. Am. J. Psychology 69, 1-25.

Working Group on Communication Aids for the Hearing Impaired (1991) Speech-perception aids for hearing-impaired people: Current status and needed research. J. Acoust. Soc. Am. 90, 637-685

Zwicker, E. (1960) Ein Verfahren zur Berechnung der Lautstärke. Acustica 10, 304-308.

Zwicker, E. (1977) Procedure for calculating loudness of temporally variable sounds. J. Acoust. Soc. Am. 62, 675-682.

Zwicker, E., Fastl, H. (1990) Psychoacoustics - Facts and Models, Springer Verlag, Berlin

Comment by M. Florentine

I was surprised to the poor fit between the calculated loudness and the categorical loudness for the impaired listeners. Florentine and Zwicker (1979) showed that Zwicker's model of loudness summation accounts well for loudness summation in impaired listeners when it is modified to take into account increased upward spread of masking, widened critical bands, and recruitment. Did you include these modifications in your calculations?

Florentine, M. and Zwicker, E. (1979): A model of loudness summation applied to listeners with noise-induced hearing loss. Hearing Research 1, 121-132

Reply

In our preliminary attempts to fit impaired patient's categorical loudness with a modified loudness model (Launer, S., Hohmann, V., Kollmeier, B. (1994): Experimente und Modellvorstellungen zur Lautheitsskalierung bei Schwerhörigen, in: Fortschritte der Akustik, DAGA'94 (in press)), at low levels most effects can be explained with the modifications of the loudness model introduced by Florentine and Zwicker (1979). At high levels, however, substantial deviations between model predictions and scaled loudness occur both for narrow-band and broadband signals. These deviations did not show up in the Florentine and Zwicker paper where only the difference between narrowband and broadband data was predicted. In addition, the reduced additivity of loudness in adjacent frequency bands can not be accounted for correctly. To predict both effects in a better way, an increased loudness growth exponent in impaired listeners should be considered.

Comment by J.W. Horst

The data in figure 6 are very promising in that they restore the maximum speech discrimination to (near) 100 %.

The shift of the speech discrimination vs. level curves of the subjects when using the compensating aid is reminiscent of the observation in audiological practice that patients often do not adjust their volume control so that they restore normal absolute threshold. Rather they usually have their speech discrimination curves shifted to higher levels than the normal curve.

Finally, it would be interesting to know about the performance under more severe conditions. Have you measured speech levels (e.g. 70 and 80 dB) and in the case of interfering noise?

Reply

The shift of the speech discrimination vs. level curve is not affected by the patient's volume control since the output level of the hearing aid processing scheme is completely determined by the input signal the individual patient's narrow-band loudness scaling data. For input levels above 60 dB, the compression characteristic of the algorithm will both limit the maximum output level and optimize the respective frequency shaping of the input spectrum. Hence, we do not expect a decrease in speech intelligibility with increasing input level. A comparison of the current algorithm with "optimum" linear frequency shaping (Hohmann and Kollmeier, Proc. ICSLP'94, in press) indicate a higher subjective quality rating for speech and music and an increased speech intelligibility in noise at 45 dB SPL input level. At 65 dB input level, however, no significant improvement was obtained by the algorithm. In all conditions tested, the current algorithm performed better than a multiband dynamic compressor with independent bands.

Comment by B. Scharf

Our experience with subjects from universities has been that most listeners do not simply rank order loudness. They assign numbers on a ratio scale. If most subjects did no more than rank order, the sone scale would be a great deal flatter than it is. Although subjects from a clinical setting are more apt to rank order, that can often be avoided by giving them brief practice in judging perceived line length.

I also point out that we seldom ask subjects to estimate the loudness of one sound relative to another, standard sound. The most valid procedure is to ask subjects to match number magnitude to loudness, without attempting to achieve consistency among successive judgments.

Reply

Although a better resolution of our procedure especially at low levels is desirable, the conditions "subjects from universities" and "brief practice" unfortunately are rarely met in practice, e.g., when fitting hearing aids to patients. Heller (1991) found the same average exponents as Stevens (i.e., no flattening of the sone scale) if the random computer trials preserve the rank order of the stimuli and the total range of responses. He argues that magnitude estimations both with and without a reference stimulus ("anchor") require a similar mathematical operation that most subjects are not able to perform. Hellbrück ("Hören - Physiologie, Psychologie und Pathologie", Hogrefe, 1993) compared magnitude estimation and categorical scaling and found a logarithmic relation similar to the one found here. Comparisons between categorical scaling and judgements of perceived line length were performed by Elberling (Danavox Symposium, 1993) and did not show substantial differences between the procedures

Pitch perception

Pitch of the Zwicker-tone and masking patterns

H. Fastl and G. Krump

Institute of Man-Machine-Communication, Technical University München
Arcisstraße 21, D-80333 München, Germany

1 Introduction

When sounds with a spectral gap are switched off, a short faint tone may be audible with a pitch corresponding to the frequency region of the spectral gap. This phenomenon was described by Zwicker (1964) as "negative afterimage" in hearing, while Lummis and Guttman (1972) proposed to call it in honor of its discoverer a Zwicker-tone. Neelen (1967) studied the Zwicker-tone of incomplete line spectra by filtering the spectra produced by DC-pulses. With the advent of digital signal synthesis, experiments on the Zwicker-tone could be performed with a large variety of spectral patterns (Fastl 1986, 1989, Zwicker and Fastl 1990). In addition, by varying the phase spectrum for constant amplitude spectrum, effects of the temporal envelope on the Zwicker-tone were studied (Krump 1992).

In this paper, data on the existence region and the bandwidth necessary to produce a Zwicker-tone are described. The dependence of the Zwicker-tone on the depth of the spectral gap as well as the level of the Zwicker-tone-exciter (ZTE) are given. A new effect (Krump 1994) is described: Not only a spectral gap, but also a spectral enhancement can elicit a Zwicker-tone.

The pitch of the Zwicker-tone can be described by means of the Zwicker-tone-exciter's masking pattern (Fastl 1989, Fig. 8). This model is considerably extended (Krump 1993a) and modified that it accounts also for the pitch of the Zwicker-tone produced by spectral enhancement.

Finally results from a pilot study (Kössl 1993) on possible physiological correlates of the Zwicker-tone are discussed.

2 Experiments

Six subjects with normal hearing ability (age 26... 47 years) took part in the experiments. Subjects were seated in a sound proof booth. Sounds were presented monaurally via an electrodynamic earphone (Beyer DT 48) with freefield equalizer (Zwicker and Fastl 1990, p.7).

The pitch of the Zwicker-tone was measured as follows: The subject had command of a switch with three positions. In position 1, the Zwicker-tone-exciter (ZTE) was presented for 5... 10 seconds. In position 2, the ZTE was switched off abruptly, and usually the Zwicker-tone was audible for 1... 3 sec. In position 3, a pure tone at approximately 10 dB SL was presented. The task of the subject was to adjust the frequency of this tone in such a way that its pitch matched the pitch of the Zwicker-tone. The frequency of the comparison tone was adjusted by the subject via a helical 10-turns potentiometer connected to a VCO. The subject had no information about the adjusted frequency and was free to operate the switch several times until a final pitch match was reached.

Within a session, each Zwicker-tone-exciter was presented four times in random order. From the resulting four data points, for each subject an individual median was calculated. These medians are displayed in the figures by different symbols for different subjects. The asterisks in all figures illustrate calculated pitch values of the Zwicker-tone, derived from masking patterns.

If not specified otherwise, the Zwicker-tone-exciters are computer generated harmonic line spectra with 16 kHz bandwidth, 1 Hz line spacing, constant amplitude, and random phase of the spectral lines.

3 Results and discussion

3.1 Pitch range of Zwicker-tones

To elicit a well defined Zwicker-tone, Zwicker-tone-exciters with a spectrum level around 0 dB (overall level around 40 dB) and a gap width of 2.5 Bark are preferred (Zwicker 1964, Fastl 1989, Krump 1993a). With this configuration, a Zwicker-tone can be produced by line spectra with a spectral gap in a region between about 8.5 Bark (1000 Hz) and 19.5 Bark (6000 Hz). In Figure 1 this region is hatched from upper left to lower right. The solid curve in Figure 1 represents the threshold of hearing for comparison. The area hatched from lower left to upper right illustrates the region between about 13 Bark (2000 Hz) to 19 Bark (5300 Hz) in which Zwicker-tones can be produced by sounds with

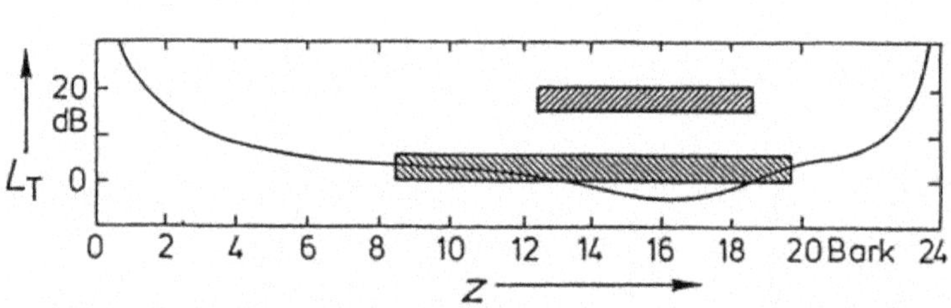

Figure 1. Pitch range of Zwicker tones. Solid line: Threshold of hearing; level L_T of just audible test tone. Area hatched from upper left to lower right: Range of Zwicker-tones elicited by line spectra at 0 dB spectrum level with 1 Hz line spacing and spectral gaps of 2.5 Bark width. Area hatched from lower left to upper right: Range of Zwicker-tones elicited by line spectra as above, however without spectral gap but with additional pure tone at 60 dB.

a spectral enhancement. In this case, a broadband line spectrum with 1 Hz line spacing and 0 dB spectrum level (about 40 dB overall level) is combined with a pure tone at 60 dB (Krump 1993a, 1994). The results displayed in Figure 1 suggest that Zwicker-tones occur predominantly in a region, in which the hearing system is most sensitive.

3.2 Bandwidth of Zwicker-tone-exciter

In previous studies (Fastl 1989, Zwicker and Fastl 1990) it was shown that a minimal bandwidth of the spectral gap is necessary to produce a Zwicker-tone. In turn, the minimal bandwidth of bands flanking a spectral gap necessary for the production of a Zwicker-tone was studied (Krump 1993b). Results are displayed in Figure 2. The total bandwidth Δz_{ZTE} of the Zwicker-tone-exciter is given as a function of the critical-band rate z. The width of the spectral gap of 2.5 Bark centered around 17 Bark was kept constant. The shaded areas illustrate the spectral distributions of the Zwicker-tone-exciters. Open symbols represent pitch matches by individual subjects, asterisks indicate calculated values of the Zwicker-tone's pitch.

The data displayed in Figure 2 show that a total bandwidth of at least 4 Bark (2 Bark at each side of the spectral gap) of the Zwicker-tone-exciter is necessary to produce a Zwicker-tone for all six subjects. With 2 Bark bandwidth of the Zwicker-tone-exciter, four subjects can hear a Zwicker-tone, with 1 Bark bandwidth, however, only one subject. In line with data from the literature (Fastl 1989), for 0 dB spectrum level of the Zwicker-tone-exciter, the Zwicker-tone lies approximately 1 Bark above the lower edge of the spectral gap. The values calculated on the basis of masking patterns (asterisks) are in line with the pitch matches for the Zwicker-tones (open symbols).

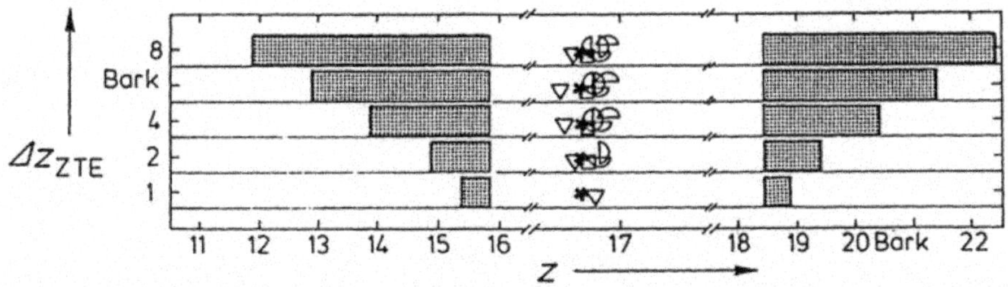

Figure 2. Zwicker-tones for different bandwidths of the Zwicker-tone-exciter. Open symbols: Individual pitch matches. Asterisks: Pitch values derived from masking patterns. Shaded areas: Illustration of spectral distributions of Zwicker-tone-exciters with 0 dB spectrum level.

3.3 Level and depth of spectral gap

Results displayed in Figure 3 show the dependence of the pitch z_{ZT} of the Zwicker-tone on the level L_{ZTE} of the Zwicker-tone-exciter as well as the depth ΔL of the spectral gap. The range of pitch matches is indicated by the shaded areas, the asterisks denote pitches derived from masking patterns. The dark areas illustrate the region of the spectral gap.

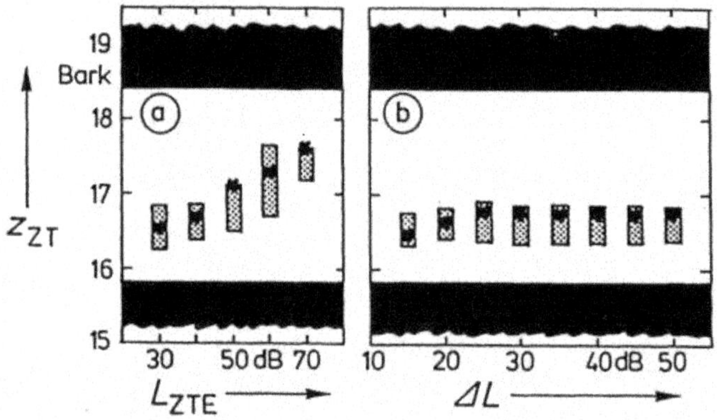

Figure 3. Pitch of the Zwicker-tone as a function of the Zwicker-tone-exciter's level L_{ZTE} or the depth of its spectral gap ΔL. Shaded areas: Range of pitch matches. Asterisks: Pitch values derived from masking patterns. Dark areas: Illustration of spectral gap. (a) depth of spectral gap ΔL = 50 dB. (b) overall level L_{ZTE} = 40 dB.

Data displayed in Figure 3a suggest in line with data from the literature (e.g. Zwicker 1964, Fastl 1989, Krump 1990) that the pitch of the Zwicker-tone increases with increasing level of the Zwicker-tone-exciter. There is good agreement between subjectively measured data (shaded areas) and data derived from masking patterns (asterisks). Most distinct Zwicker-tones are obtained for overall levels around 40 dB (spectrum level around 0 dB).

Results displayed in Figure 3b show that the depth ΔL of the spectral gap has to be at least 15 dB to produce a Zwicker-tone. The distinctness of the Zwicker-tone increases with increasing depth of the gap up to ΔL = 30 dB (Krump 1993a). Again, there is good agreement between subjectively measured and predicted pitches of the Zwicker-tone.

3.4 Spectral enhancement

Not only spectral gaps, but also spectral enhancements can produce a Zwicker-tone (Krump 1993a, 1994). Figure 4 shows results for the combination of broadband line spectra plus a pure tone. The shaded areas indicate the range of subjective pitch matches, the asterisks denote pitch values derived from masking patterns. Hatched areas illustrate broadband line spectra and circles pure tones at 15.6 Bark (3000 Hz).

The results displayed in Figure 4a suggest that a broadband line spectrum with 1 Hz line spacing and a spectrum level of -2 dB plus a pure tone with a level of 50... 80 dB can elicit a Zwicker-tone, which lies below the pure tone. With increasing level of the pure tone there seems to occur a slight shift of the Zwicker-tone towards lower pitches.

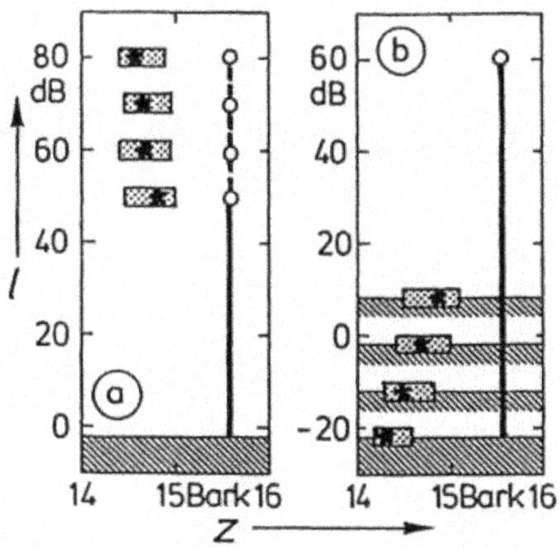

Figure 4. Zwicker-tones elicited by spectral enhancements. Shaded areas: Range of subjectively evaluated Zwicker-tones. Asterisks: Pitch of the Zwicker-tones derived from masking patterns. Hatched areas: Illustration of broadband line spectra. Circles: Illustration of pure tones added to the broadband line spectra. (a) Spectrum level of broadband line spectrum fixed. (b) Level of pure tone fixed.

Figure 4b shows the results obtained if the level of the pure tone is kept constant at 60 dB and the spectrum level l of the broadband line spectrum varied between -22 dB and +8 dB. With increasing level of the broadband line spectrum, the pitch of the Zwicker-tone increases significantly.

Again, there is good agreement between subjectively evaluated data (shaded areas) and data predicted from the Zwicker-tone-exciter's masking pattern (asterisks).

3.5 Zwicker-tone and masking patterns

The description of hearing sensations on the basis of masking patterns has proven very effective (e.g. Zwicker and Feldtkeller 1967, Fastl 1982, Zwicker and Fastl 1990). This concept can also be applied to describe the pitch of Zwicker-tones (Zwicker 1964, Fastl 1989, Krump 1993a). An elaborated model (Krump 1993a) can be illustrated by means of data displayed in Figure 5. The main feature of the model is that the pitch of the Zwicker-tone can be predicted on the basis of the Zwicker-tone-exciter's masking pattern.

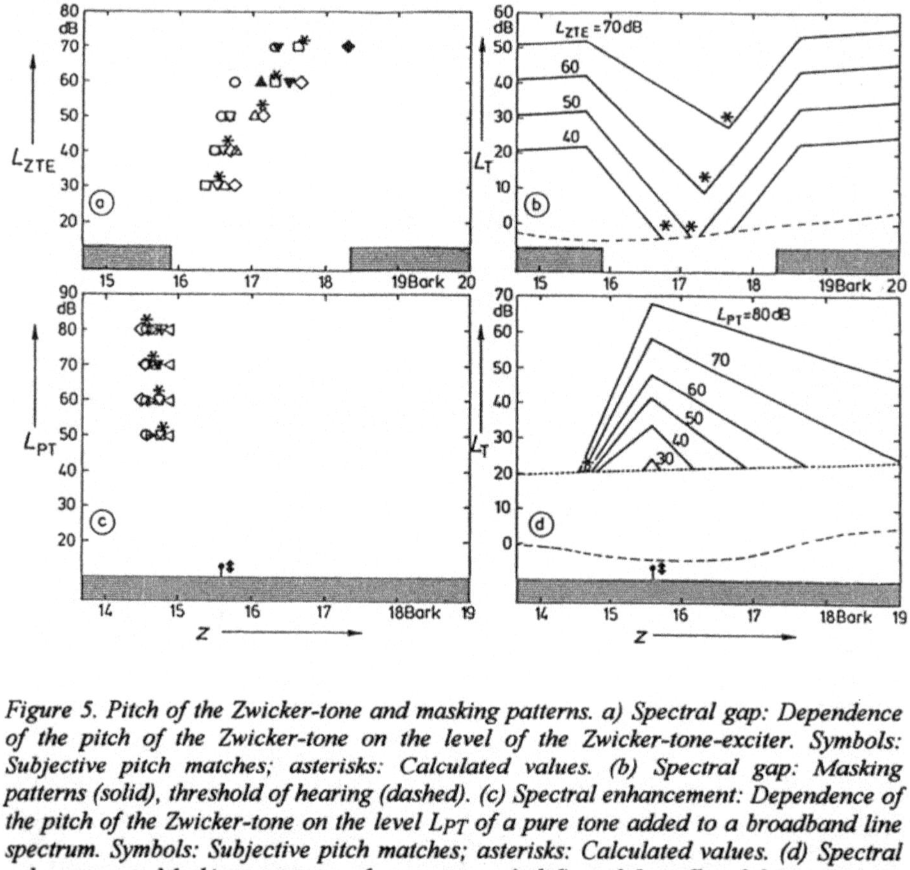

Figure 5. Pitch of the Zwicker-tone and masking patterns. a) Spectral gap: Dependence of the pitch of the Zwicker-tone on the level of the Zwicker-tone-exciter. Symbols: Subjective pitch matches; asterisks: Calculated values. (b) Spectral gap: Masking patterns (solid), threshold of hearing (dashed). (c) Spectral enhancement: Dependence of the pitch of the Zwicker-tone on the level L_{PT} of a pure tone added to a broadband line spectrum. Symbols: Subjective pitch matches; asterisks: Calculated values. (d) Spectral enhancement: Masking patterns of pure tones (solid) and broadband line spectrum (dotted). Dashed: Threshold of hearing. Shaded areas and double arrows: Illustrations of spectral distributions.

As an example Figure 5b shows masking patterns for a broadband line spectrum with a spectral gap at different levels L_{ZTE} of the Zwicker-tone-exciter. The solid lines clearly show that with increasing L_{ZTE} the steepness of the masking pattern at the lower edge of the gap decreases, whereas the steepness of the slope at the upper edge remains constant. Hence, with decreasing L_{ZTE} the minimum of the masking pattern is shifted towards lower critical-band rate z. The following hypothesis is put forward (Krump

1993a): The pitch of the Zwicker-tone (asterisks) corresponds to the minimum of the masking pattern or to the crossing point of masking pattern and hearing threshold (dashed). The data displayed in Figure 5a suggest that this hypothesis is valid: All calculated values (asterisks) are within the range of Zwicker-tones measured by subjects (symbols).

Data displayed in Figure 5d illustrate the hypothesis for Zwicker-tones elicited by spectral enhancements: The crossing of the lower slope of the masking pattern (solid) of the added pure tone with the masking pattern of the broadband line spectrum (dotted) indicates the pitch of the Zwicker-tone. However, a Zwicker-tone occurs only, if the masking pattern of the additional tone is at least 15 dB above the masking pattern of the broadband line spectrum. Corresponding subjective (symbols) and calculated (asterisks) data displayed in Figure 5c again confirm the hypothesis.

A more detailed description of the relations between the pitch of the Zwicker-tone and the Zwicker-tone-exciter's masking pattern is given in the literature (Krump 1993a, chap. 4). The data shown in Figure 2 to 5 indicate that the pitch of the Zwicker-tone can indeed be predicted on the basis of the correlated masking patterns.

4 Conclusion

The pitch of the Zwicker-tone can be predicted on the basis of the Zwicker-tone-exciter's masking pattern with an accuracy of about 0.3 Bark. If instead of <u>average</u> masking patterns (e.g. Zwicker and Fastl 1990) <u>individual</u> masking patterns are taken as starting point of the calculations, the accuracy of the predictions increases to about 0.15 Bark (Krump 1993a). This means that a useful descriptive model for the pitch of the Zwicker-tone is available.

However, the mechanism underlying the Zwicker-tone phenomenon is still unclear. In particular, a physiological correlate of Zwicker-tones is not yet at hand. Pilot studies in the colliculus inferior of laboratory mamals (Kössl 1993) so far were not successful. Therefore further physiological studies in the cochlear nucleus of mamals are planned.

In addition, psychoacoustic studies on the Zwicker-tone will be continued. Interestingly, the pitch of Zwicker-tones can be described on the basis of spectral features of the Zwicker-tone-exciters, whereas temporal features like envelope fluctuations may influence the quality of the Zwicker-tone. So far it was not possible to elicit Zwicker-tones on the basis of temporal features alone without spectral gaps or spectral enhancements.

5 Acknowledgement

This work was supported by Deutsche Forschungsgemeinschaft, SFB 204 Gehör, München.

6 References

Fastl, H. (1982) Beschreibung dynamischer Hörempfindungen anhand von Mithörschwellen-Mustern. Hochschul-Verlag, Freiburg.

Fastl, H. (1986) Auditory after-images produced by complex tones with a spectral gap. In: Proc. 12. ICA Toronto, Vol.I, B 2-5.

Fastl, H. (1989) Zum Zwicker-Ton bei Linienspektren mit spektralen Lücken. Acustica 67, 177-186.

Kössl, M. (1993) personal communication.

Krump, G. (1990) Zum akustischen Nachton bei Linienspektren. In: Fortschritte der Akustik, DAGA'90, Verl.: DPG-GmbH, Bad Honnef, 767-770.

Krump, G. (1992) Zum Zwicker-Ton bei Linienspektren unterschiedlicher Phasenlagen. In: Fortschritte der Akustik, DAGA'92, Verl.: DPG-GmbH, Bad Honnef, 825-828.

Krump, G. (1993a) Beschreibung des akustischen Nachtones mit Hilfe von Mithörschwellenmustern. Dissertation TU München.

Krump, G. (1993b) Zum Zwicker-Ton bei unterschiedlicher Bandbreite der Anregung. In: Fortschritte der Akustik, DAGA '93, Verl.: DPG-GmbH, Bad Honnef, 808-811.

Krump, G. (1994) Zum Zwicker-Ton bei Linienspektren mit spektraler Überhöhung. In: Fortschritte der Akustik, DAGA'94, Verl.: DPG-GmbH, Bad Honnef.

Lummis, R. C. und Guttman, N. (1972) Exploratory Studies of Zwicker's "Negative Afterimage" in Hearing. J. Acoust. Soc. Amer. 51, 1930-1944.

Neelen, J. J. M. (1967) Auditory Afterimages Produced by Incomplete Line Spectra. IPO Progress Report 2, 37-43.

Zwicker, E. (1964) "Negative Afterimage" in Hearing. J. Acoust. Soc. Am. 36, 2413-2415.

Zwicker, E., and Fastl, H. (1990) Psychoacoustics - Facts and Models. Springer-Verlag, Heidelberg, New York 1990.

Zwicker, E. and Feldtkeller, R. (1967) Das Ohr als Nachrichtenempfänger. 2. erw. Auflage, Hirzel-Verlag, Stuttgart 1967.

Comment by S. Buus

Your description of the Zwicker tone in terms of masking patterns implies that Zwicker tones also should be elicited by high-pass noises. Have you found Zwicker tones elicited by high-pass noise?

Reply

We could not find a Zwicker-tone for high-pass noise. Obviously, a rising slope in the masking pattern has to be preceeded by some "pedestal" excitation as we have it e.g. for a combination of broadband line spectrum plus a pure tone.

Comment by H. Duifhuis

How abruptly do you have to switch off the exciter? A rectangular on-off would optimize relatively broad band offset ringing over several cycles, and this might initiate the percept.

Reply

We have not yet studied the influence of the gating signal systematically. In our experiments we used a switch operated manually.

Comment by E. F. Evans

It is not easy to hear the Zwicker tone unless the parameters of stimulation are optimized.
a) What is the effect of the slope of the noise band cut-off?
b) What is the optimal combination of stimulus parameters to obtain the most salient pitch?

Reply

a) With steeper slopes the Zwicker-tone becomes more salient. While usually almost infinitely steep slopes are used, spectral gaps with slopes of only 24 dB/oct also can elicit Zwicker-tones.

b) As optimal combination we found:

- overall level: 40 dB
- center frequency: 4000 Hz
- width of spectral gap: 2.5 Bark
- depth of spectral gap: at least 30 dB

Comment by B. Scharf

How does the saliency of the Zwicker-tone depend on the duration of the excitation? Does that dependency interact with exciter level?

Reply

When increasing the duration of single exciter impulses from about 800 ms to over 3200 ms, the saliency of the Zwicker-tone also increases nearly independent of exciter level. Interestingly, pulsed exciters with e.g. 10 ms on-time and 10 ms off-time also can produce rather salient Zwicker-tones.

Comment by J.P. Wilson

I have always felt that a transiently evoked SOAE is the most probable explanation for Zwicker tones in view of their tonal nature and low level of optimal stimulus. However I believe Zwicker failed to find evidence of SOAEs as we have ourselves. Do you feel that this explanation can be ruled out?

Reply

Although an interpretation of the Zwicker-tone in terms of SOAEs looks very attractive, we could not measure a physical correlate to the Zwicker-tone in the closed ear canal despite a sensitivity of the setup down to -20 dB (Krump, 1993).

Krump, G. (1993) Beschreibung des akustischen Nachtones mit Hilfe von Mithörschwellenmustern. Dissertation TU München.

Aspects of pitch perception in the ultrasonic range

Sabine Schmidt, Annemarie Preisler and Heinz Sedlmeier

Zoologisches Institut der Universität München
Luisenstraße 14, 80333 München, Germany

1 Introduction

Psychoacoustic experiments reveal two essential aspects of audition in humans: pitch is attributed as a primary sensory quality to almost all auditory signals, and different pitches are perceived in terms of their frequency intervals rather than as absolute magnitudes. Thus, on two levels of abstraction, pitch and pitch intervals sum up the multitude of spectral stimulus characteristics. In comparative investigations with echolocating bats, we addressed the question to what extent these perceptual features reflect common processing mechanisms in mammals.

Echolocating bats rely on acoustical cues as a main source of information about their environment. Their sonar system not only provides information about the location of objects in space, but also on object properties such as their size, shape, and texture (for references, see Schnitzler and Henson, 1980). There is evidence that objects are recognized by the changes in the spectral composition of the echoes (Schmidt, 1992). Pitch and timbre may be the decisive perceptual dimensions in these discriminations. Most bat species use harmonically structured sonar calls, similar to speech vowels in humans, suggesting a comparable significance of pitch formation. Furthermore, as the range of the sonar calls extends to frequencies of more than 100 kHz, comparative studies in bats permit the evaluation of different models of pitch perception in mammals developed for the low frequency hearing range.

Several aspects of pitch perception were studied in the Indian False Vampire, *Megaderma lyra*, in two-alternative, forced-choice behavioural tests (see Fig.1). *M. lyra* emits brief (< 1 ms), slightly downward modulated sonar calls of low intensity (65-80 dB SPL) comprising five harmonics based on a significantly attenuated fundamental between 19 and 26 kHz. The behavioural audiogram is broadly tuned, with thresholds below 0 dB SPL between 16 and 90 kHz (Schmidt et al., 1983).

2 Absolute versus relative pitch

It has been shown in a series of experiments using falling and rising two-tone sequences that *M. lyra* can classify such sequences with respect to both absolute and relative pitch, depending on the training procedure.

In the first experiment (Sedlmeier, 1992a, 1992b), the frequency of one of the pure tones was kept constant at 23 kHz (reference frequency), while the frequency of the other

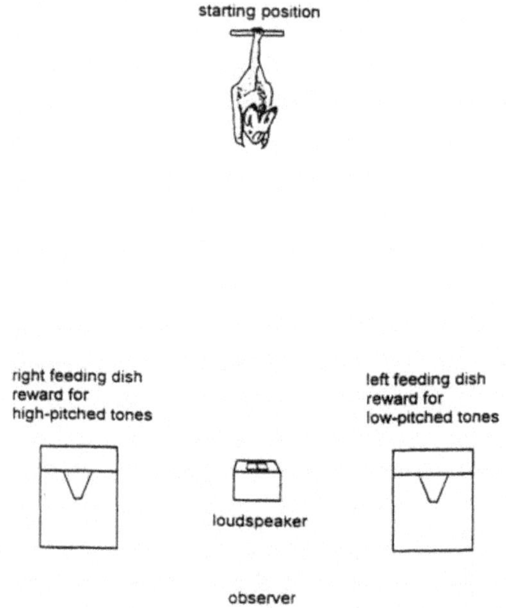

Figure 1: Experimental setup for the pitch perception experiments. In absolute pitch classifications, the bats classified the pitch of tones as higher or lower than a memorized pure tone reference by flying to the right, or left feeding dish, respectively. In relative pitch perception experiments, the right feeding dish was associated with rising, and the left with falling two-tone sequences. Stimuli were presented while the bat was at the starting position. Correct choices were rewarded with mealworms.

tone was varied. When the reference frequency was omitted in later experimental sessions, all five bats tested continued to classify the variable tones as higher or lower than the memorized reference, i.e. according to their absolute pitch. In addition, the bats were able to transfer this behaviour to classify the pitch of complex tones. Absolute pitch discrimination thresholds for pure tones and complex tones comprising four harmonics amounted to about 300 Hz, corresponding to a Weber ratio of 0.013 and thus ranging among the most sensitive values described for mammals (Fay, 1988) other than man.

In our recent experiments to establish relative pitch perception, three *M. lyra* were trained to discriminate tone pairs with a constant frequency ratio of 2:3, and their lower frequencies between 13 and 18 kHz as "rising" or "falling". Then, control experiments were performed in which tone pairs of the same frequency ratio were used retaining the frequency of one tone of the known pairs while extending the other to new frequency ranges. Only one bat developed a concept of "falling" and "rising" without referring to the absolute pitch of the first or second tones of the training pairs. Even in this animal, the maximal transfer region for relative pitch was limited to frequencies of the lower tone between 7.6 and 20.4 kHz.

Thus, *M. lyra* can easily be trained to discriminate absolute pitch with high precision, whereas it is difficult and time consuming to train the bats to rely on relative pitch. A corresponding prevalence of absolute pitch has been reported for other mammals (*Macaca fuscata*: May et al., 1989; albino rats and *Cebus apella*: D'Amato, 1988) and for various songbirds (Hulse and Cynx, 1985). In addition, the transfer regions for relative pitch have a comparable extent in *M. lyra* and the starling (*Sturnus vulgaris*: Hulse et al., 1984; Page et al., 1989). The preference for absolute pitch in echolocating bats may be supported by the necessity to identify prey objects on the basis of complex echo spectra with a defined frequency content. In contrast, absolute pitch perception is found in far less than 1% of adult humans (Bachem, 1955). However, about 50% of the musicians beginning to play an instrument at an age of less than three years are able to perceive absolute pitch (Miyazaki, 1988), which may indicate that they retain an evolutionarily ancient capacity usually suppressed by relative pitch perception in the course of speech acquisition.

3 Virtual versus spectral pitch

In humans, complex tones are known to elicit a pitch perception at their fundamental. As this pitch is perceived regardless of the actual physical presence of the

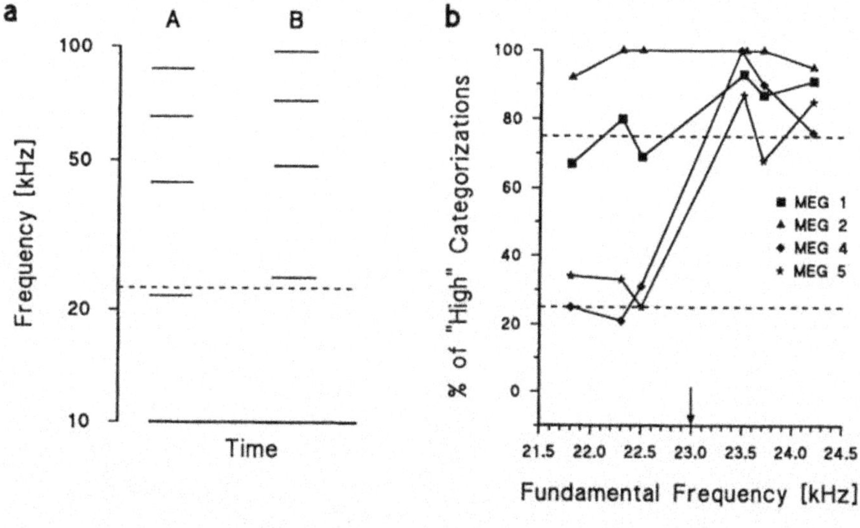

Figure 2: Spontaneous pitch classification for complete complex tones. a. Examples for complex tones used in this experiment comprising four harmonics (level of each component: 60±3 dB SPL) with their fundamental below (A) and above (B) a 23-kHz pure tone reference (dashed line). All harmonics were presented at the same level. b. The performance of four M. lyra (% of "High" Categorizations) is plotted as a function of the fundamental frequency of the complete complex tones. The arrow marks the reference frequency. The dashed lines indicate 25% and 75% "High" categorizations.

fundamental, it is also referred to as virtual pitch. Three experiments addressed the question of whether *M. lyra* also perceives the virtual pitch of its echoes.

In the first experiment (Sedlmeier, 1992a), four bats were initially trained to categorize pure tone pulses as higher or lower than a 23 kHz pure tone memory reference. Then, complete complex tones comprising four harmonics (cf. Fig.2.a) were interspersed with the pure tone pulses with a probability of 25%. All individuals spontaneously classified the complete complex tones as high when all harmonics were above the reference. For ambiguous complex stimuli, with their fundamentals below and their higher harmonics above the reference frequency (i.e. type A in Fig.2.a), two individuals (MEG 1, MEG 2) took into account the spectral pitches of the higher harmonics and classified the complex tones as high. The other two bats (MEG 4, MEG 5) referred to the fundamental pitch of the complex tones and classified the ambiguous stimuli as low (Fig.2.b). These

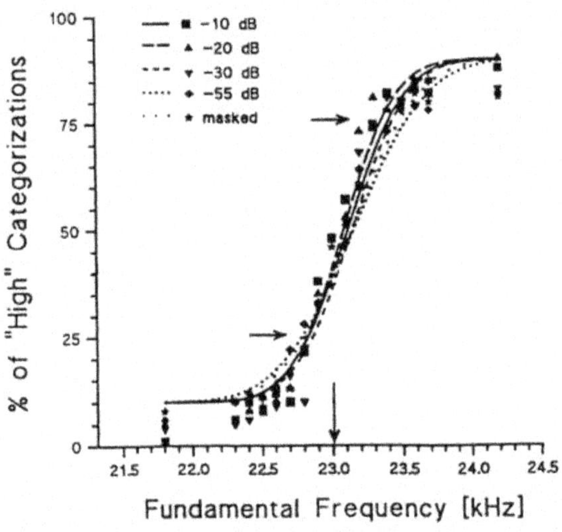

Figure 3: Fundamental pitch perception for complex tones comprising four harmonics with gradually attenuated fundamentals (level at 0 dB attenuation: 60±3 dB SPL). The performance of the bats (% of "High" Categorizations) is plotted as a function of the fundamental frequency of the complex tones. Different symbols characterize the data points obtained for different attenuations of the fundamental relative to the other harmonic components (see insert). In the masked condition, white noise of 30 dB SPL was added to the stimuli with fundamentals attenuated by 55 dB. Each data point represents the mean performance of five individuals. Please note the similar psychometric functions describing the performance at different attenuations of the fundamental.

results suggest that *M. lyra* may derive virtual as well as spectral pitches from complex tones.

In the second experiment (Sedlmeier, 1992c), five *M. lyra* were trained to pay attention to the pitch of the fundamental of complete complex tones with four harmonics by gradually increasing the intensities of the second to fourth harmonic. These bats, in later trials, generally referred to the fundamental pitch of the complex tones, even if the fundamental was drastically attenuated and additionally masked (Fig.3). This finding may be considered as evidence that the bats can be *trained* to form a virtual pitch at ultrasonic frequencies.

Finally, we tested whether *M. lyra* is also able to perceive missing fundamentals *spontaneously* (Preisler and Schmidt, 1994). Three animals were trained to classify complete complex tones (types A and B in Fig.4.a) as higher or lower than a 33-kHz pure tone memory reference. As a critical test, then, the decision behaviour for complex tones without the fundamental (types C-E in Fig.4.a, interspersed with the complete complex tones with a probability of 25%) was investigated. In these test trials, all decisions of the bat were rewarded in order to avoid training effects. Two animals classified all ambiguous stimuli (type C) as higher than the reference (Fig.4.d-e). The third bat, however, classified 22 of 23 ambiguous stimuli with missing fundamentals between 5.3 and 28.3 kHz as low (Fig.4.b-c), and only the control stimuli (type D) as high. As, at least for the lower stimulus level, the nonlinear distortions caused by the complex tones in the cochlea of *M. lyra* can be expected to be below the auditory threshold (Kössl, 1992), we conclude that this bat spontaneously referred to virtual pitch.

Thus, like humans and some other mammals (Heffner and Whitfield, 1976; Tomlinson and Schwarz, 1988) and birds (Cynx and Shapiro, 1986), bats can pay attention to either virtual or spectral pitches of complex tones. Unlike in humans, however, where a virtual pitch exists only at frequencies below 2 kHz (Ritsma, 1967), virtual pitch in *M. lyra* extends to ultrasonic frequencies. This has important implications for current models of pitch perception.

4 Implications of the occurrence of virtual pitch at ultrasonic frequencies for models of pitch perception

Acoustical events can be described in terms of their spectral content as well as their time structure. Both representations may constitute a basis for pitch extraction in the mammalian auditory system. Purely spectral theories assume that the pitch of complex tones is derived from the loci of maximal excitation, varying as a function of frequency on the basilar membrane of the inner ear (Terhardt, 1978; Wightman, 1973). The competing temporal theories postulate an additional time analysis of neuronal discharge patterns: The pitch of complex tones is thought to arise as the difference frequency of the superimposed, unresolved harmonics of the tone (Schouten, 1940), or from an analysis of its spectrally resolved components (DeBoer, 1976; Moore, 1982; Houtsma and Smurzynski, 1990), e.g. by a temporal autocorrelation across the excitation patterns at different cochlear loci (Meddis and Hewitt, 1991). Thus, temporal theories require a neuronal phase coupling to

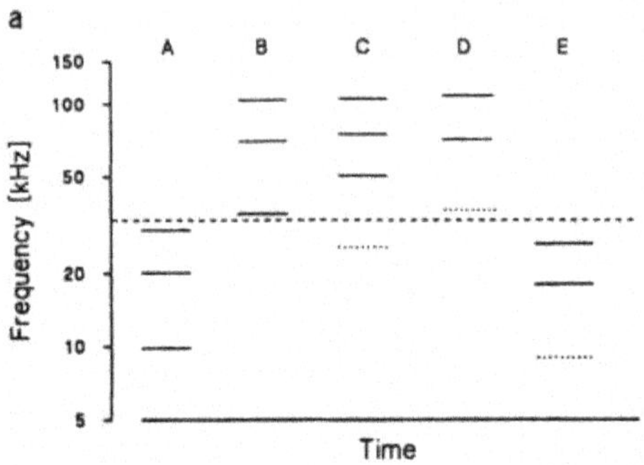

Figure 4. Spontaneous pitch classification for incomplete complex tones. a. Example for low (A) and high (B) complete complex tones, ambiguous incomplete test tones (C) and unambiguous incomplete controls (D,E). Continuous lines indicate physically present, dotted lines missing harmonics; the dashed line marks the 33-kHz reference. b.-e. Performance of two M. lyra at two test tone levels. Open squares represent data points for stimuli of type A and B, downward triangles for type C and upward triangles for type D (bat 1) and E (bat 2); for further explanations see Fig. 2.b.

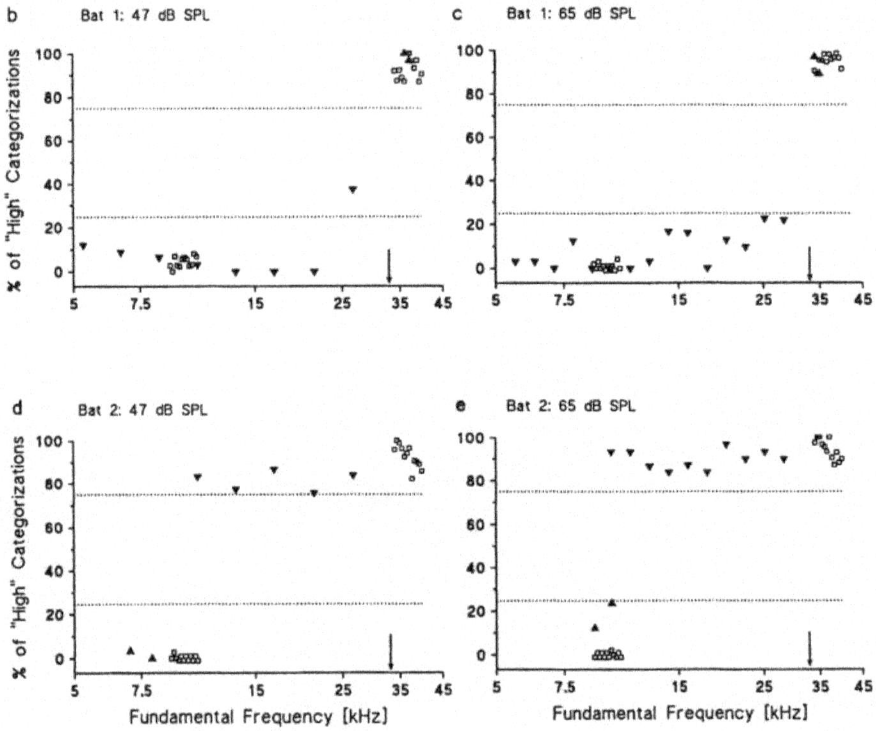

the compound signal envelope or to the single sinusoidal components of the complex tone. If temporal theories were to account for virtual pitch perception in *M. lyra*, phase coupling to steady state signals would have to be postulated at ultrasonic frequencies. However, phase-locked neuronal responses have only been found for frequencies below 5 kHz in mammals (Hind et al., 1967; Javel, 1986), including bats (Suga et al., 1975; Vater, 1982). This renders it improbable that a temporal mechanism accounts for virtual pitch perception in *M. lyra*.

Spectral theories, on the other hand, also account for virtual pitch perception at higher frequencies, provided that the harmonics of the complex tones can be spectrally resolved. This brings up the question of whether this requirement for virtual pitch perception is met by the auditory system of *M. lyra* at ultrasonic frequencies.

5 Frequency resolution and auditory filter shape

Two experiments were performed to characterize the width and the shape of the auditory filters in *M. lyra*, which are defined by the frequency range within which simultaneously present spectral components are analyzed together and can mask each other.

The width of the auditory filters was assessed by determining masked thresholds for pure tones in wideband noise, i.e. critical ratios (CR; Sedlmeier and Schmidt, 1989). The

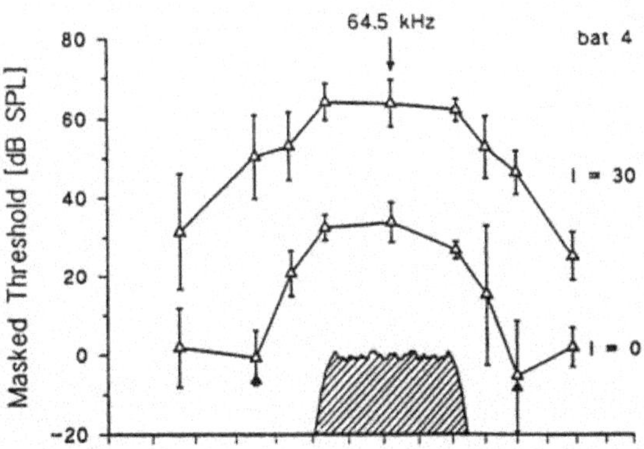

Figure 5: Auditory filter shape in M. lyra. Masked thresholds [dB SPL] for pure tone pulses in narrow-band noise of two spectrum levels (l = 0 dB, l = 30 dB) are plotted as a function of test-tone frequency [kHz]. Open symbols represent masked thresholds, closed symbols thresholds in quiet obtained from the same animal. The error bars give the standard error of the threshold values. The arrow marks the center frequency of the masker, which is indicated by the hatched area (-3 dB bandwidth: 7.5 kHz).

CR widths increased monotonically (steepness: about 6 dB/octave) as a function of test tone frequency from about 1.5 kHz at 25 kHz to about 13.5 kHz at 90 kHz. A recent determination of the critical band (CB) around a center frequency of 64.5 kHz by the method of band-narrowing yielded a bandwidth identical to the CR-value at that frequency. In this species, therefore, the CR-values can be considered to represent the CB.

Auditory filter shape was characterized by determining masked thresholds for pure tones shifted in frequency around a masker of an approximate width of one CB (Schmidt et al., 1992; Schmidt, 1993). Data were obtained at several masker levels for maskers with center frequencies of 23, 30, 40, and 64.5 kHz, i.e. in the region of the first three harmonics of the sonar calls of *M. lyra*. The filter shapes obtained (cf. Fig.5) were symmetrical around the masker center frequency at all masker levels tested, their slopes were between 40 and 100 dB/CB. Thus, in contrast to man (cf. Zwicker and Fastl, 1990), the filter slopes in *M. lyra* are exceedingly steep, and the symmetry of the auditory filters is preserved at high masker spectrum levels.

Both characteristics may result from a central sharpening of the frequency tuning reported for *M. lyra* (Rübsamen et al., 1988), and, in combination with the narrow CBs, guarantee the clear spectral separation of the harmonic components of the echoes required for virtual pitch formation. Our results in *M. lyra* may thus be taken as evidence that spectral theories are sufficient to account for virtual pitch formation in the mammalian auditory system.

6 Acknowledgements

This study was funded by the Deutsche Forschungsgemeinschaft, SFB 204/TP 8 "Gehör", München. We thank Professor E. Terhardt for stimulating discussions, and Professor G. Neuweiler for his constant support.

7 References

Bachem, A. (1955) Absolute pitch. J. Acoust. Soc. Am. 27, 1180-1185.

Cynx, J. and Shapiro, M. (1986) Perception of missing fundamental by a species of songbird (*Sturnus vulgaris*). J. Comp. Psychol. 100, 356-360.

De Boer, E. (1976) On the "residue" and auditory pitch perception. In: W.D. Keidel and W.D. Neff (Eds.), Handbook of sensory physiology V/3, Springer Verlag, Berlin, Heidelberg, New York, pp. 480-583.

D'Amato, M.R. (1988) A search for tonal pattern perception in cebus monkeys: why monkeys can't hume a tune. Music perception 5, 453-480.

Fay, R.R. (1988) Hearing in vertebrates. A psychophysics data book. Hill and Fay Associates, Winnetka, IL.

Heffner, H. and Whitfield, I.C. (1976) Perception of the missing fundamental by cats. J. Acoust. Soc. Am. 59, 915-919.

Hind, J.E., Anderson, D.J., Brugge, J.F. and Rose, J.E. (1967) Coding of information pertaining to paired low-frequency tones in single auditory nerve fibers of the squirrel monkey. J. Neurophysiol. 30, 794-816.

Houtsma, A.J.M. and Smurzynski, J. (1990) Pitch identification and discrimination for complex tones with many harmonics. J. Acoust. Soc. Am. 87, 304-310.

Hulse, H.H. and Cynx, J. (1985) Relative pitch perception is constrained by absolute pitch in songbirds (Mimus, Molothrus, and Sturnus). J. Comp. Psychol. 99, 176-196.

Hulse, H.H., Cynx, J. and Humpal, J (1984) Absolute and relative pitch discrimination in serial pitch perception by birds. J. Exp. Psychol.: General 113, 38-54.

Javel, E. (1986) Basic response properties of auditory nerve fibers. In: R.A. Altschuler, D.W. Hoffman and R.P. Bobbin (Eds.), Neurobiology of Hearing: The Cochlea, Raven Press, New York, pp. 213-245.

Kössl, M. (1992) High frequency distortion products from the ears of two bat species, *Megaderma lyra* and *Carollia perspicillata*. Hear. Res. 60, 156-164.

May, B., Moody, D.B. and Stebbins, W.C. (1989) Categorial perception of conspecific communication sounds by japanese macaques, *Macaca fuscata*. J. Acoust Soc. Am. 85, 837-847.

Meddis, R. and Hewitt, M.J. (1991) Virtual pitch and phase sensitivity of a computer model of the auditory periphery. I:Pitch identification. J. Acoust. Soc. Am. 89, 2866-2882.

Miyazaki K. (1988) Musical pitch identification by absolute pitch possessors. Percept. Psychophys. 44, 501-512.

Moore, B. (1982) An introduction to the psychology of hearing. Academic Press, London.

Page, S.C., Hulse, S.H. and Cynx J. (1989) Relative pitch perception in the European starling (*Sturnus vulgaris*): Further evidence for an elusive phenomenon. J. Exp. Psychol.: Animal behavior processes 15, 137-146.

Preisler, A. and Schmidt, S. (1994) Perception of the missing fundamental in the echolocating bat, *Megaderma lyra*. In: Elsner, N. and Breer. H.: Proc. 22th Göttingen Neurobiol. Conf., Georg Thieme Verlag, Stuttgart, (in press)

Ritsma, R.J. (1967) Existence region of the tonal residue. I. J. Acoust. Soc. Am. 42, 191-198.

Rübsamen, R., Neuweiler, G. and Sripathi, K. (1988) Comparative collicular tonotopy in two bat species adapted to movement detection, *Hipposideros speoris* and *Megaderma lyra*. J. Comp. Physiol. 163, 271-285.

Schmidt, S. (1992) Perception of structured phantom targets in the echolocating bat, *Megaderma lyra*. J. Acoust. Soc. Am. 91, 2203-2223.

Schmidt, S. (1993) Perspectives and problems of comparative psychoacoustics in echolocating bats. In: D.J. Lim and G.R. Popelka (Eds.) Abstracts of the 16th midwinter research meeting Ass. Res. Otolaryngol., p.145.

Schmidt, S., Gerber, P. and Pötke, M. (1992) Psychoacoustical characterization of auditory filter shape in the bat, *Megaderma lyra*. In: Abstracts ot the 15th annual meeting of the European Neuroscience Association, Supplement No.5, Europ. J. Neurosci., 141.

Schmidt, S., Türke, B. and Vogler, B. (1983) Behavioural audiogram from the bat, *Megaderma lyra* (Geoffroy, 1810; Microchiroptera). Myotis, 21-22, 62-66.

Schnitzler, H.U. and Henson, O.W. (1980) Performance of airborne animal sonar systems: I.Microchiroptera. In: R.G. Busnel and J.F. Fish (Eds.) Animal sonar systems, Plenum Press, New York, pp.109-181.

Schouten, J.F. (1940) The perception of subjective tones. Proc. Kon. Ned. Akad. v. Wetensch. 41, 1086-1093.

Sedlmeier, H. (1992a) Tonhöhenwahrnehmung beim Falschen Vampir, *Megaderma lyra*. Dissertation, Fakultät für Biologie, LMU München.

Sedlmeier, H. (1992b) Pitch sensation in the Indian false vampire bat (*Megaderma lyra*). In: Elsner, N. and Richter, D.W. (Eds.) Rhythmogenesis in neurons and networks. Proc. 20th Göttingen Neurobiol. Conf., Georg Thieme Verlag, Stuttgart, p.233.

Sedlmeier, H. (1992c) Perception of a missing fundamental in the ultrasonic range by the False Vampire Bat (*Megaderma lyra*). In: Abstracts ot the 15th annual meeting of the European Neuroscience Association, Supplement No.5, Europ. J. Neurosci., 2267.

Sedlmeier, H. and Schmidt, S. (1989) Masked auditory thresholds from the Indian False Vampire bat (*Megaderma lyra*). In: N. Elsner, W. Singer (Eds.) Dynamics and plasticity in neuronal systems. Proc. 17th Göttingen Neurobiol. Conf., Georg Thieme Verlag, Stuttgart, p.292.

Suga N., Simmons, J.A., and Jen, P.H.-S. (1975) Peripheral specialization for fine analysis of Doppler-shifted echoes in the auditory system of the "CF-FM" bat *Pteronotus parnellii*. J. Exp. Biol. 63, 161-192.

Terhardt, E. (1978) Psychoacoustic evaluation of musical sounds. Percept. Psychophys.23, 483-492.

Tomlinson, R.W.W. and Schwarz, D.W.F. (1988) Perception of the missing fundamental in nonhuman primates. J. Acoust. Soc. Am. 84, 560-565.

Vater, M. (1982) Single unit responses in cochlear nucleus of horseshoe bats to sinusoidal frequency and amplitude modulated signals. J. Comp. Physiol. A 149, 369-388.

Wightman, F.L. (1973) The pattern transformation model of pitch. J. Acoust. Soc. Am. 54, 407-416.

Zwicker, E. and Fastl, H. (1990) Psychoacoustics. Facts and Models. Springer Verlag, Berlin, Heidelberg, New York.

Repetition pitch: Auditory processing of rippled noise in the chinchilla

William P. Shofner and William A. Yost

Parmly Hearing Institute, Loyola University Chicago
6525 N. Sheridan Rd., Chicago, IL 60626, USA

1 Introduction

Pitch is a fundamental perception of many complex sounds, and a variety of complex sounds can produce the same pitch (Fastl and Stoll, 1979). Rippled noises produce the perception of pitch in human subjects, and this pitch is often referred to as repetition pitch. Since predicting the repetition pitches of rippled noises has been difficult for many models of pitch (see Yost and Hill, 1979), understanding of the processing of rippled noise is important for understanding pitch perception.

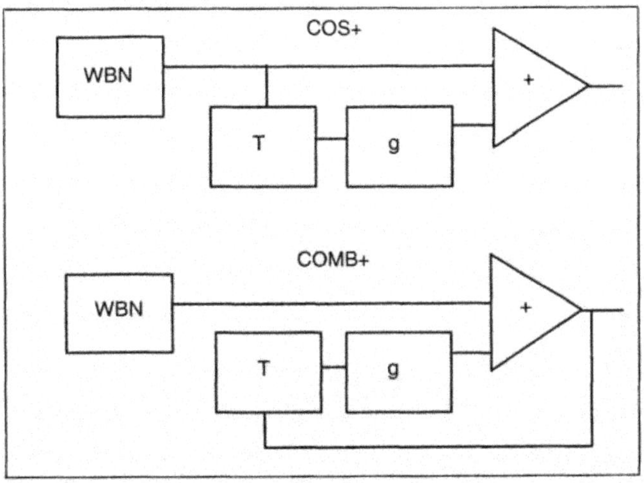

Figure 1. Comparison of the circuits used to generate cos+ rippled noise (TOP) and comb+ rippled noise (BOTTOM). WBN is wideband noise; T is the delay; g is the gain. Cos+ represents 1 iteration, while comb+ is infinitely iterated.

In general, there are two types of rippled noises, namely cosine rippled noise and comb-filtered rippled noise. Cos+ rippled noise is generated when a wideband noise is delayed and the delayed repetition of the noise is added to the undelayed noise (Figure 1).

When expressed in linear power units, cos+ rippled noise has a power spectrum given by

$$|H(f)|^2 = 1 + g^2 + 2g\cos(2\pi fT)$$

Eq. 1 (see Yost and Hill, 1979)

where g is gain and T is the delay. The resulting power spectrum has peaks which occur in a cosinusoidal manner at integer multiples of 1/T (Figure 2). Cos- rippled noise is generated when the delayed repetition is subtracted from the undelayed noise; the spectral valleys occur at integer multiples of 1/T. When the wideband noise is delayed and then positively fed back to the input, comb-filtered rippled noise is generated (Figure 1). Comb+ rippled noise has a power spectrum given by

$$|H(f)|^2 = \frac{1}{(1 + g^2 - 2g\cos(2\pi fT)}$$

Eq. 2 (see Bilsen and Raatgever, 1983)

and has sharp peaks at integer multiples of 1/T (Figure 2). If the gain of the delayed repetition of the noise is attenuated before the addition occurs, then the spectral modulation depth of the ripple decreases.

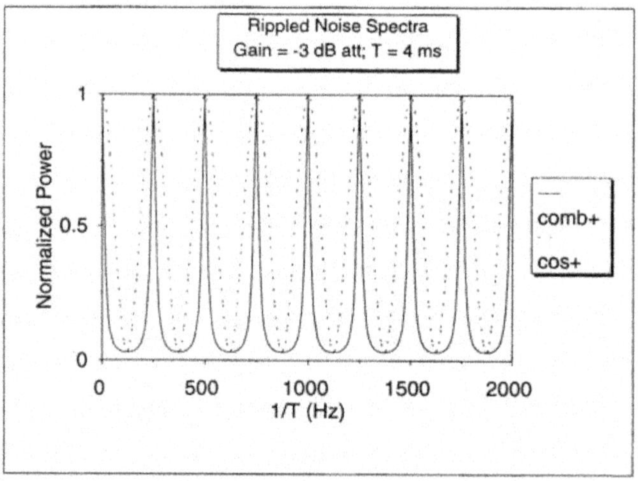

Figure 2. Comparison of the spectra for cos+ (dotted line) and comb+ (solid line) rippled noises. The gain is -3 dB and T is 4 ms for both noises.

1.1 Auditory Processing of Rippled Noise in Human Subjects

The repetition pitches of rippled noises are related to the delay. Pitch matching studies have shown that cos+ rippled noises have pitches equal to 1/T, while cos- rippled noises have ambiguous pitches approximately equal to 0.9/T and 1.1/T (Bilsen, 1970; Yost et. al., 1978). In addition to the ambiguous pitches, comb- rippled noises can give pitches equal to 0.5/T (Fastl, 1988; Raatgever and Bilsen, 1992). For both cos and comb rippled noise, the pitch strength is related to the gain of the delayed repetition of the noise. As the delayed repetition is attenuated ($g < 1$) relative to the undelayed noise, the strength of the pitch decreases. This relationship between gain and pitch strength has been used to determine how sensitive subjects are to different repetition pitches. In pitch discrimination experiments, subjects are presented with two different rippled noises having pitches that can be discriminated easily. The gain used to generate the rippled noises is decreased until the subject can no longer discriminate the pitch difference between the two rippled noises. Threshold is defined as the gain of the delayed repetition when a subject can just detect the pitch difference between the two rippled noises. Similar experiments have been carried out in which subjects discriminate spectrally flat wideband noise from rippled noise; in these coloration discrimination experiments, the threshold is the gain at which subjects can just detect the difference between rippled noise and wideband noise. In general, the results from 'pitch' and 'coloration' discriminations show that the most salient rippled noise pitches are between 100-1000 Hz, which corresponds to delays of 1-10 ms (Bilsen and Ritsma, 1970; Yost and Hill, 1978). Pitch discrimination studies using bandpass filtered noise rather than wideband noise show that there is a dominant region for repetition pitch, corresponding to the spectral peaks between 3/T to 5/T (Bilsen and Ritsma, 1970; Yost and Hill, 1978). These studies also show that above 20 dB SL, threshold is independent of the overall level (Bilsen and Ritsma, 1970; Yost and Hill, 1978).

2 Psychophysical Experiments in the Chinchilla

We obtained animal psychophysical data from experiments similar to those described above for human subjects in order to provide a behavioral framework for neurophysiological experiments. Psychophysical experiments in mammals have used rippled noise only as a masker for tonal signals in order to derive the shape of auditory filters (cat: Pickles, 1979; guinea pig: Evans et. al., 1992; chinchilla: Niemiec et. al., 1992), but have not specifically used rippled noise as a signal. Psychophysical experiments with rippled noise signals have been carried out in goldfish (Fay et al., 1983). In the experiments described below, we present behavioral data from the chinchilla using rippled noise as the signal. We have focused our initial efforts on coloration discrimination in order to establish if the chinchilla can discriminate rippled noise from wideband noise.

2.1 Procedure

Five chinchillas were trained to discriminate comb+ rippled noise from wideband noise. Comb+ rippled noise was used in order to increase the strength of the repetition pitch. In the procedure, 500-ms bursts of wideband noise were presented continuously with an inter-burst interval of 500 ms. The rise/fall time of the bursts was 10 ms. The animal initiated a trial by pressing down on the response lever and after a variable hold time of 1150-5150 ms, either a signal trial or a blank trial was presented. During a signal trial, two 500-ms bursts of comb+ rippled noise were presented; during a blank trial, two 500-ms bursts of wideband noise were presented. If the animal released the response lever before the variable hold time had elapsed, the trial was aborted. If the animal released the response lever during a signal or blank trial, the release was scored as a "yes" response. An attenuator reduced the overall level by an amount equal to the increase in overall level produced when the rippled noise was generated. Consequently, there was no confounding cue due to an increase in overall level during a signal trial.

Psychometric functions were generated using the method of constant stimuli. A block of 40 trials consisted of 4 trials at a gain of -1 dB, 4 trials each at 7 different gain values, and 8 trials at a gain of -100 dB where gain in dB is 20log g. The wideband noise was generated when the gain was set at -100 dB; these 8 trials per block (20% of the total trials) were blank trials and provided an estimate of the false alarm rate. The various gain settings were presented randomly for each block. Psychometric functions were based on a minimum of 50 blocks. In order to obtain estimates of sensitivity that were independent of response bias, psychometric functions were first fit with logistic functions having the form

$$P(yes) = F + (H_{(-1)} - F) \left(\frac{H_{(-1)}}{H_{(-1)} + \exp\left[(-k)(x - m)\right]} \right) \qquad \text{Eq. 3}$$

where F is the proportion of false alarms, $H_{(-1)}$ is the proportion of hits when the gain was set to -1 dB, k is the slope parameter and m is the mean of the function. Estimates of d' were then obtained from these best fitting logistic functions using z(H)-z(F). In addition to the 5 chinchillas, psychometric functions were obtained for 3 human subjects using the same paradigm and equipment. Stimuli were played through a Radio Shack Minimus-7 loudspeaker to chinchillas and diotically through Stax-SR5 earphones to human subjects. Animals were rewarded with food pellets for hits and correct rejections, while correct responses from human subjects were 'rewarded' by turning on a red LED.

2.2 Results

The comb+ rippled noise used in this paper had a delay set to 4 ms, resulting in a repetition pitch of 250 Hz. Psychometric functions for the discrimination of this comb+ rippled noise from wideband noise are monotonic for both human subjects (Figure 3) and chinchillas (Figure 4). Logistic functions provide excellent descriptions of behavioral performance. The coefficients of determination (R^2) are greater than 0.9 for chinchillas and human subjects. Table 1 summarizes the parameters of these logistic functions for

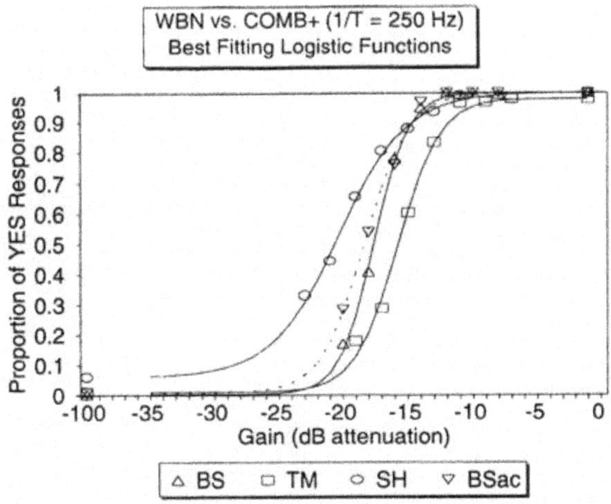

Figure 3. Psychometric functions for 3 human subjects for the discrimination of comb+ rippled noise from wideband noise. T is 4 ms.

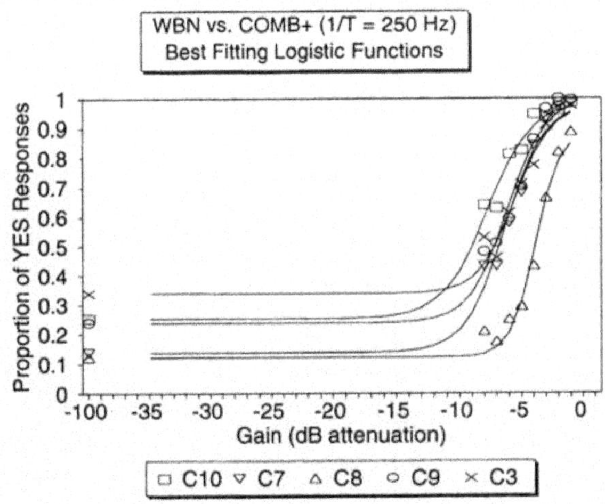

Figure 4. Psychometric functions for 5 chinchillas for the discrimination of comb+ rippled noise from wideband noise. T is 4 ms.

each subject. The average slope of the best fitting logistic functions obtained for the chinchillas is 0.707 and the average slope obtained for the human subjects is 0.583. These average slopes are not significantly different ($t = 0.956$; $t < t_{0.05(2),6}$). The rising portion

Table 1. Summary of the Parameters for the Best Fitting Logistic Functions (T = 4 ms)

Subject	# of Blocks	k	m (dB att)	R2	dB att at d'=1
BS	50	0.755	-17.6	0.9988	-22.1
SH	50	0.379	-20.3	0.9980	-23.3
TM	50	0.614	-15.8	0.9959	-19.6
C3	51	0.683	-5.6	0.9623	-5.0
C7	51	0.633	-6.4	0.9786	-7.1
C8	50	1.003	-4.0	0.9802	-4.3
C9	51	0.657	-6.2	0.9727	-6.2
C10	52	0.559	-7.8	0.9983	-7.7

of the psychometric functions occur over different ranges of gains for chinchillas and human subjects. The mean of the logistic function is the gain in dB attenuation which yields P(yes) equal to the average of $H_{(-1)}$ and F and is an estimate of sensitivity. However, the mean value will not be used to describe sensitivity, because it is dependent on the subject's criterion. The values of P(yes) that occur at a gain of -100 dB are measures of subjects' false alarm rates, and it can be observed in Figures 3 and 4 that human subjects tend to adopt higher criteria (i.e. they have lower false alarm rates) than do chinchillas. In order to obtain an estimate of sensitivity that is independent of the criterion, d' was computed.

Figure 5 compares the psychometric functions for human subjects and chinchillas with behavioral performance expressed as d'. At d' of 1, the gain in dB attenuation for human subjects ranges from -19.6 to -23.3 dB (Table 1), and these values fall within the range of gains previously reported for human subjects using cos+ rippled noise (see Yost and Hill, 1978). However, the values of gain at d' of 1 are much higher for chinchillas ranging from -4.3 to -7.7. The average gain in dB for human subjects is -21.7 dB, while the average gain is -6.1 dB for chinchillas. The average gain for chinchillas is significantly higher than that for human subjects ($t = 13.596$; $t > t_{0.0005(1),6}$).

The higher values of gain in dB obtained for the chinchillas cannot be attributed to a difference in listening environments between chinchillas and human subjects. For subject BS, the calibration microphone was placed in the position of the animal's head, and sound was played through the loudspeaker. The output of the microphone was amplified and played through the headphones. In this condition, the subject discriminated the comb+ rippled noise from the wideband noise while "listening" to the sound field produced in the animal sound-attenuating chamber. The psychometric function obtained (BSac in Figures 3 and 5) was essentially identical to this subject's original psychometric function. Thus, the behavioral performance observed for the chinchillas does reflect their sensitivity for coloration discrimination rather than a difference in the sound fields used by chinchillas and human subjects.

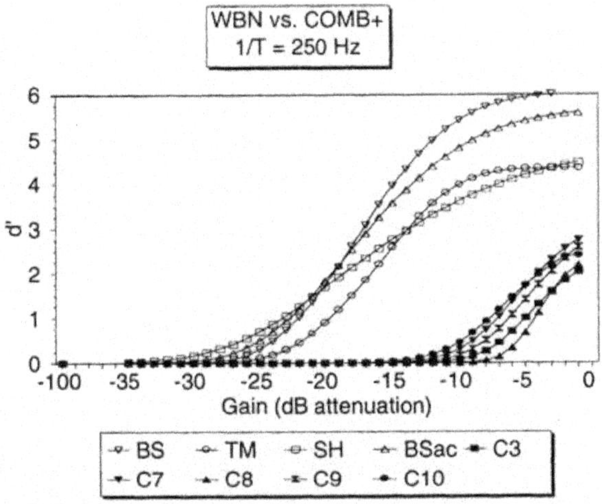

Figure 5. Comparison of psychometric functions for the discrimination of comb+ rippled noise from wideband noise for chinchillas (filled symbols) and human subjects (open symbols). Markers do not indicate actual data points, but merely are used to differentiate curves among subjects. Performance is expressed as d'.

Psychometric functions for coloration discrimination were obtained for three chinchillas at three different overall sound levels. Table 2 shows the gain at d' of 1 for each animal as a function of the overall sound level of the wideband noise. The levels tested range from 37-57 dB SL for C7 and range from 22-42 dB SL for C9 and C10. These data suggest that the sensitivity for coloration discrimination in the chinchilla is independent of level over this 20-dB range of levels.

Table 2. Effect of Overall Sound Level on Psychometric Functions (T = 4 ms)

Level of WBN:	64 dB SPL	74 dB SPL	84 dB SPL
Subject	dB att at d'=1	dB att at d'=1	dB att at d'=1
C7	-5.8	-7.1	-5.8
C9	-5.9	-6.2	-5.2
C10	-8.0	-7.7	-6.8

3 Discussion

The present results show that chinchillas can discriminate comb+ rippled noise having a repetition pitch of 250 Hz from wideband noise, but are less sensitive than human subjects. For human subjects, the average gain at d' of 1 is -21.7 and corresponds to a peak-to-valley ratio of 1.4 dB in the power spectrum. The peak-to-valley ratio, P/V in dB, is given by

$$\frac{P}{V}(dB) = 10 \log \left(\frac{(1+g)^2}{(1-g)^2}\right)$$

Eq. 4 (see Bilsen and Raatgever, 1983)

In contrast, the average gain at d' of 1 for the chinchillas is -6.1 dB and corresponds to a peak-to-valley ratio of 9.4 dB in the power spectrum. While chinchillas are less sensitive, the similarities in the slopes of the psychometric functions suggest that the underlying neural processing of the 250 Hz comb+ rippled noise may be the same between chinchillas and human subjects.

Psychophysical and neurophysiological studies of rippled noise processing in the goldfish suggest that rippled noise delay is encoded by the temporal discharge of saccular (auditory) nerve fibers (Fay et. al., 1983). For cos+ rippled noise, most saccular nerve fibers show a peak in the interspike interval histogram at the rippled noise delay. The repetition pitch is presumably encoded by the location of the peak, while pitch strength is presumably encoded by the height of the peak in the interspike interval histogram. Fay et al. (1983) suggested that similar encoding schemes may be found in mammals.

In response to cos+ rippled noise, autocorrelation functions of neural spike trains obtained from mammalian auditory nerve fibers (ten Kate and van Bekkum, 1988) and cochlear nucleus units (Shofner, 1991) can show a peak at the ripple delay. However, the presence of a peak in the neural autocorrelation function is primarily limited to low-best frequency, phase-locked units. If temporal discharge is important in pitch processing, then the weaker pitch strengths of cos rippled noises may be related to the limited number of auditory units capable of firing in a synchronous manner as well as the heights of the peaks in neural autocorrelation functions. Figure 6 shows an example of a neural autocorrelation function obtained from a primary-like-notch unit in the chinchilla cochlear nucleus in response to comb+ rippled noise with a delay of 4 ms. At a gain of -1 dB attenuation, there are peaks in the neural autocorrelation function that occur at integer multiples of the 4 ms delay. For this unit, there is a systematic increase in the height of the peak at the delay of 4 ms as the gain increases, while there is no systematic change in firing rate (Figure 7). The increase in the height of this peak as a function of gain qualitatively reflects the psychometric functions obtained for coloration discrimination. Quantitative analysis of interspike intervals as well as average firing rate of auditory neurons in response to comb+ rippled noises should provide important insights into the underlying neural mechanisms of pitch processing.

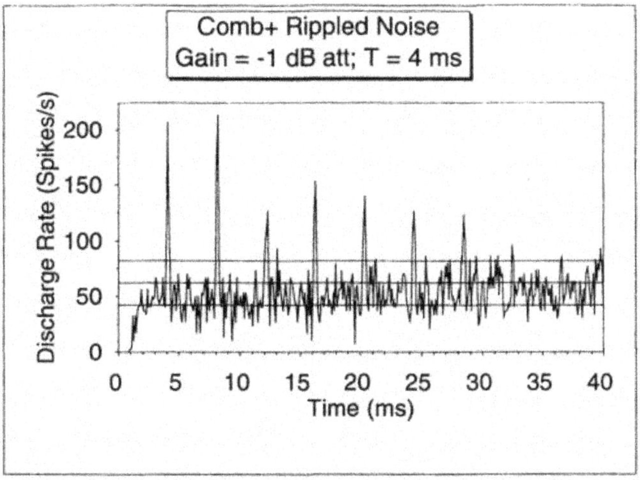

Figure 6. Neural autocorrelation function obtained from a cochlear nucleus unit in the chinchilla in response to comb+ rippled noise at 20 dB above threshold. The 3 horizontal lines show the average discharge rate ±2 S.D. as determined from the empirical spike count distribution. Gain is -1 dB; T is 4 ms. PRIMARY-LIKE-NOTCH unit; BF = 2.05 kHz.

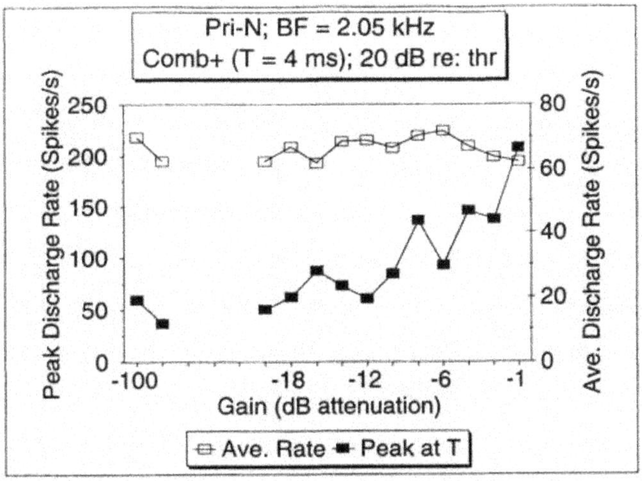

Figure 7. Comparison of discharge rate at the height of the peak at 4 ms in the neural autocorrelation function (solid squares) and average discharge rate (open squares) as a function of gain for comb+ rippled noise. T is 4 ms. The wideband noise (gain of -100 dB) was repeated twice.

4 Acknowledgements

We would like to thank Lisa Smith for her technical assistance in maintaining and running the chinchillas in the behavioral test sessions. We also thank Drs. Raymond Dye and Stanley Sheft for many helpful discussions. This research was supported by a program project grant (P50 DC00293) from the National Institute of Deafness and Other Communication Disorders.

5 References

Bilsen, F.A. (1970) Repetition pitch; Its implication for hearing theory and room acoustics. In: R. Plomp and G.F. Smoorenburg (Eds.), Frequency Analysis and Periodicity Detection in Hearing, A.J. Sijthoff, Leiden, The Netherlands, pp.292-302.

Bilsen, F.A. and Ritsma, R.J. (1970) Some parameters influencing the perceptibility of pitch. J. Acoust. Soc. Am. 47, 469-475.

Evans, E.F., Pratt, S.R., Spenner, H. and Cooper, N.P. (1992) Comparisons of physiological and behavioural properties: Auditory frequency selectivity. In: Y. Cazals, K. Horner and L. Demany (Eds.), Auditory Physiology and Perception, Pergamon Press, Oxford, pp.159-167.

Fastl, H. (1988) Pitch and pitch strength of peaked ripple noise. In: H. Duifhuis, J.W. Horst and H.P. Wit (Eds.), Basic Issues in Hearing, Academic Press, London, pp. 370-379.

Fastl, H. and Stoll, G. (1979) Scaling of pitch strength. Hearing Res. 1, 293-301.

Fay, R.R., Yost, W.P. and Coombs, S. (1983) Psychophysics and neurophysiology of repetition noise processing in a vertebrate auditory system. Hearing Res. 12, 31-55.

Kate, J.H. ten and Bekkum, M.F. van (1988) Synchrony-dependent autocorrelation in eighth-nerve-fiber response to rippled noise. J. Acoust. Soc. Am. 84, 2092-2102.

Niemiec, A.J., Yost, W.A. and Shofner, W.P. (1992) Behavioral measures of frequency selectivity in the chinchilla. J. Acoust. Soc. Am. 92, 2636-2649.

Pickles, J.O. (1979) Psychophysical frequency resolution in the cat as determined by simultaneous masking and its relation to auditory-nerve resolution. J. Acoust. Soc. Am. 66, 1725-1732.

Raatgever, J. and Bilsen, F.A. (1992) The pitch of anharmonic comb filtered noise reconsidered. In: Y. Cazals, K. Horner and L. Demany, Auditory Physiology and Perception, Pergamon Press, Oxford, pp.215-222.

Shofner, W.P. (1991) Temporal representation of rippled noise in the anteroventral cochlear nucleus of the chinchilla. J. Acoust. Soc. Am. 90, 2450-2466.

Yost, W.A. and Hill, R. (1978) Strength of the pitches associated with ripple noise. J. Acoust. Soc. Am. 64, 485-492.

Yost, W.A. and Hill, R. (1979) Models of the pitch and pitch strength of ripple noise. J. Acoust. Soc. Am. 66, 400-410.

Yost, W.A., Hill, R. and Perez-Falcon, T. (1978) Pitch and pitch discrimination of broadband signals with rippled power spectra. J. Acoust. Soc. Am. 63, 1166-1173.

Comment by J.P. Wilson

Firstly, you mentioned that you could find no data on colouration thresholds in rippled noise. We did present some data at the Driebergen Symposium (1969) which is reproduced as the downward arrows in figure 7 of our present paper corresponding with the 20-25 dB that you mention.

Secondly, it should be pointed out that when cosine noise is plotted on a dB scale it takes on a comb filter shape and is so described by many groups. Comb filtered noise is therefore not a sufficient description for your sharper peaked spectra obtained by feedback.

Thirdly, and most importantly, your claim that an autocorrelation model is favoured by your data cannot be sustained. As the two types of noise signal are both "viewed" via the auditory filter bank it is their relative peak-to-valley ratios at the output of this filter bank that should be considered not that at the input. More specifically the narrow notches of the cosine noise will be elevated to a greater extent than the peaks of the feedback noise will be flattened. But a proper comparison requires the proper convolution of the spectral shapes with the appropriate auditory filters.

Reply

With repect to your third point, our results and conclusions with regard to autocorrelation are consistent with recent data using iterated-rippled noises in human subjects (Yost et al., 1994) and auditory models (see Patterson and Akeroyd, this volume). The point I was trying to make was that autocorrelation contains sufficient information to account for the behavioral results using the simplest rule, not that autocorrelation per se was necessarily the underlying neural mechanism. It is not clear to me that at the output of a bank of critical-band filters or peripheral-weighting filters (see Yost and Hill, 1979), the narrow spectral notches of cosine rippled noise will be elevated more than the spectral peaks of comb-filtered rippled noise will be reduced. However, your point is well taken and examining these spectra at the output of an auditory filter bank is something we should do.

With respect to your second comment, the distinction that we make between cosine-rippled noise and comb-filtered rippled noise as shown in Figure 1 of our paper is between 1 iteration and an infinite number of iterations, respectively. However, when plotted on a dB scale, the spectrum of cosine-rippled noise does not take on a comb-filter shape in that the spectral peaks do not appear to be sharper; it is the spectral valleys that appear to be sharper when cosine-rippled noise is plotted on a dB scale.

Finally, in addition to your data presented at the Driebergen Symposium, there are several reports in the literature on coloration discrimination data using cosine-rippled noise. I am not aware of any published data on coloration discrimination where comb-filtered rippled noise (as we define it) was used specifically.

Yost, W.A., Sheft, S. and Patterson, R. (1994) Iterated rippled noise: Testing temporal theories of complex pitch. J. Acoust. Soc. Am. 95, 2966.

Probability distributions of the pitch of harmonic and inharmonic three tone complexes: Symmetric mistuning[1]

E. Wiersinga-Post and H. Duifhuis

Department of Biophysics, and Center for Behavioral and Cognitive Neurosciences, University of Groningen, Nyenborgh 4, Groningen. NL-9747 AG, The Netherlands.

1 Introduction

Complex tones that contain few harmonics -no fundamental- present a characteristic pitch ambiguity. The ambiguity increases with the decrease of the total number of components (Houtsma and Smurzynski, 1990) and with the increase of the lowest harmonic number (n_l) of the complex (Ritsma, 1962; Houtsma and Goldstein, 1972). In general present theories of complex tone pitch perception (e.g.: Goldstein, 1973; Wightman, 1973; Terhardt *et al.*, 1982) present an interpretation of the ambiguity. Pitch perception is interpreted as a spectral pattern recognition process which operates on the basis of *aurally resolved* frequency components. The peripheral auditory system relays information of these frequency components to the central nervous system, where a central mechanism (the central pitch processor) processes the information about the frequencies of the resolved components (the spectral pattern) and estimates their harmonic numbers (n_i). The optimum processor determines the fundamental frequency (f_0) of the complex tone. Stochastic errors occurring in the process provide the uncertainty on the basis of which the harmonic numbers, n_i, of a complex sound can be misinterpreted as $n_{i\pm1}$, $n_{i\pm2}$, etc., thus causing ambiguity of the pitch of the complex tone.

This manuscript describes experiments in which the probability distributions of the pitch of harmonic and inharmonic complex sounds are measured. The experimental data are compared with predictions from a harmonic pattern recognition model. In a series of pitch matching experiments, the subject matched a comparison sound to a stimulus, which consisted of three harmonic or inharmonic frequency components. Pitch strength is estimated on the basis of the results of numerous repetitions.

1.1 Sub-harmonic summation

A sub-harmonic summation model is used to predict the distribution of possible pitches of a single complex tone (cf., e.g., Noll, 1964; Schroeder, 1968; Parsons, 1976; Terhardt et al., 1982; Hermes, 1988). This model is closely related (see for a review:

[1]A companion paper studying the case for asymmetric mistuning has been submitted for publication (Wiersinga-Post and Duifhuis, 1994).

de Boer, 1977) to theories based on maximum likelihood estimation (Goldstein, 1973; Duifhuis *et al.*, 1982) or autocorrelation (Wightman, 1973; Brown, 1992).

The variability of the spectral pattern recognition process that operates on the aurally resolved frequency components is described by Gaussian probability distributions centred at the component frequencies. The variance of these Gaussians, a parameter of the model, is chosen to depend linearly on frequency in accordance with thevariance parameter in the optimum processor theory of Goldstein:

$$\sigma_f = \sigma \cdot f \tag{1}$$

The sub-harmonic summation procedure is schematically presented in Fig. 1. This example uses three stimulus components: f_1 = 1000 Hz, f_2 = 1200 Hz, f_3 = 1400 Hz. For each component, several sub-harmonics are computed (Fig. 1A,B,C), providing the sets of Gaussian distributions with equal widths on a logarithmic frequency scale. [Only the parts of the Gaussians with values above 0.01 are taken into account.] The areas below the Gaussians represent pitch strength and are kept constant on a linear scale. This results in higher Gaussians at lower frequencies.

In accordance with the sub-harmonic summation algorithm proposed by Hermes (Hermes, 1988), the sub-harmonics are multiplied by a second parameter W:

$$W_n = W^{n-1} \qquad n = \text{sub-harmonic number.} \tag{2}$$

A value of $W < 1$ causes higher harmonics to contribute less to the pitch perception than lower harmonics.

The sets of sub-harmonics are summed in Fig. 1D. The results are separated in Fig. 1E and 1F as peaks caused by "summation of 3 harmonics" and "summation of 2 harmonics", respectively. Since the summed curve represents a probability distribution of the pitches of the complex sound, the total area below the curve equals 1. If a subject listens synthetically to all 3 spectral components in the stimulus (Fig. 1E), then the most obvious pitch will be the pitch of 200 Hz, while the perception at ± 170 Hz (harmonic numbers 6,7,8: 1020, 1190, 1360 Hz) is also possible. A change of the parameter s will modify the width of the Gaussian sub-harmonics and thus the number and widths of pitch sidebands that occur in the sum (Fig. 1E). The higher the variance of the Gaussian, the more pitch sidebands occur in Fig. 1E. A change in the value of W affects the impact of distant sub-harmonics. In Fig. 1E a decrease in W reduces the pitch strength at 170 Hz.

2 Methods

2.1 Procedure

The subject's task was to match the pitch of the comparison tone with the pitch of the stimulus (see 2.2). Presentation of stimulus and comparison tone bursts was under the control of the subject. The f_0-value of the comparison tone could be varied in steps of 1 Hz or 10 Hz within a range of about 1 octave around f_0. In order to prevent this frequency range from affecting the matching results, roving ranges were used. The lower border of the range varied between -45% and -25% of f_0 and the upper border between +30% and +45%. The initial value of f_0 of the comparison tone varied randomly within its frequency range. No feedback was given. The data supplement related data on 4 subjects (Wiersinga-Post & Duifhuis, 1994). The data presented here are from one normal hearing subject, the first author (25 y).

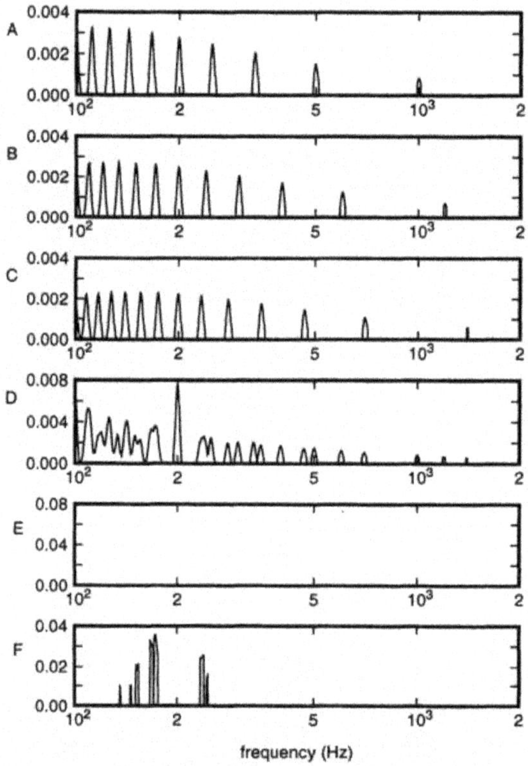

Figure 1. Sub-harmonic summation procedure, with $\sigma = 0.013$ and $W = 0.9$. (A), (B), (C): Frequency components (A: 1000 Hz, B: 1200 Hz, C: 1400 Hz) with their sub-harmonics. (D): Sum of A, B, and C. (E): Parts of D in which 3 sub-harmonics are summed. (F): Parts of D in which 2 sub-harmonics are summed.

2.2 Stimulus and comparison tone

The stimuli consisted of three harmonics -or three mistuned components- of a fundamental of 200, 225, 250, 267 or 300 Hz. In the harmonic situation, the following four sets of 3 harmonics were used: set 1: {3,4,5}, set 2: {5,6,7}, set 3: {9,10,11} or set 4: {11,12,13}. For inharmonic stimuli, similar sets were used, but the upper and lower components were mistuned by either 5% or 10% (of f_0), toward or from the central component. To indicate the different patterns of mistuning the coding ABC-x% will be used, where A, B and C refer to components 1, 2 and 3 in the complex sound. Each of these is either purely harmonic (indicated by 0), or shifted upwards (indicated by H) or downwards (indicated by L) by x= 5 or 10 %. Each stimulus set contained the following stimuli: L0H-10%, L0H-5%, 000, H0L-5% and H0L-10%.

The stimuli were generated digitally using an AT PC with a 12 bit D/A-converter (DT2812) at a sampling rate of 10 kHz. They were low-pass filtered at 5 kHz (Difa-filter; 115 dB/oct). The stimulus components were equal in amplitude and added in sinus phase.

The comparison tone was a band-stop filtered pulse. The stop band was either from 300 Hz to 2500 Hz, or from 1000 Hz to 4000 Hz, depending on the stimulus. The purpose of the filter was to prevent overlap from stimulus and comparison tone spectra.

Stimulus and comparison tone were presented at levels of approx. 20 and 12 dB above the masked threshold, respectively. At these levels the two signals were roughly equal in loudness. They were presented against a 20 dB/third-octave pink noise background. The stimulus and comparison tone had smooth rise and fall times of 20 ms and steady state durations of 330 ms. They were presented diotically through Telephonics TDH-49P earphones. The subject was seated in an Ampli-silence sound insulated chamber.

The H0L and L0H stimuli were presented in blocks containing 5 different stimuli. The data of the 000 stimuli were collected during an experiment in which beyond the 000 stimuli, HHH-x% and LLL-x% stimuli (x= 5% or 10%) were used. Within a block, each stimulus was presented twice, giving blocks of 10 trials. One block comprised of stimuli with fixed harmonic numbers, but with 5 different fundamental frequencies, and 4 different patterns of mistuning. The 10 stimuli of a block were presented in random order. All blocks were presented 3 times, except for the {11,12,13} 000 stimulus set, which was presented 6 times.

3 Results

The histograms in Fig. 2 represent the experimental data. The dashed lines in this figure are optimal theoretical fits to be described in section 4. From top to bottom results are given for stimuli with harmonic numbers {3,4,5}, {5,6,7}, {9,10,11} and {11,12,13}. From left to right the results of the different mistuning patterns, L0H-10%, L0H-5%, 000, H0L-5% and H0L-10% are shown. Each histogram contains pooled data for fundamental frequencies from 200 to 300 Hz. Therefore the pitch height of the responses is expressed as the relative deviation from the "f_0" of the stimulus. (The term "f_0" will be used to refer to the f_0 for which the harmonic numbers n_i equal the correct estimates n_i of the harmonic set.) Similar data for the 000-pattern of 3 other subjects have been presented elsewhere (Wiersinga-Post & Duifhuis, 1994).

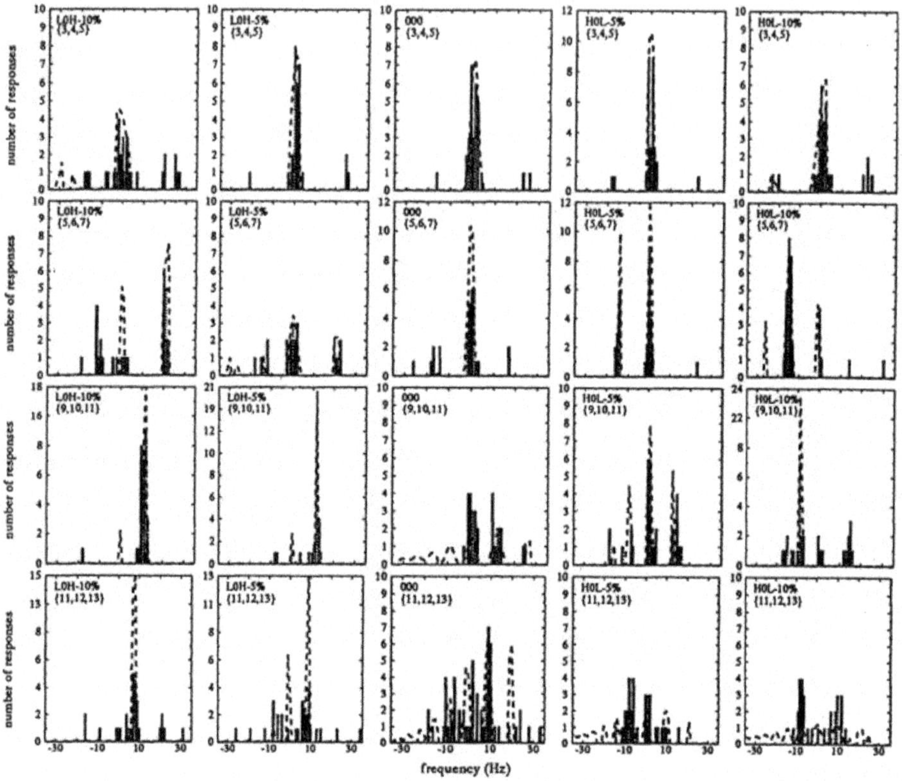

Figure 2. Experimental data (histograms) and theoretical fits (dashed lines). From top to bottom results for sets {3,4,5}, {5,6,7}, {9,10,11} and {11,12,13} are shown. Each row shows data of the different mistuning patterns: L0H-10%, L0H-5%, 000, H0L-5% and H0L-10%.

Considering the harmonic stimuli -the centre column of Fig. 2- it is obvious that pitch becomes increasingly ambiguous with the increase of n_l. The pitch of the "f_0" is by far the most prominent for stimulus sets {3,4,5} and {5,6,7}. Stimulus set {9,10,11} produces a conspicuous pitch sideband at around 12% deviation from "f_0". For stimuli with harmonics {11,12,13} separate pitches are no longer clearly distinguishable.

The L0H and H0L stimuli (columns 1, 2, 4 and 5 of Fig. 2) show that for the {3,4,5} stimuli the pitch of the "f_0" is the most prominent for as well 5% as 10% mistuning. Mistuning of the {5,6,7} stimuli causes an increased pitch ambiguity. The number of responses around "f_0" decreases, while for the H0L stimuli the number of responses at around -15% and for the L0H stimuli the number of responses at around 21% increases. For the L0H stimuli responses are also given at around -12% deviation from "f_0". Thus the pitch ambiguity is higher for the L0H stimuli than for the H0L stimuli. For stimulus sets {9,10,11} this is the other way around; here the pitch ambiguity of the H0L stimuli exceeds the ambiguity of the L0H stimuli. The L0H-10% mistuning of set {11,12,13} causes a decrease of the pitch ambiguity; a relatively large amount of the responses is given at around 8% deviation from "f_0". For the other patterns of mistuning the spread in pitch height of the responses is high, though for the H0L-10% stimuli an increase of the number of responses at around -7% deviation from "f_0" is observed.

4 Discussion

In Figure 2 the experimental results (histograms) are compared to theoretical predictions of the sub-harmonic summation (dashed lines). As a measure of the similarity between experimental and theoretical data, the coherence factor, P_{cr}, related to the correlation coefficient between experimental and theoretical data, is used:

$$P_{cr} = \frac{(\sum_i E(i-x)\cdot \sum_i T(i))^2}{\sum_i E(i-x)^2 \cdot \sum_i T(i)^2} \qquad \begin{array}{l} -45\% < i < 45\%\} \\ x = -1, 0, .. \text{ or } 3\% \\ E(i)\text{: experimental data} \\ T(i)\text{: theoretical predictions} \end{array} \qquad (3)$$

Calculations of sub-harmonics was executed for different discrete values of s and W (s=$10^{-4.0}$, $10^{-3.8}$,.., $10^{-1.0}$, W= 0.1, 0.2, .., 1.5). A third parameter, x, was introduced to correct for possible pitch shifts. The value of x was optimized over the range from -1% to 3% [1% steps]. Finally, a parameter N, indicating the number of contributing components, was optimized: either N= 3 (all components contribute to the sub-harmonic summation), or N= 2 (one component, either n_l or n_{l+1} or n_{l+2}, is excluded from the sub-harmonic summation). Table I shows optimal values for σ, W, x and N and their P_{cr}-values.

Figure 2 shows that a big part of the experimental data are well described by the theoretical predictions. However, in several cases experimental pitch sidebands are reported which are not seen in the theoretical data and vice versa. For example for the {3,4,5} L0H-10% stimuli theoretically unreported pitch sidebands are seen in the experimental data (compare the low P_{cr}-value in table I). It is possible that some of these responses are results of errors. However, the pitch of a complex tone can be determined

	{3,4,5}					{5,6,7}				
	P_{cr}	σ	W	x	N	P_{cr}	σ	W	x	N
L0H-10 %	.54	.025	.5	0	(3)	.63	.006	.1	0	(2)*
L0H-5 %	.90	.010	.7	-1	(3)	.61	.016	.7	0	(3)
000	.79	.016	.2	0	(3)	.76	.010	.1	1	(3)
H0L-5 %	.84	.025	.1	2	(3)	.83	.006	1.5	0	(3)
H0L-10 %	.75	.010	.8	1	(3)	.79	.010	1.0	1	(3)
	{9,10,11 }					{11,12,13 }				
	P_{cr}	σ	W	x	N	P_{cr}	σ	W	x	N
L0H-10 %	.61	.004	.2	0	(3)	.61	.003	.1	2	(3)
L0H-5 %	.88	.004	.1	0	(3)	.35	.004	.5	1	(3)
000	.50	.016	.7	0	(3)	.35	.010	.6	1	(3)
H0L-5 %	.56	.006	.5	0	(3)	.36	.010	.8	0	(3)
H0L-10 %	.60	.001	1.1	0	(3)	.30	.016	.8	0	(3)

Table I. Values of P_{cr}, σ, W, x and N that cause optimal fit between the theoretical results and the experimental data. (2): One harmonic (n_l) is excluded from the sub-harmonic summation. (3): Three components contribute to the sub-harmonic summation.*

by listening to one component of the complex sound (Gerson and Goldstein, 1978; Beerends and Houtsma, 1989). Therefore the responses at around 25% deviation from "f_0", which are also seen for the other mistuning patterns of set {3,4,5}, are probably due to matches to the highest component of the stimulus at 2 octaves below its actual value. It is possible that the same phenomenon caused the unpredicted pitch sidebands of the data of the L0H-10% stimuli of set {5,6,7} and the H0L-10% stimuli of set {9,10,11}. Listening to the highest component of the L0H-10% {5,6,7} complex (3 octaves below its actual value) might have caused the pitch sideband at around -11% deviation from "f_0", while the pitch sideband at around 13% deviation from "f_0" for H0L-10% {9,10,11} might be the result of listening to the lowest component of the stimulus (3 octaves below its actual value). However, interpretation of the {9,10,11} stimulus towards a complex with harmonics {8,9,10} predicts a response at around 11% deviation from "f_0". This means that for the H0L-10% stimuli of set {9,10,11} it remains unclear whether the subject has listened to the whole complex or to one component (the lowest) of the complex tone.

Theoretically predicted pitch sidebands that are not reported experimentally are seen in a number of stimulus sets (e.g.: L0H-10%, {3,4,5}; H0L-10%, {5,6,7}; 000, {9,10,11}; H0L-5% and H0L-10%, {11,12,13}). A possible explanation for this can be that the variance of the experimental data (the width of the pitch sidebands) is not only determined by the noise in the coding of frequency components, but that other factors, e.g., timbre differences between stimulus and comparison tone, play a role (Moore *et al.*, 1992). This would lead to an overestimation of the σ-parameter in the sub-harmonic summation procedure and to an overestimate of the number of pitch sidebands.

The reported differences in pitch ambiguity of the H0L stimuli compared to the L0H stimuli are easily understood for set {5,6,7}. In Fig. 3 it is seen that the H0L-10%

stimulus approaches the n_{i+1} harmonic set, while the harmonics n_l and n_{l+2} of the L0H-10% stimulus lie half-way between the n_i and n_{i-1} harmonic set.

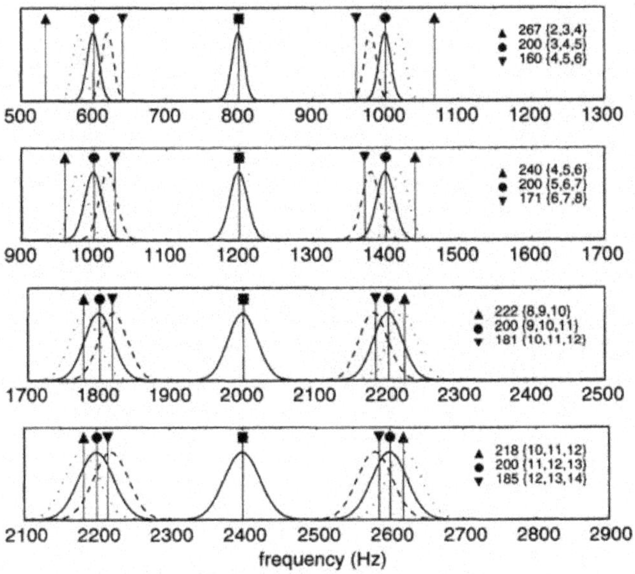

Figure 3. Illustration of stimulus representations and nearest harmonic complexes (n_i=$n_{i\pm 1}$) for stimuli with f_0= 200 Hz. The Gaussian distributions ($\sigma \approx 0.01$) reflect the stimulus representations (dotted lines: L0H-10%, solid lines: 000, dashed lines: H0L-10%). The harmonic complexes are indicated by markers: C *(n_i=n_i-1),* E *(n_i=n_i) and* S *(n_i=n_i+1). The legends in each figure give the fundamental frequencies and harmonic numbers of these complexes.*

For set {9,10,11} the reason for this difference in pitch ambiguity is not immediately clear. Fig. 3 shows that the H0L-10% stimulus fits n_{i+1} at least as well as L0H fits n_{i-1}. Apparently the subject has a tendency to interpret n_i as n_{i-1}. This preference is also well visible in the 000 stimuli of set {9,10,11}. Here a large amount of the responses are given at around 11% deviation from "f_0", for which n_i= n_{i-1}, while no responses are given below "f_0".

For set {11,12,13} the difference in pitch ambiguity between the H0L and L0H stimuli is less clear, but a tendency for interpreting n_i as n_{i-1} is seen in the fact that the total number of responses above "f_0" is higher than the total number of responses below "f_0".

The reason for the preference of interpreting n_i as n_{i-1} for high harmonic order stimuli might be that the timbre of a stimulus containing high harmonic frequency components causes a preference for pitch sidebands above "f_0". Another explanation, that only explains the data for the {9,10,11} stimuli, is that listening to a single edge component in the complex sound might influence the pitch perception. This would lead to a preference for interpreting n_i towards a complex in which one of the edge components has an octave relation with the preferred pitch.

5 Conclusions

The major part of the pitch matching data of the harmonic and inharmonic stimuli is consistent with a spectral pattern recognition model based on the strategy of sub-harmonic summation. In almost all cases best fit between theoretical and experimental data is obtained if the sub-harmonic summation procedure takes all three components into account. However, for a number of inharmonic stimuli and for stimuli of set {3,4,5}, part of the data appears to be based on listening to one of the edge components of the complex sound only.

For high harmonic stimuli there is a tendency of interpreting n_i as n_{i-1}. The sharp timbre of the high harmonic order complexes and/or an octave relation of one of the edge components with the estimated f_0 may be the cause of this phenomenon. This implies that some interesting phenomena of pitch perception are still not understood.

6 References

Beerends, J.G., and Houtsma, A.J.M. (1989). Pitch identification of simultaneous diotic and dichotic two-tone complexes, J. Acoust. Soc. Am. 85, 813-819.

de Boer, E. (1977). Pitch theories unified. In: Psychophysics and Physiology of Hearing. E.F. Evans and J.P. Wilson (Eds.) Academic Press, London, pp. 323-334.

Brown, J.C. (1992). Musical fundamental frequency tracking using a pattern recognition method. J. Acoust. Soc. Am. 92, 1394-1402.

Duifhuis, H., Willems, L.F., and Sluyter, R.J. (1982). Measurement of pitch in speech: An implementation of Goldstein's theory of pitch perception. J. Acoust. Soc. Am. 71, 1568-1580.

Goldstein, J.L. (1973). An optimum processor theory for the central formation of the pitch of complex tones. J. Acoust. Soc. Am. 54, 1496-1516.

Gerson, A., and Goldstein, J.L. (1978). Evidence for a general template in central optimal processing for pitch of complex tones. J. Acoust. Soc. Am. 63, 498-510.

Hermes, D.J. (1988). Measurement of pitch by subharmonic summation. J. Acoust. Soc. Am. 83, 257-264.

Houtsma, A.J.M., and Goldstein, J.L. (1972). The Central Origin of the Pitch of Complex Tones: Evidence from Musical Interval Recognition. J. Acoust. Soc. Am. 51, 520-529.

Houtsma, A.J.M. and Smurzynski, J. (1990). Pitch identification and discrimination for complex tones with many harmonics. J. Acoust. Soc. Am. 87, 304-310.

Moore, B.C.J., Glasberg, B.R., and Proctor, G.M. (1992) Accuracy of pitch matching for pure tones and for complex tones with overlapping or nonoverlapping harmonics. J. Acoust. Soc. Am. 91, 3443-3450.

Noll, A.M. (1964). Short-time spectrum and "cepstrum" techniques for vocal-pitch detection. J. Acoust. Soc. Am. 36, 296-302.

Parsons, T.W. (1976). Separation of speech from interfering speech by means of harmonic selection. J. Acoust. Soc. Am. 60, 911-918.

Ritsma, R.J. (1962). Existence region of the tonal residue. I. J. Acoust. Soc. Am. 34, 1224-1229.

Schroeder, M.R. (1968). Period histogram and product spectrum: New methods for fundamental-frequency measurement. J. Acoust. Soc. Am. 43, 829-834.
Terhardt, E., Stoll, G. and Seewann, M. (1982). Algorithm for extraction of pitch and pitch salience from complex tonal signals. J. Acoust. Soc. Am. 71, 679-688.
Wiersinga-Post, E., and Duifhuis, H. (1994) Probability distributions of the pitch of harmonic and inharmonic three-tone complexes. submitted.
Wightman, F.L. (1973). The pattern-transformation model of pitch. J. Acoust. Soc. Am. 54, 407-416.

Comment by J.W. Horst

It is intriguing that many of your values for σ are about an order of magnitude larger than the just noticeable frequency difference for pure tones. Can you speculate on the relation between σ and the jnd_f?

Reply

Measuring the jnd_f for pure tones is fundamentally different from measuring the pitch of the missing fundamental, in this aspect, that in the latter task a spectral pattern recognition process is needed, which compares information from different auditory channels, while for discriminating between pure tones information within one auditory channel can be used (see also: Goldstein, 1973).

Related comment by J.W. Horst

Do you agree that the jnd_f provides a lower boundary for σ.f?

Reply

Yes.

Complex spectral analysis

Shape discrimination of spectra with various bandwidths

David M. Green, Huanping Dai, and Kourosh Saberi

Psychoacoustics Laboratory, Department of Psychology
University of Florida, Gainesville, Florida 32611, U. S. A.

1 Introduction

In what we call 'profile' experiments, the listener's task is to discriminate between two sounds that differ in spectral shape (Green, 1988). One sound is the standard; the other sound is the signal plus standard. The standard sound often has a flat power spectrum with equal energy per logarithmic frequency unit (equal energy per octave). The signal-plus-standard sound is created by adding energy to some region of the standard spectrum. The sounds are pulsed on for a short duration; 100 to 500 ms is typical. In the earlier experiments, the spectra were collections of sinusoidal components which extended over several octaves in frequency. The power spectrum of the sounds, not the temporal waveforms, is clearly the critical stimulus quantity, because the same thresholds are obtained if the phase for each component is randomly chosen on each presentation (Green and Mason, 1985).

The sounds to be discriminated are presented in random order in two intervals of a forced-choice test. The listener is asked to select the interval containing the signal-plus-standard sound. Each sound is presented at a random level, chosen from a rectangular distribution; the range of the distribution is typically around 20 dB. This variation in overall level discourages the listener from attempting to discriminate between the two sounds on the basis of a *successive* comparison of absolute level in any frequency region. Rather, a *simultaneous* level comparison of different frequency regions within the same spectrum must be made to achieve good discrimination between the two spectra. These spectral discriminations share many essential features with the recognition of a speech utterance, in that the information needed for the discrimination is contained within a single sound presentation, and the phase spectrum is largely irrelevant.

In this paper, we argue that the detection of spectral changes relies on different auditory processes or cues, depending on the bandwidth of the spectrum. That different cue systems must be involved became apparent from the studies of Gilkey (1987) and Kidd (1987). They were the first to present evidence that the sensitivity to changes in spectral shape was not severely impaired if the bandwidth of the sound was greatly reduced. Sensitivity was best for spectra several octaves in width, but it decreased only slightly as the bandwidth of the spectrum was reduced to a few Hertz. The important stimulus quantity is the bandwidth of the spectrum compared to the width of the critical band. A *wide* spectrum extends over more than two critical bands. A *medium* spectrum encompasses one-half to two bands at most. A *narrow* spectrum is less than half the width of one critical band. Because the size of the critical band changes with center frequency, the number of critical bands encompassed by a fixed-bandwidth sound will change with center frequency. The majority of our research has employed spectra with center frequencies of about 1000 Hz, so most of what we will discuss is limited to that frequency. Recently, we began exploring spectra with very high frequency components, some extending above 8000 Hz. The results obtained with these high-frequency spectra are perplexing, and will be presented after our review of the three different cue systems.

2 Wide-Band Spectra

Much of our earlier work on the discrimination of spectral shape involved multitonal complexes that extended over many critical bands. We argued that discrimination of a change in the shape of such spectra involved a simultaneous measurement of the intensity level at different frequency regions of the spectrum and a subsequent comparison of those levels (Green, 1983). Such level comparisons were certainly possible, because the components of the spectrum fell into different critical bands. Each band could then provide an estimate of the level in its frequency region that was largely independent of the estimate provided at some different critical band. The channel model of Durlach, Braida, and Ito (1986) provided a quantitative analysis of such a process, and derived the optimum decision rule for the typical profile experiment. The optimum decision rule has a very simple form when the internal noise (they call it peripheral noise) associated with each channel is much smaller than the random changes in overall level. Because the peripheral noise is about 1-2 dB whereas the change in overall level, an essential control in the profile experiment, is about 20 dB, these conditions are often met. Under these conditions, the optimum decision rule is to compare the level measured in the signal channel with the average level of all the nonsignal channels. Thus, if *m* components make up the standard and the signal is an increment in one component, then the optimal decision statistic, z, is of the following form

$$z = L_s - \frac{1}{(m-1)} \sum_{i \neq s}^{m} L_i \qquad \text{Eq. 1}$$

where L_s is the level estimated in the signal channel and L_i is the level estimated in the nonsignal channels. There are m-1 such nonsignal channels. This decision statistic, z, should be near zero if the standard alone is presented and a large positive value if the signal is added to the standard. Note that such a decision statistic is not influenced by the random changes in overall intensity level, because the value of z remains the same if the levels of all components are changed by the same amount. Berg and Green (1990) used the COSS (Conditional On a Single Stimulus) procedure to estimate the weights used by listeners in an auditory profile task. COSS, developed by Berg (1989), is a new procedure used to assess the weight that an observer allocates to different components of the stimulus in a discrimination task. For a spectrum extending between 200 and 5000 Hz and containing 5, 7, or 11 components, the estimated weights were very close to the values given by Eq. 1.

While not disputing the mechanism suggested for these wide-band spectra, the research of Gilkey (1987) and Kidd (1987) raised serious questions about the generality of these results. They systematically varied the bandwidth of the spectrum from the more than five-octave range used in the research reported above to a total range of only a few Hertz (much less than 1/3 octave). Despite this enormous change in bandwidth, the threshold for detecting spectral change increased only slightly at the very small bandwidths. Clearly, with such narrow-band spectra it is impossible to make independent estimates of the levels of the different components, because they all fall within the same critical band. Other mechanisms must be responsible for the ability to hear spectral changes in these narrower spectra.

3 Medium-Width Spectra

Berg, Nguyen, and Green (1992) suggested that for spectra about the width of a critical band the detection of spectral change might be based on a pitch cue. Feth and Stover (1987) were the first to argue that profile analysis might be based on a pitch cue. They applied this idea to spectra extending over several octaves in frequency using the pitch values computed from the envelope-weighted average of the instantaneous frequency (EWAIF). They investigated a variety of conditions, and computed the change in pitch between the standard and signal-plus-standard sounds that were just discriminable. If this idea were successful, then the pitch change should be the same for all conditions. Instead, the changes in pitch value were widely different for the three-component spectra, and only moderately constant for multi-component spectra. The constant value, however, was an order of magnitude larger than what one might expect for a pure-tone stimulus. Richards, Onsan, and Green (1989) showed that a pitch change could not be an important cue for detecting changes in the shape of wide-band spectra because randomizing the rate of the digital-to-analog converter produced little change in threshold.

Berg et al. (1992) used three-tone complexes. The components were all of equal level in the standard sound, and the central component was increased in level to produce the signal-plus-standard sound. The phase of the three components was chosen at random on each presentation, so that the temporal structure of the waveform was unimportant. Because EWAIF calculations are phase dependent, it is better to use the newer procedures to calculate the pitch of a complex sound. These new procedures are called IWAIF (Anantharaman, Krishnamurthy, and Feth, 1993) for intensity or SEWAIF (Dai, 1993) for squared-envelope weighted average of the instantaneous frequency. The chief advantage of these new procedures is that the calculated pitch of a complex narrow-band spectrum is influenced only by the power spectrum of the sound, and is independent of the phase spectrum. Thus, details of the fine structure of the wave are unimportant, and the calculated pitch value is exactly equal to the center of gravity (centroid) of the power spectrum when plotted on a linear frequency scale.

The problem with the theory that pitch mediates the detection of changes in spectral shape is that if the three components are close enough in frequency to fall within the same critical band, then the spectrum is nearly symmetrical in linear frequency. The pitch of such a symmetric spectrum is simply the frequency of the central component of the complex, and it does not change when the central component is altered in level, because that does not change the symmetry. So how can changing the intensity of the central component induce a pitch change? Berg et al. argued that the listeners based their judgments on the output of a critical band whose center frequency was located at some distance from the central frequency of the complex. Such off-frequency listening (Leshowitz and Wightman, 1971) is known to occur when it will benefit the detection of a signal. In the present case, the advantage is that the spectrum at the output of the filter will be tilted, and thus highly asymmetric, if the critical band is sufficiently remote. For example, if the center frequency of the off-frequency critical-band filter is considerably above the central frequency of the complex, then the lowest frequency tone will be greatly attenuated compared to the central and highest frequency tone. The signal-plus-standard spectrum, by increasing the intensity level of the central component, would lower the center of gravity of the spectrum, and thus decrease the pitch.

Evidence for the existence of such a pitch-detection process was obtained from the COSS weights estimated from the different listeners in this task. For the wider spectra, the weights were nearly -0.5, 1, and -0.5, as would be expected on the basis of Eq. 1. For the narrower spectra, the pattern of COSS weights was quite different. Generally, one edge component had a weight of -1, the weight of the other edge was near zero, and the weight of the central component was about +0.5. The actual pattern of weights depended on the direction of the pitch cue reported by the listener. If the listener said the signal-plus-standard spectrum produced a higher pitch than the standard alone, then the lowest component had a weight near -1. If the listener reported a lower pitch, then the highest component had a weight near -1. Such differences in the direction of the pitch shift can be explained by assuming that the off-frequency critical band was located either above or below the central frequency of the complex. If the off-frequency band were above the center frequency of the complex, the level of the components would systematically increase with frequency. If the off-frequency band were below the frequency of the complex, the level of the components would systematically decrease with frequency. Raising the level of the middle component would in both cases change the pitch, decreasing it in one case and raising it in the other. For the three tones spaced at 920, 1000, and 1080 Hz, two of the four listeners said that the standard was lower in pitch than the signal-plus-standard spectrum, while the other two said the reverse.

While such a mechanism is a plausible account of the detection process for medium bandwidth spectra, it cannot operate for very narrow spectra. For narrow spectra, the components are so close in frequency that off-frequency listening would not produce any noticeable tilt in the spectrum at the output of the critical band. The output spectrum would be nearly symmetric for either an on- or off-frequency critical band. The center of gravity of such a symmetric spectrum, and hence the pitch, will not be appreciably altered by changing the central component of the spectrum. Another mechanism must be proposed to account for the remarkably good detection observed with these narrow-band spectra.

4 Narrow-Band Spectra

Narrow-band spectra have bandwidths less than half the width of a critical band. Investigators have employed spectra that are only a small fraction of the width of a critical band, for example, extending ±10 Hz about 1000 Hz. We have argued (Green, Berg, Dai, Eddins, Onsan, and Nguyen 1992) that the detection of changes in the power spectra of such narrow-band sounds is based on changes in the power spectrum of the envelope. Such detection can be accomplished even if the phases of the components that comprise the spectrum are chosen at random on each presentation. The power spectrum of the envelope of a narrow-band random process was first derived by Lawson and Uhlenbeck (1950). For audio power spectra that are rectangular in shape, such as noise or equal-amplitude sinusoids, the power spectrum of the ac part of the envelope is nearly triangular, having a base equal to the bandwidth of the audio power spectrum. Alteration in the flat audio spectrum changes the power spectrum of the envelope in different manners, depending on how the audio spectrum is altered. Figure 1 shows the envelope power spectrum of a standard, equal-amplitude audio power spectrum (solid line) and the evelope power spectrum of three different signal-plus-standard audio spectra (dotted line). In the three panels of Figure 1, a signal is added to the central component of the standard, to one end of the spectrum, or to both ends of the spectrum. In these examples, the signal component(s) is always 5 dB above the level of the other components.

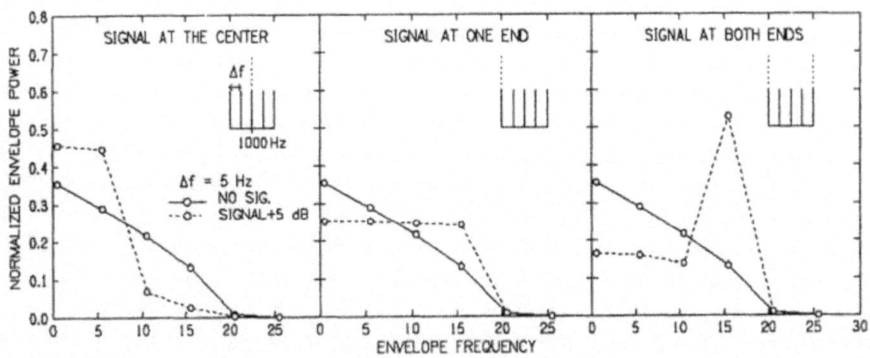

Figure 1. Average envelope power spectra for various audio spectra.

We stress again that these changes in the envelope power spectrum are averaged over different phases for the components of the audio complex, which, of course, produce different envelope waveforms. We argue that envelope power spectra that have a preponderance of low-frequency energy are heard as smooth (see left panel of Fig. 1). If the envelope power spectrum is nearly flat or has a peak at some higher frequency (see middle and right panels of Fig. 1), then the perception is of a rough envelope. In Green et al. (1992), discrimination experiments were conducted to determine the basis for discriminating between these various narrow-band spectra. The results suggest that the discrimination is based on a single, unidimensional cue system, such as the rough-smooth dimension just discussed.

5 Summary

In short, we believe that discriminating changes in spectral shape, profile analysis, depends on three different auditory processes. Each process is most appropriate for a given range of spectral bandwidth. For wide-band spectra extending over several critical bands, the detection mechanism is a simultaneous comparison of the level of different critical bands, such as that suggested in Eq. 1. For medium-band spectra, the detection mechanism is a change in pitch. This pitch value is computed at the output of a critical band located in a frequency region displaced from the central frequency of the sound. The pitch will increase or decrease when the signal is added to the standard spectrum, depending on whether the critical band is above or below the frequency region of the sound's spectrum. For narrow-band spectra, the detection mechanism is a change in the power spectrum of the envelope of the sound. The relative frequency content of the power spectrum of the envelope determines whether the sound is heard as smooth or rough. The sensitivity of all three mechanisms is very similar. Each allows a listener to detect an alteration of about 1-3 dB in the power spectrum of any sound, with changes in a wide-band spectrum being somewhat easier to detect.

6 Shape Discrimination of High-Frequency Spectra

One obvious application of the ability to discriminate changes in the power spectrum of the stimulus is to localize sounds in space. The locus of points in the sagittal plane defines what has been called a 'cone of confusion,' because the interaural differences of time and intensity are nearly the same on this cone. Disambiguating different loci on this cone can be aided by the differential filtering of the head-related transfer function. The received spectrum of a wide-band source changes as we vary the position of the source in the sagittal plane, especially for frequencies above 6 kHz. Three experiments have been conducted to measure the ability of listeners to hear changes in spectral shape at these frequencies. The results are puzzling, and more experiments are being planned. The following is a progress report on these efforts.

The goal of the first experiment was to compare the listener's ability to discriminate spectral shape in different frequency regions. Three-tone spectra with medium bandwidths were varied in center frequency f_c from 250 to 16,000 Hz. For a given center frequency, the lower and higher frequencies were $f_c/1.38$ and $1.38{\cdot}f_c$. Thus, all three components presumably fell into different critical bands. For the standard spectrum, all three components were equal in level. The median level of the standard complex was 60 dB SPL per component, and the overall level of the complex was chosen from a rectangular distribution with a 20-dB range. In the signal-plus-standard spectrum, the level of the center component was increased relative to the other two components by adding, in-phase, a component to the central component of the standard. The threshold for this added signal was determined in a two-alternative forced-choice task using an adaptive two-down one-up procedure whose equilibrium point is 70.7 % correct. The threshold values are reported as the ratio of the added signal to the standard component in decibel, 20 log (Δp/p).

Because of the problem of standing waves at the higher frequencies, the experiments were conducted using three different sound transducers: (1) a conventional headphone (Sennheiser Headphone, HD-450), (2) an insert earphone (Etymotic ER-2), and (3) a sound delivered through a long (5 meter) lossy plastic tube with a diameter of about 1 cm. The subjects listened binaurally with the phones in phase for the conventional headphone. For the other conditions, the listening was monaural. The long lossy tube provides a nearly perfect impedance match at the entrance of the ear canal, and, by decreasing reflections at this point minimizes changes in pressure level as a function of frequency at the eardrum (Zhou and Green, 1994). For some of the higher frequency conditions, some nonlinear distortion products were audible, thus for $f_c > 5$ kHz, a lowpass noise band was used extending below 4 kHz, and having a spectrum level of 24 dB.

Figure 2 shows the mean results obtained with three normal-hearing subjects. The signal-to-standard ratio at threshold is plotted as a function of the center frequency f_c. The circles represent the thresholds obtained with the conventional headphones, the triangles with the insert phone, and the squares with the long tube (two subjects). The results obtained with the three transducers are nearly the same. Profile discrimination of the three-tone complex deteriorates markedly once the center frequency is above about 5000 Hz. When the signal level is very large, it is possible that the discrimination is based on differences in overall level measured successively in the two intervals. In that case, the level of the signal-plus-standard spectrum will reliably exceed the level of the standard spectrum, despite the 20-dB randomization of presentation level. The dotted line shows the threshold value achievable for an ideal detector listening to only changes in overall level during the two intervals of the forced-choice task. Many of the measured thresholds exceed this level. We interpret this to mean that the listeners continued to listen for the simultaneous changes in spectral shape, even when the successive differences between overall level provided a potentially stronger cue. No attempt was made to instruct the observers to listen to the successive changes in overall level.

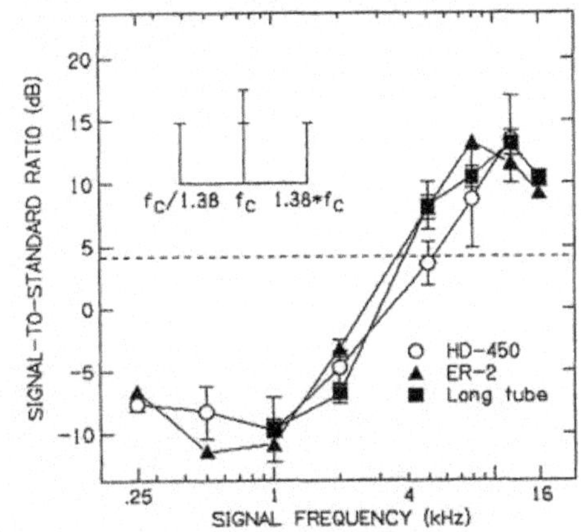

Figure 2. Profile discrimination for a 3-tone complex.

Two more experiments were conducted in the free field, which provides an experimental setting very similar to that used to study sound localization. In the first free-field experiment, we used a stimulus similar to that used in the headphone experiment, except that the number of components was increased from three to seven. The seven components were spaced in frequency at equal intervals on a logarithmic scale extending from 2327 to 16,000 Hz. Each of the seven components was set at a constant sensation level based on absolute threshold measurements for each individual listener. The median sensation level of the entire complex was about 60 dB, and the overall level was randomly varied ± 5 dB about that level.

Figure 3 presents data for this experiment. Each symbol represents data for a single listener. The dotted line again represents the performance possible for an ideal observer listening only to successive changes in absolute level. The observed thresholds nearly always exceed these levels. These data are similar to those obtained in the earlier headphone experiments. The general result is that listeners are not able to hear changes in the spectral shape of a multiple component complex at the higher frequencies. In the speech range, listeners can hear 1-dB changes in the intensity of a single component of a seven-component complex. At the higher frequencies, a change of over 20 dB is needed in some cases for the same detection accuracy.

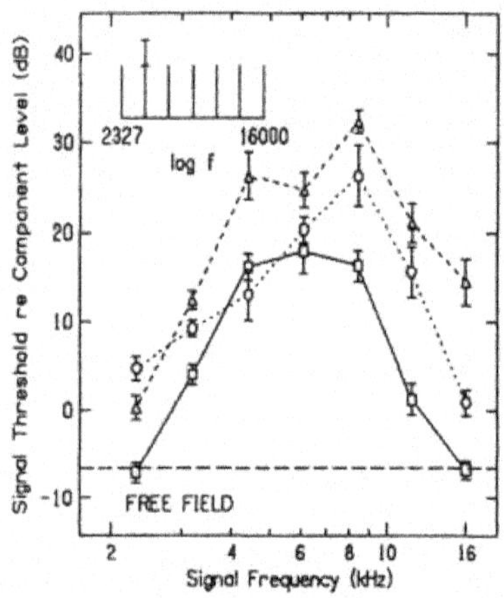

Figure 3. Profile discrimination at different frequencies of a 7-tone complex.

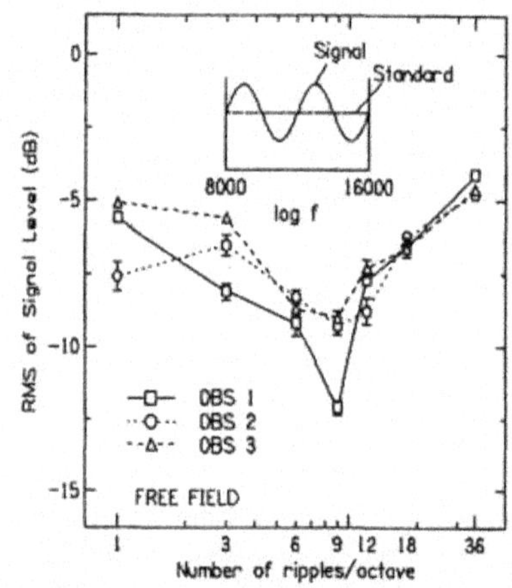

Figure 4. Profile discrimination with rippled noise at different ripple frequencies.

In the second free-field experiment, a very different stimulus was used to measure the ability to hear changes in spectral shape--what we call a rippled-noise stimulus. A nearly continuous spectrum was employed that sounded noise-like rather than tonal. The standard spectrum contained many equal-amplitude components spaced in frequency 6.25 Hz apart (the reciprocal of the duration). The phase of each component was randomized for each presentation. The components extended in frequency over the range from 8 to

16 kHz. The change in spectral shape was created by imposing a sinusoidal ripple on that flat spectrum. The ripple was sinusoidal on a logarithmic frequency scale. The phase of that ripple was randomized on each presentation to discourage detection based on the absolute level of the spectrum in any frequency region. The size of the ripple was adjusted adaptively in a three-down one-up forced-choice procedure, which produces an equilibrium point of 79.4% correct. We can think of the signal-plus-standard spectrum as the addition of a set of 'signal' components to the standard spectrum. Each 'signal' component is either in- or out-of-phase with the corresponding component in the standard spectrum, thus producing an increase or decrease in the level at that frequency. The threshold can be expressed as the rms of this 'signal' compared to the rms level of the standard components. The loudspeaker was digitally equalized to produce a standard having a flat amplitude spectrum, as measured with a sound level meter (Bruel and Kjaer Model 1613) located at the position of the listener in the sound-attenuated chamber.

Figure 4 shows discriminability data for this rippled-noise stimulus. The ordinate is the threshold rms signal-to-standard ratio in decibels. The abscissa is the number of ripples per octave. All three listeners were able to discriminate changes in the spectral shape of this noise-like stimulus. The listeners reported hearing a difference in the quality of the noise similar to that heard with noise that is time delayed and added to itself (comb filtering). The best detection occurred with about nine ripples per octave. These results are similar to those obtained for similar stimuli at the lower frequencies, except that those studies found that the best detection occurred with about three ripples per octave (Hillier, 1991; Green, 1993). Also the lowest threshold value was about -23 dB, at least for wideband spectra, 100-6400 Hz.

These results of the rippled-noise experiment are quite unlike the results obtained with the three- or seven-component complexes. For multi-tonal complexes, 30-dB changes in the level of individual components were sometimes inaudible. The reason for these differences in sensitivity changes in spectral shape at the high frequencies is not understood, and further experiments are planned to probe these very different findings.

7 Acknowledgments

This research was supported by grants from the National Institutes of Health and from the Air Force Office of Scientific Research. We thank Dr. J. Middlebrooks for the use of the free-field room in his laboratory. We also thank Drs. B. Wright and D. Eddins for their comments on an earlier draft of this paper.

8 References

Anantharaman, J. N., Krishnamurthy, A. K. and Feth, L. L. (1993) Intensity weighted average of instantaneous frequency as a model for frequency discrimination. J. Acoust. Soc. Am., 94, 723-729.

Berg, B. G. (1989) Analysis of weights in multiple observation tasks. J. Acoust. Soc. Am., 86, 1743-1746.

Berg, B. G. and Green, D. M. (1990) Spectral weights in profile listening. J. Acoust. Soc. Am., 88, 758-766.

Berg, B. G., Nguyen, Q., and Green, D. M. (1992) Discrimination of narrow-band spectra: I. Spectral weights and pitch cues. J. Acoust. Soc. Am., 92, 1911-1918.

Dai, H. (1993) On the pitch of two-tone complexes. J. Acoust. Soc. Am., 94, 730-734.

Durlack, N. I., Braida, L. D., and Ito, Y. (1986) Toward a model for discrimination of broadband signals. J. Acoust. Soc. Am., 80, 63-72.

Feth, L. L. and Stover, L. J. (1987) Demodulation processes in auditory perception, in Auditory Processing of Complex Sounds, edited by W. A. Yost and C. S. Watson (Erlbaum, Hillsdale,NJ), 76-86.

Gilkey, R. H. (1987) Spectral and temporal comparisons in auditory masking, in Auditory Processing of Complex Sounds, edited by W. A. Yost and C. S. Watson (Erlbaum, Hillsdale, NJ) 26-36.

Green, D. M. (1988) Profile Analysis: Auditory Intensity Discrimination (Oxford U. P., New York).

Green, D. M. (1983) Profile analysis: a different view of auditory intensity discrimination. Am. Psychologist, 38, 133-142.

Green, D. M. (1993) Detecting changes in spectral shape of complex auditory signals: Profile Analysis. Invited paper at the 125th meeting: Acoustical Society of America, J. Acoust. Soc. Am., 93, 2294.

Green, D. M., Berg, B. G., Dai, H., Eddins, D. A., Onsan, Z. A., and Nguyen, Q. T. (1992) Spectral shape discrimination of narrow-band sounds. J. Acoust. Soc. Am., 92, 2586-2597.

Green, D. M. and Mason, C. R. (1985) Auditory profile analysis: Frequency, phase, and Weber's Law. J. Acoust. Soc. Am., 77, 1155-1161.

Hillier, D. A. (1991) Auditory processing of sinusoidal spectral envelopes. Dissertation, Sever Institute of Technology, Washington University, St. Louis, Missouri.

Kidd, G. Jr. (1987). The effects of amplitude perturbations on spectral shape, in Auditory Processing of Complex Sounds, edited by W. A. Yost and C. S. Watson, (Erlbaum, Hillsdale, NJ) 26-36.

Kidd, G. Jr., Mason, C. R., Brantley, M. A., and Owen, G. A. (1989) Roving-level tone-in-noise detection. J. Acoust. Soc. Am., 86, 1310-1317.

Lawson, J. L. and Uhlenbeck, G. E. (1950) Threshold Signals (McGraw-Hill, New York).

Leshowitz, B. and Wightman, F. L. (1971) On-frequency masking with continuous sinusoids. J. Acoust. Soc. Am., 49, 1180-1190.

Richards, V. M., Onsan, Z. A., and Green, D. M. (1989) Auditory profile analysis: Potential pitch cues. Hearing Research, 39, 27-36.

Zhou, B. and Green, D. M. (1994) Effect of standing waves on high-frequency threshold. Submitted for publication in J. Acoust. Soc. Am.

Comment by P.W.J. van Hengel

As you showed in figure 4 of your manuscript, your subjects have a threshold minimum for detection of rippled noise at a ripple frequency of about 9 ripples per octave. If this ripple frequency is "translated" to distance along the cochlea using an exponential place-frequency map it corresponds to a periodic spatial distribution with a periodic of approximately 0.4 mm. As I have shown in my presentation (van Hengel, this volume) this distance follows from our cochlea model as an ideal separation of SOAE's that is also found in measurements.

Do you think there might be a relationship between the phenomena?

Reply

This is an interesting speculation. Unfortunately the common finding at *lower* frequencies (f < 8000) is that the minimum occurs at 3 ripples per octave rather than 9 ripples per octave, for example Hillier (1991) and Green (1993).

In short, for there to be a real relationship, the periodic spatial distribution should be *wider* at lower frequency regions of the cochlea - which is inconsistent with SOAE data.

Auditory communication in Japanese macaques: Salience of acoustic stimulus features

David B. Moody, Colleen M. Garbe, and Andrew J. Niemiec

Kresge Hearing Research Institute, University of Michigan Medical School, Ann Arbor, Michigan 48109, USA

1 Introduction

When animals communicate vocally, certain elements of the signals convey relevant information while variation in other elements may represent random or individual-specific differences that are irrelevant to information transfer. One challenge in understanding nonhuman acoustic communication systems is to determine which stimulus features are relevant; that is, to what does the animal attend in deciding the "meaning" of a particular signal. One technique for attempting to infer call function has been to observe the animals in their natural surroundings and to attempt to correlate particular vocalizations with the social contexts in which they occur. Perhaps the best example of the use of this technique is the work of Green (1975) on the vocal communication system of the Japanese macaque (*Macaca fuscata*). Based on his field observations and on spectrographic analysis of the calls, Green demonstrated strong correlations between the acoustic structure of various call classes and the social context in which they occurred.

Two of Green's call classes are the smooth-early-high (SEH) coos, given primarily by juvenile individuals out of visual contact with troop members, and the smooth-late-high (SLH) coos, given by estrous females seeking mates. These calls are distinguished by the temporal position within the call of a rising-to-falling frequency transition, and the calls can be viewed as existing along a continuum of time of occurrence of this frequency transition. These calls have been extensively studied in our laboratory and by others (for a review of these studies, see Moody et al., 1990). We have shown that Japanese monkeys 1) learn discriminations based on the SEH-SLH distinction more rapidly than do heterospecific control animals, 2) show a right-ear advantage in making the discriminations implying left-hemisphere processing (verified in cortical lesioning studies by Heffner and Heffner (1986; see also Heffner and Heffner, 1990)), 3) show perceptual constancy for novel examples of the calls, 4) show categorical perception along the call continuum, and 5) classify the calls based on the patterns of frequency modulation in the call. All of these findings indicate perceptual specializations that suggest communicative relevance. For the most part, these findings were based on paradigms in which subjects were trained to make a behavioral response to one call class and to withhold responding to the other class.

The statistical technique of multidimensional scaling (MDS), as applied to the study of complex stimulus perception in animals by Dooling (1987) and others, offers the potential advantage of demonstrating perceptual groupings of communication signals without requiring explicit differential training between signal classes. Instead, these procedures require subjects to discriminate every test signal from every other signal, with the assumption being made that signals drawn from different functional categories will be more readily discriminated and that this relative increase in discriminability will result in the calls being grouped together by the MDS procedure. The experiments reported here used MDS procedures to determine the extent to which macaque monkeys would demonstrate perceptual groupings of these call classes that corresponded to the groupings derived by Green (1975). To the extent that the stimuli were not grouped according to the original classification, the experiments also allowed determination of other acoustic features that may have influenced stimulus grouping.

2 Methods

Three macaque monkeys (two *Macaca fuscata* and one *Macaca nemestrina*) were trained using positive reinforcement techniques in a standard hold-release procedure to make a reporting response whenever a repeating auditory stimulus, the standard, changed to a different stimulus (a comparison). The subjects had no previous experimental history with vocalizations. Stimuli were presented at a rate of one every 2 seconds. The dependent variable measured was the latency between the onset of the comparison stimulus and the reporting response.

Seven training stimuli, three SEH and four SLH coos, were used in the experiment. These stimuli were digitized from Green's (1975) field recordings and were drawn from the same stimuli we had used in previous experiments (Moody et al., 1990). The stimuli were selected to be similar in duration and were adjusted to have equal overall RMS levels. For determinations of the effects of variation in stimulus parameters on MDS groupings, synthetic stimuli were used. To generate these stimuli, which were based on the natural calls, Fourier analysis was used to generate power spectra at multiple time points in each call. From these spectra, frequency-time and amplitude-time contours were determined for each of the four most prominent harmonics. The frequency-time contours were then used as input to a software-implemented voltage-controlled oscillator (SIGNAL Software Package, Engineering Design, Belmont, MA). The resulting time-domain waveforms, one for each harmonic, were then multiplied by the corresponding amplitude-time waveform to produce a signal that had the same frequency and amplitude contours as the original harmonic. This procedure was repeated for each of the four harmonics, and the resulting waveforms were added to produce a four-harmonic complex. Component phase was ignored. These complexes sounded, to human observers, extremely similar to the original field recordings, with the exception of the elimination of background noise. Stimulus manipulation was carried out by modifying the amplitude contours in various ways before resynthesis.

For a given set of determinations, each stimulus was paired 20 times with every other stimulus as both a standard and a comparison. Acquisition of the necessary number of trials usually required two or more sessions. The median latency for each of these sets of 20 pairings was determined and, after a log transformation, was entered as a similarity estimate into a multidimensional scaling procedure (SINDSCAL, Bell Labs; see Kruskal & Wish, 1978). In the present experiments, "similarity" was defined as stimulus pairs that resulted in long response latencies, while "difference" resulted in shorter latencies. Multiple sets of latency determinations were obtained for each set of stimuli, and all sets in which the requirements of the MDS procedure were met were used to produce the stimulus-space solutions.

One output produced by the multidimensional scaling procedure is a stimulus-space mapping. In such mappings, stimuli judged to be similar are grouped close together, while those judged to be different are grouped apart. The SINDSCAL procedure attempts to determine a spatial arrangement of stimuli that accounts for as much of the variance as possible, with the first dimension accounting for the most variance, the second dimension accounting for the second greatest amount of variance, and so on. Although MDS solutions of greater than two dimensions account for more of the variance in the data sets, the two-dimensional solutions proved adequate for the studies reported here.

3 Results and Discussion

All subjects produced MDS stimulus spaces, such as that shown in Figure 1, in which "good" SEH stimuli were grouped separately from "good" SLH stimuli, where "goodness" is defined in terms of the acoustic properties of the stimulus. Space restrictions prevent us from presenting all of the MDS stimulus space plots, but an effort will be made to describe similarities and differences between them. Two of the subjects, one *fuscata* and one *nemestrina*, produced stimulus spaces in which the early/late distinction generally corresponded to dimension 1, while for the remaining *fuscata*, that

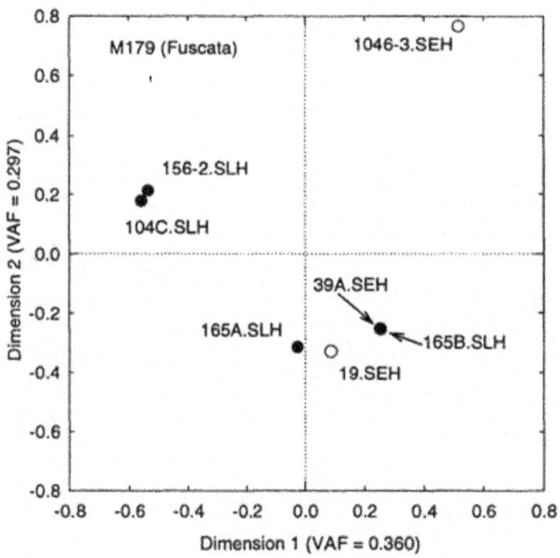

Figure 1. MDS Stimulus space from subject M179 for natural stimuli. It is assumed that stimuli that are perceived as similar to each other are grouped together in this space. "Good" SLH stimuli, such as 104C and 156-2, are to the left of dimension 1 and "Good" SEH stimuli, such as 1046-3, are to the right. For this subject, SEH 39A and SLH 165B occupy the same position in two-dimensional space. The variance accounted for by each dimension is indicated in the axis labels.

distinction corresponded to dimension 2. However, the MDS stimulus spaces for all subjects exhibited similar groupings of the calls. SLH calls 156-2 and 104C were always grouped together, and SEH 1046-3 was placed in a position well removed from the SLH calls. The lack of a species difference in the MDS spaces was somewhat surprising given our previous findings on species differences in learning the discrimination.

Although some of the stimuli were grouped as was predicted according to temporal position of the frequency inflection, other stimuli were positioned in the stimulus space in locations suggesting that they were confused with members of the other call class. For example, SLH calls 165A and 165B were frequently grouped in the vicinity of SEH call 19. These "misplaced" stimuli are particularly interesting to examine and may provide some insights into the communicatively relevant features of the calls. SLH 165B was the call that was most often placed near one or more of the SEH calls. Figure 2A illustrates the frequency-time contours for the four most prominent harmonics of this call. The

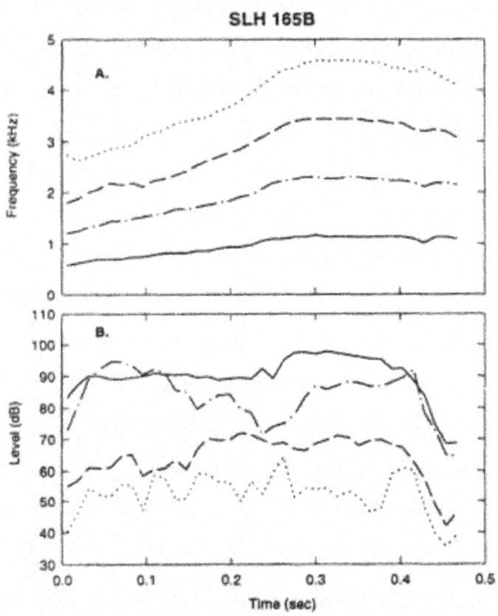

Figure 2. Frequency (A) and level (B) as a function of time for four harmonics of SLH 165B. The frequency-time plot resembles a conventional spectrogram with all level information removed.

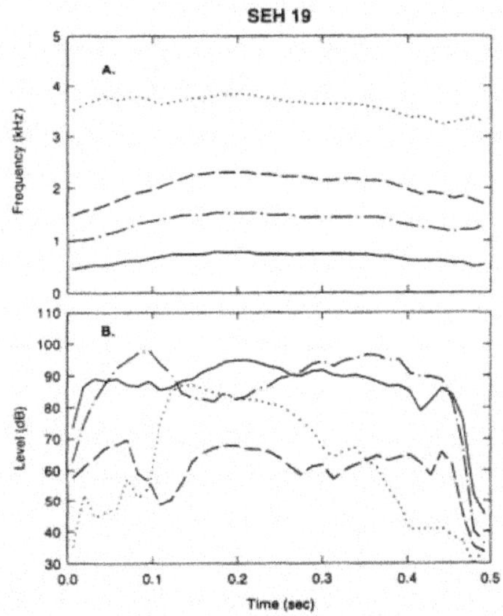

Figure 3. Frequency (A) and level (B) as a function of time for four harmonics of SEH 19. In this call, the most prominent harmonics are the first, second, third and fifth. The non-harmonic relationship of the early portion of the highest frequency component represents a failure of the algorithm used to track the energy peaks. Such anomolies were corrected before resynthesis of the calls.

amount of modulation in the frequency contours is greater than that in most calls, and the position of the frequency peak clearly qualifies it as a member of the SLH class. One hypothesis that may explain the anomalous grouping of this call is illustrated in Figure 2B which shows the levels for each of the harmonics as a function of time. Early in this call, call, the level of the second harmonic becomes greater than that of the other harmonics. If the subjects attend to the loudest harmonic at any point in time, then the maximum frequency is perceived at the point early in the call at which this increase in second harmonic amplitude occurs, thereby resulting in the perception of an SEH.

All three of the subjects grouped SLH 165A in the vicinity of SLH 165B and SEH 19 in MDS stimulus space. SLH 165A contains much less frequency modulation than SLH 165B, but early in the call there is an increase in the level of the second harmonic above that of the first, suggesting again that relative harmonic amplitude may influence perceived call similarity.

Call 19, shown in Figure 3, was the SEH that was most frequently placed by the MDS analysis in close proximity to SLH calls. This call contains a moderate amount of frequency modulation, with the frequency inflection point occurring at a time point about one third of the way through the call. Based purely on the frequency contours, this call might be expected to be an ideal example of the SEH class. Again, as with SLH calls 165A and 165B, an increase occurs in relative level of the second harmonic above that of the first, but in this example, the increase occurs in two places, once early in the call and once toward the end of the call. Applying the hypothesis that the animals are attending to the most dominant frequency, the early amplitude increase should not cause the call to be inappropriately classified, since it would tend to emphasize the early frequency inflection. The second amplitude increase, however, might be perceived as a high frequency late in the call, which could explain the ambiguous classification of the call by all subjects. It is tempting to interpret the MDS results as suggesting that the subjects may be categorizing this call as neither SEH nor SLH. There is, in fact, a call in the repertoire of Japanese macaques, the smooth-dip-high, that is characterized by frequency peaks both early and late in the call.

The remaining call, SEH 39A, was the most variable in its placement across subjects but was generally placed as an SEH. This call shows relatively little frequency modulation in the frequency-time contours and relatively little modulation in the amplitudes of at least the first two of the harmonics. Nevertheless, the cues that are available appear to be sufficient for this stimulus to be placed within the SEH portion of the stimulus space.

In all cases where calls from different classes were placed near each other in the stimulus space, analysis of relative amplitude changes of the harmonics present in the calls suggested that animals might be attending to such changes and discriminating between the calls on that basis. In other words, these results suggest that the subjects may attend to the harmonic having the greatest amplitude, or more precisely, the greatest loudness, at any point in time, and perceive that harmonic as the dominant frequency. The present data are consistent with the interpretation that discriminations between calls are based on the temporal position within the call of the highest dominant frequency.

At least two questions arise from this interpretation of the data. The first is whether monkeys are sufficiently sensitive to relative spectral amplitude to make use of the potential cue provided by changes of the magnitude seen in the calls, and the second is whether variation in relative spectral amplitude of the harmonics of these calls moves them around in MDS space. The first question asks about the sensory abilities of the monkeys; that is, what they *can* do. The second question addresses the issue of whether they actually *do* use relative spectral amplitude.

Data relevant to the first of these questions have been provided by some studies from our laboratory related to the ability of monkeys to detect a change in level of one harmonic of a multi-harmonic complex (Sommers et al, 1991; Niemiec et al, 1992). The basic stimuli used in these studies consisted of the first 20 harmonics of a 120-Hz fundamental, with the relative amplitudes modeled after the vowel /ae/, as in "bat", and having formant peaks at 480 and 1440 Hz. With these stimuli, monkeys were able to discriminate relative spectral amplitude changes of approximately 3 dB at 1440 Hz. When the stimuli consisted of 5 harmonics of a 480-Hz fundamental, more akin to the spacing of the components of these coo calls, acuity at 1440 Hz remained approximately the same. These results demonstrate that the magnitude of change in relative spectral amplitude seen in the calls should be detectable by monkeys, and support the hypothesis that relative spectral level may be a highly salient cue to monkeys discriminating communicatively relevant acoustic signals. These results were obtained with discrete stimuli in which the relative spectral amplitudes remained constant throughout the duration of each of the signals. It might be predicted that a harmonic that varied dynamically within a stimulus, as do the harmonics in the SEH and SLH calls used here, might be easier to detect, and therefore might yield lower thresholds. Experiments are underway to test this prediction.

In order to answer the question as to whether changes in relative harmonic amplitude will move calls in MDS space, some preliminary experiments are required. One of the major problems in trying to demonstrate the effects of manipulation in a single stimulus is that MDS analysis results in solutions that may be unstable. In other words, variation in one stimulus does not necessarily mean that only that particular stimulus will move. MDS analysis attempts to maximize variance accounted for with a particular spatial arrangement and, in so doing, may radically alter the spatial array from one data set to the next. It should be noted, however, that the MDS stimulus spaces from these subjects were extremely stable over time when the test stimuli were held constant. To shed some light on the question of the stability of our MDS results with variation in test stimuli, we generated synthetic versions of the two SLH calls that were consistently grouped together by all of the subjects: 104C and 156-2. The synthesis was carried out using the techniques described earlier, resulting in four-component harmonic complexes in which the frequency and level of each component varied over time in the same way as did the natural call. This experiment allowed us to examine the extent to which the two synthetic calls would retain their position in MDS space when mixed with the remaining five natural calls. The results of this experiment indicated, for all of the subjects, that the two synthetics continued to be grouped together and to retain their original spatial relations with the remaining natural calls.

The next step was to replace the five remaining original calls with synthetic versions as well in order to determine the extent to which the original MDS stimulus space

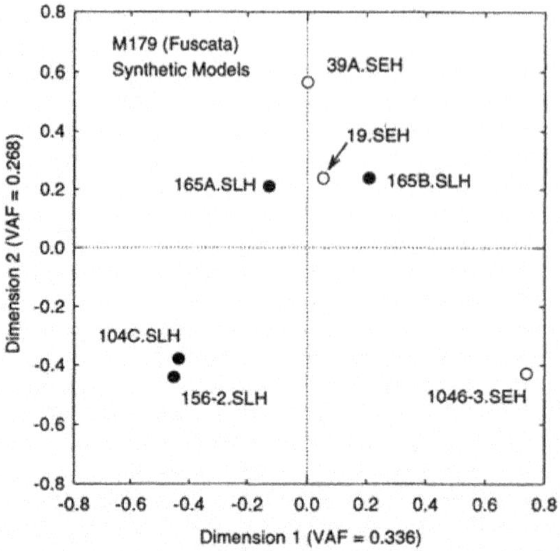

Figure 4. MDS Stimulus space from subject M179 for synthetic stimuli. The relative position of the most of the synthetic calls is remarkably similar to that of the natural calls shown in Figure 1, with the major exception that the spatial arrangement is flipped from top to bottom. SEH 39A is the only call that has substantially moved relative to the other calls.

configuration was maintained. The results of that study are illustrated in Figure 4 for the same subject presented in Figure 1. As with the natural calls, SLH 104C and SLH 156-2 are grouped together, and SEH call 1046-3 is grouped in the same half of stimulus space, but on the opposite side from the two SLH calls. In the case of the natural stimuli, these three calls occupy the positive half of dimension 2, while with the synthetic stimuli, they occupy the negative half of the dimension. It is not unusual for MDS stimulus space to flip about an axis, as in this example, and such a transformation is of little significance since the distances between the stimuli are preserved. A useful analogy is the mirror image of a road map, from which it is still possible to determine the distance between two cities, even though north and south are reversed. In Figure 4, SLH calls 165A and 165B and SEH call 19 also retain relative positions that are very similar to those seen in Figure 1. It is only call SEH call 39A that has changed its position significantly relative to the other calls. Similar stimulus space mappings were obtained from the other two subjects as well, and in all cases, SEH 39A was the call that was least stable in its relative position between the natural and synthetic conditions. A possible reason for the lack of stability noted with SEH 39A may be related to a slight click artifact that occurred near the end of the natural call. Based on the latencies obtained from this call, however, it was clear that subjects did not use this click to discriminate 39A from the other stimuli.

We consider these results extremely encouraging. They demonstrate quite unequivocally that the stimulus features used by the animals in discriminating between the stimuli, and thereby generating the data that resulted in the placement of the stimuli in MDS stimulus space, are contained within the amplitude and frequency information that was used to generate the synthetic versions of these stimuli. The relative stability of the stimulus spaces, in terms of which stimuli are grouped together, across subjects and between natural and synthetic stimuli, is an encouraging sign for future experiments that involve manipulating the presumed critical features of the stimuli — in this case, the relative level changes in the harmonics. Toward this end, subjects are currently being tested on a variant of SEH 19 in which the level contours of the second, third and fifth harmonics have been replaced with a level contour having the same temporal pattern as that of the first harmonic, but with the average level of each harmonic set to be the same as it was in the original call. Preliminary results from this manipulation indicate a disruption of discriminative performance and variability of the placement in MDS stimulus space of all of the "misplaced" calls. One of the interpretations of these initial findings is that subjects were using the cue provided by relative harmonic level, and that removal of that cue from one of the stimuli favored abandoning that discrimination strategy.

Although the final outcome of these studies is not yet known, it is nonetheless possible to consider some of the implications of the initial findings reported here. Perhaps the most important question is whether there would be any advantage to monkeys to have developed enhanced sensitivity to relative harmonic amplitude as a communicatively relevant cue. As in human speech, the relative amplitude of harmonic components in monkey vocalizations is determined by the configuration of the resonators in the vocal tract. Many of the changes in vocal tract configuration result in visible changes in facial features in the signaling animal (Hauser et al, 1993). Since primate communication systems rely heavily on visual as well as auditory signaling, it is reasonable to expect that the ability to infer facial configuration based on acoustic-only input might well be a trait that would be selected in the course of evolution.

A second issue concerns the extent to which experiments have been directed at studying the processing of relative level cues by the auditory system. A considerable body of research and theoretical interpretations exists on the ability of humans to detect relative changes in level in multi-tone complexes (see Green, 1988, for background in this area). Although it is apparent from the present data that monkeys also possess the ability to make such discriminations, it is unclear whether the ability is enhanced as a result of its potential usefulness in the communicative process. In studying the functioning of the primate auditory system, for example, by using physiological techniques, it may be important to view it as being specialized to respond to relative differences in levels of different spectral regions and to include stimuli in the testing protocol that have the potential to detect such specializations.

A third issue concerns the instrumentation that is used to study communication signals which, to a large extent, influences what we tend to view to be the critical features of those stimuli. The sound spectrogram, which formed the basis for Green's (1975) classification of the vocal repertoire of the Japanese macaque, is the most commonly used such tool. While spectrograms do an excellent job of describing the change in frequency over time of the various components of communication signals, they are less good at describing changes in the relative amplitude of the components. Analysis techniques that provide a more detailed picture of amplitude, similar to that seen in Figures 2B and 3B, may allow for a more appropriate separation of communication signals into functional groups and may help us to better understand the complexities of animal communication systems.

Earlier in this paper, we described one of the advantages of the behavioral procedure used to generate MDS data as being that it did not require that the experimenter reinforce animals for responding to a particular class of stimuli, while withholding reinforcement for responding to other stimulus classes. Although such differential reinforcement procedures have proven extremely useful in studying communication signals, they also have the potential of creating stimulus classes where none exist in nature. MDS procedures, on the other hand, are designed to avoid experimenter-generated classes by requiring the subjects to discriminate between all of the stimuli in a particular stimulus set, with the assumption being that stimuli with similar functions will end up in the same area of stimulus space. It would not be appropriate to discuss data obtained with such a procedure without at least questioning that assumption. The issue is whether requiring subjects to discriminate differences between all stimuli might have the effect of forcing them to attend to differences that were not communicatively relevant; that is, to switch into an "acoustic" mode as opposed to a "communication" mode. If such a switch occurred, then the potential would exist that the MDS groupings would represent acoustic similarities rather than communicatively relevant classes of stimuli. The potential of discriminating on an acoustic basis may be enhanced as a result of the extended training the animals receive with these stimuli, and in fact, the animals become extremely good at making the discriminations. On the other hand, the present data showing relative invariance of stimulus space with a switch from natural to synthetic stimuli demonstrate that the acoustic differences that resulted from that switch were not reflected in radical changes in MDS stimulus space. Although these findings do not guarantee that the subjects were operating in "communication" mode, they do indicate that the information conveyed by four time- and amplitude-varying harmonics was clearly relevant in the discriminations that were made between the stimuli and that other acoustic differences did not result in altered MDS stimulus spaces.

4 Conclusions

The present results demonstrate that MDS procedures can be used to derive stimulus space maps based on the latency with which an animal subject responds to a change from one communication signal to another in a series of repeating stimuli. These stimulus space maps are extremely stable over time and show a considerable consistency between subjects. When the communicative significance of the test signals is related to the temporal position of frequency peaks, then the placement of signals in MDS space is well correlated with those parameters, providing the assumption is made that the perceived frequency peak is that harmonic of the signal that has the greatest amplitude at each point in time. In other words, the evidence suggests that changes in relative harmonic levels over time determine the perceived similarity of the calls as measured by the latency of response to call difference. To test this hypothesis, synthetic calls were generated that consisted of four frequency- and amplitude-varying components modeled after the natural calls. With these synthetic calls, relative mappings remained very similar to what they were with the natural calls. In ongoing experiments, the relative amplitudes of the harmonics are being manipulated to determine the extent to which stimulus space mapping is altered.

5 Acknowledgments

This research was supported by Program Project Grant P01-DC00078 from NIDCD of NIH. Special thanks to Cathy Thompson for her assistance and patience in carrying out the tests on the subjects in these studies.

6 References

Dooling, R. J., Park, T. J., Brown, S. D., Okanoya, K., and Soli, S. D. (1987) Perceptual organization of acoustic stimuli in budgerigars (*Melopsittacus undulatus*): II. Vocal Signals. Journal of Comparative Psychology, 101:376-381.

Green, D. M. (1988) *Profile analysis: auditory intensity discrimination.* New York: Oxford University Press.

Green, S. (1975) Communication by a graded vocal system in Japanese monkeys. In L. A. Rosenblum (Ed.), *Primate Behavior* (Vol. 4). NY: Academic Press, pp 1-102.

Hauser, M. D., Evans, C. S., and Marler, P. (1993) The role of articulation in the production of rhesus monkey (*Macaca mulatta*) vocalizations. Animal Behavior, 45:423-433.

Heffner, H. E. and Heffner, R. S. (1986) Effect of unilateral and bilateral cortical lesions on the discrimination of vocalizations by Japanese macaques. J. Neurophysiol, 56: 683-701.

Heffner, H. E. and Heffner, R. S. (1990) Role of the primate auditory cortex in hearing. In W. C. Stebbins and M. A. Berkley (Eds.), *Comparative Perception: Complex Signals (Vol 2)*, New York: John Wiley, pp 279-310.

Kruskall, J. R. and Wish, M. (1978) *Multidimensional Scaling.* Beverly Hills: Sage Publications.

Moody, D. B., Stebbins, W. C., and May, B. J. (1990) Auditory perception of communication signals by Japanese monkeys. In W. C. Stebbins and M. A. Berkley (Eds.), *Comparative Perception: Complex Signals (Vol 2)*, New York: John Wiley, pp 311-343.

Niemiec, A. J., Moody, D. B., and Sommers, M. S. (1992) Discrimination of relative spectral amplitude changes for individual components of a harmonic stimulus by Japanese macaques. ARO 15th Midwinter Meeting Abstracts, p. 52.

Sommers, M. S., Moody, D. B., Prosen, C. A., and Stebbins, W. C. (1991) Spectral shape discrimination by Japanese monkeys. ARO 14th Midwinter Meeting Abstracts, p. 144.

Comment by David Moore

The degree to which animals produce and use various calls in the wild may differ from those produced and used in captivity, or their meaning may differ. Although you have to make a decision as to how these calls should be recorded, the possibility is that the animals will learn to vary their calls in response to their environment. The extent to which acoustic parameter variations affect discrimination may be modified by this type of learning. One way to address this issue would be to reassess the range of calls produced at various times before and after introduction to the laboratory housing environment.

Reply

If the ultimate concern is that of the existence of perceptual specializations that have developed in a species for dealing with communication signals, then one should be able to assume that those will be altered little, if at all, by moving the animals into a captive situation. In fact, monkeys do vocalize with considerably reduced frequency and variability in the laboratory, but even so, we continue to see robust effects when communicatively relevant stimuli are employed in a laboratory setting.

Frequency discrimination of narrowband stimuli related to vowel formants

J. Lyzenga and J.W. Horst

Institute of Audiology, Research Department, University Hospital Groningen, P.O.Box 30.001, 9700RB Groningen, The Netherlands

1 Introduction

In order to investigate the ability of humans to discriminate spectral changes in vowels, we have measured frequency discrimination for relatively simple bandlimited sounds that resemble a single vowel formant (resonance peak in the spectrum). In vowels of natural speech a number of formants can be recognized. The frequencies of the first two or three formants characterize the vowel. After investigating frequency discrimination for tones with a single peak in the spectrum, two or more of these tones can be combined to achieve a spectrum closer resembling that of a vowel. Frequency discrimination of the "formants" of such combined tones can then be studied in relation to the known frequency discrimination of the constituting tones.

The ability of humans to discriminate spectral changes in bandlimited sounds, including synthetic vowels, has been studied in a number of investigations. Frequency discrimination for the first and second formant of isolated synthetic vowels containing at least four formants has been investigated, e.g., by Flanagan (1955), Mermelstein (1978), Sinnott and Kreiter (1991) and recently Kewley-Port and Watson (1994). Mermelstein (1978) measured the jnd for a change of the first, of the second and a combined change of both these formants. He also used consonant-bound vowels. Sinnott and Kreiter (1991) investigated the jnd for a combined change of the first three formants. Whereas Flanagan (1955) and Kewley-Port and Watson (1994) used a constant fundamental, Mermelstein (1978) and Sinnott and Kreiter (1991) added a transition to the fundamental frequency in order to give the artificial vowels a more natural sound. Examples of jnds for first and second formants are shown in figure 1.

Frequency discrimination for bandlimited sounds with a single maximum in the spectrum has been investigated, e.g., by Stevens (1952), Horst et al. (1984) and Gagné and Zurek (1988). Stevens studied jnds for changes in the frequency of a single exponentially damped wave. Unfortunately, because of the dependence of the effective duration on the bandwidth, these results cannot be compared directly with frequency jnds of stimuli with fixed duration. Horst et al. (1984) used a proportional change in the center and the fundamental frequency. In the experiments of Gagné and Zurek (1988) these two parameters were independent. Horst et al. found that jnds were inversely proportional to the spectral slope, with a pure-tone jnd of .15% as the lower limit. (Wier et al. (1977) found a similar pure-tone jnd_F at 40 dB SL for 1 and 2 kHz.) Inverse proportionality between jnd and spectral slope was also found by Gagné and Zurek with a less steep slope and at higher jnds (as shown in figure 1).

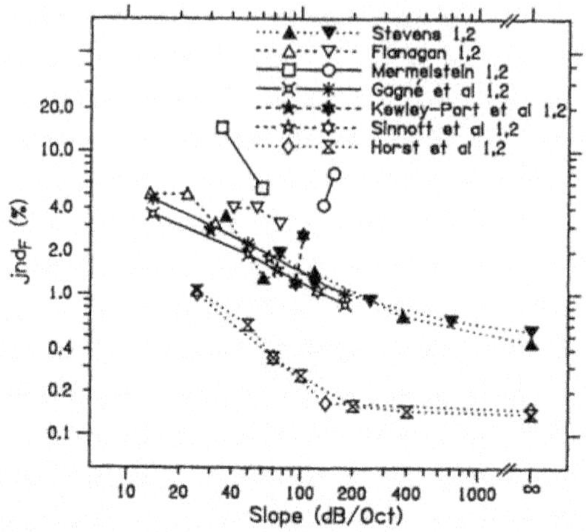

Figure 1. Jnd$_F$ for vowel-like tones. For each report two results are displayed. The numbers 1 and 2 refer to jnds for the first formant and the second formant respectively.

The reported just-noticeable differences in center frequency of complex stimuli in figure 1 show a considerable spread (about two orders of magnitude). The aim of our project is to enlarge the insight in this discrimination and to find an explanation for the large spread in the literature. Stimulus parameters were: the spectral width, the slope steepness and the center frequency. The condition of fixed fundamental frequency was held during all the jnd measurements. Later we will work on the discrimination of more natural one-formant "vowels", created by adjusting the amplitude and phase spectra. Subsequently, stimuli with more than one formant will be used to investigate the discrimination of more realistic synthetic vowels. By starting with simple harmonic tones, and increasing the complexity of the "vowels" step by step, we hope to bridge the gap in data on the discrimination of simple stimuli and that of speech.

2 Methods

Two experiments were carried out using bandlimited harmonic complexes as stimuli. All harmonic complexes had a fundamental frequency (F_0) of 100 Hz and all components were added with a starting phase of 0° (sine phase). In experiment 1 the shape of the spectral envelope was triangular on a log-log scale, in experiment 2 the envelope shape was trapezoidal with a width of the constant-level plateau of 200 Hz (i.e. twice F_0). Five values of the center frequency (F_C) were used for the triangular envelope: 2000, 2025,

2050, 2075 and 2100 Hz. For the trapezoidal envelope nine values of F_C were used; from 2000 to 2200 Hz with a 25 Hz increment. Three values for the slope steepness were employed for both spectral shapes: 100, 200 and 400 dB/oct. Figure 2 shows eight examples of stimuli with a slope steepness of 200 dB/oct.

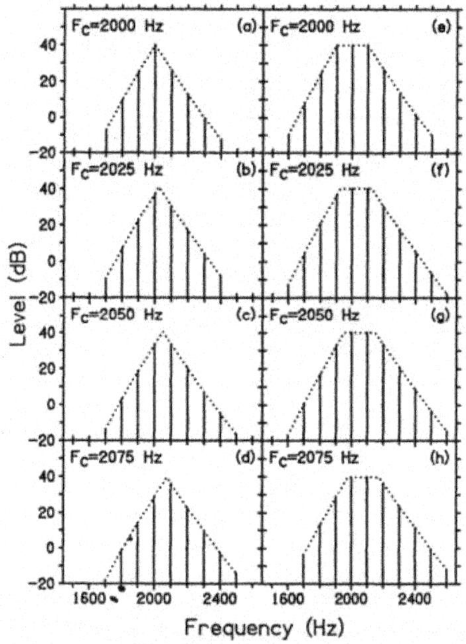

Figure 2. Eight examples of spectra of the used stimuli. Displayed in the left column are four stimuli with a triangular envelope whose slope steepness is 200 dB/oct. The F_C's are from (a) to (d): 2000, 2025, 2050 and 2075 Hz. The right column shows four stimuli with a trapezoidal envelope for the same conditions.

Jnds were estimated by comparing a reference signal with a signal that had an increased center frequency (the "target") in a 3AFC paradigm (Frijters, 1980). First an estimation of the absolute threshold of the reference tone was made, after which all stimuli were presented at a level of 40 dB above this threshold. For the target levels, relative to the level of the reference, we used two adjustments. In the first adjustment the top (or the plateau) of the spectral envelope was held at a constant level. This condition we termed "Constant Plateau" (hereafter CP). The overall level of these signals varied with the F_C. See figure 3 for the overall level of the triangular stimuli with a slope of 400 dB/oct. In the second adjustment the levels of the stimuli of a group (reference and targets) were randomized within trials, with a level rove of +/- 5 dB (Henning, 1966). This condition was termed: "Roving Level" (hereafter RL).

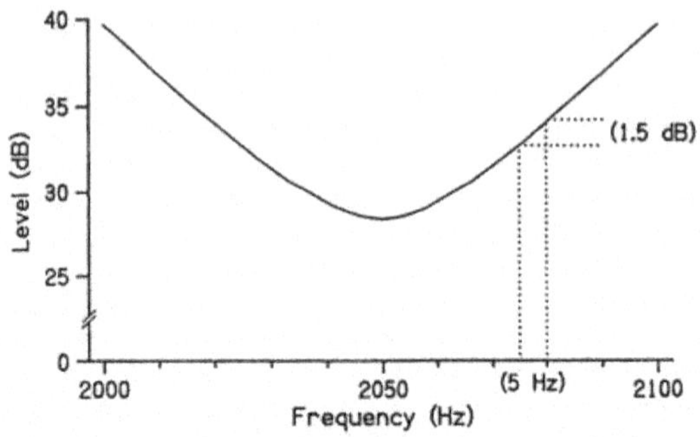

Figure 3. Overall level as a function of the center frequency, for the stimuli with a triangular spectral envelope with a slope steepness of 400 dB/oct. The dotted lines show that a change in F_C from 2075 to 2080 Hz (i.e. an increase of 0.24%) produces an overall-level change of 1.5 dB (see text).

3 Results

3.1 Results of the triangular spectral envelope

The results of the first experiment are presented in the three panels of figure 4. Each panel contains jnds for five different values of F_C and one value of the slope steepness. The averaged jnds of four subject are plotted for both the conditions "Constant Plateau" (CP: triangular symbols, dotted line) and "Roving Level" (RL: circular symbols, solid line).

Figure 4 shows, for both the CP and the RL-condition, that the jnds strongly depend on F_C (or rather on the distance of F_C to the nearest harmonics). For each slope steepness the jnds are larger at F_C=2000 and 2100 Hz than at F_C=2050 Hz. The jnds are not symmetrical around F_C=2050 Hz; this is probably due to the fact that the change of F_C in all jnd measurements was in the same (upward) direction. At F_C=2075 Hz two different values for the jnd were observed: a higher value for the RL-condition and a lower one for the CP-condition. This is particularly clear for G=400 dB/oct. We assume that an overall-level cue was used in the CP-condition. In order to check this we measured a level jnd with F_C=2000 Hz and G=400 dB/oct for three subjects (not shown in figure 4). These jnd_L's were recorded changing only the overall level of the stimulus and not the F_C. These jnd_L's ranged from 1.5 to 2.0 dB. An overall level difference of 1.5 dB would correspond for G=400 dB/oct and F_C=2075 Hz to a jnd_{Fc} of 0.24% (see figure 3), which is very close to what we find in figure 4. Therefore, the overall-level information available in the CP-condition seems to be a good explanation for the discrepancy between these CP and RL-jnds.

Figure 4 shows that in most cases the jnds of the CP-condition are somewhat below those of the RL-condition. In all cases where no overall-level information is available to the subjects, we see in the averaged results a roughly constant difference of a factor 1.5. This difference may be caused by confusion in the subjects when participating in a RL-experiment. Firstly, the random level variations produce a false cue that the subjects have to ignore. Secondly, the timbre of the used complex tones can change with the (randomized) level of the tone, when small components in the flank appear in, or disappear from, the signal spectrum above threshold. Aspects like these are likely to confuse the subject and bring down the scores (i.e. increase the jnds). Versfeld and Houtsma (1991) also found a roughly constant difference (viz. a factor 1.8) in favor of a "Constant Level" condition as compared with a "Roving Level" condition in jnds in relative component level in two-tone complexes (comparable to our stimuli with F_C=2050 Hz and G=400 dB/oct). Therefore, it seems reasonable to assume that there was no essential perceptual difference between the CP and the RL-condition.

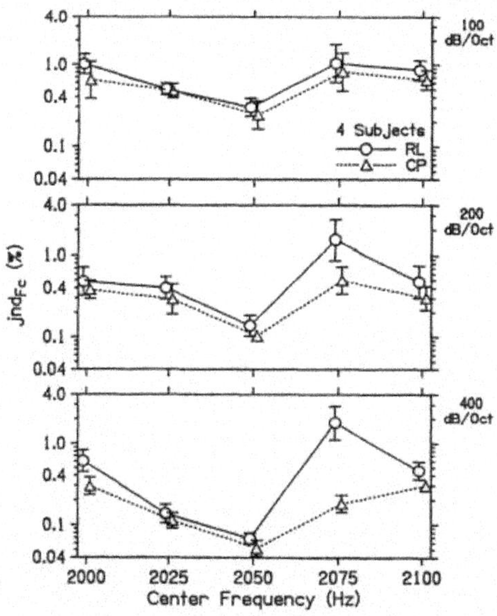

Figure 4. Jnds for the triangular envelope. Results are averaged over four subjects, the error bars indicate the standard deviation over the subjects.

At F_C=2050 Hz the stimuli with a triangular envelope have two major components that are approximately equally large (see figure 2, panel c). With an upward change of the center frequency of the spectral envelope the levels of these two components change in opposite directions. At F_C=2000 Hz the stimuli have one major component at the F_C and smaller components flanking this large one on both sides (see figure 2, panel a). With an upward change of the center frequency, the levels of the small components at the high-frequency side change compared with the level of the major component. Apparently, small changes in the spectral envelope can be heard more easily when they occur in approximately equally large components (F_C=2050 Hz), than when they occur in a large and a small component (F_C=2000 Hz).

3.2 Results of the trapezoidal spectral envelope

The results of the second experiment are presented in figure 5. Each panel contains jnds for nine values of F_C and one value of the slope steepness. The five F_C-values from 2000 to 2100 Hz are the same as those for the triangular envelope. For the F_C-values from 2100 and 2200 Hz the low-frequency slopes are the same as those for the triangular envelopes. Each panel contains the averaged results of four subjects for both the conditions "Constant Plateau" (CP: triangular symbols, dotted line) and "Roving Level" (RL: circular symbols, solid line).

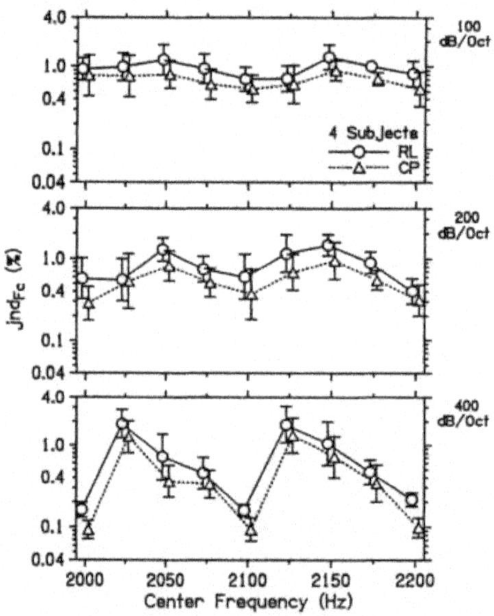

Figure 5. Jnds for the trapezoidal envelope. Results are averaged over four subjects, the error bars indicate the standard deviation over the subjects.

Figure 5 shows again that, for 200 and 400 dB/oct, the jnds strongly depend on the distance between the center frequency and the harmonics. The smallest jnds are generally found at F_C=2000, 2100 and 2200 Hz. For these three F_C-values the jnds decrease when the slope steepness increases. The results at either F_C=2025 Hz or 2050 Hz are the highest in each panel. The jnd as a function of F_C is not always locally symmetrical around F_C=2050 and 2150 Hz. As noted for the triangular envelope, this is probably due to the fact that F_C is always changed upwards. For 100 dB/oct the dependence of the jnd on the F_C has almost disappeared.

As for the triangular spectral envelope, we find a difference of about 1.5 between the CP and the RL-jnds. Moreover, for the trapezoidal envelope there is less variation in this difference than for the triangular envelope. Therefore, the results of the trapezoidal envelope indicate even more strongly that there is no essential perceptual difference between the CP and the RL-condition, as was argued for the first experiment.

At F_C=2000 Hz the stimuli with a trapezoidal envelope have three major components around F_C and smaller components flanking these large ones to both sides (see figure 2, panel e). With an upward change of the center frequency of the spectral envelope, the level of the leftmost major component changes compared with the level of the two other large components at its high-frequency side. At F_C=2050 Hz the stimuli have two major components, again with smaller components flanking these large ones to both sides (see figure 2, panel g). With a small upward change of the center frequency the levels of these two large components are unaffected and only the levels of the smaller components flanking them change. Apparently, small changes in the spectral envelope can be heard better when the changing components have levels that are similar to the unaffected components (e.g. at F_C=2000 Hz).

4 Discussion

In the previous sections we have argued that there was no essential perceptual difference between the CP and the RL-condition. The RL-condition forces the subject to perform some sort of profile comparison of the two spectra of the presented tones, instead of comparing the levels of individual frequency components from stimulus to stimulus. Because our results for the CP and the RL-condition are essentially the same, it is likely that the subjects also used this form of profile comparison during measurements with the CP-condition (at least, when no overall-level information could be used). This suggests a mechanism in which the ear compares the difference in level of neighboring components in one stimulus with the difference in level of these components in the second stimulus, rather than comparing the levels of individual frequency components in the two stimuli. In other words, the ear performs a form of profile analysis of the two stimuli under comparison (Green, 1987).

Comparing the results for both spectral shapes, as they are plotted versus F_C in the figures 4 and 5, we observe an essential difference in the general shape of the curves. For the results of the triangular spectral envelope the curves tend to show a "V"-shape in the range of F_C=2000 to 2100 Hz. The curves for the trapezoidal spectral envelope, on the contrary, tend to show a roof-like shape in the ranges of F_C=2000 to 2100 Hz and F_C=2100 to 2200 Hz. (Note that for each slope steepness the largest jnds are of about the same magnitude for both envelope shapes.) Since the smallest jnds are found at different

F_C's for both envelope shapes, it is clear that the discrimination cannot be explained by effects that take place in only one slope of the stimuli. The best jnds for the triangular envelope are smaller than the best of the trapezoidal envelope. These small jnds for the triangular envelope correspond for G=400 dB/oct with level changes in the individual components of 0.3 to 0.5 dB. This is considerably smaller than the often observed jnd_L of about 1.5 dB (e.g., Viemeister and Bacon, 1988). This suggests that in the case of the triangular envelope information from both slopes, or more specific, excitation changes with opposite signs, can be combined in the discrimination process, whereas no combining of information occurs for the trapezoidal envelope. This is illustrated in figure 6; which shows the differences in the hypothetical excitations of a place model (Patterson and Moore, 1986; Moore and Glasberg, 1987) for each spectral envelope shape. For the

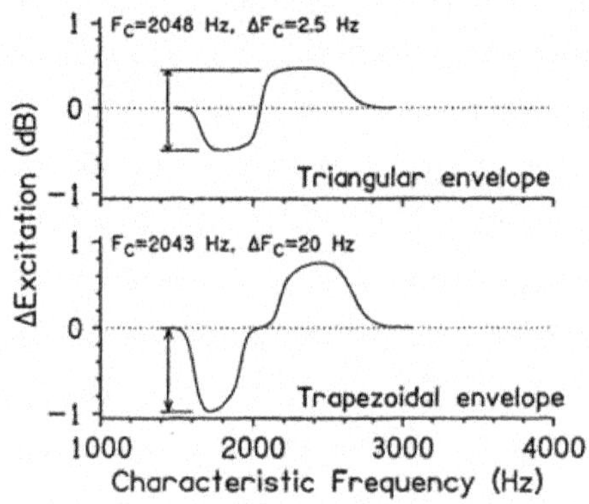

Figure 6. The difference in the hypothetical excitations for stimuli with a triangular spectral envelope (top panel) changes sign abruptly near 2050 Hz. For the trapezoidal spectral envelope (bottom panel) there is a neutral area as the excitation difference changes sign (around 2050 Hz).

trapezoidal envelope there is a small area of no excitation difference in the middle of the curve (around 2050 Hz). This area coincides with the two central components of the trapezium. Such a neutral area is not seen for the triangular envelope. It seems that this neutral area, which we find for the trapezoidal envelope, prevents subjects from combining the information of both spectral slopes, whereas combining this information in the case of the triangular envelopes boosts performance to jnds that correspond to level differences in the individual components of less than 0.5 dB. This leads us to the conclusion that the ear compares level profiles over a limited frequency range, rather than comparing individual component levels.

5 Acknowledgments

This research was supported by the Netherlands Organization for Scientific Research (NWO) through the Foundation PSYCHON.

6 References

Flanagan, J.L. (1955) A difference limen for vowel formant frequency. J.Acoust.Soc.Am. 27, 613-617.

Frijters, J.E.R. (1980) Psychophysical and psychometrical models for the triangular method. Ph.D. Thesis, Utrecht University (The Netherlands).

Gagné, J. and Zurek, P.M. (1988) Resonance-frequency discrimination. J.Acoust.Soc.Am. 83, 2293-2299.

Green, D.M. (1987) Profile Analysis: Auditory Intensity Discrimination. Oxford U.P., New York.

Henning, G.B. (1966) Frequency discrimination of random-amplitude tones. J.Acoust.Soc.Am. 39, 336-339.

Horst, J.W., Ritsma, R.J. and Wit, H.P. (1984) Frequency discrimination in quiet and noise for signals with triangular spectral envelopes. J.Acoust.Soc.Am. 76, 1067-1075.

Kewley-Port, D. and Watson, C.S. (1994) Formant-frequency discrimination for isolated English vowels. J.Acoust.Soc.Am. 95, 485-496.

Mermelstein, P. (1978) Difference limens for formant frequencies of steady-state and consonant-bound vowels. J.Acoust.Soc.Am. 63, 572-580.

Moore. B.C.J. and Glasberg, B.R. (1987) Formulae describing frequency selectivity as a function of frequency and level, and their use in calculating excitation patterns. Hearing Res. 28, 209-225.

Patterson, R.D. and Moore, B.C.J. (1986) Auditory filters and excitation patterns as representations of frequency resolution. In: B.C.J. Moore (Ed.) Frequency selectivity in hearing, Academic Press Inc, London, pp 123-177.

Sinnott, J.M. and Kreiter, N.A. (1991) Differential sensitivity to vowel continua in Old World monkeys (Macaca) and humans. J.Acoust.Soc.Am. 89, 2421-2429.

Stevens, K.N. (1952) Frequency discrimination for damped waves. J.Acoust.Soc.Am. 24, 76-79.

Versfeld, N.J. and Houtsma, A.J.M. (1991) Perception of spectral changes in multi-tone complexes. Q.J.Exp.Psychol. 43A, 459-479.

Viemeister, N.F. and Bacon, S.P. (1988) Intensity discrimination, increment detection, and magnitude estimation for 1-kHz tones. J.Acoust.Soc.Am. 84, 172-178.

Wier, C.C., Jesteadt, W. and Green, D.M. (1977) Frequency discrimination as a function of frequency and sensation level. J.Acoust.Soc.Am. 61, 178-184.

Comment by S. Buus

Have you investigated the possibility that discrimination may be based on envelope cues? It seems that the changes in relative amplitudes of the components would result in substantial changes in the envelopes of your stimuli.

Reply

We did search extensively for a correlation between our data and both the crest factor and the modulation depth of the stimuli but could not find any satisfactory correlations. This analysis could be extended with a search for possible correlations between the power spectrum of the temporal envelopes and the data. This seems worth while investigating.

Comment by L. Feth

Have you considered applying a "spectral-center-of-gravity" model such as the IWAIF model (Anantharaman et al., 1993) to your results?

Anantharaman J.N., Krishnamurthy, A.K. and Feth L.L. (1993): Intensity weighted avegage of instantaneous frequency as a model for frequency discrimination. J. Acoust. Soc. Amer. 94, 723-729

Reply

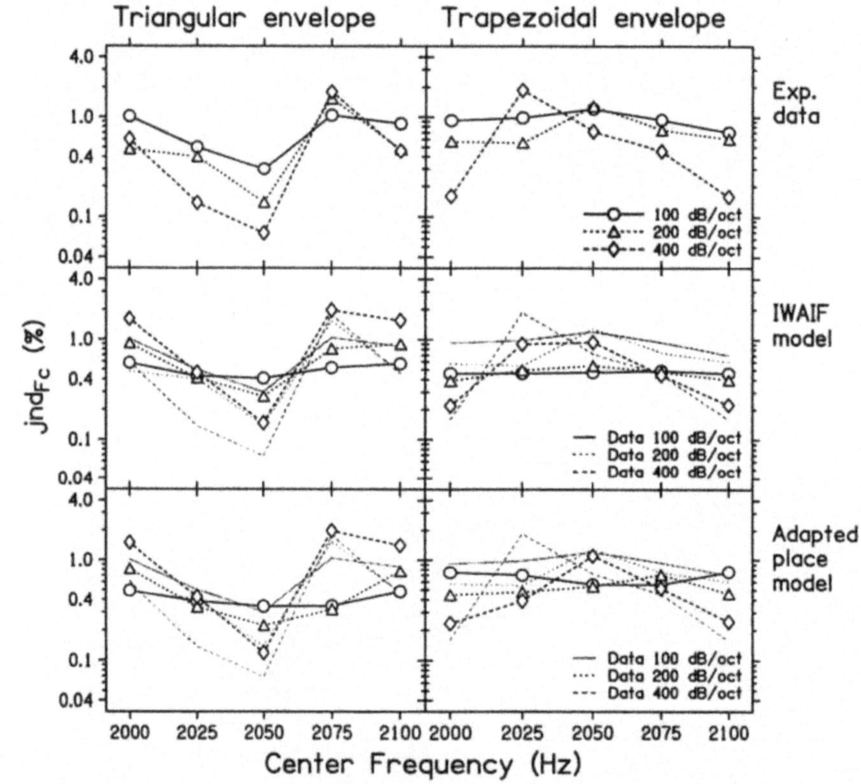

Figure 1. Experimentally determined jnds in comparison to predictions generated with IWAIF and adapted place models (for details see next page).

We have tried to describe our data with both an EWAIF and an IWAIF model (see Fig. 1). The EWAIF model performed rather poorly, particularly for the jnds measured with the trapezoidal spectral envelope. The IWAIF model produced a reasonable description of the data for both the triangular and the trapezoidal spectral envelope. This is shown in the figure for an IWAIF threshold of 10 Hz. However, in order to obtain a good description of all the data two different threshold values (7 Hz for the triangular versus 15 Hz for the trapezoidal envelope) had to be used. Therefore, a constant difference in the center of gravity of the frequency does not appear to provide an adequate description of the data. For this reason we proposed the adapted place model as described in the discussion. In the future we plan to do a more thorough quantative comparison of EWAIF, IWAIF and place models.

Representation of spectral profiles in the auditory system: Theory, physiology, and psychoacoustics

Shihab A. Shamma, Svetlana Vranic-Sowers and Huib Versnel

A.V. Williams Building, Institute for Systems Research,
Department of Electrical Engineering, University of Maryland,
College Park, MD 20742, U.S.A.

1 Introduction

The shape of the acoustic spectrum plays a fundamental role in the perception and recognition of complex sounds. It is uncertain, however, how this spectral profile is represented at the central stages of auditory processing. Several representations have been inspired by a wide range of psychoacoustical tests such as the profile analysis experiments and discriminations of simultaneous vowels (Durlach et at., 1986; Bernstein and Green, 1987; Feth et al., 1982; Klatt 1982; Assmann and Summerfield, 1989). All these models share the same fundamental starting point that the spectral profile is represented by the acoustic spectrum on a logarithmic frequency axis. Relative to this profile, various operations are defined to predict perceptual thresholds.

An alternative model is proposed here in which the perception of the spectral shape is based upon the Fourier transformation of the profile. Inspired by physiological findings in the primary auditory cortex, it is hypothesized that an arbitrary spectral profile is explicitly represented in the auditory system by a collection of weighted elementary spectral profiles - called ripples, which are sinusoidal in shape (against the logarithmic frequency axis) with different frequencies and phases. The idea that the brain performs such a ripple analysis on its sensory input patterns is relatively common in the vision literature, where it has been variously called multi-resolution or multi-scale representation, and spatial frequency analysis (Campbell and Robson, 1968; De Valois and De Valois, 1990).

A computational model for the ripple analysis is presented in Sec. 2. Physiological evidence for this kind of analysis in the primary auditory cortex is discussed in Sec. 3. In Sec. 4 several important psychoacoustical predictions of the model are tested and validated. Finally, broader implications of the ripple analysis hypothesis are discussed in Sec. 5.

2 The ripple analysis model

2.1 Terminology and notation

The following terms are frequently used here to describe the ripple analysis representation of profiles: **Ripple**: a sinusoidal spectral profile, $p(\omega) = \sin(2\pi\Omega\omega + \Phi)$, on the logarithmic frequency axis ω. A ripple has a ripple frequency Ω (in cycle/octave) and a ripple phase Φ (in radians or degrees); **Ripple analysis filter,**

$H(\Omega;\Omega_o,\Phi_o,\omega_o)$: a bandpass filter tuned to a characteristic ripple frequency, Ω_o, and phase, Φ_o, and located at ω_o on the tonotopic axis ω. Its impulse response (or the inverse Fourier transform) is denoted by $h(\omega;\Omega_o,\Phi_o,\omega_o)$. **Ripple transform,** $r(\cdot)$: the output of a bank of ripple analysis filters.

2.2 Computing the ripple transform of a spectral profile

The transformation of the input spectral profile $p(\omega)$ into different ripple components is assumed to be performed by a bank of ripple analysis filters (Fig. 1). Each filter operates only locally around a particular point along the tonotopic axis (e.g., ω_o). The impulse response of such a filter, $h(\omega;\Omega_o,\Phi_o,\omega_o)$, is modeled as a Gaussian shaped ripple (Fig. 1A). For instance, the filter centered around $\omega_o = 0$ is given by: $h(\omega;\Omega_o,\Phi_o,\omega_o=0) = 2\ g_o(\omega)\cos(2\pi\Omega_o\omega - \Phi_o)$, where $g_o(\omega) = \sqrt{2\pi}\sigma\ e^{-\frac{(2\pi\omega\sigma)^2}{2}}$ and σ determines the width of the Gaussian envelope. In the Fourier transform domain, these filters are Gaussian shaped (Fig. 1B) and are given by:

$$H(\Omega;\Omega_o,\Phi_o) = H(\Omega;\Omega_o)\cos(\Phi_o) + \hat{H}(\Omega;\Omega_o)\sin(\Phi_o) = H(\Omega;\Omega_o)\ e^{-\jmath\ sign(\Omega)\Phi_o},$$

where $\hat{H}(\Omega;\Omega_o)$ is the Hilbert transform of $H(\Omega;\Omega_o)$ and $H(\Omega;\Omega_o)$ is the Fourier transform of $2\ g_o(\omega)\cos(2\pi\Omega_o\omega)$.

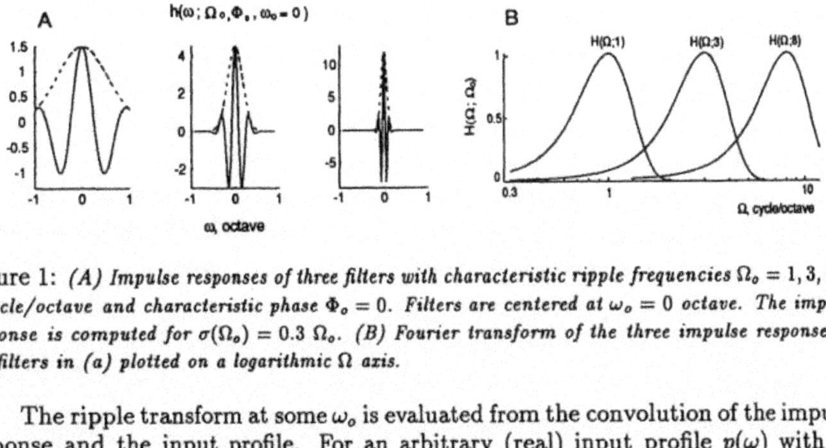

Figure 1: *(A) Impulse responses of three filters with characteristic ripple frequencies $\Omega_o = 1, 3$, and 8 cycle/octave and characteristic phase $\Phi_o = 0$. Filters are centered at $\omega_o = 0$ octave. The impulse response is computed for $\sigma(\Omega_o) = 0.3\ \Omega_o$. (B) Fourier transform of the three impulse responses of the filters in (a) plotted on a logarithmic Ω axis.*

The ripple transform at some ω_o is evaluated from the convolution of the impulse response and the input profile. For an arbitrary (real) input profile $p(\omega)$ with its Fourier transform $P(\Omega) = |P(\Omega)|e^{\jmath\Phi(\Omega)}$, the response is:

$$r(\Omega_o,\Phi_o,\omega_o) = \int_{-\infty}^{\infty} h(\omega_o-\omega;\Omega_o,\Phi_o)p(\omega)d\omega = \int_{-\infty}^{\infty} H(\Omega;\Omega_o,\Phi_o)P(\Omega)e^{+\jmath 2\pi\Omega\omega_o}d\Omega$$

$$= 2\int_{0}^{\infty} H(\Omega;\Omega_o)\ |P(\Omega)|\cdot\cos(\Phi_o - \Phi(\Omega) - 2\pi\Omega\omega_o)d\Omega. \quad (1)$$

This equation can be simplified for profiles which are even or odd symmetric around their center (arbitrarily designated at ω_o), or otherwise have a constant phase Φ_c

around it so that $\Phi(\Omega) = sign(\Omega)\Phi_c - 2\pi\Omega\omega_o$. This assumption applies approximately to all profiles discussed here. The ripple transform computed at such a point ω_o is:

$$r(\Omega_o, \Phi_o) = \cos(\Phi_o - \Phi_c) \int_{-\infty}^{\infty} H(\Omega; \Omega_o)\ |P(\Omega)| d\Omega = \cos(\Phi_o - \Phi_c)\ r(\Omega_o), \qquad (2)$$

where $r(\Omega_o) = \int_{-\infty}^{\infty} H(\Omega; \Omega_o)\ |P(\Omega)| d\Omega$ is a "magnitude" part and $\Phi_o - \Phi_c$ is a "phase" part of the ripple transform. The majority of profile analysis tasks reported in the literature and considered here can be effectively described either as a change in the magnitude or in the phase of the ripple transform, as discussed later in Sec. 4.

2.3 Parameters of the model

The input profile $p(\omega)$ is taken to be the normalized amplitude spectrum of the stimulus. The filter bank depicted in Fig. 1B is assumed to be a constant-Q bank, i.e., its filters have constant widths on a logarithmic Ω axis or, equivalently, have linearly increasing widths (σ's) with Ω_o. This choice is primarily justified by data from adaptation experiments (both with ripples (Hillier, 1991) and visual gratings (De Valois and De Valois, 1990)) and neurophysiological experiments (Shamma et al., 1994), in which filter tuning was estimated around various Ω_o's to be about 1 octave (measured at the half amplitude points). This corresponds approximately to $\sigma(\Omega_o) = 0.3\ \Omega_o$.

3 Physiological evidence for ripple analysis in AI

In this section we present responses to ripple profiles in the primary auditory cortex (AI) in the ferret. The experimental procedures, stimuli, and data analysis are described in Shamma et al. (1993, 1994). Briefly, the stimuli used were ripple profiles as illustrated in Fig. 2A. For each ripple frequency Ω, the responses to eight different ripple phases Φ were recorded. Responses of a single unit as a function of Φ are shown in Fig. 2B. Note the response changes from maximum to minimum with a 180° shift, reflecting a strong ripple-phase following. At each Ω the phase following component of the spike counts was determined, and is illustrated by the sinusoidal fit curves in Fig. 2C. On the basis of the phase-locking component the magnitude and phase of the transfer function were derived: $|T(\Omega)|$ and $\Phi(\Omega)$. The *impulse response* of a cell, termed here the response field (RF), was obtained by inverse Fourier transforming the ripple transfer function.

3.1 AI units are tuned to different ripple frequencies and phases

Figure 3 illustrates that AI cells are tuned around specific (characteristic) ripple frequencies, Ω_o. They also exhibit a linear phase function of the ripple frequency ($\Phi(\Omega)$), in addition to a constant phase delay, the characteristic phase Φ_o, evaluated at the intercept ($\Phi(0)$). The slope of the phase function reflects the location of the RF along the tonotopic axis. The parameters Ω_o and Φ_o are interpreted, respectively, as the best ripple frequency and phase to drive the cell.

In general, Ω_o reflects the width or scale of the RF: a higher Ω_o usually implies a finer or narrower RF (compare Figs. 3A and 3B), while Φ_o reflects the asymmetry of RF: e.g., RF is symmetric for $\Phi_o \approx 0$ and strongly asymmetric for $\Phi_o \approx \pm 90°$

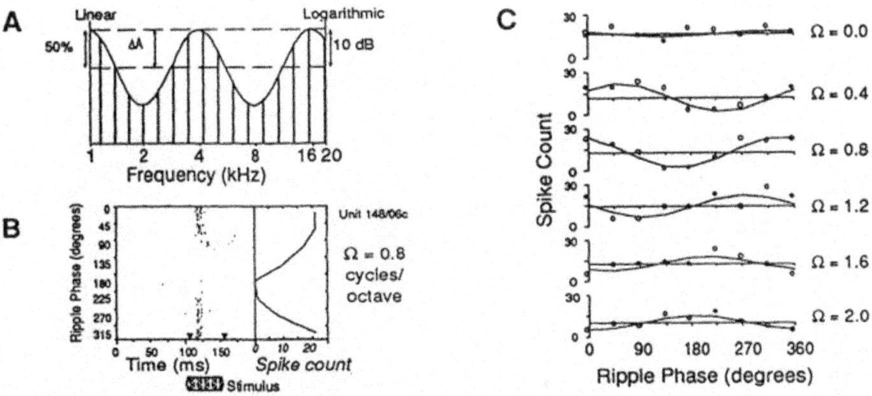

Figure 2: *(A) Rippled complex stimulus composed of 101 tones equally spaced along the logarithmic frequency axis between 1 and 20 kHz. The envelope is sinusoidally modulated on a logarithmic frequency axis either on a linear (left ordinate) or a logarithmic (right ordinate) amplitude scale. The ripple phase is defined relative to the start of a ripple (i.e., low-frequency edge). The ripple stimuli were varied in ripple frequency Ω (0 – 4 cycle/octave in steps of 0.2 or 0.4) or ripple phase Φ (0–$7\pi/4$ in $\pi/4$ steps). The stimulus duration was 50 ms. (B) Dot display of responses of an AI cell ($BF = 7.5$ kHz) to a ripple of a fixed Ω at various ripple phases. The stimuli were started at 100 ms. Spike counts are computed over a 50 ms window as indicated by the bold arrows, and are displayed in the inset plot to the right. (C) Spike counts as a function of ripple phase for various ripple frequencies Ω. The spike counts are indicated by the circles, and for each Ω the abscissa is placed at the spike count averaged over all phases. The solid line is the best mean-square-error fit to a sinusoid.*

(compare Figs. 3A and 3C). The distributions of Ω_o and Φ_o in the ferret AI are shown in Fig. 3D.

The RF of a cell closely corresponds to the response area measured with two-tone stimuli (Shamma et al., 1992, 1993): Ω_o is inversely correlated with the tonal excitatory bandwidth; Φ_o is correlated with the asymmetry of the response area; and the best frequencies (BFs) measured from the peak of the RF or with a single tone are very similar.

3.2 Columnar and topographic distribution of the Ω_o and Φ_o

AI units exhibit a uniform columnar organization with respect to their characteristic ripple and phase (Shamma et al., 1994; Versnel et al., 1994), much like that seen for the BF and the symmetry of the response area (Shamma et al., 1993). They also have an ordered and clustered topographic distribution along the isofrequency planes of AI. This is demonstrated in Figs. 4: (A) Ω_o is usually highest near the center of AI and decreases gradually towards the edges; (B) Φ_o tends to be negative near the caudal end of AI in the ferret, it gradually changes to symmetric ($\Phi_o \approx 0$) near the middle, and finally becomes positive towards the rostral end. In some animals, these trends are repeated near the edges (Fig. 4A). The distribution of the two parameters

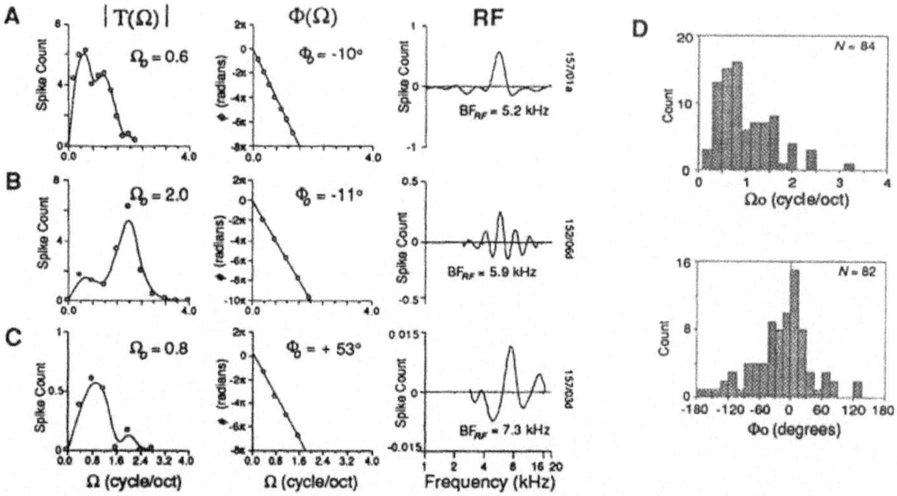

Figure 3: *(A-C) Examples of ripple responses from three cells. Left: magnitude transfer function $|T(\Omega)|$; middle: phase transfer function $\Phi(\Omega)$; right: response field (inverse Fourier transform of transfer function). Note that width of $|T(\Omega)|$ is about 1 octave. (D) Distribution of Ω_o and phase Φ_o of single units in different experiments in ferret AI.*

mirrors closely that of the response area bandwidth (Schreiner and Mendelson, 1990; Versnel et al., 1994) and asymmetry (Shamma et al., 1993).

3.3 Functional significance of the ripple responses

The ripple responses in AI including the distributions and topographic organization support the notion that the auditory system is capable of performing the ripple analysis as proposed in Sec. 2. Cells with low Ω_o respond best to the gross (slowly varying) features of the profile, whereas units with high Ω_o detect fine (rapidly varying) features. Similarly, the ripple phase sensitivity can be seen as explicitly encoding the local asymmetry of the profile. Therefore, the strength of a cell's output reflects both the ripple frequency content (near its Ω_o) and the local asymmetry (relative to its Φ_o) of a region of the profile where the cell is located (at some ω_o). Finally, an array of AI cells with different ω_o's (or BFs), Ω_o's, and Φ_o's performs the complete ripple analysis, i.e., the transformation of the profile into its ripple transform.

4 Psychoacoustical evidence for ripple analysis

The ability of the ripple analysis model to account for perceptual thresholds of various spectral profile manipulations can be psychoacoustically tested. Three broad categories of such profile manipulations will be considered below: detection of a profile against a flat background (Sec. 4.1); dilation (stretching or compressing) of a spectral profile (Sec. 4.2); and a change in the phase of the ripple transform of a profile (Sec. 4.3). For the last two cases, the profiles are well above their detection thresholds. We first define detection procedures for the three tests on the basis of perceptual experiments with single ripples. Next, we use the model to account for

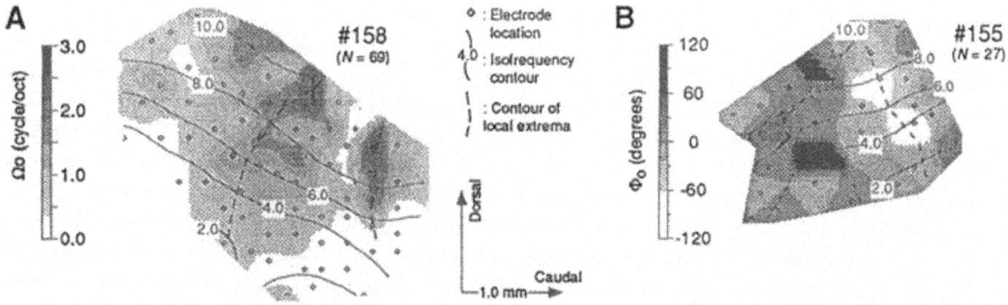

Figure 4: *Cortical maps of Ω_o (A) and Φ_o (B) for multiunit recordings in ferrets #158 and #155. The scaling bar on the left indicates the values represented by the grey intensities. A Gaussian weighted filling was applied to obtain the values between penetration locations (marked by circles). Original values at the electrode locations were preserved. The map is made on the basis of responses where $|\Phi_o| \leq 100°$. The dashed lines connect local maxima of Ω_o, and maxima and minima of Φ_o, across isofrequency planes.*

thresholds of more complex profiles.

4.1 Profile detection tests

To predict detection thresholds for any arbitrary profile, we first incorporate into the model (as a baseline) the detection thresholds obtained with single ripple profiles (Hillier, 1991). These are denoted by the dashed line $K(\Omega_o)$ in Fig. 5A. The model predicts that detection of a profile occurs when its ripple transform magnitude $r(\Omega_o)$ exceeds the perceptual baseline $K(\Omega_o)$. This prediction is confirmed for the three profiles shown in Fig. 5B. In each case, when the profile is set at its just-detectable amplitude (Bernstein and Green, 1987), the ripple transform of the profile approximately reaches the perceptual threshold curve $K(\Omega_o)$.

4.2 Profile dilation tests

As with profile detection tests above, thresholds for dilating an arbitrary profile can be predicted from dilation thresholds of single ripple profiles. Dilating a single ripple profile corresponds to changing its ripple frequency, and hence dilation tests have been called ripple frequency-difference-limen (ripple-fdl) tests (Hillier, 1991). The ripple-fdl data are reproduced by the dashed curve in Fig. 6A and denoted by fdl (right ordinate). In general, dilating a profile $p(\omega)$ by a factor α (about its center ω_o), i.e., $p(\omega) \longrightarrow p(\alpha\,\omega)$ or $P(\Omega) \longrightarrow 1/\alpha P(\Omega/\alpha)$ translates $r(\Omega_o)$ by $\Delta = \log_2 \alpha$ octaves along the logarithmic Ω_o axis, leaving the shape of the ripple transform unaltered. This shift is demonstrated for the ripple profile in Fig. 6B. We assume that in order to detect a profile dilation, subjects sense the shift (Δ) in the steepest lowpass edge of a ripple transform. The ripple-fdl curve can therefore be re-expressed in terms of the equivalent Δ shifts as (solid line and left ordinate in Fig. 6A):

$$\Delta(\Omega_o) = \log_2(1 + \text{fdl}(0.8\ \Omega_o)), \tag{3}$$

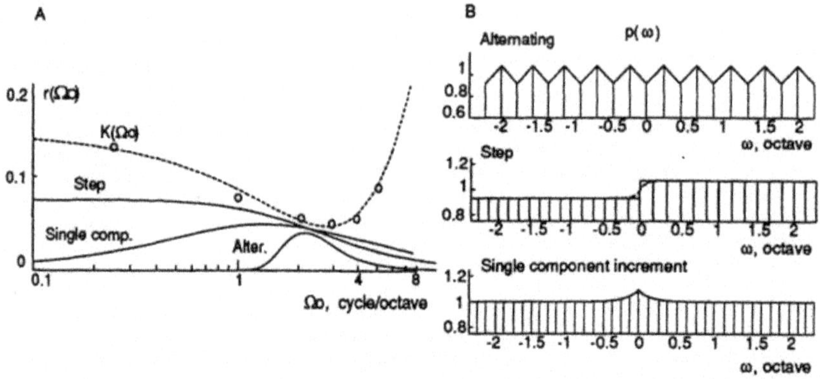

Figure 5: *Profile detection tests in the ripple analysis model. (A) The dashed line is a polynomial approximation to the perceptual thresholds measured with single ripples (reproduced from Fig. 3.27 in Hillier, 1991). Each data point (denoted by circles) represents the peak amplitude of $r(\Omega_o)$ due to a just-detectable ripple with frequency Ω_o. The solid lines represent $r(\Omega_o)$ computed for the profiles shown in (B). (B) The alternating, step, and single component increment profiles at their just-detectable amplitudes according to Bernstein and Green (1987).*

where $\Delta(\Omega_o)$ (in octave) is the same as fdl(Ω_o) but translated by approximately 0.3 octaves (i.e., $\log_2 \frac{\Omega_1}{\Omega_1'}$, where $\Omega_1 = 0.8\,\Omega_1'$, Fig. 6B) to compensate for the misalingment between the location of the lowpass edge of $r(\Omega_o)$ relative to the ripple frequency Ω.

Therefore, the model predicts that for any spectral profile whose ripple transform magnitude $r(\Omega_o)$ is large relative to the perceptual threshold $K(\Omega_o)$ and has a lowpass edge approximately in the range 0.85–7 cycle/octave, dilation thresholds will be constant at 20%, or $\Delta = 0.25$ octave.

This prediction was tested for spectral peak profiles with bandwidths (BWFs) ranging from 0.1-0.4 octaves (Fig. 7A), and different asymmetries (Sec. 4.3 below). All these peaks have ripple transforms with lowpass edges in the range 0.85-4 cycle/octave (Fig. 7B), and hence dilation thresholds were expected to yield $\Delta \approx 0.25$ octave regardless of the peak shape. These predictions are confirmed by the perceptual data (reported in Vranić-Sowers and Shamma, 1994a), where the percentage change in BWF (δBWF/BWF) needed for detection was measured at 0.22 regardless of the starting peak's bandwidth and asymmetry. This corresponds to a dilation factor of $\alpha = 0.82$, or a $\Delta = \log_2 \alpha = -0.29$ octave (downward) shift in $r(\Omega_o)$, approximately as predicted.

4.3 Detection of ripple transform phase shifts

It is also possible to predict sensitivity to phase shifts in the ripple transform of arbitrary profiles from phase-difference-limens (pdl) measured with single ripple profiles. Such measurements are shown in Fig. 8A. They reveal that for low ripple frequencies ($< 1 - 2$ cycles/octave) ripple-pdl thresholds are approximately constant

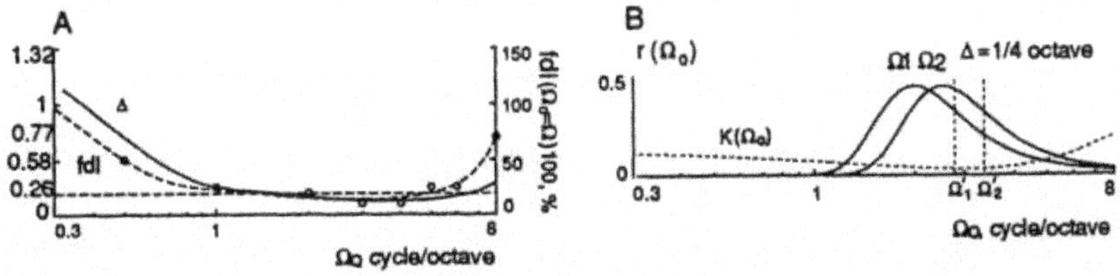

Figure 6: *Dilation thresholds for single ripples. (A) The dashed line represents the interpolated ripple-fdl or the just-detectable percentage change in ripple frequency (right ordinate) for single ripples (reproduced from Fig. 3.30 in Hillier, 1991). The solid line, Δ, is the shifted version of the ripple-fdl curve (see Eq. 3). (B) The shift Δ in $r(\Omega_o)$ due to dilating a ripple profile from $\Omega_1 = 2$ cycle/octave to $\Omega_2 = 2.4$ cycle/octave. The vertical dashed lines denote the locations of the steepest lowpass edges in $r(\Omega_o)$ (Ω_1' and Ω_2'). The ripple-fdl for a 2 cycle/octave ripple is 20%, which corresponds to a dilation factor of $\alpha = 1.2$ or a translation of $r(\Omega_o)$ by $\Delta = \log_2 \alpha \approx 1/4$ octave. Note that the ripple amplitude is large (i.e., $r(\Omega_o)$ maxima significantly exceed $K(\Omega_o)$).*

at 6°-7°; they begin to rise linearly above 2 cycles/octave. Based on these results the model predicts that, for any spectral profile whose ripple transform magnitude $r(\Omega_o)$ contains low frequency ripples (< 1 cycle/octave), phase sensitivity is expected to be approximately 6°.

This prediction was confirmed in the case of the peak profiles shown in Fig. 7 (Vranić-Sowers and Shamma, 1994a). For peaks with BWF>0.1 octave, detection thresholds were measured at approximately 6° regardless of the starting peak's shape. For the narrowest peaks (BWF=0.1), thresholds were slightly higher (10°) presumably reflecting the higher ripple frequency content of the peak as illustrated by its ripple transform in Fig. 7B.

5 Discussion

It is proposed that the central auditory system represents the spectral profile by its local Fourier transform, or more accurately, by its ripple transform. A computational model of this ripple analysis is presented (Sec. 2). It consists of a bank of filters tuned to different ripple frequencies and phases, which transform the profile into its ripple domain. An important aspect of the ripple representation is its locality with respect to the tonotopic axis. Computationally, this is implied by the relatively broad bandwidths of the ripple filters or, equivalently, the limited extent of the impulse response of the filters (Fig. 1A). The ripple analysis model is supported by physiological responses recorded in ferret AI, i.e., AI cells are found to behave like ripple filters (Sec. 3). Psychoacoustical implications of the model are explored in Sec. 4, where manipulations of various spectral profiles are interpreted and detected in this domain (Sec. 4). For the profiles considered in Sec. 4, a simplified, one-dimensional version of the model (see Eq. 2) is used. In general, a comparison between two profiles must be done along all three dimensions (Ω_o, Φ_o, and ω_o) (according to Eq. 1), since the changes along all three axes are perceptually detectable.

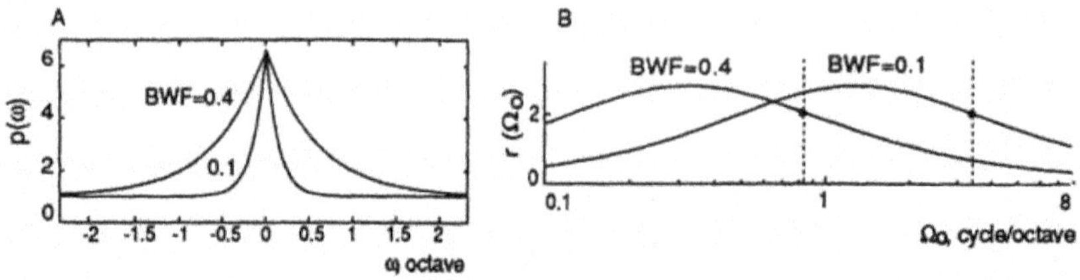

Figure 7: *(A) Profiles of two symmetric peaks (described in detail in Vranić-Sowers and Shamma 1994a). The BWF measures the 3dB-bandwidth of a peak. (B) The ripple transform magnitudes, $r(\Omega_o)$, of the peaks in (A). The dashed lines denote the locations of the steepest low pass edges in $r(\Omega_o)$. The effect of a BWF change is a shift (and not a change in shape) of the ripple transform along the logarithmic Ω_o axis. For example, a four-fold increase in BWF (from 0.1 to 0.4 octaves), i.e., $\delta BWF/BWF$=3 or $\alpha = 0.25$ results in a ($\Delta = \log_2 \alpha =$) 2 octave downward shift in $r(\Omega_o)$.*

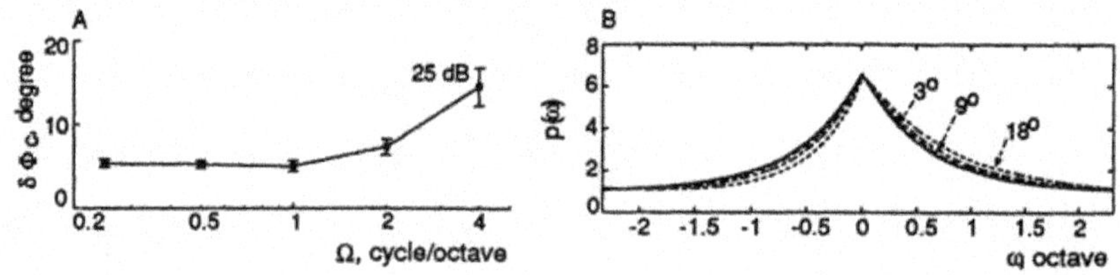

Figure 8: *(A) Perceptual phase difference, $\delta\Phi_c$, at threshold (reproduced from Vranić-Sowers and Shamma, 1994b) for various ripple frequencies Ω, for 161 frequency components and at 25 dB peak-to-valley amplitude. The task is to detect a change in the phase of a ripple while keeping the ripple frequency constant. (B) Shifting the phase of the ripple transform phase of the peak profile by a constant angle simply changes the symmetry of the profile. Solid line is a symmetric peak (BWF = 0.4 octave) with ripple transform phase = 0. Dashed lines are the skewed peaks resulting from adding three different angles to the ripple transform phase (Vranić-Sowers and Shamma, 1994a).*

The notion of a Fourier transformation of a spectrum is common in engineering speech applications and is known as convolutional homomorphic processing. It involves computing Fourier-like coefficients of the spectral profile known as cepstral coefficients (Oppenheim and Schafer, 1990). While quite different in details, the cepstral coefficients encode roughly similar types of information about the shape of the spectrum as the ripple transform, and have been found especially useful in automatic speech recognition systems.

Finally, an appealing aspect of the ripple analysis model is that it shares the conceptual framework of *spatial frequency analysis* that has long been prevalent in visual processing. While having its critics, this approach has been supported by substantial anatomical, neurophysiological, and psychophysical evidence (see reviews in De Valois and De Valois, 1990). The correspondence between the auditory ripple analysis and the visual spatial frequency analysis is in fact deeper than a mere analogy.

As evidence, consider the closely matched values of the filter parameters and detection thresholds measured in the auditory and visual systems, e.g., roughly constant-Q and 1 octave wide filters, and the constant 6° phase sensitivity which increases at higher ripple frequencies (Table 6.1 and Figs. 6.11 and 8.3 in De Valois and De Valois, 1990). These remarkable equivalences may simply reflect modality-independent limitations imposed by identically structured sensory areas in the central nervous system. For instance, the resolution of the analysis filters may be dictated by developmental rules limiting the minimum divergence or convergence of dendritic fields along the sensory epithelium. Clearly, exploring further equivalences and differences between similarly defined psychophysical measures would shed considerable light on the underlying functional organization of both systems.

ACKNOWLEDGEMENTS

This work is supported by the Air Force Office of Scientific Research, The Office of Naval Research, and the National Science Foundation ERC Grant (NSFD CDR8803012).

REFERENCES

Assmann, P.F. and Summerfield, Q. (1989) Modeling the perception of concurrent vowels: Vowels with the same fundamental frequency. J. Acoust. Soc. Am. 85, 327–338.

Bernstein, L.R. and Green, D.M. (1987) Detection of simple and complex changes of spectral shape. J. Acoust. Soc. Am. 82, 1587–1592.

Campbell, F.W. and Robson, J.G. (1968) Application of Fourier Analysis to the visibility of gratings. J. Physiol. 197, 551–566.

De Valois, R.L. and De Valois, K.K. (1990) Spatial Vision, Oxford University Press, New York.

Durlach, N.I., Braida, L.D. and Ito, Y. (1986) Towards a model for discrimination of broadband signals. J. Acoust. Soc. Am. 80, 63–72.

Feth, L.L., O'Malley, H. and Ramsey, J.J. (1982) Pitch of unresolved two-component complex tones. J. Acoust. Soc. Am. 72, 1403–1412.

Hillier, D.A. (1991) Auditory processing of sinusoidal spectral envelopes. Ph.D. Dissertation, The Washington University and Severn Institute.

Klatt, D.H. (1982) Prediction of perceived phonetic distance from critical-band spectra: A first step. Proceedings ICASSP 2, 1278–1281.

Oppenheim, A. and Schafer, R. (1990) Digital Signal Processing. Prentice Hall, New Jersey.

Schreiner, C.E. and Mendelson, J.R. (1990) Functional topography of cat primary auditory cortex: Distribution of integrated excitation. J. Neurophysiol. 64, 1442–1459.

Shamma, S.A., Fleshman, J.W., Wiser, P.R. and Versnel, H. (1993) Organization of response areas in ferret primary auditory cortex. J. Neurophysiol. 69, 367–383.

Shamma, S.A., Versnel, H. and Kowalski, N. (1994) Ripple analysis in ferret primary auditory cortex. I. Response characteristics of single units to sinusoidally rippled spectra. ISR Technical Report 94-20, Univ. of Maryland.

Shamma, S.A., Vranić S. and Wiser, P.R. (1992) Spectral gradient columns in primary auditory cortex: Physiological and psychoacoustical correlates. In: Y. Cazals, L. Demany, K.C. Horner (Eds.) Auditory physiology and perception, Advances in the Biosciences, Vol. 83, Pergamon Press, Oxford, pp. 387–496.

Versnel, H., Kowalski, N. and Shamma, S.A. (1994) Ripple analysis in ferret primary auditory cortex. II. Topographic and columnar distribution of ripple response parameters. ISR Technical Report 94-21, Univ. of Maryland.

Vranić-Sowers S. and Shamma, S.A. (1994a) Representation of spectral profiles in the auditory system. II: Detection of spectral peak shape changes. ISR Technical Report 94-15, Univ. of Maryland.

Vranić-Sowers S. and Shamma, S.A. (1994b) Modeling and predicting perception of spectral profile changes. Proceedings of the 28th Annual Conference on Information Sciences and Systems, Princeton, NJ.

Time-interval patterns and sound quality

Roy D. Patterson and Michael A. Akeroyd

MRC Applied Psychology Unit
15 Chaucer Road, Cambridge, CB2 2EF, U.K.

1 Introduction

We have known for 50 years that the firing of auditory nerve fibers is phase locked to the motion of the basilar membrane at frequencies up to 4-5 kHz (Galambos and Davis, 1943). But relatively little progress has been made in understanding the role of this fine-grain timing information in perception. Most perceptual models either begin with a spectral representation of the stimuli, in which case the fine-structure in the auditory nerve is completely ignored (e.g. Green, 1988), or they begin with a cochlea simulation that generates the fine structure and then promptly remove it in the course of constructing a spectrographic representation of the sound (e.g. Giguerre and Woodland, 1994). We have also known for almost 50 years that the relative phases of the components of a sound often affect the timbre of the sound (Mathes and Miller, 1947). Helmholtz' (1885, 1954, p 127) phase rule has been disproven repeatedly (see Patterson, 1987, for a review). But, little progress has been made in understanding the role of phase in auditory perception. Indeed, it is still commonly assumed that Helmholtz was essentially correct, that phase is of little importance, and that timbre is largely determined by the distribution of energy across the spectrum (e.g. Moore, 1989, p. 230).

In this paper we argue that the lack of progress in understanding the role of phase locking in perception and the lack of an adequate model of sound quality are related; both arise from the continued implicit use of the Fourier transform as a model of auditory processing. The Fourier transform is most appropriate in applications where the important aspect of the signal is the distribution of energy across a range of frequencies, *and* where the fine-grain temporal information in the signal is irrelevant. The non-energy information in Fourier analysis occurs as a spectrum of time shifts between the sinusoids that carry the energy. The auditory system performs a spectral analysis which is like the Fourier analysis inasmuch as the energy of the sound is distributed along the basilar membrane in accordance with its frequency, but which is unlike Fourier analysis insofar as the remainder of the information does not occur in the form of time shifts between channels containing unmodulated sinusoids. Rather, it occurs within channels as time intervals of varying duration which encode non-sinusoidal aspects of the driving wave as well as the level of activation.

In this paper it is argued that the auditory system converts the temporal information in the auditory nerve into some form of multi-channel post-stimulus-time (PST) histogram, and that this form of the 'phase information' provides insight into sound quality that the Fourier phase spectrum does not. The discussion focuses on three new timbre discriminations that are difficult to explain in spectral terms (Section 2). An Auditory Image Model (AIM) of hearing is introduced to convert the sounds into dynamic, multi-channel, PST histograms (Section 3) by means of a simple cochlea simulation and a form of strobed temporal integration. The histograms reveal that there is a time-interval basis for the timbre discriminations, and that the simulated auditory images provide a basis for understanding the sound qualities associated with these stimuli.

2 Timbre Experiments with Tonal Sounds and Noisy Sounds

2.1 Damped and Ramped Sinusoids

The first timbre contrast involves the sound quality associated with a sinusoid and the effect of asymmetric amplitude modulation on the strength of that quality. The 'damped' sinusoid shown in Figure 1a was produced by applying an exponential decay to a short segment of a sinusoid and then repeating the segment to produce a stationary sound. The frequency of the sinusoid is 800 Hz, the period of the segment is 25 ms, and the half life of the exponential damping function is 4 ms. The 'ramped' sinusoid in Figure 1b was produced simply by reversing the damped sinusoid in time. The damped sinusoid is heard as a unitary source, something like a drum roll on a hollow, resonant object. The ramped sinusoid is heard as a co-ordinated pair of sounds, one of which is like a roll on a non-

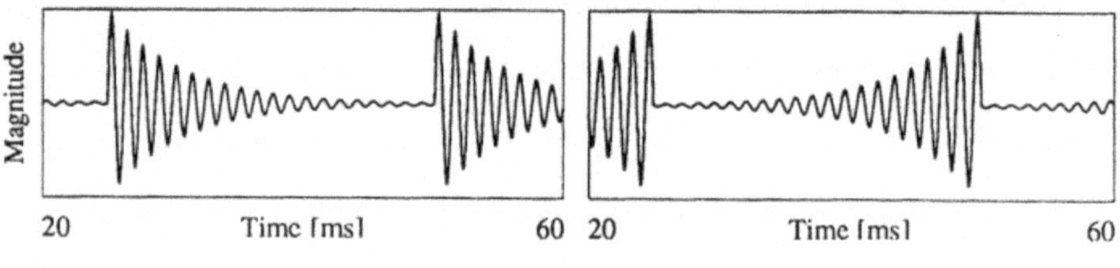

Figure 1. Waveforms of (a) damped and (b) ramped sinusoids with 4-ms half lives and 800-Hz carriers.

resonant surface, and the other of which is *a continuous sinusoid.* The drum role components of the perceptions derive from the streams of transients in these sounds. It is not clear, however, why the ramped sound should carry the distinctive character of the sinusoid and the damped sound not. Patterson (1994a,b) demonstrated the discriminability of damped and ramped sinusoids by presenting listeners with pairs that had the same half life and asking them to choose the member of the pair with the stronger sinusoidal sound quality. The listeners are able to perform the discrimination without difficulty for half lives ranging from 2-16 ms, for carrier frequencies ranging from 400 to 4800 Hz, and for envelope periods ranging from 10 to 100 ms.

The Fourier Energy (FE) spectra of damped and ramped sinusoids contain one, well defined, peak rising out of a broad plateau (produced by the stream of transients), and the pitch of the sound is that appropriate to the peak in the spectrum. But, the FE spectra of damped and ramped sounds with the same half life are identical, and so models based on the FE spectrum provide no basis for even distinguishing pairs of damped and ramped sounds, let alone explaining the pronounced difference in sound quality that we hear. The phase of the damped sinusoid has the opposite sign to that of the ramped sinusoid throughout the phase spectrum, but this provides little insight into why the damped sound does not have the quality of a sinusoid.

Auditory models designed to simulate cochlear processing can be used to simulate internal, or auditory, spectra of complex sounds by measuring the level of activity in each channel at a given point in time and plotting the values as a function of channel frequency. Provided the measure is *not* the energy of the filtered wave, the auditory spectra of damped and ramped sinusoids will differ, and if the system is compressive, the peak in the auditory spectrum of the damped sinusoid will be narrower than the peak in the spectrum of the ramped sinusoid. The difference arises because of the way the damped and ramped sinusoids drive off-frequency filters. The damped sinusoid hits the filter with a large pulse of energy which initially causes a strong response. At the same time, however, it causes the filter to try to ring at its centre frequency. Over the course of a few cycles, the ringing energy builds up and, at the same time, the level of the input sinusoid decreases. Since the two terms are associated with different frequencies (the carrier frequency and the filter centre frequency), they eventually drift out of phase and this causes partial cancellation of the output. The ramped sinusoid puts much less energy into the filter initially and when this ringing energy returns to oppose the forcing function, the level of the input sinusoid has increased. The ringing term is small relative to the input throughout the rising portion of the ramped sinusoid. Thus, in a wide range of off-frequency channels, the ramped sinusoid generates more activity at the output when measured in terms of, for example, the average peak-to-trough level, and this difference is preserved in the output of the cochlea simulation. Thus, a model of sound quality based on auditory spectra of this type predicts that damped and ramped sinusoids are discriminable, and that the *damped* member of the pair will sound more like a sinusoid because its spectral peak is narrower and more like that of an unmodulated sinusoid. Nevertheless, the listeners consistently chose the *ramped* sinusoid as the one with the stronger sinusoidal quality.

2.2 Wideband noise versus Iterated Rippled Noise

The second timbre contrast involves the sound of noise. It is the contrast between the sound of a bandpass random noise and that of a bandpass Iterated Rippled Noise (IRN). Rippled noise is constructed from a random noise by delaying a copy of the random noise and adding it back to the original. The delay-and-add process introduces ripples into the spectrum of the IRN, with peaks at multiples of the reciprocal of the delay and valleys midway between them. The rippled noise sounds like a pair of concurrent sources, a weak low-pitched complex tone in a prominent broadband noise. When the delay-and-add process is repeated, or iterated, the tonal component of the perception grows stronger and the noise component grows weaker, and by about 10 iterations the noise component of the perception is barely noticeable. When the delay is long (say 16 ms), the spectral peaks are closely packed (every 62.5 Hz) and, in the region above about ten times the peak spacing, the auditory spectrum of the IRN is quite similar to that of the random noise. Thus, a spectral model of hearing would suggest that if random and iterated noises are highpass filtered and equated for energy, they will not be discriminable. Nevertheless, they are perfectly discriminable; one has the *shshsh* of noise and the other sounds like a buzzy musical note. Their phase spectra are complex, random functions that do not provide any obvious explanation for the sound qualities we hear.

The timbre contrast between random and iterated noises led us to suspect that IRN would be more detectable in random noise than in IRN, and that random noise would be more detectable in iterated noise than in random noise. To test this hypothesis, a standard, two-interval forced-choice experiment was performed to determine the signal level required to detect both a random noise and a IRN with 256 iterations in each of five maskers, a random noise and IRNs with 1, 4, 16 and 256 iterations. The IRN was produced using the method described by Yost *et. al.* (1993). To reduce the value of loudness cues and promote the use of timbre cues, we used a roving level paradigm with a range of 10 dB (Green, 1988). This has the effect of making it considerably more difficult to detect the random noise in random noise and the IRN in IRN, because the only cue available to the listeners is the loudness of the sounds. In conditions where there is a timbre contrast, the listeners can ignore the roving level and use the relative level of the tonal and noisy components of the perception. All of the signals and maskers were bandpass filtered between 800 and 4500 Hz and so their long-term auditory spectra all had the same shape. In a spectral model of masking, then, the two signals should be about equally detectable in all of the maskers.

Three normal hearing listeners took part in the experiment and the pattern of results was similar for all three. The average data showed that the random noise was about 4 dB more difficult to detect than the IRN with 256 iterations when the masker was a random noise or an IRN with one iteration. As the number of iterations in the masker increased, however, the IRN signal became about 6 dB harder to detect while the random noise became about 14 dB easier to detect! Thus, the timbre contrasts lead to a 20-dB interaction in masking threshold where few, if any, differences should exist at all.

2.3 Damped and Ramped Noises

The third timbre contrast also involves the sound of a noise. When the sinusoidal carrier of the damped and ramped sounds is replaced by a wideband noise, the perception produced by the ramped noise contains more of the *shshsh* and *hissss* associated with random noise sources than does the perception produced by the damped noise. As with damped and ramped tones, the FE spectra of damped and ramped noises are identical and, since the carrier is a broadband noise, there is no difference (e.g. the width of the passband) to distinguish their auditory spectra. Akeroyd and Patterson (1994) have demonstrated the discriminability of damped and ramped noises by presenting listeners with pairs that had the same half life and asking them to choose the member of the pair with the "most drum-like" sound quality. At the shortest half lives (less than 2 ms) performance was not quite as good as that with damped and ramped sinusoids. But with half lives greater than 8 ms, performance was as good or better for the noise stimuli. The discrimination of damped and ramped sinusoids falls off as the half life increases beyond 16 ms because eventually the damped sinusoid develops a strong sinusoidal component and the two versions of the sinusoid become indistinguishable. With a noise carrier, however, increasing the half life makes the ramped version noisier *but not the damped version*, and so discrimination performance remains high for half lives up to, at least, 32 ms. Moreover, extending the period of the envelope of the sound increases the difference between the perceptions of ramped and damped noise; again, the ramped version becomes noisier but not the damped version. Both of these findings run contrary to what one might expect either from a consideration of forward and backward masking, or from the envelope differences at the output of a set of leaky integrators.

In summary, this section has presented three timbre contrasts involving the most basic auditory perceptions -- those associated with pure tones, complex tones and broadband noises. The data show that timbre discriminations occur where power spectrum models predict no discrimination. Moreover, the phase spectra of the stimuli do not provide any obvious explanations for the sound quality differences that we hear in these sounds.

3 The Auditory Image Model and Sound Quality

A computational model of peripheral auditory processing has been developed to explain the auditory images we hear when presented with sounds -- the Auditory Image Model of Patterson *et. al.*, (1992a). The image is constructed in three stages, each of which involves filtering, or sorting, the components of the sound in some way, and arranging the products of the process along a space-like dimension. The first two stages simulate the frequency analysis and the laterality analysis performed by the peripheral auditory system in the usual way. Together they produce a frequency-laterality plane like that shown in the centre of Figure 2; in this particular case, it illustrates the separation of a source 40 degrees to the right with energy in the mid-frequencies, from a source 20 degrees to the left with energy at higher and lower frequencies. The frequency-laterality analysis is often presented as if it represented peripheral processing in its entirety. At this point, however, it would be difficult to tell whether the sound was a low-pitched bassoon note or a bandpass filtered noise with a similar spectral shape, because information about regularity in the fine-structure of the sound is not available in the frequency-laterality plane. The complex sound qualities we hear in tonal sounds indicates that there is a third stage of analysis involving the temporal fine-structure of the neural activity flowing from the cochlea. It is as if the system maintained a two-dimensional array of dynamic PST histograms behind the frequency-laterality plane, one histogram for each frequency-laterality combination. The set of histograms activated by a wideband point source would form a vertical plane at a given angle, like the planes shown in Figure 2. When the sound is periodic, the plane contains a set of regular and related histograms; when the sound is irregular, the plane contains irregular and unrelated histograms. In the Auditory Image

Model (AIM), the space described in Figure 2 is the basic space of auditory perception. The images that form in this space are the first internal representation of the sound that we are aware of, and subsequent processing is based on these auditory images.

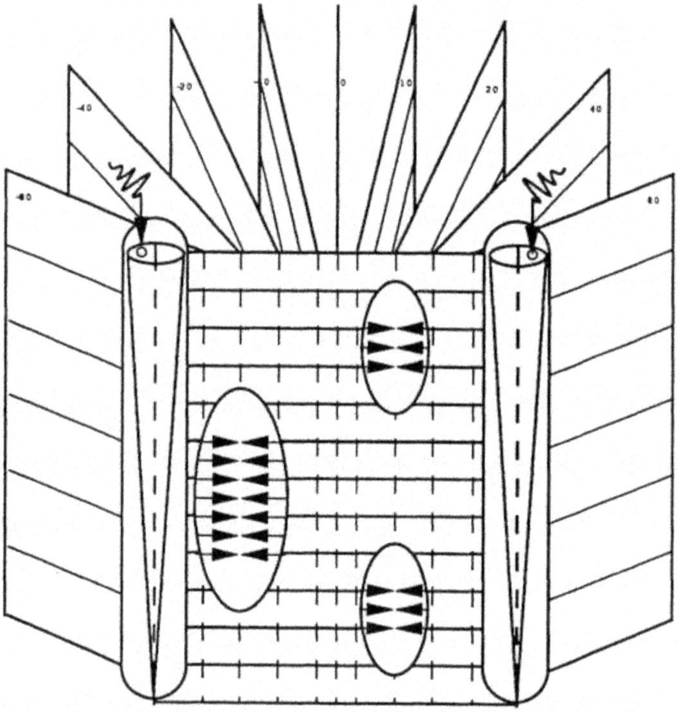

Figure 2. The space of auditory perception in the auditory image model.

The mechanism that constructs the histogram from phase-locked neural activity is a new form of temporal integration that is intended to stabilise repeating time-interval patterns from quasi-periodic sounds without smearing their fine-structure. Briefly, a bank of delay lines is used to form a buffer store for the neural activity flowing from the cochlea; the activity level decays as it flows down the buffer at the rate of 1.5-2.5 percent/ms. Each channel has a strobe unit which monitors the instantaneous activity level and when it encounters a large peak it transfers the entire record in that channel of the buffer to the corresponding channel of a static image buffer, where the record is added, point for point, with whatever is already in that channel of the image buffer. Information in the image buffer decays exponentially with a half-life of about 30 ms. In the case of periodic and quasi-periodic sounds, the strobe unit tends to synchronise to the period of the sound and so generates a regular stream of pulses that initiate temporal integration in synchrony with the repeating neural pattern. This process stabilises repeating patterns in the simulated neural activity in much the same way as a PST histogram reveals a recurring neural pattern. The one innovation in AIM is that the pulses that reset time in the construction of the PST histogram are derived from the activity pattern itself, without prior knowledge of the sound. For a point source, the activity is restricted to one vertical plane of histograms which is AIM's representation of our auditory image of the sound. When the sound is periodic, or quasi-periodic, this process performs temporal integration over cycles without smearing the fine-structure within the period of the pattern. One can think of the strobed temporal integration in AIM as a better way of handling the "phase" information in the sound. The traditional leaky integration process removes the majority of the non-energy information from the output of the cochlea simulation. Strobed temporal integration preserves the time-interval patterns of periodic sounds while removing between-channel phase differences and some order-of-arrival information. It is argued that the stabilised patterns provide a better basis for analysing sound quality and identifying sources than do spectra, spectrograms or cochleograms (Patterson, *et. al.*, 1992b).

3.1 Auditory Images of Damped and Ramped Sinusoids

The auditory images of the damped and ramped sinusoids with 4-ms half lives and 800-Hz carriers are presented in Figures 3a and 3b, respectively. The figures show the frequency region from 1.5 octaves below, to 1.5 octaves above, 800 Hz (9.3-19.2 ERBs). In the upper section of each sub-figure, the activity in each channel is essentially an impulse response produced by the abrupt change in amplitude of the stimulus once per

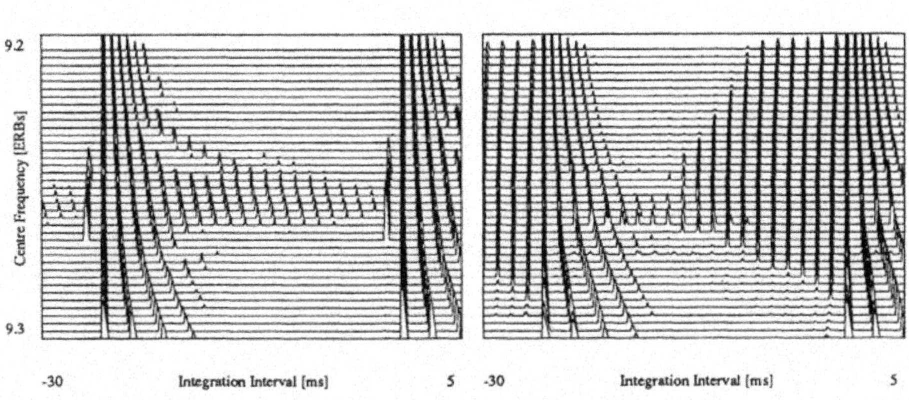

(a) (b)

Figure 3. Auditory images of (a) damped and (b) ramped sinusoids with 4-ms half lives. The time interval between the parallel vertical ridges in ramped image is 1.25 ms -- the period of the carrier.

cycle of the sound. The response to the carrier frequency is shown in the central section of each panel. The ramped sinusoid (Figure 3b) activates a broader frequency region than the damped sinusoid (Figure 3a). The phase alignment induced by strobed temporal integration reveals that the carrier activity of the ramped sinusoid is mainly composed of time intervals at the period of the carrier, even when the activity is in channels well above or below the carrier channel. This sound has the quality of a sinusoid. The response to the damped sinusoid reveals time intervals characteristic of the carrier only in the channel at the centre of the carrier response. As the channel frequency decreases below that of the carrier, the time intervals in the response lengthen, and as the channel frequency increases above that of the carrier, the time intervals shorten. This behaviour is characteristic of a set of resonators struck by an acoustic pulse; each rings at its own centre frequency. This sound has a hollow quality rather than a sinusoidal quality.

Damped and ramped sounds produce relatively simple auditory images composed either of time intervals at the carrier period or at the period of the centre frequency of the channel. For these simple images, it is possible to segregate and measure the carrier period activity, and so test the hypothesis that the sound of a sinusoid is associated with a concentration of time intervals at the carrier period rather than with a concentration of energy in the carrier channel. Auditory images were produced for a range of damped and ramped sounds and time-interval histograms were calculated for each channel of each image. (The calculations were limited to time-intervals between adjacent pulses for simplicity.) The multi-channel time-interval histograms confirmed that the ramped sinusoid produces a substantial number of 1.25-ms intervals in off-frequency channels whereas the damped sinusoid does not. The number of 1.25-ms intervals was calculated for each auditory image and pairs of values for damped and ramped sinusoids with the same half life were compared. Broadly speaking, for all carrier frequencies, the number of carrier periods was substantially higher for the ramped sinusoid in the range of half lives where discrimination performance was good, that is, between 2 and 16 ms. For the higher carrier frequencies (3200 and 4800 Hz), the model also produced more carrier periods for the ramped sinusoid at half lives less than 2 ms, where the listeners could not hear a difference. This presumably reflects a loss of phase locking at short time-intervals in the auditory system; a loss which is not simulated in the current version of AIM. Despite its obvious limitations, the quantitative analysis of carrier period activity suggests that it is the presence of time intervals at the carrier period rather than energy in the carrier channels *per se* that gives a sound the quality associated with a sinusoid.

3.2 Auditory Images of Wideband noise and Iterated Rippled Noise

The second timbre contrast was between the sound of a bandpass random noise and the sound of a bandpass IRN. Auditory images of a white noise and a ripple noise with 256 iterations and a 16-ms delay are presented in Figure 4a and 4b. The frequency region is once again 9.3-19.2 ERBs. Both images show regularity at the shortest time intervals, since even white noise is correlated with itself in the short term. Beyond a few cycles, however, there are no stable features in the white noise image (Figure 4a). In the IRN, there are vertical ridges at 16 and 32 ms (Figure 4b) indicating temporal regularity both within and across channels at these time intervals. The auditory images provide a basis for understanding the timbre of these sounds. The *shshsh* of noise arises when the image contains regions where there is no structure and the rate of change in the detail is relatively high. In contrast, a tonal sensation arises when the image contains regions where the time-interval pattern is orderly and the rate of change in the detail is relatively low. If the auditory system performs an analysis of time-interval patterns like that implied by

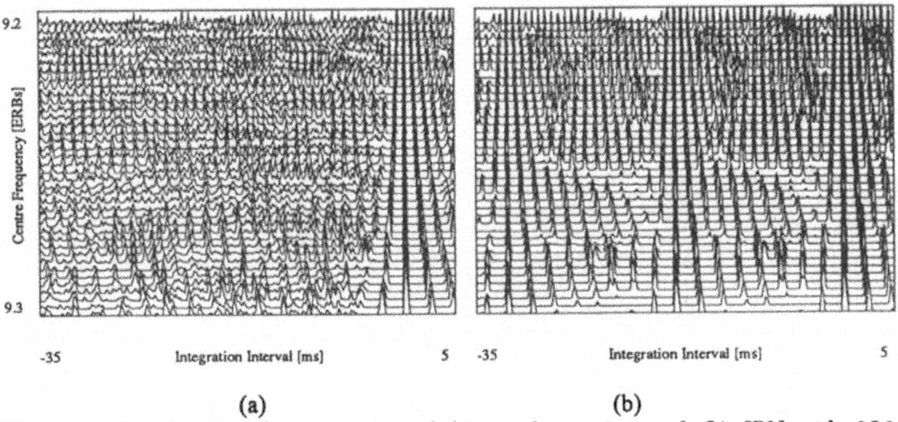

Figure 4. Simulated auditory images of (a) random noise and (b) IRN with 256 iterations.

these simulated auditory images, and if it is able to analyse the images and separate the orderly regions (i.e. figures) from the unordered regions (i.e. background noise), then the ratio of the level of activity in the figure to the level of activity in the background would provide a basis for the timbre discrimination data from the IRN experiment. When the signal and masker have the same number of iterations adding the signal to the noise does not alter the form of the auditory image; there is nothing but a level difference to distinguish the interval with the signal, and the roving level paradigm makes this difficult. But when the signal has no iterations and the masker has many, the signal can be detected by the irregularity that it introduces into the auditory image associated with the signal interval (Figure 4b). The roving level paradigm does not interfere with detection in this case because the listener is using the figure/ground ratio as the cue to the presence of the signal. We do not yet have an algorithm for identifying and segregating regular and irregular regions of auditory images, and so we do not have a quantitative measure of the figure/ground ratio to compare with the data from the experiment. Nevertheless, this qualitative explanation of the timbre discrimination would appear to be better than what could be expected from a spectrographic model of sound quality for these stimuli.

3.3 Auditory Images of Damped and Ramped Noises

The final timbre contrast was that associated with damped and ramped noises; whereas, all of the ramped stimuli carry the *shshsh* of noise, many of the damped stimuli do not. The monitor units in AIM's temporal integration mechanism have an asymmetric temporal response, introduced to ensure that the temporal asymmetries produced by everyday sounds in the neural activity pattern were preserved in the auditory image. Fine-structure peaks occurring just after a transient in the damped noise are less likely to cause integration than pulses of similar size occurring an equal time before a transient in the corresponding ramped noise. As a result, integration occurs somewhat more frequently for the ramped noise and the level of activity level in its auditory image is somewhat greater than that in the corresponding damped image. This difference could be used to explain the discriminability of damped and ramped noises. However, the images of damped and ramped noise both show irregular activity throughout the image and the degree of irregularity does not appear to differ substantially. In its current form then, AIM only predicts that the ramped noise will sound louder that the damped noise. It does not explain why the *shshsh* component of the sound is absent from many of the damped noises. It is as if the strobe process, and thus temporal integration, is inhibited during periods when the slope of the envelope of the neural activity is negative. It is possible that the information in onsets is more important in some way than the information in offsets, and that temporal asymmetry in strobe sensitivity helps prevent the details of offsets from interfering with the perception of onsets.

4 Summary

The auditory image model has been used to convert the phase-locked time-interval patterns of some tonal and noisy sounds into dynamic PST histograms, and to relate the patterns in the histograms to three timbre discriminations. The first discrimination involved the strength of the sinusoidal quality produced by asymmetrically modulated sinusoids, which was found to vary with the direction of the asymmetry. The model explains that the onsets of sinusoids drive off-frequency auditory filters in a temporally synchronous mode whereas the offsets of sinusoids do not. The auditory images of damped and ramped sinusoids suggest that it is these time-intervals at the carrier period that give rise to the sound of a sinusoid rather than energy in the carrier channel *per se*. The second discrimination involved the difference between the *shshsh* of random noise and the tonal buzz of iterated rippled noise. It led to a masking experiment where the timbre contrast was found to support a 20-dB interaction in masking levels that would not have been anticipated from the spectra of the sounds. The discrimination was explained in terms of the variability of the time intervals in the multi-channel histograms of the sounds. The third discrimination involved the lack of *shshsh* in the perception of damped noises. It appears to indicate that the auditory system suppresses the fine-structure of offsets. Together the model and experiments suggest that the timbre of sounds is closely related to the time-interval patterns produced by sounds in the auditory nerve, and that even simple models of the production and processing of these time-interval patterns are sufficient to support productive research into the perception of sound quality.

5 Acknowledgements

The authors thank W. Yost for assistance with the IRN generators; J. Datta and S. Handel for contributions to the IRN experiment and comments on an earlier draft of the paper; M. Allerhand for continuing support of the AIM software; and M. d'Souza for help with the postscript figures. The research was supported by DRA grant FRNIC/U/759 and an MRC studentship to author M. A.

6 References

Akeroyd, M.A. and Patterson, R.D. (1994) Discrimination of time-asymmetric modulated noise. J. Acoust. Soc. Am. MIT meeting, (in press).

Giguerre, C. and Woodland, P.C. (1994) A computational model of the auditory periphery for speech and hearing research: I. Ascending path. J. Acoust. Soc. Am. 331-342.

Galambos, R. and Davis, H. (1943) The response of single auditory nerve fibers to acoustic stimulation. J. Neurophysiology, 6, 39-57.

Green, D.M. (1988) Profile Analysis: auditory intensity discrimination, Oxford University Press, New York.

Helmholtz, H. (1885, 1954) On the sensations of tone. (English translation), Dover, New York.

Mathes, R.C. and Miller, R.L. (1947) Phase effects in monaural percpetion. J. Acoust. Soc. Am. 18, 780-797.

Moore, B.C.J. (1989) An introduction to the psychology of hearing. Academic Press, London.

Patterson, R.D. (1987) A pulse ribbon model of monaural phase perception. J. Acoust. Soc. Am. 82, 1560-1586.

Patterson, R.D. (1994a) The sound of a sinusoid: Spectral models. J. Acoust. Soc. Am. (in press).

Patterson, R.D. (1994b) The sound of a sinusoid: Time-interval models. J. Acoust. Soc. Am. (in press).

Patterson, R.D., Holdsworth, J. and Allerhand M. (1992b) 'Auditory Models as preprocessors for speech recognition', In: *The Auditory Processing of Speech: From the auditory periphery to words,* M. E. H. Schouten (Ed), Mouton de Gruyter, Berlin, 67-83.

Patterson, R., Robinson, K., Holdsworth, J., McKeown, D., Zhang, C. and Allerhand, M. (1992a) Complex sounds and auditory images. In: Auditory physiology and perception. Eds. Y Cazals, L. Demany, K. Horner, (Pergamon, Oxford), 429-446.

Yost, W.A., Allerhand, M., Robinson, K., and Patterson, R.D. (1993) The pitch and pitch strength of iterated rippled noise. Abstract of the 16th meeting of the Association. for Research in Otolaryngology, No. 186.

Comment by A.J.M. Houtsma

Some years ago Rossing and I published pitch matching data for 40 ms damped and ramped sinusoids and for 40 ms square dated sinusoids. One of the findings was that both ramps and damps shifted the pitch upwards compared with the gated comparison tone. What prediction does your model make for this situation?

Rossing, T.D. and Houtsma, A.J.M. (1986) Effects of signal envelope on the pitch of short sinusoidal tones. J. Acoust. Soc. Am. 79, 1926-1933.

Reply

While it is interesting to consider the effects of the damped and ramped envelopes on the pitches of our stimuli, pitch perception was not the focus of our research and so we did not measure the pitches of our stimuli. We were concerned with the timbre of the sounds, and in particular, the strength of the sinusoidal quality of the perception. The intriguing point is that the sound whose energy is concentrated in the carrier channel has less of the sound of a sinusoid.

With regard to pitch, informal listening led me to conclude that the pitches of damped and ramped sounds did not vary significantly from the pitch of the carrier.

Adaptation to unidirectional sweeping spectral peaks

J. P. Wilson, D. Frost and G.D. Wilkes

Keele University, Department of Communication & Neuroscience, Keele, Staffordshire, ST5 5BG, U.K.

1 Introduction

Physiological experiments have demonstrated neurones in various parts of the brain responsive to specific types of stimulus modulation (Whitfield & Evans, 1965; Nelson et al, 1966; Suga, 1973). Attempts to replicate these findings by psychophysical techniques in humans have led to the concept of feature specific channels (Kay & Matthews, 1972; Green & Kay, 1973, 1974; Gardner & Wilson, 1979; Regan & Tansley, 1979; Tansley & Regan, 1979; Davidson et al, 1981; Suffield & Tansley, 1983). The nature of this specificity is that exposure to one type of modulation, e.g. FM, subsequently raises the threshold for this type of modulation (by a factor of 2 or 3) but not for other types of modulation. Kay & Matthews (1972) were able to show that this adaptation effect was specific to the carrier frequency region used and to the modulation rate. Gardner & Wilson (1979) showed that the FM adaptation was directionally specific so that upsweep adaptors raised the threshold for upsweeps but not for downsweeps, and vice versa. Tansley & Regan (1979) confirmed this and also found that intensity upsweeps and downsweeps did likewise. In 1981 Diehl cast doubts on the selective channel hypothesis for speech signals. Supporting these doubts, Wakefield & Viemeister (1984) repeated the experiment of Gardner & Wilson (1979) showing that the adaption factor of 1.7 represented only a small detectability drop from 75% to 65%, and that this might be explained by cognitive factors which affect the subject's view of the reference signal. Moody et al (1984) also questioned the selective channel hypothesis by showing that with repeated testing, the difference between adapted and unadapted thresholds gradually disappeared. They thought it possible, however, that their subjects learned to use another cue that was unaffected by adaptation. Their use of feedback of results would enhance this possibility. No other study has found this decrement of adaptation even though some experiments have lasted appreciably longer.

One of the shortcomings of the unidirectional sweep experiments was that the nature of threshold determination was such that the rate of change of frequency of the test stimulus can be very different from that of the adaptor, which may be inappropriate for the channel hypothesis. In view of these various difficulties and of the relevance of such studies to the recognition of speech signals, it was decided to investigate directional adaptation using a different type of stimulus and a different type of threshold determination. The stimuli were to be multiple-peaked noise signals somewhat akin to multiple-formant speech signals and the thresholds were to be obtained (again using a forced-choice technique to minimise non-sensory factors) by reducing spectral peak-to-valley ratios rather than by altering the rates of change of frequency.

2 Methods

2.1 Stimulus Generation

The frequency-sweeping adaptation and test stimuli were derived from two identical pseudorandom-sequence noise generators set to a relative delay, T, of 1 ms in experiment 1 and 0.125 to 16 ms in experiment 2. Addition of such signals gives a comb-filtered noise with a power density spectrum of $A^2(1+\cos 2\pi fT)$. Therefore, for T = 1 ms, the peaks are spaced at 1 kHz intervals and have half-power bandwidths of 500 Hz. In order to cause continuous upwards or downwards motion of the peaks, the phases of all the components of one of the signals have to be set in rotation by a low-frequency modulating signal before addition to the other signal. This is achieved by passing the signal through two phase-shifting networks (ø and ø+90°) which produce outputs differing by 90°±1° over the audible range. These outputs are multiplied by the in-phase and quadrature outputs from a low-frequency oscillator (see Fig. 1). The sum and difference between these products represent signals whose phases are rotating clockwise and anti-clockwise, respectively, at the rate of the modulating signal, but which still have flat spectra and sound identical to the original pseudorandom sequence. A similar arbitrary phase function, ø, is applied to the delayed signal before adding it to the rotating vector signals. These final additions give the high peak-valley-ratio (PVR) upward and downward sweeping spectra used as adapting stimuli.

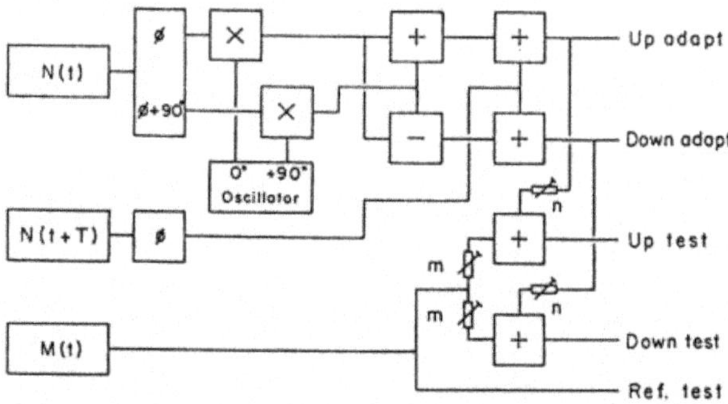

Figure 1. Stimulus generation system, N(t) and N(t+T) are two pseudorandom noise generators with a relative delay, T=0.125 - 16ms, and M(t) is an analogue noise generator, ø and ø+90° are all pass networks with a relative phase difference of 90°±1° from 4 Hz to80 kHz. X,+,- represent analogue multipliers, adders and a subtractor, respectively. The quadrature oscillator was set at 3 Hz for one subject and 8 Hz for the others.

To produce the lower PVR signals required for the test signals an independent analogue noise, M(t), is added to reduce the contrast. The attenuation factors, m and n are set to give both the required PVR and also a mean spectral density equal to that of the adapting stimulus. Fig. 2 shows a representation of a downward sweeping test stimulus with a PVR of 1.7 (2.3dB).

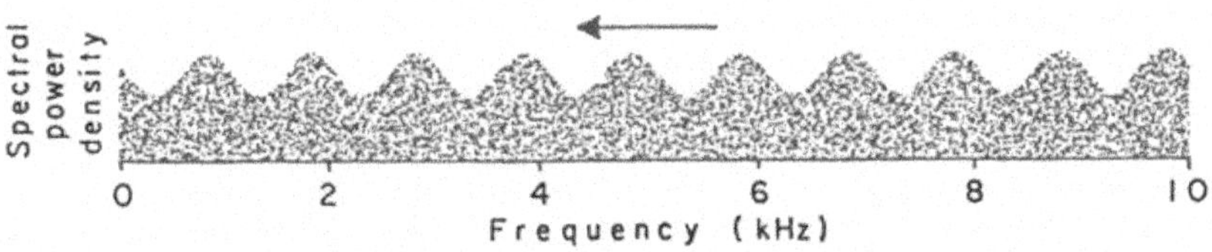

Figure 2. A representation of the stimulus spectrum for a PVR of 1.7 (2.3 dB). The arrow is intended to indicate that all the ripples are moving downward in frequency. The adapting stimulus has a PVR > 30 dB.

2.2 Psychophysical Method

A two-interval forced-choice (2-IFC) technique is used to determine the ear's sensitivity to sweeping spectral peaks. To obtain the threshold a series of stimulus pairs (1 and 2) is presented, one containing the target stimulus and the other a neutral comparison signal of white noise. Indicator lights define the intervals for the subject and prompt him to respond by pressing a key to indicate in which interval the target stimulus occurred. The target stimulus is presented at one of four possible PVRs in order to bracket threshold, preferably between the two lowest levels. As the subject's response is recorded, randomisers determine the sequence of the stimulus-pair, the PVR level, and restart the stimulus sequence. Each threshold determination consists of about 100 stimulus pairs and the percentage correct at each level is plotted on a probability scale. Threshold is taken as the interpolated stimulus value that would give a 75% correct response.

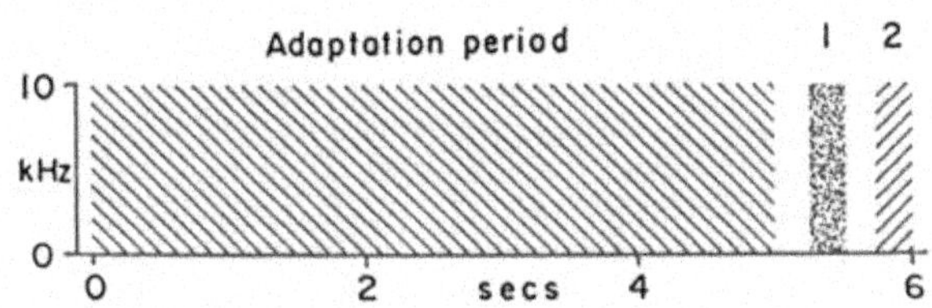

Figure 3. The stimulus sequence is shown as a frequency-time pattern where the diagonal lines represent spectral peaks and the grain pattern represents white noise. The task of the subject was to decide whether interval 1 or 2 contained the sweep-frequency stimulus.

2.3 Experimental Procedure

Stimuli were presented diotically via a filter to equalise the Sennheiser HD 414 phones in a sound attenuating enclosure. The overall level of the stimuli was set at 50 dB above absolute threshold for each subject. The experimental stimulus sequence is illustrated in Fig. 3 for a downward sweeping adapting stimulus and an upward sweeping test stimulus in interval 2. The diagonal lines represent the frequency-time paths for the spectral peaks at 8 Hz modulating frequency, producing a temporal pattern of 8 peaks per second, or a spectral velocity of 8 kHz per second. The overall bandwidth, however, was not restricted to 10 kHz. The test stimulus durations and intervening intervals were all 0.25 s and the adapting stimuli lasted for 5 s. All combinations of upward and downward test and adapting stimuli were used. As the stimuli were all noise signals, rectangular gating functions were used. Starting phases of the adapting and test stimuli were random. Four of the subjects used 8 Hz modulation rate whereas the other used 3 Hz. For JPW the tests were done alternately in the order shown and then in reverse order but for the other subjects a random sequence was used. All subjects had normal hearing thresholds.

3 Results

Results are shown for five subjects in Figs. 4, 5 and 6. Fig. 4 shows data for three subjects which were presented in preliminary form in Wilson et al, 1991. All had a

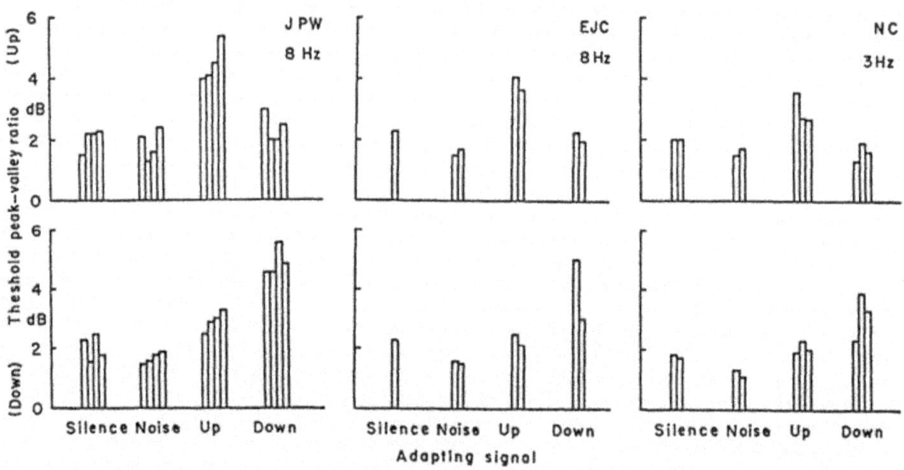

Figure 4. Threshold PVR plotted for adapting signals of silence, white noise, and upward and downward sweeping spectral peaks. Upper and lower plots are for upsweep and downsweep test signals respectively. All stimuli were for T=1ms (1 kHz peak spacing) with modulation rates of 8 Hz (8 peaks/s) for subjects JPW and EJC and 3 Hz for NC.

spectral peak spacing of 1 kHz and two of the subjects, JPW & EJC used an 8 Hz modulation giving a sweep rate of 8 kHz/s and the other, NC, used 3 Hz giving 3 kHz/s. For each test condition the lowest threshold PVR was obtained with a white noise adaptor, followed by no adaptor, then the case when adaptor and test sweeps were of opposite sign, and finally the case showing the biggest increment and highest threshold occurred when adaptor and test were in the same direction. The latter represents the

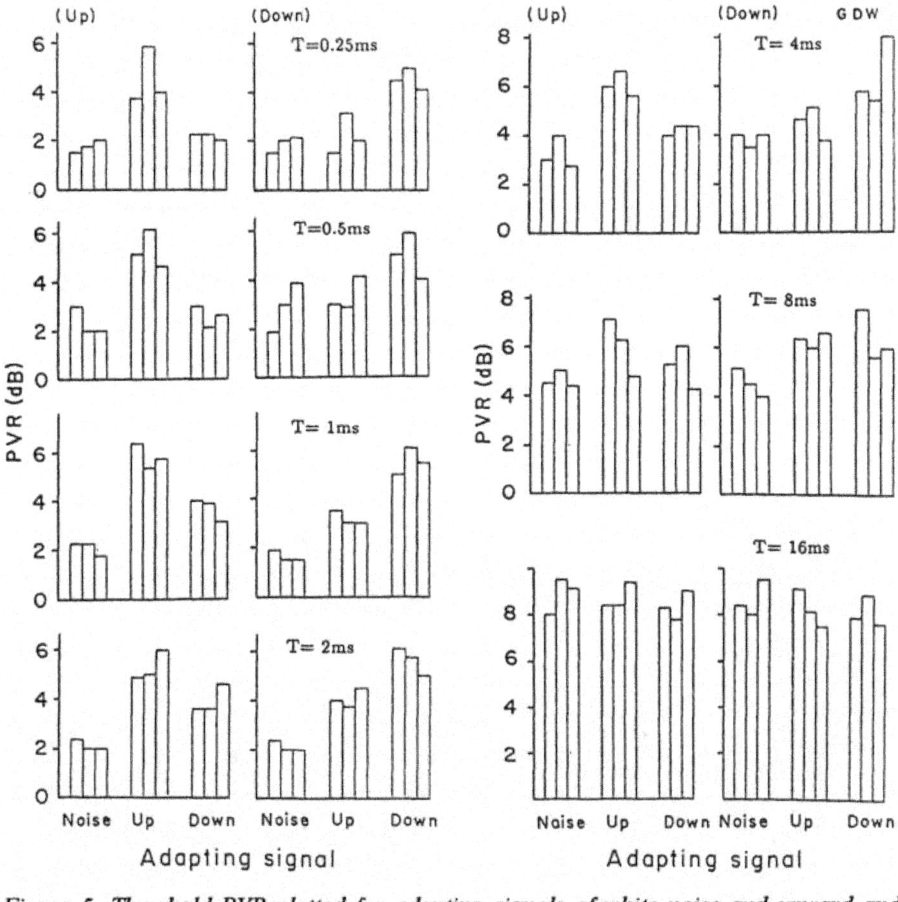

Figure 5. Threshold PVR plotted for adapting signals of white noise and upward and downward sweeps with T as parameter. Upward test signals are shown on the left of each pair and downward on the right. The spectral peak spacing ranges from 4 kHz at 0.25 ms to 62.5 Hz at 16 ms. Modulation rate 8 Hz.

principal outcome of the experiment, directionally specific adaptation. These observations were confirmed by statistical analysis using the Mann-Whitney test and pooling the two subjects at 8 Hz. Firstly, there was no significant difference between the detectability of upsweeps and downsweeps in the control conditions. At 8 Hz a noise adaptor gave a just significantly lower threshold than silence ($p<0.05$). Same versus different, the directional effect, was highly significant ($p<0.0001$ at 8 Hz, $p<0.01$ at 3 Hz) as was same versus noise, the main adapting condition ($p<0.0001$ at 8 Hz and $p<0.001$ at 3 Hz). More surprisingly different versus noise, representing non direction specific adaptation, was also significant at 8 Hz ($p<0.01$) but not at 3 Hz.

In Figs. 5 and 6 the tests were repeated using two other subjects with relative time delay, T, as parameter in order to see whether directional specificity of adaptation depends upon spectral analysis of the signal by the auditory system. The first control condition

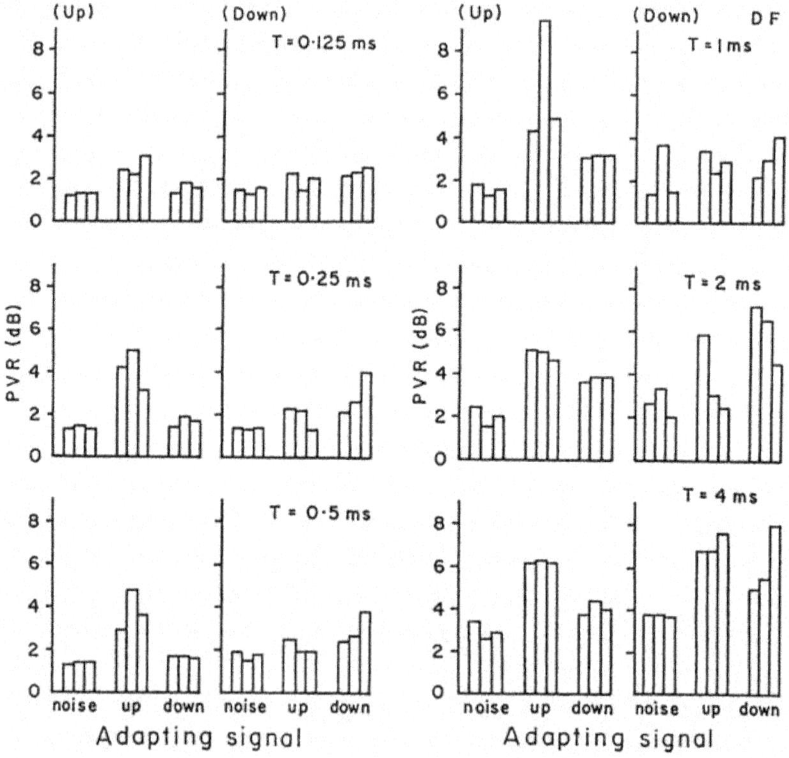

Figure 6. As Fig. 5 for a different subject with spectral peak spacing ranging from 8 kHz at 0.125 ms to 250 Hz at 4 ms.

without adaptor, was however omitted as this appeared less appropriate than white noise. For subject GDW (Fig. 5) the results appeared similar to the previous experiment for the 0.25, 0.5, 1, 2 and 4 ms conditions, but were equivocable for the 8 ms condition and at 16 ms there appeared to be no difference between any of the conditions with all thresholds high at about 8 dB PRV. Statistical analysis revealed no differences between upsweeps and downsweeps in the white noise condition, differences at $p<0.01$ between same and different (the directional effect) for T=0.25, 0.5, 1, 2 and 4 ms and N.S. at 8 or 16 ms, significance at $p<0.01$ for same versus noise at all except T=16ms (N.S.). For different versus noise (non specific adaptation) significance was found at 1-8 ms but not at 0.25, 0.5 or 16 ms. Pooling the data across the 0.5-2 ms range increased the three significances to $p<0.0001$ but upsweep versus downsweep remained N.S.

For subject DF (Fig. 6) the results appeared similar but rather more variable. Despite many attempts he was not able to obtain consistent thresholds at 8 or 16 ms. Statistical significance was obtained at $p<0.05$ for all conditions except same versus different at 1 and 4 ms and different versus noise at 0.5 and 1 ms. Again all upsweep versus downsweep results were N.S. Pooling data across time delays increased significance to $p<0.01$ for the three comparisons.

In order to see the influence of spectral peak spacing more clearly the average values of PVR for noise (N), same (S) and different (D) were plotted as a function of T for the two subjects in Fig. 7 (upper). To ascertain the corresponding adaptation ratios the quotiants S/N, S/D and D/N were calculated and plotted below.

In both subjects the threshold PVRs increased with T, i.e., as the spectral peak spacings became less. For GDW it became high and the functions converged at 16 ms. Over the range 0.25 to 2 ms the adaptation ratios remained approximately constant and then decreased systematically above. 2 ms corresponds to a 500 Hz peak spacing or a 250 Hz half-power bandwidth.

4 Discussion

4.1 Upsweeps versus Downsweeps

Previous studies have sometimes revealed a difference in sensitivity for upward versus downward sweeps. In particular Gardner & Wilson (1979) found the sensitivity to sinusoidal frequency upsweeps to be nearly twice that for downsweeps. In the present study none of the five subjects showed any significant difference between upward and downward sweeps for broadband signals.

4.2 Direction-Specific Adaptation

In all five subjects there was clear evidence for directional adaptation at least over the range of peak spacings for which spectral resolution of the peaks should be possible. Thus the psychophysical channel hypothesis receives further support and can be seen to apply to broadband stimuli which simulate speech formants. The adaptation ratio S/D amounts to about 1.5-2 in all subjects.

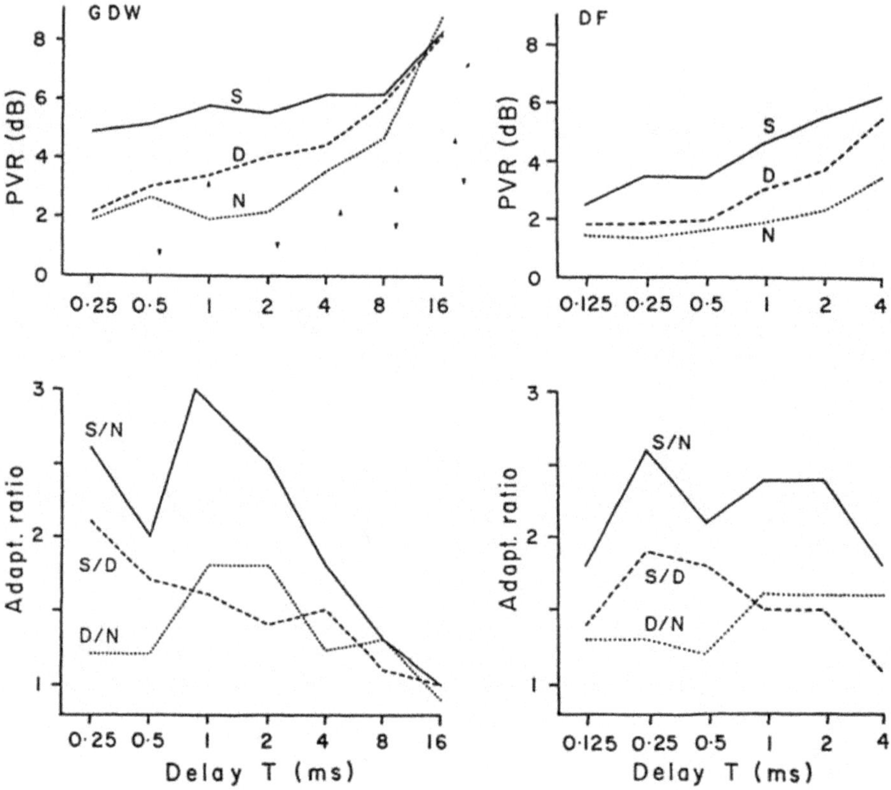

Figure 7. Data from Figs. 5 (left) and 6 (right) plotted as PVR (above) and adaptation ratio (below) where N represents noise adaptor, S represents test and adaptor in the same direction, and D represents the opposite direction. S/N represents the main adapting condition, S/D represents the direction specific component alone and D/N represents a non-specific adaptation component. The triangular dots represent threshold PVRs for static stimuli from (upright) Bilsen, 1968, and (inverted) Wilson, 1969.

4.3 Non-Specific Adaptation

In the cases where there were sufficient data, a small but significant degree of adaptation was also found when the directions of adaptation and test were opposite. In this respect the results are different from earlier studies using sinusoidal signals where no such adaptation was found. An alternative possible outcome might have been an enhancement of sensitivity following opposite sweeps corresponding to various forms of negative afterimage. The present results represent a non-direction specific component of adaptation.

4.4 Spectral Resolution of the Stimuli

A low-pitched sensation can be obtained from noise plus delayed noise up to a delay of about 25 ms. As this would require auditory filters of about 20 Hz bandwidth to resolve, the sensation would appear to be due to temporal analysis mechanisms. The question addressed above is whether the adaptation effect could occur in similar circumstances or whether it is restricted to conditions explicable by spectral analysis channels alone. For both subjects in Fig. 7 threshold PVRs begin to rise consistently for T>1 ms and the adaptation ratios fall for T>2 ms. Above 4 ms one subject was unable to obtain thresholds and the other obtained much high thresholds. It would appear from this that the detectability is indeed being limited by the spectral resolution of the stimuli and that adaptation ratio declines as the threshold PVR increases. The threshold PVRs for static stimuli (upward and downward triangles in Fig. 7) do not show such a strong dependency upon T.

4.5 Rates of Change of Frequency

The modulation rate of 8 Hz was chosen to correspond with that used in most of the sine wave studies. At T=1ms this gives a linear rate of 8 kHz/s which in octave terms corresponds to 3.8 oct./s at 3 kHz and 38 oct./s at 300 Hz. For comparison, formant transitions in speech and sweep-sensitive neurones in animals both cover the range from 1 to 5 oct./s (Whitfield and Evans, 1965, Nelson et al., 1966, Suga, 1973). In the present study this would implicate the 2-3 kHz region for 1 ms and correspondingly lower or higher as T is increased or reduced respectively. Thus at 8 ms, the point at which directional effects disappear, this would be in the 300 Hz region. This suggests the possibility that a lower rate than 8 Hz could give better results, although those at 3 Hz were very comparable.

4.6 Decrement in Adaptation with Extended Testing

Moody et al (1984) claimed that the degree of adaptation decreased with repeated testing. No evidence for this claim was found in the present study even though tests extended over the range over which most of their decrement occurred. For any one condition shown in Figs. 4, 5 and 6 the bars indicate the sequence in which results were obtained. There is no tendency for later results to be any different from the earlier ones.

4.7 Change of Criterion

Wakefield and Viemeister (1984) claimed that although the degree of adaptation appeared to be large the actual change in subject performance in their experiments was not large and might easily be affected by cognitive factors. This does not appear to be the case in the present experiments. Firstly, the psychometric functions upon which the thresholds are based appear to be steeper so that the observed change of detectability, d', corresponding to adaptation is about 1.1 compared with their value of 0.41. Secondly, at 8 Hz it is not readily apparent to the subject for either the adaptor or the test signal whether the spectral sweeps are upward or downward. It would be necessary to detect this for it to have an influence on criterion. In spite of this, of course, the results show that the system is sensitive to the direction of the stimuli.

5 References

Bilsen, F.A. (1968) On the interaction of sound with its repetitions. Ph D Thesis, University of Delft.

Davidson, L.M., Stebbins, W.C., Moody, D.B. and Cole, D.M. (1981) Detection of frequency modulation (FM) following FM adaptation. J. Acoust. Soc. Am. 69 Supp 1, S105.

Diehl, R.L. (1981) Feature detectors for speech: A critical reappraisal. Psychol. Bull. 89, 1-18.

Gardner, R.B. and Wilson, J.P. (1979) Evidence for direction-specific channels in the processing of frequency modulation. J. Acoust. Soc. Am. 66, 704-709.

Green, G.G.R. and Kay, R.H. (1973) The adequate stimuli for channels in the human auditory pathways concerned with the modulation present in frequency-modulated tones. J. Physiol. 234, 50-52P.

Green, G.G.R. and Kay, R.H. (1974) Channels in the human auditory system concerned with the waveform of the modulation present in amplitude and frequency-modulated tones. J. Physiol. 241, 29-30P.

Kay, R.H. and Matthews, D.R. (1972) On the existence of human auditory pathways of channel selectivity tuned to the modulation present in frequency-modulated tones. J. Physiol. 225, 657-677.

Moody, D.B., Cole, D., Davidson, L.M. and Stebbins, W.C. (1984) Evidence for a reappraisal of the psychophysical selective adaptation paradigm. J. Acoust. Soc. Am. 76, 1076-1079.

Nelson, P.G., Erulkar, S.D. and Bryan J.S. (1966) Responses of units of the inferior colliculus to time-varying acoustic stimuli. J. Neurophysiol. 29, 834-860.

Regan, D. and Tansley, B.W. (1979) Selective adaptation to FM tones: Evidence for information-processing channel selectivity sensitive to frequency changes. J. Acoust. Soc. Am. 65, 1249-1257.

Scharf, B. (1970) Critical bands. In: J.V. Tobias (Ed), Foundations of Modern Auditory Theory I, Academic Press, New York, pp. 159-202.

Suffield, J.B. and Tansley, B.W. (1983) Time course of adaptation and recovery of human auditory channels selectively sensitive to amplitude and frequency modulation. J. Acoust. Soc. Am. 73, 765-775.

Suga, N. (1973) Feature extraction in the auditory system of bats. In: A.R. Moller (Ed), Basic Mechanisms of Hearing, Academic Press, New York, pp. 675-742.

Tansley, B.W. and Regan, D. (1979) Separate auditory channels for unidirectional frequency modulation and unidirectional amplitude modulation. Sens. Proces. 3, 132-140.

Wakefield, G.H. and Viemeister, N.F. (1984) Selective adaptation to linear frequency-modulated sweeps: Evidence for direction-specific FM channels? J. Acoust. Soc. Am. 75, 1588-1592.

Whitfield, I.C. and Evans, E.F. (1965) Responses of auditory cortical neurones to stimuli or changing frequency. J. Neurophysiol. 28, 655-672.

Wilson, J.P., Crampin, E.J. and Cann, N. (1991) Directional adaptation to formant-like frequency sweeps. Proc. Inst. Acoust. 13, (2), 535-541.

Wilson, J.P. (1969) An auditory after-image. In: R. Plomp and G.F. Smoorenburg (Eds) Frequency Analysis and Periodicity Detection in Hearing, Sijthoff, Leiden, pp. 303-318.

An evaluation of the detection of a tone added to modulated noise based on reproducible noise samples

V. M. Richards and E. Buss

Department of Psychology, University of Pennsylvania
3815 Walnut Street, Philadelphia, PA/19104, USA

1 Introduction

Hall, Haggard and Fernandes (1984) were the first to compare detection thresholds for a tone added to a bandlimited noise that had either been amplitude modulated or not. They found that for unmodulated maskers, detection thresholds initially grew with increasing bandwidth, and then remained relatively constant for bandwidths greater than approximately a critical bandwidth. For the modulated masker, however, thresholds initially grew with increasing bandwidth, and then fell for bandwidths exceeding a critical bandwidth. Hall et al. suggested that observers were comparing amplitude fluctuations across frequencies, and that these across-frequency temporal comparisons allowed reliable signal detection at lower signal levels. In the absence of coherent amplitude modulations, it was assumed that detection depended on the level at the output of a single auditory filter.

More recently, work has indicated an effect of amplitude modulation even for narrow bands of noise, where across frequency comparisons of temporal pattern are not available (at least at the output of statistically independent auditory filters). For example, Schooneveldt and Moore (1988; and Carlyon et al., 1989) have demonstrated reduced detection thresholds for narrow bands of noise amplitude modulated at low rates. Other experiments have suggested that the detection of a tone added to unmodulated narrow bands of noise may also depend in part on the modulation pattern inherent in narrow bands of noise (c.f., Hall and Grose, 1988). These results are consistent with Hall et al.'s original proposal -- if across-frequency comparisons of temporal patterns contribute to detection when the stimuli span independent auditory filters, why would the temporal information be discarded when the stimuli are constrained to a single critical bandwidth?

In recent experiments, we have begun to examine three questions concerning the observers' decision processes for the detection of a tone added to noise. First, for narrowband maskers is the decision process associated with the detection of a tone different for amplitude modulated and unmodulated maskers? A single decision scheme may be used, but the scheme may be better suited to modulated maskers than to unmodulated maskers.

Second, this question may also be asked in the case of wideband maskers. Does the improvement in detection associated with amplitude modulation reflect a shift from a single-channel to a multiple-channel detection scheme? Third, what are the effects of bandwidening? As the masker bandwidth increases, does the observer employ different decision strategies? For example, as the masker bandwidth is increased from 100 to 900 Hz, is the information contained in the 100-Hz region surrounding the signal frequency processed in the same way?

The experiments described below examined the detection of a 1-kHz tone added to either an unmodulated or a sinusoidally amplitude modulated masker. Three masker bandwidths were tested: 100, 300 and 900 Hz. The experimental procedures were based on past experiments (e.g., Hall et al., 1984; Schooneveldt and Moore, 1988; Carlyon et al., 1989; Haggard et al., 1990). Unlike previous experiments, however, these experiments employed a large number of reproducible masker and signal-plus-masker tokens. Thus, not only were thresholds estimated, but responses to particular stimulus tokens were recorded and used for data analysis. Here, an initial analysis of the data is presented and the results compared with results of other experiments in which wider-band stimuli were used.

The use of reproducible stimulus tokens allowed observers' responses to be analyzed with respect to the spectral properties of the stimuli. The data were analyzed in terms of correlation coefficients between the magnitude of the Fourier spectral components and the observers' responses. For example, consider a Fourier component in the region of the signal frequency. When the magnitude of this component is large, the observer is likely to respond "signal present". When the magnitude is small, a response "no signal" is more likely. In this case, a positive correlation between the magnitude of the spectral component and the observers' binary responses (coded as 0s and 1s, where 1 indicates a "signal present" response) is expected. In contrast, for a spectral component with a frequency much lower than the signal frequency, no correlation would be expected if the observer depends on information limited to frequencies in the region of the signal (e.g., within an auditory filter bandwidth). The function relating frequency to the correlation coefficients will be referred to as the correlation function.

Richards and Zhu (1994) showed that if the observer's responses reflect a linear combination of normally distributed spectral magnitudes, and if the spectral components are independent of one another, the correlation coefficient for each component is proportional to the corresponding linear combination weight. That is, for a linear model, the correlation function indicates the relative contribution of each frequency region to the detection of a tone added to noise. Thus, comparing correlation functions for modulated and unmodulated maskers allows a comparison of the underlying decision rules. Even if the decision processes are not actually linear, a comparison of the linear approximations (i.e., the correlation functions) might still indicate similarities or differences of decision processes. Likewise, comparing the correlation functions as the masker bandwidths increase allows a qualitative evaluation of the consistency of decision rules. If the correlation functions change with bandwidth, it would seem likely that the change reflects a change in the observers' decision process.

2 Experimental Methods

For the main experiment described below, six experimental conditions were examined. The maskers were either amplitude modulated or not, and were one of three bandwidths -- 100, 300 and 900 Hz. When modulated, 100 percent sinusoidal amplitude modulation at 30 Hz was used. The signal was a 1-kHz tone added in-phase to the signal component of the masker. The maskers were arithmetically centered on 1 kHz, and the noise spectrum level was on average 40 dB SPL.

The signal level was adjusted for each observer so as to allow approximately 70 percent correct responses in a single-interval, two-alternative forced-choice task. In an effort to ensure stable performance in the single-interval task, practice trials using a two-interval, two-alternative forced choice task were frequently completed.

A total of 250 masker and 250 signal-plus-masker stimuli were generated for each experimental condition. The generation algorithm for the amplitude modulated bands was as follows. A wide band of noise was generated using magnitudes drawn from a uniform distribution with a range that was +/- 90 percent of the mean. Phases were assigned randomly from a uniform distribution ranging from 0 to 2π. Maskers were then amplitude modulated, and the range of frequencies restricted to 900-Hz, 300-Hz, and 100-Hz bands arithmetically centered at 1 kHz. For signal-present maskers, the phase of the signal component was randomly re-assigned. Finally, a signal with the same phase as the signal component was generated and added to the masker. For the unmodulated bands of noise the procedure was identical, except that following the application of amplitude modulation the phases of each spectral component were randomly re-assigned, thereby removing the coherent temporal modulation.

Four aspects concerning the stimulus generation method should be noted. First, the middle of the power spectra of the wider bands of noise contained the power spectra of the narrower bands of noise. Thus, any differences in correlation functions associated with band widening could not be attributed to the differences in power spectra. Second, the magnitude of the spectral components were drawn from a population of equal variance. Third, due to amplitude modulation, the Fourier components were not mutually independent, regardless of whether the temporal aspects of the amplitude modulation were retained. Thus, the correlations across spectral components will be present in the correlation functions (partial correlations were not estimated). Fourth, the assumption that the spectral components had normally distributed magnitudes was violated. Because the analysis depended on within-observer, across-condition comparisons, and because the power spectra were similarly distributed across conditions, these violations were not significant. Additionally, computer simulations indicated that the effects of across-frequency correlations in the stimulus and the failure to use normal distributions did not greatly compromise the computational method.

Richards and Tian (1994) have applied a similar analysis to the detection of a tone masked by a wideband noise. In that experiment, the spectral components were mutually independent. When the signal was present, the signal-frequency correlation coefficient was elevated relative to the other correlation coefficients. Richards and Tian attributed that result to a mismatch between the variance of the external stimulus and the internal representation of the stimulus (e.g., due to a nonlinearity, the change in mean became a change in variance). Similar elevations were anticipated for the current experiments.

Observers heard each stimulus token eight times. The eight replications were used to generate eight correlation functions. Then, the replicate functions were averaged, and lowpass filtered at 60 percent of the Nyquist rate so as to accentuate the relatively low-frequency aspects of the functions.

3 Results

Figure 1 plots the correlation functions for one of the three observers, Obs 1. For each panel, correlation coefficients are plotted as a function of frequency. Error bars indicate an estimate of the standard deviation of the correlation coefficients when the correlations are zero. The left panels show results for the unmodulated maskers and the right panels show the results for the modulated maskers. The top panels are for the 100-Hz wide maskers, the middle panels for the 300-Hz wide maskers, and the bottom panels for the 900-Hz wide maskers. In the upper left corner of each panel the signal level used and the percent correct responses are indicated. To a large degree, the correlation functions derived for Obs 1 are representative of the functions derived for the other observers. Figure 2 shows the correlation function obtained for Obs 1 when the masker was a wideband noise lowpass filtered at 3 kHz. These results are taken from an experiment in which the magnitudes of the spectral components were mutually independent draws from a uniform distribution (Richards and Tian, 1994). For the 900-Hz wide masker, the correlation functions obtained for Obs 2 differed from Obs 1's. Obs 2's correlation functions are shown in Fig. 3.

First consider the effects of amplitude modulation for the narrowest masker. Thresholds did not depend on whether or not the masker was amplitude modulated. As an example, for the observer shown, approximately equal signal levels led to approximately equal detection performance. The top two panels of Fig. 1 also show that negative correlations were obtained. Negative correlations were found for two of the three observers. Ahumada and Lovell (1970), Ahumada et al. (1975), and Gilkey and Robinson (1986), who used a similar approach to that used here, also found negative weights for the detection of a tone added to noise. The existence of negative correlation coefficients allows the rejection of detection models that depend solely on changes in level at the output of a single linear filter.

In an effort to quantify the degree of similarity between the correlation functions derived for modulated and unmodulated maskers, two sequences of computations were completed. First, for each experimental condition and each observer, the eight replicate correlation functions were separated into two sets of four. For each set, an averaged, lowpass filtered correlation function was generated. Then, the proportion of variance that one function could account for in the other function was computed. That value was taken as an estimate of the amount of variance in the correlation functions that was due to features of the detection process that are stable across trials (i.e., not due to internal noise). For Obs 1 these "split-half" (S/H) values are indicated in the upper right corner for each panel in Fig. 1. Next, the proportion of the variance in the correlation functions for the modulated masker that could be accounted for by unmodulated correlation functions was computed. These "across-condition" (A/C) values are indicated in the upper right corner of the right panels of Fig. 1. A comparison of these two values, S/H and A/C, allows an estimate of the degree to which the reproducible features in the correlation functions for modulated maskers can be accounted for using the correlation functions for unmodulated maskers.

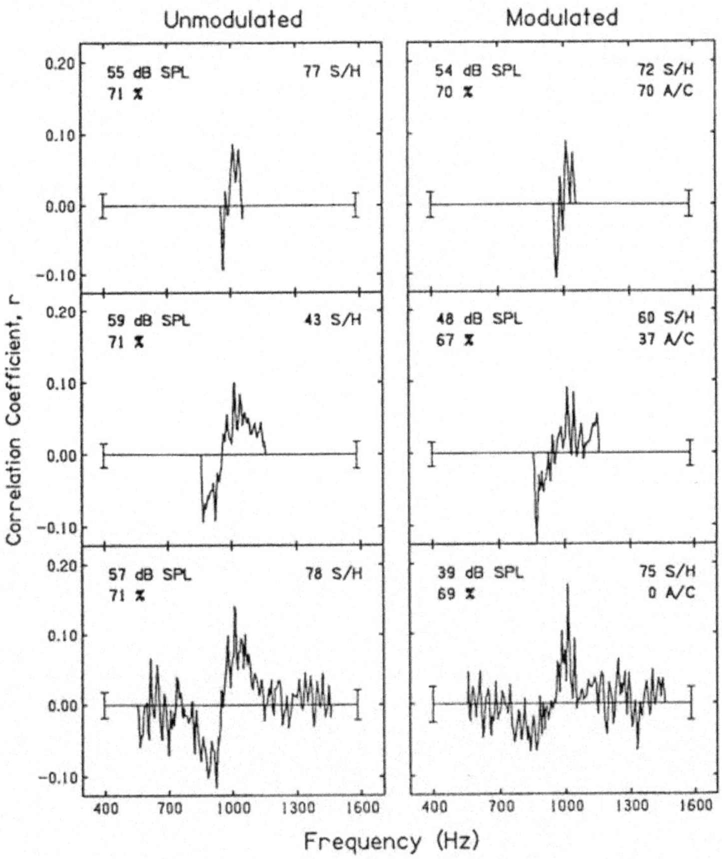

Figure 1. Correlation coefficients are plotted as a function of frequency for unmodulated (left) and modulated (right) maskers. Masker bandwidths are 100 Hz (top), 300 Hz (middle), and 900 Hz (bottom). The data are for Obs 1. Signal levels, percent correct responses, split-half values (S/H, as a percent of variance), and across-condition values (A/C, as a percent of variance) are indicated.

For the narrow bands of noise, the shape of the correlation functions are largely independent of amplitude modulation. Like Obs 1, Obs 2's data showed a high degree of similarity. For Obs 3, the correlation functions were elevated but flat, and so there was no reproducible variance to account for (i.e., the mean was a good predictor of the correlation function).

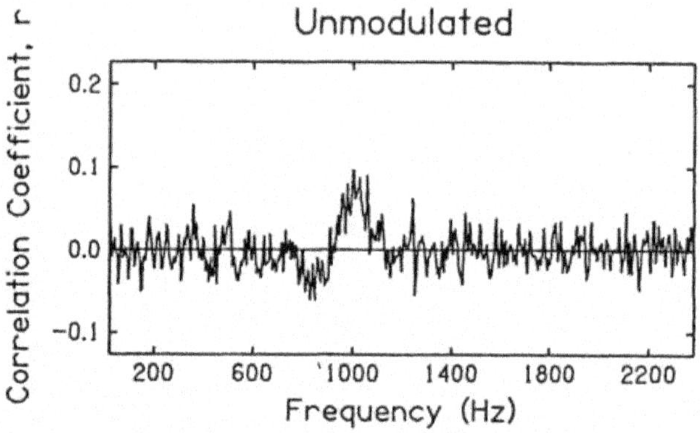

Figure 2. Correlation coefficients are plotted as a function of frequency for wideband noise (Richards and Tian, 1994). The observer is the same as in Fig. 1.

For the 300-Hz wide bands of noise, thresholds were lower when the masker was amplitude modulated. The 11 dB shift in signal level indicated in Fig. 1 is typical. Nonetheless, the correlation functions are somewhat similar. For Obs 1 and 3, approximately 50 percent of the estimated reproducible variance is shared by correlation functions derived for the modulated and unmodulated maskers. For Obs 2, the functions are less similar, so much so that the mean of the modulated correlation function was as good a predictor as the unmodulated correlation function. Thus, the change in signal level required for detectability is marginally mirrored in the correlation functions. For both the unmodulated and modulated correlation functions, restricting the analysis to the central 100-Hz portion of the correlation functions, the reproducible variance in the correlation function for the 300-Hz wide maskers could not be accounted for by the correlation functions obtained for the 100-Hz wide maskers. To the degree that the data are free of stimulus artifacts, this result suggests that dissimilar decision processes are followed for the 100- and 300-Hz wide maskers, regardless of the presence or absence of amplitude modulation.

For the 900-Hz wide maskers, effects of amplitude modulation were readily apparent in both thresholds and correlation functions. The approximately 18 dB reduction in signal level associated with the introduction of amplitude modulation indicated in Fig. 1 (bottom panels) is typical of the other observers. The data also indicate that the unmodulated correlation functions were relatively more stable than the modulated correlation functions (split-half values of 78 vs. 75; 48 vs. 33; and 79 vs. 50 for Obs 1-3, respectively).

For 900-Hz wide unmodulated maskers, and for Obs 1 and 3, the central 300-Hz portion of the correlation functions were similar to the pattern obtained for the 300-Hz wide masker. For these two observers, the similarity of patterns was poorer for the amplitude modulated maskers. For Obs 2, little similarity was present for either the modulated or unmodulated maskers. At least for Obs 1 and 3, then, the effects of widening the masker from 300- to 900-Hz appears to depend on the type of masker employed. Additionally, comparing the left panel of Fig. 1 and Fig. 2, it is apparent that further bandwidening is unlikely to significantly alter the correlation functions when the masker is unmodulated.

For the 900-Hz wide unmodulated maskers, one of the observers' correlation functions (Obs 2) deviated from the functions derived for the other two observers. Her results are shown in Fig. 3. For the unmodulated masker, it appears that Obs 2 depended on information drawn from a wide range of frequencies. For example, it appears that Obs 2 'attended' to information at higher frequencies as well as information in the region of the signal. Similar findings have been obtained for this observer in other experiments.

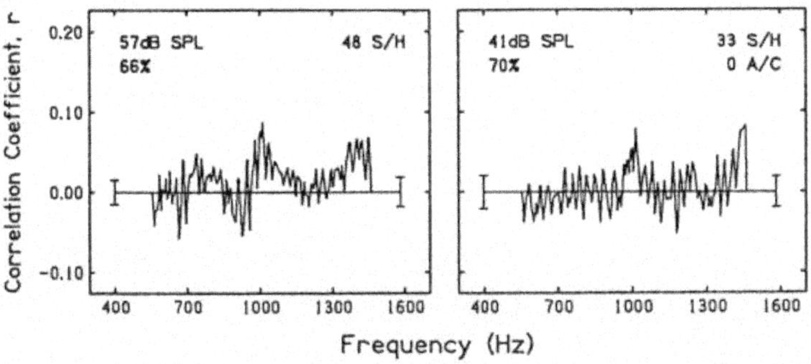

Figure 3. Correlation coefficients are plotted as a function of frequency for the 900-Hz wide unmodulated (left) and modulated (right) maskers. The data are for Obs 2 (compare with Fig. 1, bottom).

In comparison with the results obtained at the narrower bandwidths, the degree of similarity of correlation functions for the unmodulated and modulated maskers was diminished for the 900-Hz wide maskers. For all three observers, the modulated correlation function was as well described by its mean as by the unmodulated correlation function. For two of the three observers (one shown in Fig. 1), the modulated and unmodulated functions appear somewhat similar. For Obs 2, whose results are plotted in Fig. 3, the similarity is lacking. It seems unlikely that the detection of a tone added to a wide band of modulated noise depends on the same detection scheme as when the noise is unmodulated.

For an across-frequency detection scheme, such as has been proposed by Hall et al. (1984) for the detection of a tone added to modulated noise, each frequency region would contribute to detection. As a result, each frequency region would account for only a small amount to the total variance in the responses. Thus, the lack of reliable correlation functions for the wideband modulated maskers is consistent with a shift to, or the inclusion of, a detection scheme that depends on information pooled across a larger range of frequencies.

4 Summary and Conclusions

For the 100- and 300-Hz wide bands of noise, the data do not provide evidence for the hypothesis that the detection of a tone added to noise depends on different detection processes, regardless of whether or not the masker was amplitude modulated. It is possible that observed differences in threshold that are associated with amplitude modulation reflect the degree to which the stimulus and detection process are matched. For 900-Hz wide unmodulated maskers, the data do not suggest a difference in detection scheme relative to that employed for moderate bandwidths. For the 900-Hz wide amplitude-modulated masker, the correlation functions were compressed relative to the unmodulated functions. That result is consistent with a suggestion originally made by Hall et al. (1984) that observers rely on an across-frequency comparison of information when coherent modulation is present. Although it seems plausible that observers would employ across frequency information as it becomes available, robust differences in correlation functions were not obtained using moderate bandwidth maskers.

5 Acknowledgments

This work was supported by a grant from the National Institutes of Health. Lijun Tian and Shunping Zhu assisted in programming the stimulus generation, data collection, and data analysis routines.

6 References

Ahumada, A., Jr. and Lovell, J. (1970). Stimulus features in signal detection. J. Acoust. Soc. Am., 49, 1751-1756.

Ahumada, A., Jr., Marken, R., and Sandusky, A. (1975). Time and frequency analyses of auditory signal detection. J. Acoust. Soc. Am., 57, 385-390.

Carlyon, R. P., Buus, S., and Florentine, M. (1989). Comodulation masking release for three types of modulators as a function of modulation rate. Hear. Res., 42, 37-45.

Gilkey, R. H., and Robinson, D. E. (1986). Models of auditory masking: A molecular approach. J. Acoust. Soc. Am., 79, 1499-1510.

Hall, J. W. III, and Grose, J. H. (1988). Comodulation masking release: Evidence for multiple cues. J. Acoust. Soc. Am., 84, 1669-1675.

Hall, J. W., Haggard, M. P., and Fernandes, M. A. (1984). Detection in noise by spectro-temporal pattern analysis. J. Acoust. Soc. Am., 76, 50-56.

Haggard, M. P., Hall, J. W. III, and Grose, J. H. (1990). Comodulation masking release as a function of bandwidth and test frequency. J. Acoust. Soc. Am., 88, 113-118.
Richards, V. M., and Zhu, S. (1994). Relative estimates of combination weights, decision criteria, and internal noise based on correlation coefficients. J. Acoust. Soc. Am., 85, 243-234.
Richards, V. M. and Tian, L. J. (1994). Examination of power-based and envelope-based models for the detection of a tone added to noise. Abstract, 17th midwinter meeting of the Association for Research in Otolaryngology.
Schooneveldt, G. P., and Moore, B. C. J. (1988). Comodulation masking release (CMR) as a function of masker bandwidth, modulator bandwidth, and signal duration. J. Acoust. Soc. Am., 85, 273-281.

Comment by H. Dai

It would be interesting to try to predict the threshold differences, or the CMR effect, based on the obtained correlation functions. To a first approximation, it may be assumed the observers' decision statistics are linearly weighted sum of the levels of the spectral components, where the weights can be derived from the obtained correlation coefficients. Then the performances of the estimated decision rules may be compared.

Reply

As you indicate, the correlation coefficients are proportional to weights for a weighted linear model. Indeed, the correlation functions are essentially multiple regression solutions relating features of the stimuli to the observers' responses. Thus, one may use the resulting correlation (weighting) functions to predict thresholds, to predict psychometric functions, or even to predict responses to individual stimuli. However, there are several limitations that should be kept in mind:

(a) The correlation functions provide a "model" of detection which consumes a large portion of the degrees of freedom available. It is important to test the "model" using novel stimuli, not those used to estimate the model parameters (otherwise, a goodness of fit to the data is being estimated). In practice, we use half of the stimuli to generate the correlation functions, and the other half to test the model by predicting thresholds, predicting responses to particular stimuli, etc.

(b) For the current experiment, there is evidence that the linear model is not completely successful. In particular, the correlation obtained at the signal frequency is higher for correlation functions based on signal-present than signal-absent stimuli. Were the linear model correct, changes in mean would not result in changes in correlation coefficients. While we take that failure to indicate a "mismatch" between the physical and subjective scales, it may reflect a larger problem with the linear approach used here.

Across-channel contributions to auditory enhancement

Beverly A. Wright

Psychoacoustics Laboratory, Department of Psychology
University of Florida, Gainesville, Florida 32611, U. S. A.

1 Introduction

A fundamental feature of the auditory system is its capacity to filter sounds into their component frequencies. This property is often demonstrated in psychophysical masking experiments, in which the ability to detect an audio signal is degraded by the presence of another, "masking," sound. Such experiments have repeatedly shown that, in steady-state conditions, only the sounds presented within a relatively narrow frequency range around the signal are effective maskers. The standard interpretation of this result is that the auditory system is composed of an array of frequency filters, channels, or "critical bands."

The primary purpose of this paper is to describe a particular set of apparently related effects which indicate that signal detectability can also be influenced by masking energy presented to critical bands remote from the signal frequency. We will call these phenomena "enhancement" effects because, in all but one of them, a component of the stimulus, either the signal or the masker, is made more effective by delaying its onset. In signal enhancement, a signal is easier to detect when its onset is delayed from masker onset. In masker enhancement, certain frequency components cause more masking when the onset of these components is delayed relative to the onset of the rest of the masker. As will be illustrated in section 2, all of the enhancement effects appear to depend primarily upon frequency components presented above about 1.2 times the signal frequency (f_S). We will refer to the frequency region above $1.2f_S$ as the "enhancement region." The dependence of enhancement effects upon components in this region suggests the existence of an across-channel process through which masking energy in remote critical bands acts on the signal. The idea that such a process exists was first advanced by Elliott (1965, 1967), and has recently been revived by a number of investigators (e.g., Carlyon, 1987; Kimberley et al., 1989; Bacon and Smith, 1991; Wright, 1991). Proposed explanations of auditory enhancement are reviewed in section 3.

2 Enhancement Effects and Frequencies above $1.2f_S$

This section describes the various signal- and masker-enhancement effects and provides evidence showing the dependence of each particular effect on masking components above $1.2f_S$.

2.1 Signal Enhancement

Forward signal enhancement: In simultaneous masking, a signal becomes easier to detect as its onset is delayed from masker onset. This widely studied effect has been variously referred to as "overshoot" (e.g., Zwicker, 1965), "auditory enhancement" (e.g., Viemeister, 1980), or "the temporal decline of masking" (e.g., McFadden and Wright, 1990). Here we will use the term "forward signal enhancement" or simply "signal enhancement" to emphasize that it is the signal that is enhanced by delaying its onset. We will define the amount of signal enhancement as the threshold for signals either gated on and off with the masker (*burst condition*) or presented at the onset of a longer masker (*backward-fringe condition*) minus that for signals presented with some relatively long signal delay (*forward-fringe condition*; see schematic diagrams at the top of Fig. 1).

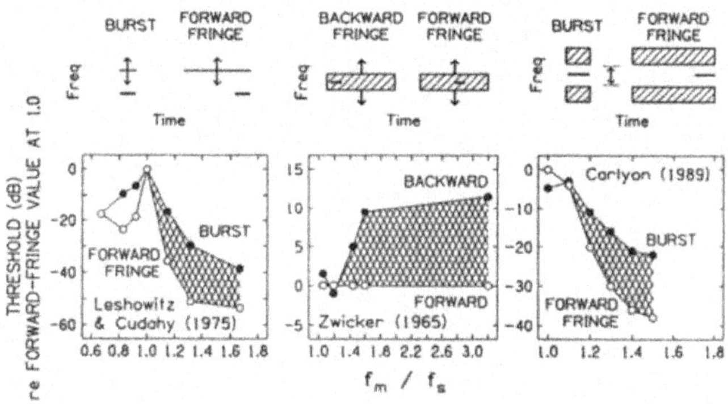

Figure 1. Forward Signal Enhancement (shaded areas) with tonal maskers [left panel; f_m = masker frequency (Hz)], band-pass noise maskers [middle panel; f_m = upper edge of noise (Hz)], and notched-noise maskers [right panel; f_m = upper edge of notch (Hz)].

That signal enhancement depends strongly upon masking components remote from the signal frequency is most clearly evident in data obtained by manipulating the spectral shape of the masker. The three panels in Fig. 1 show schematic diagrams of the basic conditions, and the corresponding results, of a representative set of such experiments. The amount of signal enhancement (indicated by the shaded areas in each panel) is always greatest when a tonal masker, or the edge of a noise masker, is above $1.2f_s$. This is true regardless of whether the masker is a pure tone of variable frequency (left panel), a band-pass noise of variable width centered at f_s (middle panel), or a noise having a spectral notch of variable width centered at f_s (right panel). [The signal enhancement measured with tonal maskers (left panel) when the masker frequency (f_m) is less than f_s appears to result from the detection of combination products that are discernible only in the forward-fringe condition (Leshowitz and Cudahy, 1975; Bacon and Viemeister, 1985) and will be ignored in this discussion.].

The importance of remote frequency components to signal enhancement is also demonstrated in experiments designed to investigate how long it takes for threshold to return to its unenhanced value following stimulation. McFadden (1989) attempted to reset the signal-enhancement process by inserting, immediately before signal onset, temporal gaps into various spectral regions of an otherwise continuous wideband masker. He reported resetting only when the temporal gap was introduced into frequency regions remote from the signal. Remarkably, there was no resetting when the temporal gap was introduced into a band of masking components centered at the signal frequency.

Signal enhancement in forward masking: There is also evidence for signal enhancement in forward masking. Parallel to the signal enhancement observed in simultaneous masking, shorter forward maskers appear to produce more masking than longer ones when the closest masking component is above about $1.2f_S$. Elliott (1967) reported this for narrowband maskers and we recently observed the same result with notched-noise maskers (Wright, 1992). Schematic diagrams of the basic conditions used in these experiments, and the resulting data, are shown in the left panel of Fig. 2 (see shaded areas).

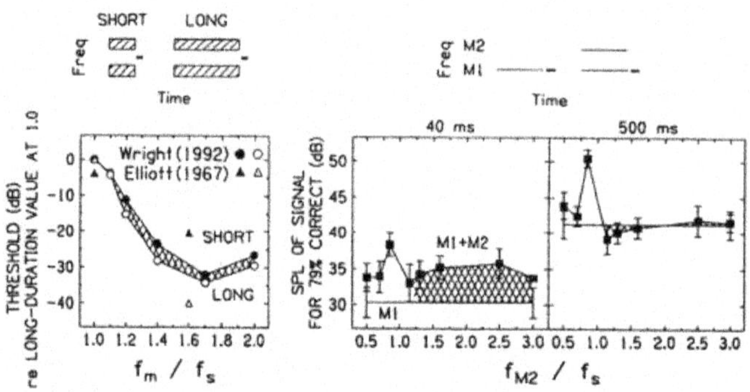

Figure 2. Signal Enhancement in Forward Masking with notched-noise maskers [left panel (shaded areas); f_m = upper edge of notch (Hz)], and two-tone maskers [middle and right panels (compare shaded areas above M1 lines)]. Note also psychophysical suppression [right panel (shaded area below M1 line)].

We also have new data showing a similar result for two-tone forward maskers. Using the standard paradigm for measuring psychophysical two-tone suppression (e.g., Houtgast, 1972; Shannon, 1975), we fixed the frequency of one tone (M1) at the signal frequency of 1000 Hz and varied the frequency of the second tone (M2). The level of M1 was 50 dB SPL and the level of M2 was 70 dB SPL. The middle and right panels of Fig. 2 show the amount of forward masking of the 20-ms signal as a function of the frequency of M2, for two stimulus durations: 40 ms (middle panel) and 500 ms (right panel). All stimuli were gated with cosine-squared rise-fall envelopes of 10 ms. Each point indicates the mean signal threshold and standard error across five highly-trained subjects.

The results obtained when the masker duration was long (right panel) were consistent with previous reports of psychophysical suppression (Houtgast, 1972; Shannon, 1975). Adding M2 to M1 reduced the amount of masking slightly when M2 was presented at about $1.15f_s$ (see small shaded area below the M1 line), and performance when M2 was added at other frequencies can be explained simply by the amount of masking produced when either M1 or M2 was presented alone (M2-alone data not shown). In contrast, when the masker duration was short (middle panel), adding M2 to M1 always increased the amount of masking, particularly when M2 was in the frequency range above about $1.2f_s$ (see shaded area above the M1 line). This threshold increase occurred even though the thresholds obtained when M2 was presented alone (not shown) were around 21 dB for all M2 frequencies above $1.2f_s$. Thus, as the stimulus duration was increased, the amount of suppression increased, and the amount of masking from the enhancement region decreased. A similar trend is evident in the data of Shannon (1975, Fig. 20).

Backward signal enhancement: Surprisingly, we recently observed that a signal presented at the onset of a brief notched-noise masker can also be made easier to hear by allowing the masker to last after signal offset. We will refer to this effect as "backward signal enhancement," and will define its magnitude as the threshold difference across the burst and backward- fringe conditions. Schematic representations of the experimental conditions and the corresponding data are provided in Fig. 3. The signal was either a narrowband noise that filled the masker notch (left panel) or a tone centered in the notch (right panel). As with the other enhancement effects, backward signal enhancement is greatest when the upper edge of the spectral notch in a notched-noise masker is at a frequency greater than $1.2f_s$ (see shaded areas). We have replicated this unusual result in several experiments and in two different laboratories (Wright, 1991, 1992; Kidd and Wright, 1994).

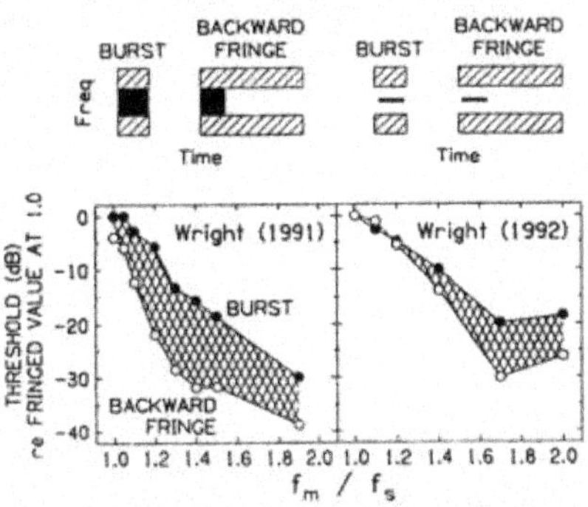

Figure 3. Backward Signal Enhancement (shaded areas) with notched-noise maskers [f_m = upper edge of notch (Hz)].

2.2 Masker Enhancement

Forward-masker enhancement: A signal forward masked by a brief tonal-complex masker is harder to hear when that masker is preceded by an "enhancer" that is a longer version of the masker, but with the component at the signal frequency deleted (e.g., Viemeister and Bacon, 1982). We will refer to this effect as "forward-masker enhancement" to emphasize that, here, the effectiveness of the masker component at the signal frequency is enhanced by delaying its onset relative to the enhancer onset. The basic conditions used to measure forward-masker enhancement are schematically illustrated at the top of Fig. 4. We will define the amount of forward-masker enhancement as the threshold difference between signals presented with enhanced and unenhanced maskers.

As with signal enhancement, forward-masker enhancement also appears to depend upon masking components quite remote from the signal frequency. We recently reported that the amount of forward-masker enhancement was greatest for a wideband-noise masker when the upper edge of the spectral notch in the notched-noise enhancer was above about $1.2f_S$ (Wright et al., 1993). Those data are plotted in Fig. 4 (see shaded areas).

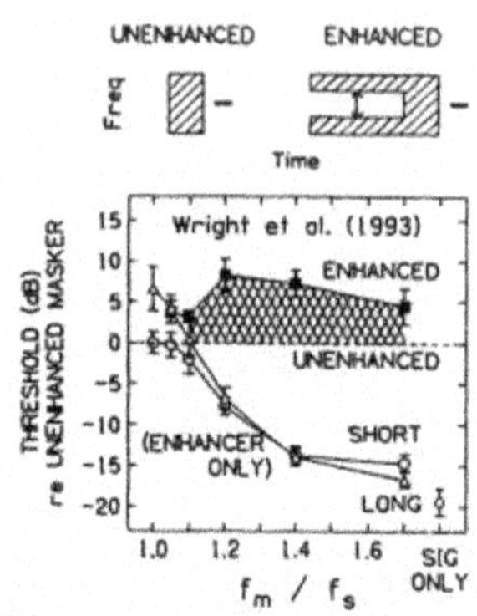

Figure 4. Forward-masker Enhancement (shaded areas) with a notched-noise enhancer [fm = upper edge of notch (Hz)].

<u>Simultaneous-masker enhancement:</u> Another interesting enhancement effect appeared in a recent experiment in which we used the basic paradigm for measuring forward-masker enhancement, but presented the signal simultaneously with the masker. The basic conditions are schematically illustrated at the top of Fig. 5. In this experiment, the signal was a 50-ms tone at 1000 Hz, the unenhanced masker was a 51-ms wideband noise, and the enhancer was a 350-ms wideband noise having a spectral notch of variable width centered on the signal. Signal offset coincided with masker offset. The spectrum level of the masker and enhancer was 33 dB SPL. The results for seven subjects are shown in the left panel of Fig. 5. The amount of masking clearly depended upon the notch width in the enhancer. When the frequency of the upper edge of the notch was less than about $1.2f_S$, the enhancer reduced the amount of masking. However, when the frequency of the upper edge of the notch was greater than $1.2f_S$, the enhancer actually increased the amount of masking (see shaded areas). We will refer to this increase in masking as "simultaneous-masker enhancement." A similar pattern is evident in the data of Bacon and Smith (1991; see right panel of Fig. 5), although not discussed by them. Viemeister (1980) and Carlyon (1987) also reported a masking release for a narrow notch width under similar conditions, but neither varied the notch width to reveal the masking increase.

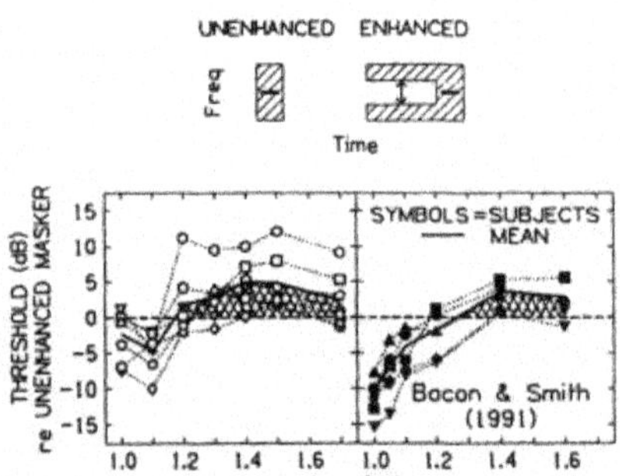

Figure 5. Simultaneous-masker Enhancement (shaded areas) with a notched-noise enhancer [fm = upper edge of notch (Hz)].

3 Proposed Explanations for Enhancement Effects

This section summarizes the proposed explanations for auditory enhancement. All of the explanations were originally suggested to account for forward signal enhancement (see Fig. 1), and all but one of the proposals (Section 3.4) deal solely with that phenomenon.

3.1 Spectral Splatter

When a pure tone is gated with an instantaneous rise/fall time, over 90% of the total energy in the tone is contained in a band 2/T cycles wide centered at the tonal frequency, where T is the duration of the tone in seconds. Thus, for a brief tone or at the onset of a longer-duration tone, where T is small, the energy of the tone is spread or "splattered" over a wide range of frequencies. Green (1969) suggested that, in forward signal enhancement, the signal is least detectable when its onset is coincident with masker onset because that is when the most energy is splattered from the masker into the frequency region of the signal. It appears that masker splatter can exaggerate the estimated magnitude of signal enhancement, but cannot entirely account for the effect. For example, there is still 10-20 dB of signal enhancement when the splatter from a remote tonal masker has been minimized (e.g., Bacon and Viemeister, 1985), and when splatter is not a factor, as with wideband maskers (e.g., Zwicker, 1965).

3.2 Narrowing Auditory Filter

Scholl (1962) was the first to propose that signal enhancement could result from a narrowing of the auditory filter ("critical band") over time (see also, e.g., Elliott, 1965, 1967; Green, 1969). According to this hypothesis, if the width of the auditory filter were to narrow over time, then more masking noise would be allowed through the filter at masker onset, when the filter was widest, than after the masker had been on for a while and the filter was narrower. Signal detectability would thus be worst at masker onset, and would improve over the course of masker presentation, just as is seen in signal enhancement. In support of this idea, all of the enhancement effects are greater for maskers remote from, than for those near, the signal frequency (see section 1, particularly Fig. 1). It has been argued, however, that this temporal improvement in filtering does not necessarily reflect a change in filtering at the auditory periphery (e.g., Moore et al., 1987). The proposed explanations for signal enhancement treated in the remaining sections are related to this argument. These explanations can therefore be evaluated on the basis of their ability to predict temporal improvements in filtering, and can be viewed as acting at sites central to the peripheral auditory filter.

3.3 Adaptation of Excitation

In response to a sound of constant intensity, the firing rate of a single auditory nerve fiber is at its maximum at the onset of a stimulus, and then decays or adapts to a steady-state level. This decrease in firing rate is referred to as adaptation. One widely cited hypothesis about the origins of signal enhancement appeals to short-term adaptation, a particular stage of adaptation that has a time constant of about 60 ms (e.g., Bacon and Viemeister, 1985; Kimberley et al., 1989). The foundation of this explanation is that, neurophysiologically, the absolute increase in firing rate introduced by an increment in intensity added during the presentation of an adapting pedestal is the same, regardless of the temporal position of the increment in the adapting pedestal (e.g., Smith and Zwislocki, 1971). Thus, the ratio of the response to an increment (signal) relative to the response to an adapting pedestal (masker) improves as the onset of the signal is delayed. If this signal-to-masker ratio at the neural level determines signal detectability psychophysically, the argument goes, adaptation of the masker would improve detectability, and hence produce signal enhancement (e.g., Smith and Zwislocki, 1971).

While short-term adaptation in the auditory nerve is likely involved in the production of signal enhancement, there are two primary reasons why it cannot completely account for the effect. First, from the few data available, it appears that physiological adaptation does not depend upon the relative frequency of the "signal" and "masker" (e.g., Harris and Dallos, 1979), as psychophysical signal enhancement does. Second, Smith and Zwislocki (1971) estimated that the increase in the signal-to-masker ratio during the course of adaptation could only account for a 3-5 dB improvement in detectability. This is consistent with the typically small amount of signal enhancement obtained when the masker is a tone or narrowband noise at or near the signal frequency, but it almost certainly cannot explain the 10-20 dB of signal enhancement seen when the masker is in the enhancement region (see Fig. 1).

Another explanation of signal enhancement invokes adaptation of excitation as an across-channel process. According to this proposal, each peripheral channel adapts independently, but masking occurs at a stage following the convergence of the outputs of the peripheral channels (Viemeister, 1980; Viemeister and Bacon, 1982; McFadden and Wright, 1990). The sites of these two stages are, hypothetically, the auditory nerve and cochlear nucleus. McFadden and Wright (1990) suggested that channel-specific adaptation could account for the frequency dependence of signal enhancement. They argued that with maskers in the enhancement region there would be more adaptation in the peripheral channel(s) primarily processing the masker than in the channel primarily processing the signal. Hence, at the second stage, where the peripheral channels converge, there would be less masking with a long signal delay because then the unadapted signal would be masked by an adapted masker. In contrast, with maskers near the signal frequency, there would be less opportunity for differential adaptation of the signal and masker because the masker would contribute to adaptation in the signal channel. Hence, there would be less signal enhancement. Viemeister (1980) made a related argument.

One shortcoming of this explanation is that, if, as is implied, all of the channels converging on the second stage adapt by the same amount, then simply combining the signal and masker channels would not produce a signal-enhancement effect greater than 3-5 dB [Smith and Zwislocki's (1971) estimate of the amount of adaptation in the peripheral channels]. Thus, the proposal does not account for the 10-20 dB effects observed with maskers in the enhancement region (see Fig. 1). This difficulty could be overcome by modifying the proposal so that the amount of adaptation in the remote channels converging on the second stage would be amplifed at the second stage.

3.4 Adaptation of Suppression

Viemeister and Bacon (1982) suggested that signal enhancement was the result, not of the reduced masking ability of adapted maskers, but rather of a gain in the effective level of the delayed signal, caused by adaptation of the suppressive effect of the masker on that signal. According to this hypothesis, the psychophysical level of the masker remains unchanged throughout its time course, but its suppressive power declines over time. Hence, a delayed signal is more detectable because it is introduced into a partially, or completely, unsuppressed region. In support of their hypothesis, Viemeister and Bacon presented the first demonstration of forward-masker enhancement (see section 2.2).

As for the adaptation-of-excitation proposals, adaptation of suppression could account for signal enhancement only if (1) the adapting suppression were an across-channel process activated by maskers in the enhancement region ($f_m>1.2f_s$), and (2) the amount of adaptation in each peripheral channel were amplified at the suppressive synapse to account for the 10-20 dB of enhancement that is often observed. Thus, the adapting suppression which is proposed to account for signal enhancement seemingly would have to be a type other than that standardly referred to as psychophysical two-tone suppression, which is greatest when the ratio between the signal and suppressor frequencies is 1.15 (e.g., Houtgast, 1972; Shannon, 1975).

3.5 Transient Masking

Bacon and Moore (1987) proposed that the high thresholds at signal onset in simultaneous masking might be partially accounted for if a centrally-mediated onset response to the signal, purported to facilitate signal detection, were obscured by a corresponding onset response to the masker. According to their definition, unlike excitation-based masking, "transient masking" of the onset response of the signal has occurred if the masked threshold of a signal is increased by the addition of a "transient masker" that is gated on and off with the signal and does not mask the signal when it is presented without the primary masker. In apparent support of this idea, Bacon and Moore reported that the level of a long 1250-Hz masker needed to just mask a 20-ms, 1000-Hz signal was reduced by as much as 20-25 dB by a 500-Hz transient masker presented at a very low level. Due to the slower growth of masking for remote maskers, this 20-25 dB change in masker level probably corresponds to about a 6-dB change in signal threshold. Thus, the transient-masking effect probably cannot account for the entire amount of signal enhancement.

To explain the frequency dependence of signal enhancement, Bacon and Moore suggested that transient responses to the signal might be most important for detection when the listener is forced to attend to a small portion of the overall excitation pattern (signal plus masker). They further reasoned that transient responses to the masker might be particularly detrimental to detection when transient responses to the signal were most important. These assumptions successfully predict that the influence of the transient masker, and thus the amount of signal enhancement, would be largest when $f_m > f_s$. Unfortunately, Bacon and Moore only employed a single masker frequency ($f_m > f_s$) in their experiments, so their proposal remains largely untested.

3.6 Grouping

Finally, Carlyon (1989) suggested that signal enhancement could be explained by assuming that the outputs of auditory filters processing stimuli with similar envelopes are irreversibly grouped together prior to detection. This proposal appears to have been strongly influenced by his use of a masker that had the same duration as the signal for his estimate of detectability with a short signal delay. Carlyon reasoned that this "burst" masker had an envelope similar to that of his signal because they were both very brief (approximately 5 ms), and were gated on and off together. Thus, according to his proposal, signal detectability is worse with a short signal delay because the signal is grouped with the burst masker, but is better with a long signal delay because the signal is not grouped with the masker. It is not clear how this hypothesis could explain the frequency dependence of enhancement, nor how it could be applied to cases in which there was no complete common gating envelope, as when the signal is presented at the onset of a long masker.

4 Summary

A set of effects were described in which a stimulus component, either the signal or the masker, is made more effective by delaying its onset. All of these "enhancement" effects depend primarily upon frequency components presented above about $1.2f_s$, suggesting the existence of an across-channel process through which masking energy in remote critical bands acts on the signal. Proposed explanations for enhancement were reviewed, but none is sufficiently detailed to account for all of the data.

5 Acknowledgments

This research was supported by a grant from the National Institute of Health. I thank Drs. H. Dai, D.M. Green, and K. Saberi for their comments on an earlier draft of this paper, and Z. Onsan for her assistance in preparing the figures.

6 References

Bacon, S.P., and Moore, B.C.J. (1987) Transient masking and the temporal course of simultaneous tone-on-tone masking. J. Acoust. Soc. Am., 81, 1073-1077.

Bacon, S.P., and Smith, M.A. (1991) Spectral, intensive, and temporal factors influencing overshoot. Q. J. Exp. Psychol., 43A, 373-399.

Bacon, S.P., and Viemeister, N.F. (1985) Simultaneous masking by gated and continuous sinusoidal maskers. J. Acoust. Soc. Am., 78, 1220-1230.

Carlyon, R.P. (1987) A release from masking by continuous, random, notched noise. J. Acoust. Soc. Amer., 81, 418-426.

Carlyon, R.P. (1989) Changes in the masked threshold of brief tones produced by prior bursts of noise. Hear. Res. 81, 223-236.

Elliott, L.L. (1965) Changes in the simultaneous masked threshold of brief tones. J. Acoust. Soc. Am., 38, 738-746.

Elliott, L.L. (1967) Development of auditory narrow-band frequency contours. J.Acoust. Soc.Am., 42, 143-153.

Green, D.M. (1969) Masking with continuous and pulsed sinusoids. J. Acoust. Soc.Am.,46, 939-946.

Harris, D.M., and Dallos, P. (1979) Forward masking of auditory nerve fiber responses. J. Neurophys.,42, 1083-1107.

Houtgast, T. (1972) Psychophysical evidence for lateral inhibition in hearing. J. Acoust. Soc. Am., 51, 1885-1894.

Kidd, G., Jr., and Wright, B.A. (1994) Improving the detectability of a brief tone in noise using forward and backward masker fringes: Monotic and dichotic presentations. J. Acoust. Soc. Am., 95, 962-967.

Kimberley, B.P., Nelson, D.A., and Bacon, S.P. (1989) Temporal overshoot in simultaneous-masked psychophysical tuning curves from normal and hearing-impaired listeners. J. Acoust. Soc. Am., 85, 1660-1665.

Leshowitz, B., and Cudahy, E. (1975) Masking patterns for continuous and gated sinusoids. J. Acoust. Soc. Am., 58, 235-242.

McFadden, D. (1989) Spectral differences in the ability of temporal gaps to reset the mechanisms underlying overshoot. J. Acoust. Soc. Am., 85, 254-261.

McFadden and Wright, B.A. (1990) Temporal decline of masking and comodulation detection differences. J. Acoust. Soc. Am., 88, 711-724.

Moore, B.C.J., Poon, P.W.F., Bacon, S.P., and Glasberg, B.R. (1987) The temporal course of masking and the auditory filter shape, J. Acoust. Soc. Am., 81, 1873-1880.

Scholl, H. (1962). Das dynamische Verhalten des Gehors bei der Unterteilung des Schallspektrums in Frequenzgruppen. Acustica, 12, 101-107.

Shannon, R.V. (1975). Suppression of forward masking. Unpublished doctoral dissertation, University of California at San Diego, pp. 149.

Smith, R.L., and Zwislocki, J.J. (1971) Responses of some neurons of the cochlear nucleus to tone-intensity increments. J. Acoust. Soc. Am., 50, 1520-1525.

Viemeister, N.F. (1980) Adaptation of masking. In: G. van den Brink and F.A. Bilsen (Eds.), Psychophysical, Physiological and Behavioural Studies in Hearing, Delft University Press, Delft, pp. 190-197.

Viemeister, N.F., and Bacon, S.P. (1982) Forward masking by enhanced components in harmonic complexes. J. Acoust. Soc. Am., 71, 1502-1507.

Wright, B.A. (1991) Contributions of stimulus bandwidth, the reference condition, and individual differences to the auditory temporal effect: Evidence for within- and across-channel mechanisms. Unpublished doctoral dissertation, University of Texas, pp. 277.

Wright, B.A. (1992) Masker duration affects frequency resolution in simultaneous and nonsimultaneous masking. J. Acoust. Soc. Am., 92, 2364 (A).

Wright, B.A., McFadden, D.M., and Champlin, C.A. (1993) Adaptation of suppression as an explanation of enhancement effects. J. Acoust. Soc. Am., 84, 72-82.

Zwicker, E. (1965) Temporal effects in simultaneous masking and loudness. J. Acoust. Soc. Am., 38, 132-141.

Comment by R.P. Carlyon

I agree with your conclusion that none of the proposed explanations can account for all of the data. In particular, the "grouping by common envelope" hypothesis has trouble in accounting for some of the masker enhancement experiments that you describe, as well as the "flat spectrum vowel" phenomenon described by Summerfield and his colleagues (1984). However, it *can* account for both the frequency selectivity of some of the "signal enhancement" data (e.g., those of Carlyon, 1989), as well as the effects of having only a backward fringe, in contrast to your statement in section 3.6.

Consider first the masking release phenomenon described by Carlyon, and shown schematically in your Fig. 1 (top right). When the masker and precursor have a very narrow, or no, notch, there is substantial masker energy within the auditory filter centered on the signal. This masking is determined by peripheral processes and cannot be reduced by a precursor. At intermediate notch widths, masker energy occurs in bands flanking the auditory filter centered on the signal. Here, the common masker and signal envelopes cause the output of filters adjacent to the signal frequency to be grouped with the signal, thereby resulting in increased masking in the burst condition. This relatively central form of masking *can* be reduced by the precursor. Finally, at very wide notch widths, very little central or peripheral masking takes place, even in the burst condition. Hence the masking release is greatest at intermediate notch widths.

Second, consider the literature on the effects of onset and offset asynchronies on grouping. The data show that onset asynchronies are the most effective for segregation, but that offset asynchronies also have an effect. Thus, although forward fringes should be most effective in perceptually segregating the masker and signal, backward fringes should also have some effect.

Summerfield, Q., Haggard, M., Foster, J., and Gray, S. (1984). "Perceiving vowels from uniform spectra: Phonetic exploration of an auditory aftereffect," Perception and Psychophysics, 35, 203-213.

Reply

I concur that higher-level processes such as grouping probably influence measures of signal enhancement as well as many other psychophysical phenemona. The similarity in the frequency dependence of both signal and masker enhancement, however, appears to indicate that all of the enhancement effects are produced by common processes and thus that any grouping explanation would also have to account for the masker-enhancement results. Again, what is clearly lacking on all sides of this issue is a rigorous, quantitative model of enhancement effects.

Finally, I would like to point out that your comment that there is very little enhancement for wideband maskers with no notch is generally true at lower signal frequencies (< 2 kHz), but that substantial amounts of enhancement are obtained at higher signal frequencies under similar conditions. For example, see the results of Zwicker in the middle panel of Fig. 1, tested at 4.8 kHz.

Comment by E.F. Evans

Physiological evidence seems more consistent with the virtually instantaneous availability of cochlear filtering: Measurement of frequency selectivity of single cochlear nerve fibres obtained in terms of the filter weighting of individual harmonics of multicomponent stimuli, measured from their temporal discharge patterns, gives similar filter shapes for both impulsive stimuli (click trains) and continuous signals (harmonic series, broadband noise), and the pure tone frequency threshold curve (Evans, 1989).

Evans, E. F. (1989) Cochlear filtering: a view seen through the temporal discharge patterns of single cochlear nerve fibres. In: J. P. Wilson and D. T. Kemp (Eds.), *Cochlear Mechanisms - Structure, Function and Models*, Plenum Publ., NY, 241-250.

Reply

Your data fit in nicely with the idea that enhancement is an across-channel, and thus post-cochlear, effect.

Comment by A.R. Palmer

We have recently completed (Palmer et al., 1994) a study of the responses of cochlear nerve fibres in the guinea pig to stimuli consisting of an harmonic series missing components around 2 kHz followed by the same series with the 2-kHz component present. We analysed the responses for any evidence that responses to the 2-kHz component were enhanced. While the data are subject to certain caveats, (the appropriateness of the sound levels used and the paucity of fibres with low spontaneous activity in our sample), we found no evidence of an enhancement in the representation of the 2-kHz component at this peripheral level.

Palmer, A.R., Summerfield, Q. and Fantini, D.A. (1994) Responses of auditory nerve fibers to stimuli producing psychophysical enhancement. J. Acoust. Soc. Am. (under review).

Comment by S. Wartini

In your paper you state that enhancement by tonal maskers below the testtone is caused by detection of the cubic difference tone. So this case can be reduced to a situation where the masker is spectrally above the signal (the cubic difference tone).

According to unpublished data I found enhancement of a single tone by a harmonic complex tone below this signal. The cubic difference tone will coincide with a component of the masker because the test-tone was a harmonic of the masker's fundamental. The level of the cubic difference tone is to be expected 10dB below the level of the coinciding component, so it´s unlikely that subjects can use beats to detect the test-tone.

Reply

Thank you for raising this issue. My dismissal of signal-enhancement effects obtained when fm < fs was misleading. It was intended to refer only to cases involving single tonal maskers. In addition to your data, signal enhancement has also been obtained using low-pass maskers having upper cutoff frequencies below the signal frequency (Carlyon, 1989; Wright, 1991; Hicks and Bacon, 1992). Such maskers likewise preclude the detection of the cubic difference tone. In the paper I emphasize the frequency region above the signal frequency both because it seems to be the most important and because its role in an across-channel process is clearer than for the region below the signal frequency, where within-channel process are more likely to also contribute to the results.

Carlyon, R.P. (1989) Changes in the masked threshold of brief tones produced by prior bursts of noise. Hear. Res. 41, 223-236.

Hicks, M.L., and Bacon, S.P. (1992) Factors influencing temporal effects with notched-noise maskers. Hear. Res. 64, 123-132.

Wright, B.A. (1991) Contributions of stimulus bandwidth, the reference condition, and individual differences to the auditory temporal effect: Evidence for within- and across-channel mechanisms. Unpublished doctoral dissertation, University of Texas, pp. 277.

Author Index

www.ingramcontent.com/pod-product-compliance
Lightning Source LLC
Chambersburg PA
CBHW040911170826
49827CB00002B/4
* 9 7 8 9 8 1 0 2 2 2 6 0 4 *